A Researcher's Guide to Basic References in Bartonellosis, Babesiosis and Borreliosis or Lyme Disease

A Voluminous Citation Guide to Move Beyond Terse Guidelines And Reviews

James Schaller, M.D., M.A.R.

and

Kimberly Mountjoy, M.S.

International University Infectious Disease Press
Bank Towers • Newgate Center (305)
5150 Tamiami Trail North [Highway 41]
Naples, Florida 34103

Cover Art: Derek Murphy

Lead Research and Research Study Acquisitions: Randal Blackwell

Copy Editing by Kimberly Mountjoy, Lindsay Gibson, Kathleen Snyder
and anonymous patients from all over the world

The cover image is FL1953 protozoa from a forty to fifty year old male patient from Germany and is presented with full permission, courtesy of Stephen Fry, M.S., M.D. and Dr. Ellis of Fry Laboratories in Arizona. Their exceptional assistance in furnishing images, discussing staining, genetics sequencing science, and genetic databases with us is deeply appreciated.

Wholesale discount requires purchase of at least twenty copies and can be in five book units. Fax request to (239) 304-1987 and (239) 263-6760.

Library of Congress Cataloging Data

Schaller, J.L; Mountjoy, K.

ISBN: 9780985669270

A researcher's guide to basic references in bartonellosis, babesiosis
and borreliosis or lyme disease: a voluminous citation guide to
move beyond terse guidelines and reviews / J.L. Schaller and K. Mountjoy.

1. Bartonellosis 2. Babesiosis 3. Borreliosis 4. Research 5. Lyme disease
6. Bartonella 7. Babesia 8. Citations

Manufactured in the United States of America

First Edition

10 9 8 7 6 5 4 3 2 1

To Those Who Thirst For Liberty

To the Dalits or Untouchables of India
and the Slaves of India
Numbering Together 600-700 Million—
Clearly Hinduism Has No Credibility.

To The Followers of Islam,
Living Under the Rule of Mohammed,
a Slave Owner, I Hope You Will See Freedom.

The Definitive Collection of Academic References on Bartonella and the Pathology of Bartonellosis

Introduction — Bartonella

I have been studying Bartonella almost full-time for many years. While I know some very select agents for treating Bartonella, we still have many issues that limit application of effective care throughout the world.

The number of true experts on Bartonella, and who have read most of the publications in English print, is possibly under a dozen individuals.

Bartonella has huge impacts in human biochemistry, hormones, sleep, sleep quality, personality, insight, hatred, agitation, rigidity, sadness, body sensations, tissue and organs. You cannot do one test and determine if Bartonella is present in either an animal or a human. I wish such a comfortable myth was true, but it is just old and ineffective medicine.

The references that follow are a small sample of materials related to this infection.

This book is written for individuals who have a master's degree, a Ph.D. or M.D. in the medical sciences. It is also only for those doing research on these infections.

Abandeh FI, Bazan JA, Davis JA, Zaidi AN, Daniels CJ, Firstenberg MS. Bartonella henselae Prosthetic Valve Endocarditis in an Adult Patient with Congenital Heart Disease: Favorable Outcome After Combined Medical and Surgical Management. J Card Surg. 2012 Mar 1. [Epub ahead of print]. PMID:22381119

Abbot P, Aviles AE, Eller L, Durden LA. Mixed infections, cryptic diversity, and vector-borne pathogens: evidence from Polygenis fleas and Bartonella species. Appl Environ Microbiol. 2007 Oct;73(19):6045-52. Epub 2007 Aug 10. PMID:17693558

Abdel-Haq N, Abuhammour W, Al-Tatari H, Asmar B. Disseminated cat scratch disease with vertebral osteomyelitis and epidural abscess. South Med J. 2005 Nov;98(11):1142-5. PMID:16351038

Abdollahi-Roodsaz S, Joosten LA, Roelofs MF, Radstake TR, Matera G, Popa C, van der Meer JW, Netea MG, van den Berg WB. Inhibition of Toll-like receptor 4 breaks the inflammatory loop in autoimmune destructive arthritis. Arthritis Rheum. 2007 Sep;56(9):2957-67. PMID:17763416

Abgueguen P, Chennebault JM, Achard J, Cottin J, Pichard E. [Cat scratch disease. Clinical study of 26 patients. Role and importance of PCR].[Article in French]. Rev Med Interne. 2001 Jun;22(6):522-9. PMID:11433560

Abino JF, Peraldi R, Lepidi H, Luciani M, Girard PM. Bacillary splenitis (Bartonella henselae) during immune restoration in an HIV-infected patient. AIDS. 2002 Jul 5;16(10):1429-30. PMID:12131223

Aboudharam G, Fournier PE, Drancourt M, Raoult D, Foucault C, Brouqui P. Molecular detection of Bartonella quintana DNA in the dental pulp of a homeless patient. Eur J Clin Microbiol Infect Dis. 2004 Dec;23(12):920-2. PMID:15558347

Aboudharam G, Vu DL, Davoust B, Drancourt M, Raoult D. Molecular detection of Bartonella spp. in the dental pulp of stray cats buried for a year. Microb Pathog. 2005 Jan;38(1):47-51. Epub 2004 Dec 8. PMID:15652295

Abstracts for the 4th International Conference on Bartonella as Emerging Pathogens, 26-28 August 2005, Uppsala, Sweden. Ups J Med Sci Suppl. 2005;(57):1-46. PMID:16100842

Accorinti M. Ocular bartonellosis. Int J Med Sci. 2009;6(3):131-2. Epub 2009 Mar 19. PMID:19319232

Acosta SC. Case 5-2005: a man with depression and shortness of breath. N Engl J Med. 2005 May 26;352(21):2248-9; author reply 2248-9. PMID:15917395

Acquitter M, Fleuret C, Kupfer-Bessaguet I, Tanguy C, Plantin P. [Groove sign in cat-scratch disease].[Article in French]. Ann Dermatol Venereol. 2011 Nov;138(11):757-8. Epub 2011 Jul 14. PMID:22078038

Adamska M. [Bartonella spp. as a zoonotic pathogens transmitting by blood-feeding arthropods].[Article in Polish]. Wiad Parazytol. 2010;56(1):1-9. PMID:20450002

Adelson ME, Rao RV, Tilton RC, Cabets K, Eskow E, Fein L, Occi JL, Mordechai E. Prevalence of Borrelia burgdorferi, Bartonella spp., Babesia microti, and Anaplasma phagocytophila in Ixodes scapularis ticks collected in Northern New Jersey. J Clin Microbiol. 2004 Jun;42(6):2799-801. PMID:15184475

Agan BK, Dolan MJ. Laboratory diagnosis of Bartonella infections. Clin Lab Med. 2002 Dec;22(4):937-62. PMID:12489289

Aguirrebengoa K, Blanco R, Llorente A, Pérez-Irezabal J, Montejo M, Anda P. [Endocarditis due to Bartonella henselae on a native valve. A new case with some notable aspects].[Article in Spanish]. Enferm Infecc Microbiol Clin. 2002 Oct;20(8):415-7. PMID:12372243

Al-Attar N, Ruimy R, Baron F, Hvass U. Bartonella endocarditis complicating congenital heart disease. BMJ Case Rep. 2009;2009. pii: bcr06.2008.0092. Epub 2009 Mar 17. PMID:21686936

Albini TA, Lakhanpal RR, Foroozan R, Holz ER. Macular hole in cat scratch disease. Am J Ophthalmol. 2005 Jul;140(1):149-51. PMID:16038666

Albrich WC, Kraft C, Fisk T, Albrecht H. A mechanic with a bad valve: blood-culture-negative endocarditis. Lancet Infect Dis. 2004 Dec;4(12):777-84. PMID:15567127

Alcantara V, Rolain JM, Eduardo AG, Raul MJ, Raoult D. Molecular detection of Bartonella quintana in human body lice from Mexico City. Clin Microbiol Infect. 2009 Dec;15 Suppl 2:93-4. Epub 2009 Sep 28. PMID:19793127

Al-Daraji WI, Prescott RJ, Abdellaoui A, Khan MM, Kulkarni K, Youssef MM, Zelger BG, Zelger B. Cutaneous epithelioid angiomatous nodule: different views or interpretations in the analysis of ten new cases. Dermatol Online J. 2009 Mar 15;15(3):2. PMID:19379646

Alejandro del Río Vizoso M, Riera Jaume M, Salvá F, Bonnin O. [Endocarditis by Bartonella in a patient with human immunodeficiency virus infection].[Article in Spanish]. Med Clin (Barc). 2001 Feb 17;116(6):238. PMID:11333726

Al-Kappany YM, Lappin MR, Kwok OC, Abu-Elwafa SA, Hilali M, Dubey JP. Seroprevalence of Toxoplasma gondii and concurrent Bartonella spp., feline immunodeficiency virus, feline leukemia virus, and Dirofilaria immitis infections in Egyptian cats. J Parasitol. 2011 Apr;97(2):256-8. Epub 2010 Oct 14. PMID:21506874

Al-Majali AM, Al-Qudah KM. Seroprevalence of Bartonella henselae and Bartonella quintana infections in children from Central and Northern Jordan. Saudi Med J. 2004 Nov;25(11):1664-9. PMID:15573198

Al-Majali AM. Seroprevalence of and risk factors for Bartonella henselae and Bartonella quintana infections among pet cats in Jordan. Prev Vet Med. 2004 Jun 10;64(1):63-71. PMID:15219970

Al-Matar MJ, Petty RE, Cabral DA, Tucker LB, Peyvandi B, Prendiville J, Forbes J, Cairns R, Rothstein R. Rheumatic manifestations of Bartonella infection in 2 children. J Rheumatol. 2002 Jan;29(1):184-6. PMID:11824958

Alozie A, Yerebakan C, Westphal B, Podbielski A. Bartonella quintana Endocarditis of the Tricuspid and Mitral Valves. Thorac Cardiovasc Surg. 2011 May 9. [Epub ahead of print]. PMID:21557164

Al-Rahawan MM, Gray BM, Mitchell CS, Smith SD. Thoracic vertebral osteomyelitis with paraspinous mass and intraspinal extension: an atypical presentation of cat-scratch disease. Pediatr Radiol. 2012 Jan;42(1):116-9. Epub 2011 May 19. PMID:21594549

Alsmark CM, Frank AC, Karlberg EO, Legault BA, Ardell DH, Canbäck B, Eriksson AS, Näslund AK, Handley SA, Huvet M, La Scola B, Holmberg M, Andersson SG. The louse-borne human pathogen Bartonella quintana is a genomic derivative of the zoonotic agent Bartonella henselae. Proc Natl Acad Sci U S A. 2004 Jun 29;101(26):9716-21. Epub 2004 Jun 21. PMID:15210978

Alves AS, Milhano N, Santos-Silva M, Santos AS, Vilhena M, de Sousa R. Evidence of Bartonella spp., Rickettsia spp. and Anaplasma phagocytophilum in domestic, shelter and stray cat blood and fleas, Portugal. Clin Microbiol Infect. 2009 Dec;15 Suppl 2:1-3. Epub 2009 Mar 26. PMID:19416279

Amóra SS, Bevilaqua CM, Feijó FM, D Alves N, do V Maciel M. Control of phlebotomine (Diptera: Psychodidae) leishmaniasis vectors. Neotrop Entomol. 2009 May-Jun;38(3):303-10. PMID:19618043

Amsbaugh S, Huiras E, Wang NS, Wever A, Warren S. Bacillary angiomatosis associated with pseudoepitheliomatous hyperplasia. Am J Dermatopathol. 2006 Feb;28(1):32-5. PMID:16456322

Anan'ina IuV. [Bacterial zoonoses with natural focality: current trends in epidemic manifestation].[Article in Russian]. Zh Mikrobiol Epidemiol Immunobiol. 2002 Nov-Dec;(6):86-90. PMID:12506638

Anbu AT, Foulerton M, McMaster P, Bakalinova D. Basal ganglia involvement in a child with cat-scratch disease. Pediatr Infect Dis J. 2003 Oct;22(10):931-2. PMID:14579820

Andersen-Nissen E, Smith KD, Strobe KL, Barrett SL, Cookson BT, Logan SM, Aderem A. Evasion of Toll-like receptor 5 by flagellated bacteria. Proc Natl Acad Sci U S A. 2005 Jun 28;102(26):9247-52. Epub 2005 Jun 13. PMID:15956202

Anderson B. The interactions of Bartonella with endothelial cells and erythrocytes. Trends Microbiol. 2001 Nov;9(11):530-2. PMID:11825706

Andersson SG, Alsmark C, Canbäck B, Davids W, Frank C, Karlberg O, Klasson L, Antoine-Legault B, Mira A, Tamas I. Comparative genomics of microbial pathogens and symbionts. Bioinformatics. 2002;18 Suppl 2:S17. PMID:12385978

Andersson SG, Dehio C. Rickettsia prowazekii and Bartonella henselae:differences in the intracellular life styles revisited. Int J Med Microbiol. 2000 May;290(2):135-41. PMID:11045918

Andersson SG, Kempf VA. Host cell modulation by human, animal and plant pathogens. Int J Med Microbiol. 2004 Apr;293(7-8):463-70. PMID:15149019

Angelakis E, Billeter SA, Breitschwerdt EB, Chomel BB, Raoult D. Potential for tick-borne bartonelloses. Emerg Infect Dis. 2010 Mar;16(3):385-91. PMID:20202411

Angelakis E, Biswas S, Taylor C, Raoult D, Rolain JM. Heterogeneity of susceptibility to fluoroquinolones in Bartonella isolates from Australia reveals a natural mutation in gyrA. J Antimicrob Chemother. 2008 Jun;61(6):1252-5. Epub 2008 Mar 10. PMID:18334491

Angelakis E, Diatta G, Abdissa A, Trape JF, Mediannikov O, Richet H, Raoult D. Altitude-dependent Bartonella quintana genotype C in head lice, Ethiopia. Emerg Infect Dis. 2011 Dec;17(12):2357-9. PMID:22172306

Angelakis E, Edouard S, La Scola B, Raoult D. Bartonella henselae in skin biopsy specimens of patients with cat-scratch disease. Emerg Infect Dis. 2010 Dec;16(12):1963-5. PMID:21122232

Angelakis E, Khamphoukeo K, Grice D, Newton PN, Roux V, Aplin K, Raoult D, Rolain JM. Molecular detection of Bartonella species in rodents from the Lao PDR. Clin Microbiol Infect. 2009 Dec;15 Suppl 2:95-7. Epub 2009 Apr 3. PMID:19374642

Angelakis E, Lepidi H, Canel A, Rispal P, Perraudeau F, Barre I, Rolain JM, Raoult D. Human case of Bartonella alsatica lymphadenitis. Emerg Infect Dis. 2008 Dec;14(12):1951-3. PMID:19046532

Angelakis E, Pulcini C, Waton J, Imbert P, Socolovschi C, Edouard S, Dellamonica P, Raoult D. Scalp eschar and neck lymphadenopathy caused by Bartonella henselae after Tick Bite. Clin Infect Dis. 2010 Feb 15;50(4):549-51. PMID:20070235

Angelakis E, Raoult D, Rolain JM. Molecular characterization of resistance to fluoroquinolones in Bartonella henselae and Bartonella quintana. J Antimicrob Chemother. 2009 Jun;63(6):1288-9. Epub 2009 Apr 15. PMID:19369272

Angelakis E, Rolain JM, Raoult D, Brouqui P. Bartonella quintana in head louse nits. FEMS Immunol Med Microbiol. 2011 Jul;62(2):244-6. Epub 2011 May 5. PMID:21477003

Angelakis E, Roux V, Raoult D, Rolain JM. Real-time PCR strategy and detection of bacterial agents of lymphadenitis. Eur J Clin Microbiol Infect Dis. 2009 Nov;28(11):1363-8. Epub 2009 Aug 14. PMID:19685089

Angel-Moreno A, Hernández-Cabrera M, Pérez-Arellano JL. Kikuchi's disease or Kikuchi's syndrome? Clin Infect Dis. 2006 Feb 15;42(4):578-9; author reply 579-80. PMID:16421809

Angibaud G, Balagué JP, Lafontan JF. [Bartonella hensalae encephalopathy].[Article in French]. Presse Med. 2005 Feb 26;34(4):297-8. PMID:15798550

Antoniou M, Economou I, Wang X, Psaroulaki A, Spyridaki I, Papadopoulos B, Christidou A, Tsafantakis E, Tselentis Y. Fourteen-year seroepidemiological study of zoonoses in a Greek village. Am J Trop Med Hyg. 2002 Jan;66(1):80-5. PMID:12135274

Aragão RE, Ramos RM, Bezerra AF, Cavalcanti Júnior RB, Albuquerque TL. Optic neuropathy secondary to cat scratch disease: case report. Arq Bras Oftalmol. 2010 Nov-Dec;73(6):537-8. PMID:21271032

Arnez M, Luznik-Bufon T, Avsic-Zupanc T, Ruzic-Sabljic E, Petrovec M, Lotric-Furlan S, Strle F. Causes of febrile illnesses after a tick bite in Slovenian children. Pediatr Infect Dis J. 2003 Dec;22(12):1078-83. PMID:14688569

Arvand M, Feil EJ, Giladi M, Boulouis HJ, Viezens J. Multi-locus sequence typing of Bartonella henselae isolates from three continents reveals hypervirulent and feline-associated clones. PLoS One. 2007 Dec 19;2(12):e1346. PMID:18094753

Arvand M, Ignatius R, Regnath T, Hahn H, Mielke ME. Bartonella henselae-specific cell-mediated immune responses display a predominantly Th1 phenotype in experimentally infected C57BL/6 mice. Infect Immun. 2001 Oct;69(10):6427-33. PMID:11553587

Arvand M, Kazak I, Jovanovic S, Foss HD, Liesenfeld O. Cervical cat scratch disease lymphadenitis in a patient with immunoglobulin M antibodies to Toxoplasma gondii. Clin Diagn Lab Immunol. 2002 Mar;9(2):496-8. PMID:11874902

Arvand M, Klose AJ, Schwartz-Porsche D, Hahn H, Wendt C. Genetic variability and prevalence of Bartonella henselae in cats in Berlin, Germany, and analysis of its genetic relatedness to a strain from Berlin that is pathogenic for humans. J Clin Microbiol. 2001 Feb;39(2):743-6. PMID:11158141

Arvand M, Raoult D, Feil EJ. Multi-locus sequence typing of a geographically and temporally diverse sample of the highly clonal human pathogen Bartonella quintana. PLoS One. 2010 Mar 19;5(3):e9765. PMID:20333257

Arvand M, Schäd SG. Isolation of Bartonella henselae DNA from the peripheral blood of a patient with cat scratch disease up to 4 months after the cat scratch injury. J Clin Microbiol. 2006 Jun;44(6):2288-90. PMID:16757642

Arvand M, Schubert H, Viezens J. Emergence of distinct genetic variants in the population of primary Bartonella henselae isolates. Microbes Infect. 2006 Apr;8(5):1315-20. Epub 2006 Mar 15. PMID:16697237

Arvand M, Viezens J, Berghoff J. Prolonged Bartonella henselae bacteremia caused by reinfection in cats. Emerg Infect Dis. 2008 Jan;14(1):152-4. PMID:18258096

Arvand M, Viezens J. Evaluation of pulsed-field gel electrophoresis and multi-locus sequence typing for the analysis of clonal relatedness among Bartonella henselae isolates. Int J Med Microbiol. 2007 Jul;297(4):255-62. Epub 2007 Mar 30. PMID:17398157

Asano T, Ichiki K, Koizumi S, Kaizu K, Hatori T, Fujino O. High prevalence of antibodies against Bartonella henselae with cervical lymphadenopathy in children. Pediatr Int. 2010 Aug;52(4):533-5. PMID:20059723

Asensio-Sánchez VM, Rodríguez-Delgado B, García-Herrero E, Cabo-Vaquera V, García-Loygorri C. [Serous macular detachment as an atypical sign in cat scratch disease].[Article in Spanish]. Arch Soc Esp Oftalmol. 2006 Dec;81(12):717-9. PMID:17199167

Asharaf M, Letha S. Cutaneous bacillary angiomatosis. Indian J Pediatr. 2002 Nov;69(11):1003-5. PMID:12503674

Assarasakorn S, Veir JK, Hawley JR, Brewer MM, Morris AK, Hill AE, Lappin MR. Prevalence of Bartonella species, hemoplasmas, and Rickettsia felis DNA in blood and fleas of cats in Bangkok, Thailand. Res Vet Sci. 2012 Apr 20. [Epub ahead of print]. PMID:22521739

Astudillo L, Dahan S, Escourrou G, Sailler L, Carreiro M, Ollier S, Arlet P. Cat scratch responsible for primary cutaneous Nocardia asteroides in an immunocompetent patient. Br J Dermatol. 2001 Oct;145(4):684-5. PMID:11703311

Atamanyuk I, Raja SG, Kostolny M. Bartonella henselae endocarditis of percutaneously implanted pulmonary valve: a case report. J Heart Valve Dis. 2011 Jan;20(1):94-7. PMID:21404904

Atenstaedt RL. The response to the trench diseases in World War I: a triumph of public health science. Public Health. 2007 Aug;121(8):634-9. Epub 2007 May 30. PMID:17540420

Atenstaedt RL. Trench fever: the British medical response in the Great War. J R Soc Med. 2006 Nov;99(11):564-8. PMID:17082300

Aupy B, Conessa C, Clement P, Roguet E, Poncet JL. [Cat scratch disease: a diagnosis to be aware of!].[Article in French]. Rev Laryngol Otol Rhinol (Bord). 2008;129(1):53-6. PMID:18777770

Avidor B, Giladi M. The right answer. Lancet. 2004 Aug 28-Sep 3;364(9436):758. PMID:15337400

Avidor B, Graidy M, Efrat G, Leibowitz C, Shapira G, Schattner A, Zimhony O, Giladi M. Bartonella koehlerae, a new cat-associated agent of culture-negative human endocarditis. J Clin Microbiol. 2004 Aug;42(8):3462-8. PMID:15297484

Avidor B, Varon M, Marmor S, Lifschitz-Mercer B, Kletter Y, Ephros M, Giladi M. DNA amplification for the diagnosis of cat-scratch disease in small-quantity clinical specimens. Am J Clin Pathol. 2001 Jun;115(6):900-9. PMID:11392888

Ayllón T, Diniz PP, Breitschwerdt EB, Villaescusa A, Rodríguez-Franco F, Sainz A. Vector-borne diseases in client-owned and stray cats from Madrid, Spain. Vector Borne Zoonotic Dis. 2012 Feb;12(2):143-50. Epub 2011 Oct 24. PMID:22022820

Ayoub EM, McBride J, Schmiederer M, Anderson B. Role of Bartonella henselae in the etiology of Henoch-Schönlein purpura. Pediatr Infect Dis J. 2002 Jan;21(1):28-31. PMID:11791094

Azevedo ZM, Higa LY, Boechat PR, Boechat MB, Klaplauch F. [Cat-scratch disease caused by Bartonella quintana in an infant: an unusual presentation].[Article in Portuguese]. Rev Soc Bras Med Trop. 2000 May-Jun;33(3):313-7. PMID:10967601

Backert S, Meyer TF. Type IV secretion systems and their effectors in bacterial pathogenesis. Curr Opin Microbiol. 2006 Apr;9(2):207-17. Epub 2006 Mar 9. PMID:16529981

Backert S, Selbach M. Tyrosine-phosphorylated bacterial effector proteins: the enemies within. Trends Microbiol. 2005 Oct;13(10):476-84. PMID:16099656

Badger JL, Wass CA, Kim KS. Identification of Escherichia coli K1 genes contributing to human brain microvascular endothelial cell invasion by differential fluorescence induction. Mol Microbiol. 2000 Apr;36(1):174-82. PMID:10760174

Badiaga S, Brouqui P, Raoult D. Autochthonous epidemic typhus associated with Bartonella quintana bacteremia in a homeless person. Am J Trop Med Hyg. 2005 May;72(5):638-9. PMID:15891141

Badiaga S, Brouqui P. Human louse-transmitted infectious diseases. Clin Microbiol Infect. 2012 Apr;18(4):332-7. Epub 2012 Feb 23. PMID:22360386

Badiaga S, Paganelli F, Parola P, Beghin M, Barrau K, Eb F, Brouqui P. Chlamydia pneumoniae, but not Bartonella quintana, is associated with coronary heart disease: results of a French case-control study. Clin Microbiol Infect. 2003 Apr;9(4):315-8. PMID:12667243

Badiaga S, Raoult D, Brouqui P. Preventing and controlling emerging and reemerging transmissible diseases in the homeless. Emerg Infect Dis. 2008 Sep;14(9):1353-9. PMID:18760000

Bai HM, Yang FL, Yang H, Zhang Q. [Study on Bartonella species in rodents in western Yunnan, China].[Article in Chinese]. Zhonghua Liu Xing Bing Xue Za Zhi. 2005 Nov;26(11):868-70. PMID:16676607

Bai Y, Calisher CH, Kosoy MY, Root JJ, Doty JB. Persistent infection or successive reinfection of deer mice with Bartonella vinsonii subsp. arupensis. Appl Environ Microbiol. 2011 Mar;77(5):1728-31. Epub 2011 Jan 14. PMID:21239553

Bai Y, Cross PC, Malania L, Kosoy M. Isolation of Bartonella capreoli from elk. Vet Microbiol. 2011 Mar 24;148(2-4):329-32. Epub 2010 Sep 29. PMID:20961711

Bai Y, Kosoy M, Martin A, Ray C, Sheff K, Chalcraft L, Collinge SK. Characterization of Bartonella strains isolated from black-tailed prairie dogs (Cynomys ludovicianus). Vector Borne Zoonotic Dis. 2008 Spring;8(1):1-5. PMID:18237261

Bai Y, Kosoy M, Recuenco S, Alvarez D, Moran D, Turmelle A, Ellison J, Garcia DL, Estevez A, Lindblade K, Rupprecht C. Bartonella spp. in Bats, Guatemala. Emerg Infect Dis. 2011 Jul;17(7):1269-72. PMID:21762584

Bai Y, Kosoy MY, Boonmar S, Sawatwong P, Sangmaneedet S, Peruski LF. Enrichment culture and molecular identification of diverse Bartonella species in stray dogs. Vet Microbiol. 2010 Dec 15;146(3-4):314-9. Epub 2010 May 12. PMID:20570065

Bai Y, Kosoy MY, Cully JF, Bala T, Ray C, Collinge SK. Acquisition of nonspecific Bartonella strains by the northern grasshopper mouse (Onychomys leucogaster). FEMS Microbiol Ecol. 2007 Sep;61(3):438-48. Epub 2007 Aug 2. PMID:17672850

Bai Y, Kosoy MY, Lerdthusnee K, Peruski LF, Richardson JH. Prevalence and genetic heterogeneity of Bartonella strains cultured from rodents from 17 provinces in Thailand. Am J Trop Med Hyg. 2009 Nov;81(5):811-6. PMID:19861616

Bai Y, Kosoy MY, Ray C, Brinkerhoff RJ, Collinge SK. Temporal and spatial patterns of Bartonella infection in black-tailed prairie dogs (Cynomys ludovicianus). Microb Ecol. 2008 Aug;56(2):373-82. Epub 2008 Jan 5. PMID:18176820

Bai Y, Montgomery SP, Sheff KW, Chowdhury MA, Breiman RF, Kabeya H, Kosoy MY. Bartonella strains in small mammals from Dhaka, Bangladesh, related to Bartonella in America and Europe. Am J Trop Med Hyg. 2007 Sep;77(3):567-70. PMID:17827381

Bajer A, Pawelczyk A, Behnke JM, Gilbert FS, Sinski E. Factors affecting the component community structure of haemoparasites in bank voles (Clethrionomys glareolus) from the Mazury Lake District region of Poland. Parasitology. 2001 Jan;122 Pt 1:43-54. PMID:11197763

Balakrishnan N, Menon T, Fournier PE, Raoult D. Bartonella quintana and Coxiella burnetii as causes of endocarditis, India. Emerg Infect Dis. 2008 Jul;14(7):1168-9. PMID:18598654

Baneth G, Bourdeau P, Bourdoiseau G, Bowman D, Breitschwerdt E, Capelli G, Cardoso L, Dantas-Torres F, Day M, Dedet JP, Dobler G, Ferrer L, Irwin P, Kempf V, Kohn B, Lappin M, Little S, Maggi R, Miro G, Naucke T, Oliva G, Otranto D, Penzhorn B, Pfeffer M, Roura X, Sainz A, Shaw S, Shin S, Solano-Gallego L, Straubinger R, Traub R, Trees A, Truyen U, Demonceau T, Fitzgerald R, Gatti D, Hostetler J, Kilmer B, Krieger K, Mencke N, Mendao C, Mottier L, Pachnicke S, Rees B, Siebert S, Stanneck D, Tarancon Mingote M, von Simson C, Weston S. Vector-Borne Diseases - constant challenge for practicing veterinarians: recommendations from the CVBD World Forum. Parasit Vectors. 2012 Mar 20;5(1):55. [Epub ahead of print]. PMID:22433172

Barankin B, Houston S, Alanen K, Ting PT, Lauzon G. Crusted plaques in an immunocompromised host. Arch Dermatol. 2005 Feb;141(2):263-8. PMID:15724025

Barber RM, Li Q, Diniz PP, Porter BF, Breitschwerdt EB, Claiborne MK, Birkenheuer AJ, Levine JM, Levine GJ, Chandler K, Kenny P, Nghiem P, Wei S, Greene CE, Kent M, Platt SR, Greer K, Schatzberg SJ. Evaluation of brain tissue or cerebrospinal fluid with broadly reactive polymerase chain reaction for Ehrlichia, Anaplasma, spotted fever group Rickettsia, Bartonella, and Borrelia species in canine neurological diseases (109 cases). J Vet Intern Med. 2010 Mar-Apr;24(2):372-8. PMID:20102497

Barbian KD, Minnick MF. A bacteriophage-like particle from Bartonella bacilliformis. Microbiology. 2000 Mar;146 (Pt 3):599-609. PMID:10746763

Barbier F, Fournier PE, Dauge MC, Gallien S, Raoult D, Andremont A, Ruimy R. Bartonella quintana coinfection in Staphylococcus aureus endocarditis: usefulness of screening in high-risk patients? Clin Infect Dis. 2009 May 1;48(9):1332-3. PMID:19344260

Barie PS. Forensic microbiology and the reinterpretation of history. Surg Infect (Larchmt). 2008 Aug;9(4):413-4. PMID:18759677

Barnes A, Bell SC, Isherwood DR, Bennett M, Carter SD. Evidence of Bartonella henselae infection in cats and dogs in the United Kingdom. Vet Rec. 2000 Dec 9;147(24):673-7. PMID:11132671

Baron C, OCallaghan D, Lanka E. Bacterial secrets of secretion: EuroConference on the biology of type IV secretion processes. Mol Microbiol. 2002 Mar;43(5):1359-65. PMID:11918819

Barquero-Calvo E, Conde-Alvarez R, Chacón-Díaz C, Quesada-Lobo L, Martirosyan A, Guzmán-Verri C, Iriarte M, Mancek-Keber M, Jerala R, Gorvel JP, Moriyón I, Moreno E, Chaves-Olarte E. The differential interaction of Brucella and ochrobactrum with innate immunity reveals traits related to the evolution of stealthy pathogens. PLoS One. 2009 Jun 16;4(6):e5893. PMID:19529776

Barr YR, Qiu S. A 16-year-old adolescent boy with unilateral cervical lymphadenopathy suspicious for malignancy. Arch Pathol Lab Med. 2005 Aug;129(8):1065-6. PMID:16048405

Barrs VR, Beatty JA, Wilson BJ, Evans N, Gowan R, Baral RM, Lingard AE, Perkovic G, Hawley JR, Lappin MR. Prevalence of Bartonella species, Rickettsia felis, haemoplasmas and the Ehrlichia group in the blood of cats and fleas in eastern Australia. Aust Vet J. 2010 May;88(5):160-5. PMID:20529020

Batard ML, Cheret A, Muller P, Sarrouy J, Mareel A, Lamaury I. [Bacillary angiomatosis associated with AIDS].[Article in French]. Ann Dermatol Venereol. 2006 May;133(5 Pt 1):498-9. PMID:16760847

Bathelier E, Balme B. [Kaposi's sarcoma].[Article in French]. Ann Dermatol Venereol. 2006 Aug-Sep;133(8-9 Pt 1):728-30. PMID:17053753

Battisti JM, Minnick MF. Laboratory maintenance of Bartonella quintana. Curr Protoc Microbiol. 2008 Aug;Chapter 3:Unit 3C.1.1-3C.1.13. PMID:18729057

Battisti JM, Sappington KN, Smitherman LS, Parrow NL, Minnick MF. Environmental signals generate a differential and coordinated expression of the heme receptor gene family of Bartonella quintana. Infect Immun. 2006 Jun;74(6):3251-61. PMID:16714552

Battisti JM, Smitherman LS, Sappington KN, Parrow NL, Raghavan R, Minnick MF. Transcriptional regulation of the heme binding protein gene family of Bartonella quintana is accomplished by a novel promoter element and iron response regulator. Infect Immun. 2007 Sep;75(9):4373-85. Epub 2007 Jun 18. PMID:17576755

Batts S, Demers DM. Spectrum and treatment of cat-scratch disease. Pediatr Infect Dis J. 2004 Dec;23(12):1161-2. PMID:15626957

Baty G, Lanotte P, Hocqueloux L, Prazuck T, Bret L, Romano M, Mereghetti L. [PCR rDNA 16S used for the etiological diagnosis of blood culture negative endocarditis].[Article in French]. Med Mal Infect. 2010 Jun;40(6):358-62. Epub 2009 Sep 30. PMID:19796889

Bayliss DB, Steiner JM, Sucholdolski JS, Radecki SV, Brewer MM, Morris AK, Lappin MR. Serum feline pancreatic lipase immunoreactivity concentration and seroprevalences of antibodies against Toxoplasma gondii and Bartonella species in client-owned cats. J Feline Med Surg. 2009 Aug;11(8):663-7. Epub 2009 Jun 26. PMID:19560385

Baylor P, Garoufi A, Karpathios T, Lutz J, Mogelof J, Moseley D. Transverse myelitis in 2 patients with Bartonella henselae infection (cat scratch disease). Clin Infect Dis. 2007 Aug 15;45(4):e42-5. Epub 2007 Jul 5. PMID:17638185

Beard AW, Maggi RG, Kennedy-Stoskopf S, Cherry NA, Sandfoss MR, DePerno CS, Breitschwerdt EB. Bartonella spp. in feral pigs, southeastern United States. Emerg Infect Dis. 2011 May;17(5):893-5. PMID:21529405

Beati L, Cáceres AG, Lee JA, Munstermann LE. Systematic relationships among Lutzomyia sand flies (Diptera: Psychodidae) of Peru and Colombia based on the analysis of 12S and 28S ribosomal DNA sequences. Int J Parasitol. 2004 Feb;34(2):225-34. PMID:15037108

Becker JL. Vector-borne illnesses and the safety of the blood supply. Curr Hematol Rep. 2003 Nov;2(6):511-7. PMID:14561396

Beerlage C, Varanat M, Linder K, Maggi RG, Cooley J, Kempf VA, Breitschwerdt EB. Bartonella vinsonii subsp. berkhoffii and Bartonella henselae as potential causes of proliferative vascular diseases in animals. Med Microbiol Immunol. 2012 Mar 27. [Epub ahead of print]. PMID:22450733

Bejarano EE, Rojas W, Uribe S, Vélez ID. [Systematics of the Lutzomyia species of the verrucarum Theodor group, 1965 (Diptera: Psychodiadae)].[Article in Spanish]. Biomedica. 2003 Mar;23(1):87-102. PMID:12696402

Beldomenico PM, Chomel BB, Foley JE, Sacks BN, Baldi CJ, Kasten RW, Gardner IA. Environmental factors associated with Bartonella vinsonii subsp. berkhoffii seropositivity in free-ranging coyotes from northern California. Vector Borne Zoonotic Dis. 2005 Summer;5(2):110-9. PMID:16011426

Belgard S, Truyen U, Thibault JC, Sauter-Louis C, Hartmann K. Relevance of feline calicivirus, feline immunodeficiency virus, feline leukemia virus, feline herpesvirus and Bartonella henselae in cats with chronic gingivostomatitis. Berl Munch Tierarztl Wochenschr. 2010 Sep-Oct;123(9-10):369-76. PMID:21038808

Bellissimo-Rodrigues F, da Fonseca BA, Martinez R. Bacillary angiomatosis in a pregnant woman. Int J Gynaecol Obstet. 2010 Oct;111(1):85-6. Epub 2010 Jul 21. PMID:20650456

Belongia EA. Epidemiology and impact of coinfections acquired from Ixodes ticks. Vector Borne Zoonotic Dis. 2002 Winter;2(4):265-73. PMID:12804168

Bemis DA, Kania SA. Isolation of Bartonella sp. from sheep blood. Emerg Infect Dis. 2007 Oct;13(10):1565-7. PMID:18258009

Ben Slama L, Hasni W, Royer B. [Cat-scratch disease localisation in the parotid gland].[Article in French]. Rev Stomatol Chir Maxillofac. 2008 Jun;109(3):183-6. Epub 2008 Jun 3. PMID:18533210

Ben-Ami R, Ephros M, Avidor B, Katchman E, Varon M, Leibowitz C, Comaneshter D, Giladi M. Cat-scratch disease in elderly patients. Clin Infect Dis. 2005 Oct 1;41(7):969-74. Epub 2005 Aug 30. PMID:16142661

Benesch M, Kerbl R, Wirnsberger A, Stünzner D, Mangge H, Schenkeli R, Deutsch J. [Peripheral lymphadenopathy in childhood--recommendations for diagnostic evaluation].[Article in German]. Klin Padiatr. 2000 Sep-Oct;212(5):277-82. PMID:11048289

Bennett AD, Gunn-Moore DA, Brewer M, Lappin MR. Prevalence of Bartonella species, haemoplasmas and Toxoplasma gondii in cats in Scotland. J Feline Med Surg. 2011 Aug;13(8):553-7. Epub 2011 May 13. PMID:21570883

Benslimani A, Fenollar F, Lepidi H, Raoult D. Bacterial zoonoses and infective endocarditis, Algeria. Emerg Infect Dis. 2005 Feb;11(2):216-24. PMID:15752438

Bentzel DE, Espinosa BJ, Canal E, Blazes DL, Hall ER. Susceptibility of owl monkeys (Aotus nancymaae) to experimental infection with Bartonella bacilliformis. Comp Med. 2008 Feb;58(1):76-80. PMID:19793460

Bergh K, Bevanger L, Hanssen I, Løseth K. Low prevalence of Bartonella henselae infections in Norwegian domestic and feral cats. APMIS. 2002 Apr;110(4):309-14. PMID:12076266

Berghoff J, Viezens J, Guptill L, Fabbi M, Arvand M. Bartonella henselae exists as a mosaic of different genetic variants in the infected host. Microbiology. 2007 Jul;153(Pt 7):2045-51. PMID:17600049

Berglund EC, Ehrenborg C, Vinnere Pettersson O, Granberg F, Näslund K, Holmberg M, Andersson SG. Genome dynamics of Bartonella grahamii in micro-populations of woodland rodents. BMC Genomics. 2010 Mar 4;11:152. PMID:20202191

Berglund EC, Ellegaard K, Granberg F, Xie Z, Maruyama S, Kosoy MY, Birtles RJ, Andersson SG. Rapid diversification by recombination in Bartonella grahamii from wild rodents in Asia contrasts with low levels of genomic divergence in Northern Europe and America. Mol Ecol. 2010 Jun;19(11):2241-55. Epub 2010 May 6. PMID:20465583

Berglund EC, Frank AC, Calteau A, Vinnere Pettersson O, Granberg F, Eriksson AS, Näslund K, Holmberg M, Lindroos H, Andersson SG. Run-off replication of host-adaptability genes is associated with gene transfer agents in the genome of mouse-infecting Bartonella grahamii. PLoS Genet. 2009 Jul;5(7):e1000546. Epub 2009 Jul 3. PMID:19578403

Berguiga M, Abouzeid H, Bart PA, Guex-Crosier Y. Severe occlusive vasculitis as a complication of cat scratch disease. Klin Monbl Augenheilkd. 2008 May;225(5):486-7. PMID:18454406

Bermas H, Fenoglio ME, Haun W, Moore JT. Hand-assisted laparoscopic splenectomy: indications and technique. JSLS. 2004 Jan-Mar;8(1):69-71. PMID:14974668

Bermond D, Boulouis HJ, Heller R, Van Laere G, Monteil H, Chomel BB, Sander A, Dehio C, Piémont Y. Bartonella bovis Bermond et al. sp. nov. and Bartonella capreoli sp. nov., isolated from European ruminants. Int J Syst Evol Microbiol. 2002 Mar;52(Pt 2):383-90. PMID:11931146

Bermond D, Heller R, Barrat F, Delacour G, Dehio C, Alliot A, Monteil H, Chomel B, Boulouis HJ, Piémont Y. Bartonella birtlesii sp. nov., isolated from small mammals (Apodemus spp.). Int J Syst Evol Microbiol. 2000 Nov;50 Pt 6:1973-9. PMID:11155970

Bernabeu-Wittel J, Luque R, Corbi R, Mantrana-Bermejo M, Navarrete M, Vallejo A, Bernabeu-Wittel M. Bacillary angiomatosis with atypical clinical presentation in an immunocompetent patient. Indian J Dermatol Venereol Leprol. 2010 Nov-Dec;76(6):682-5. PMID:21079313

Bernard L, Ghez D, Perronne C. Isolated splenic cat scratch disease. Clin Infect Dis. 2003 Sep 15;37(6):860; author reply 860-1. PMID:12955654

Bernit E, Veit V, La Scola B, Tissot-Dupont H, Gachon J, Raoult D, Harlé JR. Bartonella quintana and Mycobacterium tuberculosis coinfection in an HIV-infected patient with lymphadenitis. J Infect. 2003 May;46(4):244-6. PMID:12799150

Bernscherer G. [Carrión-disease--history of a long-forgotten malady]. [Article in Hungarian]. Orv Hetil. 2004 Jan 25;145(4):197-9. PMID:14978887

Berrich M, Kieda C, Grillon C, Monteil M, Lamerant N, Gavard J, Boulouis HJ, Haddad N. Differential effects of Bartonella henselae on human and feline macro- and micro-vascular endothelial cells. PLoS One. 2011;6(5):e20204. Epub 2011 May 27. PMID:21637717

Berry D. History of cardiology: Wilhelm His, Jr, MD. Circulation. 2006 May 9;113(18):f72. PMID:16688857

Berryessa NA, Johnson LR, Kasten RW, Chomel BB. Microbial culture of blood samples and serologic testing for bartonellosis in cats with chronic rhinosinusitis. J Am Vet Med Assoc. 2008 Oct 1;233(7):1084-9. PMID:18828717

Besada E, Woods A, Caputo M. An uncommon presentation of Bartonella-associated neuroretinitis. Optom Vis Sci. 2002 Aug;79(8):479-88. PMID:12199539

Besson-Leaud L, Mancel E, Missotte I, Morlat C, Menager C. [Sudden sight impairment revealing a cat-scratch disease: report of three cases].[Article in French]. Arch Pediatr. 2004 Oct;11(10):1209-11. PMID:15475278

Bettenay SV, Lappin MR, Mueller RS. An immunohistochemical and polymerase chain reaction evaluation of feline plasmacytic pododermatitis. Vet Pathol. 2007 Jan;44(1):80-3. PMID:17197627

Bevins SN, Carver S, Boydston EE, Lyren LM, Alldredge M, Logan KA, Riley SP, Fisher RN, Vickers TW, Boyce W, Salman M, Lappin MR, Crooks KR, VandeWoude S. Three pathogens in sympatric populations of pumas, bobcats, and domestic cats:implications for infectious disease transmission. PLoS One. 2012;7(2):e31403. Epub 2012 Feb 8. PMID:22347471

Bhansali P, Sekaran A, Sikora MM, Mancao MY, Carnahan GE, Silver FM, Foley T, Fury M, Adler S. Index of suspicion. Pediatr Rev. 2005 Apr;26(4):143-7. PMID:15805237

Bharti DR, Mehta AV. Constrictive pericarditis following cat-scratch disease in a 12-year-old female: a rare association. Tenn Med. 2003 Nov;96(11):509-10. PMID:14635359

Bhatti MT, Asif R, Bhatti LB. Macular star in neuroretinitis. Arch Neurol. 2001 Jun;58(6):1008-9. PMID:11405817

Bhatti Z, Berenson CS. Adult systemic cat scratch disease associated with therapy for hepatitis C. BMC Infect Dis. 2007 Feb 23;7:8. PMID:17319959

Bhengsri S, Baggett HC, Peruski LF Jr, Morway C, Bai Y, Fisk TL, Sitdhirasdr A, Maloney SA, Dowell SF, Kosoy M. Bartonella spp. infections, Thailand. Emerg Infect Dis. 2010 Apr;16(4):743-5. PMID:20350414

Bhengsri S, Baggett HC, Peruski LF, Morway C, Bai Y, Fisk TL, Sitdhirasdr A, Maloney SA, Dowell SF, Kosoy M. Bartonella seroprevalence in rural Thailand. Southeast Asian J Trop Med Public Health. 2011 May;42(3):687-92. PMID:21706948

Bianda JC, Dedes W. [Positive polymerase chain reaction for Bartonella henselae in conjunctival granuloma].[Article in German]. Klin Monbl Augenheilkd. 2009 Apr;226(4):347. Epub 2009 Apr 21. PMID:19384797

Biddinger PD, Isselbacher EM, Fan D, Shepard JA. Case records of the Massachusetts General Hospital. Weekly clinicopathological exercises. Case 5-2005. A 53-year-old man with depression and sudden shortness of breath. N Engl J Med. 2005 Feb 17;352(7):709-16. PMID:15716566

Bilavsky E, Amit S, Avidor B, Ephros M, Giladi M. Cat scratch disease during pregnancy. Obstet Gynecol. 2012 Mar;119(3):640-4. PMID:22353964

Billeter SA, Blanton HL, Little SE, Levy MG, Breitschwerdt EB. Detection of Rickettsia amblyommii in association with a tick bite rash. Vector Borne Zoonotic Dis. 2007 Winter;7(4):607-10. PMID:18052716

Billeter SA, Breitschwerdt EB, Levy MG. Invasion of canine erythrocytes by Bartonella vinsonii subsp. berkhoffii. Vet Microbiol. 2012 Apr 23;156(1-2):213-6. Epub 2011 Oct 20. PMID:22071179

Billeter SA, Cáceres AG, Gonzales-Hidalgo J, Luna-Caypo D, Kosoy MY. Molecular detection of Bartonella species in ticks from Peru. J Med Entomol. 2011 Nov;48(6):1257-60. PMID:22238888

Billeter SA, Diniz PP, Battisti JM, Munderloh UG, Breitschwerdt EB, Levy MG. Infection and replication of Bartonella species within a tick cell line. Exp Appl Acarol. 2009 Nov;49(3):193-208. Epub 2009 Feb 26. PMID:19242658

Billeter SA, Gundi VA, Rood MP, Kosoy MY. Molecular detection and identification of Bartonella species in Xenopsylla cheopis fleas (Siphonaptera: Pulicidae) collected from Rattus norvegicus rats in Los Angeles, California. Appl Environ Microbiol. 2011 Nov;77(21):7850-2. Epub 2011 Sep 9. PMID:21908631

Billeter SA, Hayman DT, Peel AJ, Baker K, Wood JL, Cunningham A, Suu-Ire R, Dittmar K, Kosoy MY. Bartonella species in bat flies (Diptera: Nycteribiidae) from western Africa. Parasitology. 2012 Mar;139(3):324-9. Epub 2012 Feb 6. PMID:22309510

Billeter SA, Kasten RW, Killmaster LF, Breitschwerdt EB, Levin ML, Levy MG, Kosoy MY, Chomel BB. Experimental infection by capillary tube feeding of Rhipicephalus sanguineus with Bartonella vinsonii subspecies berkhoffii. Comp Immunol Microbiol Infect Dis. 2012 Jan;35(1):9-15. Epub 2011 Nov 5. PMID:22062313

Billeter SA, Levy MG, Chomel BB, Breitschwerdt EB. Vector transmission of Bartonella species with emphasis on the potential for tick transmission. Med Vet Entomol. 2008 Mar;22(1):1-15. PMID:18380649

Billeter SA, Miller MK, Breitschwerdt EB, Levy MG. Detection of two Bartonella tamiae-like sequences in Amblyomma americanum (Acari: Ixodidae) using 16S-23S intergenic spacer region-specific primers. J Med Entomol. 2008 Jan;45(1):176-9. PMID:18283962

Biousse V. [Optic neuritis in cat scratch disease].[Article in French]. Rev Neurol (Paris). 2005 May;161(5):571-3. PMID:16106808

Birtles RJ, Fry NK, Ventosilla P, Cáceres AG, Sánchez E, Vizcarra H, Raoult D. Identification of Bartonella bacilliformis genotypes and their relevance to epidemiological investigations of human bartonellosis. J Clin Microbiol. 2002 Oct;40(10):3606-12. PMID:12354853

Birtles RJ, Hazel S, Bown K, Raoult D, Begon M, Bennett M. Subtyping of uncultured bartonellae using sequence comparison of 16 S/23 S rRNA intergenic spacer regions amplified directly from infected blood. Mol Cell Probes. 2000 Apr;14(2):79-87. PMID:10799268

Birtles RJ, Hazel SM, Bennett M, Bown K, Raoult D, Begon M. Longitudinal monitoring of the dynamics of infections due to Bartonella species in UK woodland rodents. Epidemiol Infect. 2001 Apr;126(2):323-9. PMID:11349984

Birtles RJ, Laycock G, Kenny MJ, Shaw SE, Day MJ. Prevalence of Bartonella species causing bacteraemia in domesticated and companion animals in the United Kingdom. Vet Rec. 2002 Aug 24;151(8):225-9. PMID:12219899

Birtles RJ. Bartonellae as elegant hemotropic parasites. Ann N Y Acad Sci. 2005 Dec;1063:270-9. PMID:16481527

Biswas S, Maggi RG, Papich MG, Breitschwerdt EB. Molecular mechanisms of Bartonella henselae resistance to azithromycin, pradofloxacin and enrofloxacin. J Antimicrob Chemother. 2010 Mar;65(3):581-2. Epub 2009 Dec 18. PMID:20022937

Biswas S, Maggi RG, Papich MG, Keil D, Breitschwerdt EB. Comparative activity of pradofloxacin, enrofloxacin, and azithromycin against Bartonella henselae isolates collected from cats and a human. J Clin Microbiol. 2010 Feb;48(2):617-8. Epub 2009 Dec 9. PMID:20007401

Biswas S, Raoult D, Rolain JM. A bioinformatic approach to understanding antibiotic resistance in intracellular bacteria through whole genome analysis. Int J Antimicrob Agents. 2008 Sep;32(3):207-20. Epub 2008 Jul 10. PMID:18619818

Biswas S, Raoult D, Rolain JM. Molecular characterisation of resistance to rifampin in Bartonella quintana. Clin Microbiol Infect. 2009 Dec;15 Suppl 2:100-1. Epub 2009 Dec 24. PMID:19929979

Biswas S, Raoult D, Rolain JM. Molecular characterization of resistance to macrolides in Bartonella henselae. Antimicrob Agents Chemother. 2006 Sep;50(9):3192-3. PMID:16940128

Biswas S, Raoult D, Rolain JM. Molecular mechanism of gentamicin resistance in Bartonella henselae. Clin Microbiol Infect. 2009 Dec;15 Suppl 2:98-9. PMID:20584166

Biswas S, Raoult D, Rolain JM. Molecular mechanisms of resistance to antibiotics in Bartonella bacilliformis. J Antimicrob Chemother. 2007 Jun;59(6):1065-70. Epub 2007 Apr 21. PMID:17449882

Biswas S, Rolain JM. Bartonella infection: treatment and drug resistance. Future Microbiol. 2010 Nov;5(11):1719-31. PMID:21133691

Bitam I, Dittmar K, Parola P, Whiting MF, Raoult D. Fleas and flea-borne diseases. Int J Infect Dis. 2010 Aug;14(8):e667-76. Epub 2010 Mar 1. PMID:20189862

Bitam I, Rolain JM, Kernif T, Baziz B, Parola P, Raoult D. Bartonella species detected in rodents and hedgehogs from Algeria. Clin Microbiol Infect. 2009 Dec;15 Suppl 2:102-3. Epub 2009 Dec 24. PMID:19929978

Bitam I, Rolain JM, Nicolas V, Tsai YL, Parola P, Gundi VA, Chomel BB, Raoult D. A multi-gene analysis of diversity of bartonella detected in fleas from Algeria. Comp Immunol Microbiol Infect Dis. 2012 Jan;35(1):71-6. Epub 2011 Dec 5. PMID:22153359

Biviji AA, Paiement GD, Steinbach LS. Musculoskeletal manifestations of human immunodeficiency virus infection. J Am Acad Orthop Surg. 2002 Sep-Oct;10(5):312-20. PMID:12374482

Blanco Badillo A, Telenti Asensio M, Anda P, Figueroa Fábregas E. [Carrión disease: two centuries later].[Article in Spanish]. Med Clin (Barc). 2005 Jul 9;125(6):239. PMID:16022842

Blanco JR, Jado I, Marín M, Sanfeliu I, Portillo A, Anda P, Pons I, Oteo JA. [Microbiological diagnosis of emerging bacterial pathogens: Anaplasma, Bartonella, Rickettsia, and Tropheryma whipplei].[Article in Spanish]. Enferm Infecc Microbiol Clin. 2008 Nov;26(9):573-80. PMID:19100178

Blanco JR, Pérez-Martínez L, Vallejo M, Santibáñez S, Portillo A, Oteo JA. Prevalence of rickettsia felis-like and Bartonella Spp. in Ctenocephalides felis and Ctenocephalides canis from La Rioja (Northern Spain). Ann N Y Acad Sci. 2006 Oct;1078:270-4. PMID:17114721

Blanco JR, Raoult D. [Diseases produced by Bartonella].[Article in Spanish]. Enferm Infecc Microbiol Clin. 2005 May;23(5):313-9; quiz 320. PMID:15899181

Bloch KC, Glaser C. Diagnostic approaches for patients with suspected encephalitis. Curr Infect Dis Rep. 2007 Jul;9(4):315-22. PMID:17618552

Boggs SR, Fisher RG. Bone pain and fever in an adolescent and his sibling. Cat scratch disease (CSD). Pediatr Infect Dis J. 2011 Jan;30(1):89, 93-4. PMID:21513084

Bogumiła S, Adamska M. [Capreolus capreolus and Ixodes ricinus as a reservoir of Bartonella in north-western Poland].[Article in Polish]. Wiad Parazytol. 2005;51(2):139-43. PMID:16838623

Boillat N, Greub G. [Cat scratch disease and other human infections caused by Bartonella species].[Article in French]. Rev Med Suisse. 2008 Apr 9;4(152):901-7. PMID:18578430

Boiron E, Soto B, Zimmermann B, Jullien M. [Atypical presentation of hepatosplenic cat scratch disease in a 3-year-old child].[Article in French]. Arch Pediatr. 2012 May 4. [Epub ahead of print]. PMID:22561046

Bolton JG, Galeckas KJ, Satter EK. Inoculation bartonellosis in an adult: a case report. Cutis. 2010 Jan;85(1):37-42. PMID:20184210

Bonatti H, Mendez J, Guerrero I, Krishna M, Ananda-Michel J, Yao J, Steers JL, Hellinger W, Dickson RC, Alvarez S. Disseminated Bartonella infection following liver transplantation. Transpl Int. 2006 Aug;19(8):683-7. PMID:16827686

Bonhomme CJ, Nappez C, Raoult D. Microarray for serotyping of Bartonella species. BMC Microbiol. 2007 Jun 25;7:59. PMID:17593301

Bonilla DL, Kabeya H, Henn J, Kramer VL, Kosoy MY. Bartonella quintana in body lice and head lice from homeless persons, San Francisco, California, USA. Emerg Infect Dis. 2009 Jun;15(6):912-5. PMID:19523290

Bonza S, McDougle L, McConaghy JR. Progressive lymphadenopathy and intractable pain in an immunocompetent African-American adult with cat-scratch disease. J Natl Med Assoc. 2008 Oct;100(10):1231-4. PMID:18942286

Bookman I, Scholey JW, Jassal SV, Lajoie G, Herzenberg AM. Necrotizing glomerulonephritis caused by Bartonella henselae endocarditis. Am J Kidney Dis. 2004 Feb;43(2):e25-30. PMID:14750122

Boonjakuakul JK, Gerns HL, Chen YT, Hicks LD, Minnick MF, Dixon SE, Hall SC, Koehler JE. Proteomic and immunoblot analyses of Bartonella quintana total membrane proteins identify antigens recognized by sera from infected patients. Infect Immun. 2007 May;75(5):2548-61. Epub 2007 Feb 16. PMID:17307937

Boralevi F, Léauté-Labrèze C, Lepreux S, Barbarot S, Mazereeuw-Hautier J, Eschard C, Taïeb A; Groupe de Recherche Clinique en Dermatologie Pédiatrique. Idiopathic facial aseptic granuloma: a multicentre prospective study of 30 cases. Br J Dermatol. 2007 Apr;156(4):705-8. PMID:17493068

Borboli S, Afshari NA, Watkins L, Foster CS. Presumed oculoglandular syndrome from Bartonella quintana. Ocul Immunol Inflamm. 2007 Jan-Feb;15(1):41-3. PMID:17365807

Borker A, Gardner R. Severe thrombocytopenic purpura as a complication of cat scratch disease. Clin Pediatr (Phila). 2002 Mar;41(2):117-8. PMID:11931328

Botelho-Nevers E, Raoult D. Fever of unknown origin due to rickettsioses. Infect Dis Clin North Am. 2007 Dec;21(4):997-1011, ix. PMID:18061086

Bouchon A, Facchetti F, Weigand MA, Colonna M. TREM-1 amplifies inflammation and is a crucial mediator of septic shock. Nature. 2001 Apr 26;410(6832):1103-7. PMID:11323674

Bouchouicha R, Boulouis HJ, Berrich M, Monteil M, Chomel B, Haddad N. Comparison of the performances of MLVA vs. the main other typing techniques for Bartonella henselae. Clin Microbiol Infect. 2009 Dec;15 Suppl 2:104-5. Epub 2009 Sep 28. PMID:19793125

Bouchouicha R, Durand B, Monteil M, Chomel BB, Berrich M, Arvand M, Birtles RJ, Breitschwerdt EB, Koehler JE, Maggi R, Maruyama S, Kasten R, Petit E, Boulouis HJ, Haddad N. Molecular epidemiology of feline and human Bartonella henselae isolates. Emerg Infect Dis. 2009 May;15(5):813-6. PMID:19402978

Boudebouch N, Sarih M, Beaucournu JC, Amarouch H, Hassar M, Raoult D, Parola P. Bartonella clarridgeiae, B. henselae and Rickettsia felis in fleas from Morocco. Ann Trop Med Parasitol. 2011 Oct;105(7):493-8. PMID:22185943

Boulouis HJ, Barrat F, Bermond D, Bernex F, Thibault D, Heller R, Fontaine JJ, Piémont Y, Chomel BB. Kinetics of Bartonella birtlesii infection in experimentally infected mice and pathogenic effect on reproductive functions. Infect Immun. 2001 Sep;69(9):5313-7. PMID:11500400

Boulouis HJ, Chang CC, Henn JB, Kasten RW, Chomel BB. Factors associated with the rapid emergence of zoonotic Bartonella infections. Vet Res. 2005 May-Jun;36(3):383-410. PMID:15845231

Boulouis HJ, Chomel B. [Bartonellosis: emerging infection].[Article in French]. Rev Prat. 2004 Nov 30;54(18):1982-6. PMID:15673067

Boulouis HJ, Haddad N, Vayssier-Taussat M, Maillard R, Chomel B. [Persistent Bartonella infection: epidemiological and clinical implications].[Article in French]. Bull Acad Natl Med. 2007 Jun;191(6):1037-44; discussion 1047-9. PMID:18402163

Bouvresse S, Socolovshi C, Berdjane Z, Durand R, Izri A, Raoult D, Chosidow O, Brouqui P. No evidence of Bartonella quintana but detection of Acinetobacter baumannii in head lice from elementary schoolchildren in Paris. Comp Immunol Microbiol Infect Dis. 2011 Dec;34(6):475-7. Epub 2011 Oct 5. PMID:21974965

Bowen BE, Manning RA, Foster JB, Kurup SK, Ramaiya KJ, Shah GK. Diagnostic and therapeutic challenges. Retina. 2011 Oct;31(9):1967-71. PMID:21866076

Bowman DD. Introduction to the alpha-proteobacteria: Wolbachia and Bartonella, Rickettsia, Brucella, Ehrlichia, and Anaplasma. Top Companion Anim Med. 2011 Nov;26(4):173-7. PMID:22152604

Bown KJ, Bennet M, Begon M. Flea-borne Bartonella grahamii and Bartonella taylorii in bank voles. Emerg Infect Dis. 2004 Apr;10(4):684-7. PMID:15200860

Bown KJ, Ellis BA, Birtles RJ, Durden LA, Lello J, Begon M, Bennett M. New world origins for haemoparasites infecting United Kingdom grey squirrels (Sciurus carolinensis), as revealed by phylogenetic analysis of bartonella infecting squirrel populations in England and the United States. Epidemiol Infect. 2002 Dec;129(3):647-53. PMID:12558350

Boyer JD. Molecular and immunological approaches to controlling parasitic infection. DNA Cell Biol. 2003 Jun;22(6):355-6. PMID:12906731

Bradbury CA, Lappin MR. Evaluation of topical application of 10% imidacloprid-1% moxidectin to prevent Bartonella henselae transmission from cat fleas. J Am Vet Med Assoc. 2010 Apr 15;236(8):869-73. PMID:20392182

Braden B, Helm B, Fabian T, Dietrich CF. [Bacillary angiomatosis of the liver, a suspected ultrasound diagnosis?].[Article in German]. Z Gastroenterol. 2000 Sep;38(9):785-9. PMID:11072674

Bradley PJ. Benign salivary gland disease. Hosp Med. 2001 Jul;62(7):392-5. PMID:11480124

Braekeveld R, Verstraete K, Deprest K, Van Hecke E, Kunnen M. Bacillary angiomatosis in a patient with AIDS. JBR-BTR. 2002 Jun-Jul;85(3):124-5. PMID:12152714

Branley J. Cat scratch disease. A cause of regional lymphadenitis. Aust Fam Physician. 2001 Aug;30(8):751-4. PMID:11681146

Bravo F, Sanchez MR. New and re-emerging cutaneous infectious diseases in Latin America and other geographic areas. Dermatol Clin. 2003 Oct;21(4):655-68, viii. PMID:14717406

Bray DP, Bown KJ, Stockley P, Hurst JL, Bennett M, Birtles RJ. Haemoparasites of common shrews (Sorex araneus) in Northwest England. Parasitology. 2007 Jun;134(Pt 6):819-26. Epub 2007 Feb 9. PMID:17288633

Brecht A, Stiegler T, Lange J, de Groot K. [Generalized lymphadenitis associated with Hashimoto's thyroiditis].[Article in German]. Dtsch Med Wochenschr. 2007 Apr 20;132(16):874-7. PMID:17443443

Breitkopf C, Hammel D, Scheld HH, Peters G, Becker K. Impact of a molecular approach to improve the microbiological diagnosis of infective heart valve endocarditis. Circulation. 2005 Mar 22;111(11):1415-21. Epub 2005 Mar 7. PMID:15753218

Breitschwerdt EB, Blann KR, Stebbins ME, Muñana KR, Davidson MG, Jackson HA, Willard MD. Clinicopathological abnormalities and treatment response in 24 dogs seroreactive to Bartonella vinsonii (berkhoffii) antigens. J Am Anim Hosp Assoc. 2004 Mar-Apr;40(2):92-101. PMID:15007043

Breitschwerdt EB, Hegarty BC, Maggi R, Hawkins E, Dyer P. Bartonella species as a potential cause of epistaxis in dogs. J Clin Microbiol. 2005 May;43(5):2529-33. PMID:15872304

Breitschwerdt EB, Kordick DL. Bartonella infection in animals: carriership, reservoir potential, pathogenicity, and zoonotic potential for human infection. Clin Microbiol Rev. 2000 Jul;13(3):428-38. PMID:10885985

Breitschwerdt EB, Maggi RG, Cadenas MB, de Paiva Diniz PP. A groundhog, a novel Bartonella sequence, and my father's death. Emerg Infect Dis. 2009 Dec;15(12):2080-6. PMID:19998749

Breitschwerdt EB, Maggi RG, Chomel BB, Lappin MR. Bartonellosis: an emerging infectious disease of zoonotic importance to animals and human beings. J Vet Emerg Crit Care (San Antonio). 2010 Feb;20(1):8-30. PMID:20230432

Breitschwerdt EB, Maggi RG, Duncan AW, Nicholson WL, Hegarty BC, Woods CW. Bartonella species in blood of immunocompetent persons with animal and arthropod contact. Emerg Infect Dis. 2007 Jun;13(6):938-41. PMID:17553243

Breitschwerdt EB, Maggi RG, Farmer P, Mascarelli PE. Molecular evidence of perinatal transmission of Bartonella vinsonii subsp. berkhoffii and Bartonella henselae to a child. J Clin Microbiol. 2010 Jun;48(6):2289-93. Epub 2010 Apr 14. PMID:20392912

Breitschwerdt EB, Maggi RG, Lantos PM, Woods CW, Hegarty BC, Bradley JM. Bartonella vinsonii subsp. berkhoffii and Bartonella henselae bacteremia in a father and daughter with neurological disease. Parasit Vectors. 2010 Apr 8;3(1):29. PMID:20377863

Breitschwerdt EB, Maggi RG, Nicholson WL, Cherry NA, Woods CW. Bartonella sp. bacteremia in patients with neurological and neurocognitive dysfunction. J Clin Microbiol. 2008 Sep;46(9):2856-61. Epub 2008 Jul 16. PMID:18632903

Breitschwerdt EB, Maggi RG, Robert Mozayeni B, Hegarty BC, Bradley JM, Mascarelli PE. PCR amplification of Bartonella koehlerae from human blood and enrichment blood cultures. Parasit Vectors. 2010 Aug 24;3:76. PMID:20735840

Breitschwerdt EB, Maggi RG, Sigmon B, Nicholson WL. Isolation of Bartonella quintana from a woman and a cat following putative bite transmission. J Clin Microbiol. 2007 Jan;45(1):270-2. Epub 2006 Nov 8. PMID:17093037

Breitschwerdt EB, Maggi RG, Varanat M, Linder KE, Weinberg G. Isolation of Bartonella vinsonii subsp. berkhoffii genotype II from a boy with epithelioid hemangioendothelioma and a dog with hemangiopericytoma. J Clin Microbiol. 2009 Jun;47(6):1957-60. Epub 2009 Apr 15. PMID:19369441

Breitschwerdt EB, Maggi RG. A confusing case of canine vector-borne disease: clinical signs and progression in a dog co-infected with Ehrlichia canis and Bartonella vinsonii ssp. berkhoffii. Parasit Vectors. 2009 Mar 26;2 Suppl 1:S3. PMID:19426442

Breitschwerdt EB, Maggi RG. Comparative medical features of canine and human bartonellosis. Clin Microbiol Infect. 2009 Dec;15 Suppl 2:106-7. Epub 2009 Apr 30. PMID:19438635

Breitschwerdt EB, Mascarelli PE, Schweickert LA, Maggi RG, Hegarty BC, Bradley JM, Woods CW. Hallucinations, sensory neuropathy, and peripheral visual deficits in a young woman infected with Bartonella koehlerae. J Clin Microbiol. 2011 Sep;49(9):3415-7. Epub 2011 Jul 6. PMID:21734026

Breitschwerdt EB, Sontakke S, Cannedy A, Hancock SI, Bradley JM. Infection with Bartonella weissii and detection of Nanobacterium antigens in a North Carolina beef herd. J Clin Microbiol. 2001 Mar;39(3):879-82. PMID:11230398

Breitschwerdt EB, Suksawat J, Chomel B, Hegarty BC. The immunologic response of dogs to Bartonella vinsonii subspecies berkhoffii antigens: as assessed by Western immunoblot analysis. J Vet Diagn Invest. 2003 Jul;15(4):349-54. PMID:12918816

Breitschwerdt EB. Feline bartonellosis and cat scratch disease. Vet Immunol Immunopathol. 2008 May 15;123(1-2):167-71. Epub 2008 Jan 19. PMID:18295347

Brenneis C, Scherfler C, Engelhardt K, Helbok R, Brössner G, Beer R, Lackner P, Walder G, Pfausler B, Schmutzhard E. Encephalitis lethargica following Bartonella henselae infection. J Neurol. 2007 Apr;254(4):546-7. Epub 2007 Mar 12. PMID:17351727

Brenner EC, Chomel BB, Singhasivanon OU, Namekata DY, Kasten RW, Kass PH, Cortés-Vecino JA, Gennari SM, Rajapakse RP, Huong LT, Dubey JP. Bartonella infection in urban and rural dogs from the tropics: Brazil, Colombia, Sri Lanka and Vietnam. Epidemiol Infect. 2012 Mar 30:1-8. [Epub ahead of print]. PMID:22459880

Brettschneider H, Bennett NC, Chimimba CT, Bastos AD. Bartonellae of the Namaqua rock mouse, Micaelamys namaquensis (Rodentia: Muridae) from South Africa. Vet Microbiol. 2012 May 25;157(1-2):132-6. Epub 2011 Dec 11. PMID:22204791

Brinar VV, Habek M. Rare infections mimicking MS. Clin Neurol Neurosurg. 2010 Sep;112(7):625-8. Epub 2010 May 2. PMID:20439131

Brinkane A, Crickx L, Leroy Terquem E, Mauger C, Akpan T, Bergheul S, Peschard S, Raheriarisoa H, Gaudin B, Levy R. [Encephalopathy during cat scratch disease in an adult].[Article in French]. Rev Med Interne. 2001 Jun;22(6):589-90. PMID:11433571

Brinkerhoff RJ, Kabeya H, Inoue K, Bai Y, Maruyama S. Detection of multiple Bartonella species in digestive and reproductive tissues of fleas collected from sympatric mammals. ISME J. 2010 Jul;4(7):955-8. Epub 2010 Mar 11. PMID:20220787

Brook I. Acute bacterial suppurative parotitis: microbiology and management. J Craniofac Surg. 2003 Jan;14(1):37-40. PMID:12544218

Brook I. Joint and bone infections due to anaerobic bacteria in children. Pediatr Rehabil. 2002 Jan-Mar;5(1):11-9. PMID:12396847

Brook I. The bacteriology of salivary gland infections. Oral Maxillofac Surg Clin North Am. 2009 Aug;21(3):269-74. PMID:19608044

Brouqui P, Bacellar F, Baranton G, Birtles RJ, Bjoërsdorff A, Blanco JR, Caruso G, Cinco M, Fournier PE, Francavilla E, Jensenius M, Kazar J, Laferl H, Lakos A, Lotric Furlan S, Maurin M, Oteo JA, Parola P, Perez-Eid C, Peter O, Postic D, Raoult D, Tellez A, Tselentis Y, Wilske B; ESCMID Study Group on Coxiella, Anaplasma, Rickettsia and Bartonella; European Network for Surveillance of Tick-Borne Diseases. Guidelines for the diagnosis of tick-borne bacterial diseases in Europe. Clin Microbiol Infect. 2004 Dec;10(12):1108-32. PMID:15606643

Brouqui P, Raoult D. Arthropod-borne diseases in homeless. Ann N Y Acad Sci. 2006 Oct;1078:223-35. PMID:17114713

Brouqui P, Raoult D. Endocarditis due to rare and fastidious bacteria. Clin Microbiol Rev. 2001 Jan;14(1):177-207. PMID:11148009

Brouqui P, Raoult D. New insight into the diagnosis of fastidious bacterial endocarditis. FEMS Immunol Med Microbiol. 2006 Jun;47(1):1-13. PMID:16706783

Brouqui P, Stein A, Dupont HT, Gallian P, Badiaga S, Rolain JM, Mege JL, La Scola B, Berbis P, Raoult D. Ectoparasitism and vector-borne diseases in 930 homeless people from Marseilles. Medicine (Baltimore). 2005 Jan;84(1):61-8. PMID:15643300

Brouqui P. Arthropod-borne diseases associated with political and social disorder. Annu Rev Entomol. 2011;56:357-74. PMID:20822446

Brown DB, Huang YC, Kannenberg EL, Sherrier DJ, Carlson RW. An acpXL mutant of Rhizobium leguminosarum bv. phaseoli lacks 27-hydroxyoctacosanoic acid in its lipid A and is developmentally delayed during symbiotic infection of the determinate nodulating host plant Phaseolus vulgaris. J Bacteriol. 2011 Sep;193(18):4766-78. Epub 2011 Jul 15. PMID:21764936

Bruneval P, Choucair J, Paraf F, Casalta JP, Raoult D, Scherchen F, Mainardi JL. Detection of fastidious bacteria in cardiac valves in cases of blood culture negative endocarditis. J Clin Pathol. 2001 Mar;54(3):238-40. PMID:11253139

Brunt J, Guptill L, Kordick DL, Kudrak S, Lappin MR; American Association of Feline Practitioners; Academy of Feline Medicine Advisory Panel. American Association of Feline Practitioners 2006 Panel report on diagnosis, treatment, and prevention of Bartonella spp. infections. J Feline Med Surg. 2006 Aug;8(4):213-26. PMID:16846781

Bryant K, Marshall GS. Hepatosplenic cat scratch disease treated with corticosteroids. Arch Dis Child. 2003 Apr;88(4):345-6. PMID:12651767

Buchko GW, Edwards TE, Abendroth J, Arakaki TL, Law L, Napuli AJ, Hewitt SN, Van Voorhis WC, Stewart LJ, Staker BL, Myler PJ. Structure of a Nudix hydrolase (MutT) in the Mg(2+)-bound state from Bartonella henselae, the bacterium responsible for cat scratch fever. Acta Crystallogr Sect F Struct Biol Cryst Commun. 2011 Sep 1;67(Pt 9):1078-83. Epub 2011 Aug 16. PMID:21904053

Buchmann AU, Kempf VA, Kershaw O, Gruber AD. Peliosis hepatis in cats is not associated with Bartonella henselae infections. Vet Pathol. 2010 Jan;47(1):163-6. PMID:20080497

Buchmann AU, Kershaw O, Kempf VA, Gruber AD. Does a feline leukemia virus infection pave the way for Bartonella henselae infection in cats? J Clin Microbiol. 2010 Sep;48(9):3295-300. Epub 2010 Jul 7. PMID:20610682

Buckles EL, McGinnis Hill E. Interaction of Bartonella bacilliformis with human erythrocyte membrane proteins. Microb Pathog. 2000 Sep;29(3):165-74. PMID:10968948

Buelvas F, Alvis N, Buelvas I, Miranda J, Mattar S. [A high prevalence of antibodies against Bartonella and Babesia microti has been found in villages and urban populations in Cordoba, Colombia].[Article in Spanish]. Rev Salud Publica (Bogota). 2008 Jan-Feb;10(1):168-77. PMID:18368229

Bureau NJ, Cardinal E. Imaging of musculoskeletal and spinal infections in AIDS. Radiol Clin North Am. 2001 Mar;39(2):343-55. PMID:11316363

Burgess AW, Paquet JY, Letesson JJ, Anderson BE. Isolation, sequencing and expression of Bartonella henselae omp43 and predicted membrane topology of the deduced protein. Microb Pathog. 2000 Aug;29(2):73-80. PMID:10906262

Burns DL. Type IV transporters of pathogenic bacteria. Curr Opin Microbiol. 2003 Feb;6(1):29-34. PMID:12615216

Bystrov IV, Ni GV. [Hematozoon cenoses of small rodents and insectivora in the Orenburg Region].[Article in Hungarian]. Med Parazitol (Mosk). 2007 Jul-Sep;(3):31-5. PMID:17912832

Cabassi CS, Farnetti E, Casali B, Taddei S, Donofrio G, Galvani G, Cavirani S. Isolation of Bartonella henselae from domestic cats in an Italian urban area. New Microbiol. 2002 Apr;25(2):253-7. PMID:12019735

Cadenas MB, Bradley J, Maggi RG, Takara M, Hegarty BC, Breitschwerdt EB. Molecular characterization of Bartonella vinsonii subsp. berkhoffii genotype III. J Clin Microbiol. 2008 May;46(5):1858-60. Epub 2008 Mar 26. PMID:18367567

Cadenas MB, Maggi RG, Diniz PP, Breitschwerdt KT, Sontakke S, Breithschwerdt EB. Identification of bacteria from clinical samples using Bartonella alpha-Proteobacteria growth medium. J Microbiol Methods. 2007 Nov;71(2):147-55. Epub 2007 Aug 24. PMID:17889384

Callison JA, Battisti JM, Sappington KN, Smitherman LS, Minnick MF. Characterization and expression analysis of the groESL operon of Bartonella bacilliformis. Gene. 2005 Oct 10;359:53-62. PMID:16126349

Calza L, Manfredi R, Chiodo F. Infective endocarditis: a review of the best treatment options. Expert Opin Pharmacother. 2004 Sep;5(9):1899-916. PMID:15330728

Campos Franco J, Mallo González N, López Rodríquez R, Pérez Pampín E. [Cat-scratch disease].[Article in Spanish]. Med Clin (Barc). 2007 Sep 8;129(8):320. PMID:17969956

Cañas-Ventura A, Esteve E, Horcajada JP, Andreu M, Knobel H, Márquez L. Systemic Bartonella henselae infection and Crohn's disease treatment with infliximab. Inflamm Bowel Dis. 2012 Jan;18(1):E197-8. Epub 2011 Sep 16. PMID:21928372

Canback B, Andersson SG, Kurland CG. The global phylogeny of glycolytic enzymes. Proc Natl Acad Sci U S A. 2002 Apr 30;99(9):6097-102. PMID:11983902

Canzano JC, Lim JI. Pars plana vitrectomy for epiretinal membrane secondary to cat scratch neuroretinitis. Retina. 2001;21(3):272-3. PMID:11421023

Capelli G, Ravagnan S, Montarsi F, Ciocchetta S, Cazzin S, Porcellato E, Babiker AM, Cassini R, Salviato A, Cattoli G, Otranto D. Occurrence and identification of risk areas of Ixodes ricinus-borne pathogens: a cost-effectiveness analysis in north-eastern Italy. Parasit Vectors. 2012 Mar 27;5:61. PMID:22452970

Capitta P, Zobba R, Masala G, Cocco R, Tola S, Parpaglia ML. Isolation and characterization of Bartonella strains in cats in Italy. Transbound Emerg Dis. 2010 Jun;57(3):201-4. Epub 2010 Mar 14. PMID:20345572

Capo C, Amirayan-Chevillard N, Brouqui P, Raoult D, Mege JL. Bartonella quintana bacteremia and overproduction of interleukin-10: model of bacterial persistence in homeless people. J Infect Dis. 2003 Mar 1;187(5):837-44. Epub 2003 Feb 24. PMID:12599058

Caponetti G, Pantanowitz L. Cat-scratch disease lymphadenitis. Ear Nose Throat J. 2007 Aug;86(8):449-50. PMID:17915663

Caponetti GC, Pantanowitz L, Marconi S, Havens JM, Lamps LW, Otis CN. Evaluation of immunohistochemistry in identifying Bartonella henselae in cat-scratch disease. Am J Clin Pathol. 2009 Feb;131(2):250-6. PMID:19141385

Carmenini E, Pitucco G, Tripodi DA, Centi M, Castelli V, Lentini P, Galdenzi R, Bologna E. [Cat scratch pneumonia: a case report].[Article in Italian]. Clin Ter. 2006 Nov-Dec;157(6):517-8. PMID:17228851

Carroll JA, Coleman SA, Smitherman LS, Minnick MF. Hemin-binding surface protein from Bartonella quintana. Infect Immun. 2000 Dec;68(12):6750-7. PMID:11083791

Carucci LR, Halvorsen RA. Abdominal and pelvic CT in the HIV-positive population. Abdom Imaging. 2004 Nov-Dec;29(6):631-42. Epub 2004 Jun 16. PMID:15520901

Carucci LR, Halvorsen RA. Hepatic peliosis (bacillary angiomatosis) in AIDS: CT findings. Abdom Imaging. 2006 Mar-Apr;31(2):253; author reply 254. PMID:16447083

Casalta JP, Gouriet F, Richet H, Thuny F, Habib G, Raoult D. Prevalence of Coxiella burnetii and Bartonella species as cases of infective endocarditis in Marseilles (1994-2007). Clin Microbiol Infect. 2009 Dec;15 Suppl 2:152-3. Epub 2009 Sep 28. PMID:19793124

Case JB, Chomel B, Nicholson W, Foley JE. Serological survey of vector-borne zoonotic pathogens in pet cats and cats from animal shelters and feral colonies. J Feline Med Surg. 2006 Apr;8(2):111-7. Epub 2006 Jan 23. PMID:16434226

Casolari C, Pecorari M, Balli F, Fabio G, Gennari W, Sabbatini AM, Nanni N, Migaldi M, Guaraldi N, Tagliazucchi S, Alù M, Bertoli G, Fabio R, Portolani M. Unusual concurrent detection by polymerase chain reaction of Bartonella henselae and parvovirus b19 in an immunocompetent child with erythema nodosum and hepatic granulomatous disease. Diagn Microbiol Infect Dis. 2007 Sep;59(1):81-4. Epub 2007 May 29. PMID:17532594

Castle KT, Kosoy M, Lerdthusnee K, Phelan L, Bai Y, Gage KL, Leepitakrat W, Monkanna T, Khlaimanee N, Chandranoi K, Jones JW, Coleman RE. Prevalence and diversity of Bartonella in rodents of northern Thailand: a comparison with Bartonella in rodents from southern China. Am J Trop Med Hyg. 2004 Apr;70(4):429-33. PMID:15100459

Cat-scratch disease in children--Texas, September 2000 to August 2001.[Article in English, French]. Can Commun Dis Rep. 2002 Apr 15;28(8):64-7. PMID:11974428

Celebi B, Carhan A, Kilic S, Babur C. Detection and genetic diversity of Bartonella vinsonii subsp. berkhoffii strains isolated from dogs in Ankara, Turkey. J Vet Med Sci. 2010 Aug;72(8):969-73. Epub 2010 Mar 16. PMID:20234114

Celebi B, Kilic S, Aydin N, Tarhan G, Carhan A, Babur C. Investigation of Bartonella henselae in cats in Ankara, Turkey. Zoonoses Public Health. 2009 May;56(4):169-75. Epub 2008 Nov 4. PMID:18990198

Celebi B, Taylan Ozkan A, Kilic S, Akca A, Koenhemsi L, Pasa S, Yildiz K, Mamak N, Guzel M. Seroprevalence of Bartonella vinsonii subsp. berkhoffii in urban and rural dogs in Turkey. J Vet Med Sci. 2010 Nov;72(11):1491-4. Epub 2010 Jun 22. PMID:20574140

Celebi B, Yalçın E, Babür C. [Fever of unknown origin and detection of Bartonella henselae IgG seropositivity: a case report].[Article in Turkish]. Mikrobiyol Bul. 2010 Jul;44(3):489-94. PMID:21064000

Celebi B. [Bartonella henselae and its infections].[Article in Turkish]. Mikrobiyol Bul. 2008 Jan;42(1):163-75. PMID:18444576

Centers for Disease Control and Prevention (CDC). Cat-scratch disease in children--Texas, September 2000-August 2001. MMWR Morb Mortal Wkly Rep. 2002 Mar 15;51(10):212-4. PMID:11922191

Cerimele F, Brown LF, Bravo F, Ihler GM, Kouadio P, Arbiser JL. Infectious angiogenesis: Bartonella bacilliformis infection results in endothelial production of angiopoetin-2 and epidermal production of vascular endothelial growth factor. Am J Pathol. 2003 Oct;163(4):1321-7. PMID:14507641

Chae JS, Yu do H, Shringi S, Klein TA, Kim HC, Chong ST, Lee IY, Foley J. Microbial pathogens in ticks, rodents and a shrew in northern Gyeonggi-do near the DMZ, Korea. J Vet Sci. 2008 Sep;9(3):285-93. PMID:18716449

Chai CL, Lu QY, Sun JM, Jiang LP, Ling F, Zhang LJ, Zheng SG, Zhang H, Ge JH. [Sero-epidemiologic investigation on tick-borne diseases of humans and domestic animals in Zhejiang province]. [Article in Chinese]. Zhonghua Liu Xing Bing Xue Za Zhi. 2010 Oct;31(10):1144-1147. PMID:21162818

Chai Y, Yamamoto S, Hirayama A, Yotsukura J, Yamazaki H. Pattern visual evoked potentials in eyes with disc swelling due to cat scratch disease-associated neuroretinitis. Doc Ophthalmol. 2005 Mar-May;110(2-3):271-5. PMID:16328936

Chaillon A, Besnier JM, Choutet P. [Pathology of inoculation].[Article in French]. Rev Prat. 2008 Jan 31;58(2):213-21. PMID:18361288

Chaloner GL, Harrison TG, Coyne KP, Aanensen DM, Birtles RJ. Multilocus sequence typing of Bartonella henselae in the United Kingdom indicates that only a few, uncommon sequence types are associated with zoonotic disease. J Clin Microbiol. 2011 Jun;49(6):2132-7. Epub 2011 Apr 6. PMID:21471345

Chaloner GL, Palmira Ventosilla, Birtles RJ. Multi-locus sequence analysis reveals profound genetic diversity among isolates of the human pathogen Bartonella bacilliformis. PLoS Negl Trop Dis. 2011 Jul;5(7):e1248. Epub 2011 Jul 19. PMID:21811647

Chamberlin J, Laughlin L, Gordon S, Romero S, Solórzano N, Regnery RL. Serodiagnosis of Bartonella bacilliformis infection by indirect fluorescence antibody assay: test development and application to a population in an area of bartonellosis endemicity. J Clin Microbiol. 2000 Nov;38(11):4269-71. PMID:11060108

Chamberlin J, Laughlin LW, Romero S, Solórzano N, Gordon S, Andre RG, Pachas P, Friedman H, Ponce C, Watts D. Epidemiology of endemic Bartonella bacilliformis: a prospective cohort study in a Peruvian mountain valley community. J Infect Dis. 2002 Oct 1;186(7):983-90. Epub 2002 Sep 3. PMID:12232839

Chan KS, Kosoy M. Analysis of multi-strain Bartonella pathogens in natural host population--do they behave as species or minor genetic variants? Epidemics. 2010 Dec;2(4):165-72. Epub 2010 Sep 9. PMID:21352787

Chang AA, Zeldovich A, Sachdev NH, Ly C, Beaumont P. Papillary vasoproliferative changes in cat scratch disease. Br J Ophthalmol. 2005 Jan;89(1):122-3. PMID:15615761

Chang CC, Chen YJ, Tseng CS, Lai WL, Hsu KY, Chang CL, Lu CC, Hsu YM. A comparative study of the interaction of Bartonella henselae strains with human endothelial cells. Vet Microbiol. 2011 Apr 21;149(1-2):147-56. Epub 2010 Oct 7. PMID:21035278

Chang CC, Chomel BB, Kasten RW, Heller RM, Ueno H, Yamamoto K, Bleich VC, Pierce BM, Gonzales BJ, Swift PK, Boyce WM, Jang SS, Boulouis HJ, Piémont Y, Rossolini GM, Riccio ML, Cornaglia G, Pagani L, Lagatolla C, Selan L, Fontana R. Bartonella spp. isolated from wild and domestic ruminants in North America. Emerg Infect Dis. 2000 May-Jun;6(3):306-11. PMID:10827123

Chang CC, Chomel BB, Kasten RW, Romano V, Tietze N. Molecular evidence of Bartonella spp. in questing adult Ixodes pacificus ticks in California. J Clin Microbiol. 2001 Apr;39(4):1221-6. PMID:11283031

Chang CC, Chomel BB, Kasten RW, Tappero JW, Sanchez MA, Koehler JE. Molecular epidemiology of Bartonella henselae infection in human immunodeficiency virus-infected patients and their cat contacts, using pulsed-field gel electrophoresis and genotyping. J Infect Dis. 2002 Dec 15;186(12):1733-9. Epub 2002 Nov 22. PMID:12447758

Chang CC, Hayashidani H, Pusterla N, Kasten RW, Madigan JE, Chomel BB. Investigation of Bartonella infection in ixodid ticks from California. Comp Immunol Microbiol Infect Dis. 2002 Jul;25(4):229-36. PMID:12135237

Chang CC, Kasten RW, Chomel BB, Simpson DC, Hew CM, Kordick DL, Heller R, Piemont Y, Breitschwerdt EB. Coyotes (Canis latrans) as the reservoir for a human pathogenic Bartonella sp.: molecular epidemiology of Bartonella vinsonii subsp. berkhoffii infection in coyotes from central coastal California. J Clin Microbiol. 2000 Nov;38(11):4193-200. PMID:11060089

Chang CC, Lee CC, Maruyama S, Lin JW, Pan MJ. Cat-scratch disease in veterinary-associated populations and in its cat reservoir in Taiwan. Vet Res. 2006 Jul-Aug;37(4):565-77. Epub 2006 Apr 28. PMID:16641017

Chang MS, Lee SS, Cunningham ET Jr. Focal retinal phlebitis as a presenting sign of systemic Bartonella henselae infection. Retina. 2001;21(3):280-1. PMID:11421028

Chausov EV, Ternovoĭ VA, Protopopova EV, Konovalova SN, Kononova IuV, Pershikova NL, Moskovitina NS, Romanenko VN, Ivanova NV, Bol'shakova NP, Moskvitin SS, Korobitsyn IG, Gashkov SI, Tiuten'kov OIu, Kuranova VN, Kravchenko LB, Suchkova NG, Agulova LP, Loktev VB. [Genetic diversity of ixodid tick-borne pathogens in Tomsk City and suburbs].[Article in Russian]. Parazitologiia. 2009 Sep-Oct;43(5):374-88. PMID:19957906

Chen L, Chen Y, Wood DW, Nester EW. A new type IV secretion system promotes conjugal transfer in Agrobacterium tumefaciens. J Bacteriol. 2002 Sep;184(17):4838-45. PMID:12169609

Chen TC, Lin WR, Lu PL, Lin CY, Chen YH. Cat scratch disease from a domestic dog. J Formos Med Assoc. 2007 Feb;106(2 Suppl):S65-68. PMID:17493900

Chen X, Remotti F, Tong GX, Gorczyca E, Hamele-Bena D. Fine-needle aspiration cytology of subcutaneous toxoplasmosis: A case report. Diagn Cytopathol. 2010 Oct;38(10):716-20. PMID:20014129

Chenoweth MR, Greene CE, Krause DC, Gherardini FC. Predominant outer membrane antigens of Bartonella henselae. Infect Immun. 2004 Jun;72(6):3097-105. PMID:15155610

Chenoweth MR, Somerville GA, Krause DC, O'Reilly KL, Gherardini FC. Growth characteristics of Bartonella henselae in a novel liquid medium: primary isolation, growth-phase-dependent phage induction, and metabolic studies. Appl Environ Microbiol. 2004 Feb;70(2):656-63. PMID:14766538

Cherinet Y, Tomlinson R. Cat scratch disease presenting as acute encephalopathy. Emerg Med J. 2008 Oct;25(10):703-4. PMID:18843081

Cherry NA, Diniz PP, Maggi RG, Hummel JB, Hardie EM, Behrend EN, Rozanski E, Defrancesco TC, Cadenas MB, Breitschwerdt EB. Isolation or molecular detection of Bartonella henselae and Bartonella vinsonii subsp. berkhoffii from dogs with idiopathic cavitary effusions. J Vet Intern Med. 2009 Jan-Feb;23(1):186-9. PMID:19175739

Cherry NA, Liebisch G, Liebisch A, Breitschwerdt EB, Jones SL, Ulrich R, Allmers E, Wolf P, Hewicker-Trautwein M. Identification of Bartonella henselae in a horse from Germany. Vet Microbiol. 2011 Jun 2;150(3-4):414-5. Epub 2011 Feb 18. PMID:21388754

Cherry NA, Maggi RG, Cannedy AL, Breitschwerdt EB. PCR detection of Bartonella bovis and Bartonella henselae in the blood of beef cattle. Vet Microbiol. 2009 Mar 30;135(3-4):308-12. Epub 2008 Sep 21. PMID:19019574

Cherry NA, Maggi RG, Rossmeisl JH, Hegarty BC, Breitschwerdt EB. Ecological diversity of Bartonella species infection among dogs and their owner in Virginia. Vector Borne Zoonotic Dis. 2011 Nov;11(11):1425-32. Epub 2011 Jul 7. PMID:21736485

Chetty R, Sabaratnam RM. Upper gastrointestinal bacillary angiomatosis causing hematemesis: a case report. Int J Surg Pathol. 2003 Jul;11(3):241-4. PMID:12894361

Cheuk W, Chan AK, Wong MC, Chan JK. Confirmation of diagnosis of cat scratch disease by immunohistochemistry. Am J Surg Pathol. 2006 Feb;30(2):274-5. PMID:16434905

Cheung VW, Moxham JP. Cat scratch disease presenting as acute mastoiditis. Laryngoscope. 2010;120 Suppl 4:S222. PMID:21225820

Chi SL, Stinnett S, Eggenberger E, Foroozan R, Golnik K, Lee MS, Bhatti MT. Clinical characteristics in 53 patients with cat scratch optic neuropathy. Ophthalmology. 2012 Jan;119(1):183-7. Epub 2011 Sep 28. PMID:21959368

Chian CA, Arrese JE, Piérard GE. Skin manifestations of Bartonella infections. Int J Dermatol. 2002 Aug;41(8):461-6. PMID:12207759

Chiaraviglio L, Duong S, Brown DA, Birtles RJ, Kirby JE. An immunocompromised murine model of chronic Bartonella infection. Am J Pathol. 2010 Jun;176(6):2753-63. Epub 2010 Apr 15. PMID:20395436

Chiller K, Selkin BA, Murakawa GJ. Skin microflora and bacterial infections of the skin. J Investig Dermatol Symp Proc. 2001 Dec;6(3):170-4. PMID:11924823

Chinga-Alayo E, Huarcaya E, Nasarre C, del Aguila R, Llanos-Cuentas A. The influence of climate on the epidemiology of bartonellosis in Ancash, Peru. Trans R Soc Trop Med Hyg. 2004 Feb;98(2):116-24. PMID:14964812

Chinnadurai SK, Birkenheuer AJ, Blanton HL, Maggi RG, Belfiore N, Marr HS, Breitschwerdt EB, Stoskopf MK. Prevalence of selected vector-borne organisms and identification of Bartonella species DNA in North American river otters (Lontra canadensis). J Wildl Dis. 2010 Jul;46(3):947-50. PMID:20688703

Chipczyńiska B, Grałek M, Kepa B. [Neuroretinitis in children—independent observations].[Article in Polish]. Ann Acad Med Stetin. 2007;53 Suppl 1:76-9; discussion 79. PMID:19425485

Chiu AG, Hecht DA, Prendiville SA, Mesick C, Mikula S, Deeb ZE. Atypical presentations of cat scratch disease in the head and neck. Otolaryngol Head Neck Surg. 2001 Oct;125(4):414-6. PMID:11593185

Chmielewski T, Fiett J, Gniadkowski M, Tylewska-Wierzbanowska S. Improvement in the laboratory recognition of lyme borreliosis with the combination of culture and PCR methods. Mol Diagn. 2003;7(3-4):155-62. PMID:15068385

Chmielewski T, Podsiadły E, Tylewska-Wierzbanowska S. Presence of Bartonella spp. in various human populations. Pol J Microbiol. 2007;56(1):33-8. PMID:17419187

Chmielewski T, Tylewska-Wierzbanowska S. Inhibition of fibroblast apoptosis by Borrelia afzelii, Coxiella burnetii and Bartonella henselae. Pol J Microbiol. 2011;60(3):269-72. PMID:22184936

Choi P, Qin X, Chen EY, Inglis AF Jr, Ou HC, Perkins JA, Sie KC, Patterson K, Berry S, Manning SC. Polymerase chain reaction for pathogen identification in persistent pediatric cervical lymphadenitis. Arch Otolaryngol Head Neck Surg. 2009 Mar;135(3):243-8. PMID:19289701

Chomel B. Tick-borne infections in dogs-an emerging infectious threat. Vet Parasitol. 2011 Jul 15;179(4):294-301. PMID:21777730

Chomel BB, Boulouis HJ, Breitschwerdt EB, Kasten RW, Vayssier-Taussat M, Birtles RJ, Koehler JE, Dehio C. Ecological fitness and strategies of adaptation of Bartonella species to their hosts and vectors. Vet Res. 2009 Mar-Apr;40(2):29. Epub 2009 Mar 14. PMID:19284965

Chomel BB, Boulouis HJ, Breitschwerdt EB. Cat scratch disease and other zoonotic Bartonella infections. J Am Vet Med Assoc. 2004 Apr 15;224(8):1270-9. PMID:15112775

Chomel BB, Boulouis HJ, Maruyama S, Breitschwerdt EB. Bartonella spp. In pets and effect on human health. Emerg Infect Dis. 2006 Mar;12(3):389-94. PMID:16704774

Chomel BB, Boulouis HJ, Petersen H, Kasten RW, Yamamoto K, Chang CC, Gandoin C, Bouillin C, Hew CM. Prevalence of Bartonella infection in domestic cats in Denmark. Vet Res. 2002 Mar-Apr;33(2):205-13. PMID:11944808

Chomel BB, Boulouis HJ. [Zoonotic diseases caused by bacteria of the genus Bartonella genus: new reservoirs ? New vectors?].[Article in French]. Bull Acad Natl Med. 2005 Mar;189(3):465-77; discussion 477-80. PMID:16149211

Chomel BB, Henn JB, Kasten RW, Nieto NC, Foley J, Papageorgiou S, Allen C, Koehler JE. Dogs are more permissive than cats or guinea pigs to experimental infection with a human isolate of Bartonella rochalimae. Vet Res. 2009 Jul-Aug;40(4):27. PMID:19272295

Chomel BB, Kasten RW, Henn JB, Molia S. Bartonella infection in domestic cats and wild felids. Ann N Y Acad Sci. 2006 Oct;1078:410-5. PMID:17114749

Chomel BB, Kasten RW, Sykes JE, Boulouis HJ, Breitschwerdt EB. Clinical impact of persistent Bartonella bacteremia in humans and animals. Ann N Y Acad Sci. 2003 Jun;990:267-78. PMID:12860639

Chomel BB, Kasten RW, Williams C, Wey AC, Henn JB, Maggi R, Carrasco S, Mazet J, Boulouis HJ, Maillard R, Breitschwerdt EB. Bartonella endocarditis: a pathology shared by animal reservoirsand patients. Ann N Y Acad Sci. 2009 May;1166:120-6. PMID:19538271

Chomel BB, Kasten RW. Bartonellosis, an increasingly recognized zoonosis. J Appl Microbiol. 2010 Sep;109(3):743-50. PMID:20148999

Chomel BB, Kikuchi Y, Martenson JS, Roelke-Parker ME, Chang CC, Kasten RW, Foley JE, Laudre J, Murphy K, Swift PK, Kramer VL, O'brien SJ. Seroprevalence of Bartonella infection in American free-ranging and captive pumas (Felis concolor) and bobcats (Lynx rufus). Vet Res. 2004 Mar-Apr;35(2):233-41. PMID:15099499

Chomel BB, Mac Donald KA, Kasten RW, Chang CC, Wey AC, Foley JE, Thomas WP, Kittleson MD. Aortic valve endocarditis in a dog due to Bartonella clarridgeiae. J Clin Microbiol. 2001 Oct;39(10):3548-54. PMID:11574571

Chomel BB, Wey AC, Kasten RW, Stacy BA, Labelle P. Fatal case of endocarditis associated with Bartonella henselae type I infection in a domestic cat. J Clin Microbiol. 2003 Nov;41(11):5337-9. PMID:14605199

Chomel BB, Wey AC, Kasten RW. Isolation of Bartonella washoensis from a dog with mitral valve endocarditis. J Clin Microbiol. 2003 Nov;41(11):5327-32. PMID:14605197

Chomel BB. Cat-scratch disease. Rev Sci Tech. 2000 Apr;19(1):136-50. PMID:11189710

Chomel BB. Lack of transovarial transmission of Bartonella by rodent fleas. Mol Ecol. 2011 Jul;20(13):2660-1. PMID:21834170

Chondrogiannis K, Vezakis A, Derpapas M, Melemeni A, Fragulidis G. Seronegative cat-scratch disease diagnosed by PCR detection of Bartonella henselae DNA in lymph node samples. Braz J Infect Dis. 2012 Jan-Feb;16(1):96-9. PMID:22358366

Chow A, Robinson JL. Fever of unknown origin in children: a systematic review. World J Pediatr. 2011 Feb;7(1):5-10. Epub 2010 Dec 30. PMID:21191771

Christiansen S, Fehske W, Autschbach R. Aortic valve endocarditis with Bartonella quintana - a rare entity. Herz. 2005 Dec;30(8):761-3. PMID:16331372

Christopher GW, Agan MB, Cieslak TJ, Olson PE. History of U.S. military contributions to the study of bacterial zoonoses. Mil Med. 2005 Apr;170(4 Suppl):39-48. PMID:15916282

Chu BC, Tam VT. A serologically proven case of cat-scratch disease presenting with neuroretinitis. Hong Kong Med J. 2009 Oct;15(5):391-3. PMID:19801700

Chung CY, Kasten RW, Paff SM, Van Horn BA, Vayssier-Taussat M, Boulouis HJ, Chomel BB. Bartonella spp. DNA associated with biting flies from California. Emerg Infect Dis. 2004 Jul;10(7):1311-3. PMID:15324557

Chung JY, Han TH, Kim BN, Yoo YS, Lim SJ. Detection of bartonella henselae DNA by polymerase chain reaction in a patient with cat scratch disease: a case report. J Korean Med Sci. 2005 Oct;20(5):888-91. PMID:16224169

Chung JY, Kim SW, Han TH, Lim SJ. Detection of the Bartonella henselae gene sequence in lymph nodes of children with Kikuchi's disease. Pediatrics. 2005 Apr;115(4):1112. PMID:15805408

Ciampolini J, Timperley J, Morgan M. Prosthetic joint infection by cat scratch. J R Soc Med. 2004 Sep;97(9):441-2. PMID:15340030

Ciceroni L, Fabbi M, Ciarrocchi S, Pinto A, Ciervo A, Kasten RW, Chomel BB. Characterization of the first Bartonella henselae strain isolated from a cat in Italy. Comp Immunol Microbiol Infect Dis. 2002 Jul;25(4):217-28. PMID:12135236

Ciceroni L, Pinto A, Ciarrocchi S, Ciervo A. Bartonella infections in Italy. Clin Microbiol Infect. 2009 Dec;15 Suppl 2:108-9. Epub 2009 Apr 30. PMID:19438634

Ciervo A, Ciceroni L. Rapid detection and differentiation of Bartonella spp. by a single-run real-time PCR. Mol Cell Probes. 2004 Oct;18(5):307-12. PMID:15294318

Ciervo A, Mastroianni CM, Ajassa C, Pinto A, Ciceroni L. Rapid identification of Bartonella henselae by real-time polymerase chain reaction in a patient with cat scratch disease. Diagn Microbiol Infect Dis. 2005 Sep;53(1):75-7. PMID:16054323

Ciervo A, Petrucca A, Ciarrocchi S, Pinto A, Bonazzi L, Fabio A, Farnetti E, Chomel BB, Ciceroni L. Molecular characterization of first human Bartonella strain isolated in Italy. J Clin Microbiol. 2001 Dec;39(12):4554-7. PMID:11724882

Cilla Eguiluz G, Montes Ros M, López García D, Iraola Sierra B, Aramburu Soraluce V. [Bartonella henselae endocarditis. Report of a case and review of the literature].[Article in Spanish]. An Med Interna. 2001 May;18(5):255-8. PMID:11496560

Cimolai N, Benoit L, Hill A, Lyons C. Bartonella henselae infection in British Columbia: evidence for an endemic disease among humans. Can J Microbiol. 2000 Oct;46(10):908-12. PMID:11068677

Cockwill KR, Taylor SM, Philibert HM, Breitschwerdt EB, Maggi RG. Bartonella vinsonii subsp. berkhoffii endocarditis in a dog from Saskatchewan. Can Vet J. 2007 Aug;48(8):839-44. PMID:17824328

Cohnstaedt LW, Beati L, Caceres AG, Ferro C, Munstermann LE. Phylogenetics of the phlebotomine sand fly group Verrucarum (Diptera: Psychodidae: Lutzomyia). Am J Trop Med Hyg. 2011 Jun;84(6):913-22. PMID:21633028

Cohnstaedt LW, Caceres AG, Beati L, Munstermann LE. The population structure of Lutzomyia verrucarum (Diptera: Psycodidae), a Bartonella bacilliformis and Leishmania peruviana vector in Peru. J Med Entomol. 2012 Jan;49(1):77-84. PMID:22308774

Colborn JM, Kosoy MY, Motin VL, Telepnev MV, Valbuena G, Myint KS, Fofanov Y, Putonti C, Feng C, Peruski L. Improved detection of Bartonella DNA in mammalian hosts and arthropod vectors by real-time PCR using the NADH dehydrogenase gamma subunit (nuoG). J Clin Microbiol. 2010 Dec;48(12):4630-3. Epub 2010 Oct 6. PMID:20926707

Coleman SA, Minnick MF. Differential expression of the invasion-associated locus B (ialB) gene of Bartonella bacilliformis in response to environmental cues. Microb Pathog. 2003 Apr;34(4):179-86. PMID:12668141

Coleman SA, Minnick MF. Establishing a direct role for the Bartonella bacilliformis invasion-associated locus B (IalB) protein in human erythrocyte parasitism. Infect Immun. 2001 Jul;69(7):4373-81. PMID:11401976

Colitz CM. Feline uveitis: diagnosis and treatment. Clin Tech Small Anim Pract. 2005 May;20(2):117-20. PMID:15948426

Colombo AP, Teles RP, Torres MC, Souto R, Rosalém WJ, Mendes MC, Uzeda M. Subgingival microbiota of Brazilian subjects with untreated chronic periodontitis. J Periodontol. 2002 Apr;73(4):360-9. PMID:11990436

Colomina J, Tomás JM, Villar J, Navarrete J. [Non henselae Bartonella neuroretinitis].[Article in Spanish]. Med Clin (Barc). 2003 Apr 12;120(13):519. PMID:12716551

Colton L, Zeidner N, Kosoy MY. Experimental infection of Swiss webster mice with four rat bartonella strains: host specificity, bacteremia kinetics, dose dependent response, and histopathology. Comp Immunol Microbiol Infect Dis. 2011 Dec;34(6):465-73. Epub 2011 Sep 9. PMID:21908045

Colton L, Zeidner N, Lynch T, Kosoy MY. Human isolates of Bartonella tamiae induce pathology in experimentally inoculated immunocompetent mice. BMC Infect Dis. 2010 Jul 30;10:229. PMID:20673363

Comer JA, Diaz T, Vlahov D, Monterroso E, Childs JE. Evidence of rodent-associated Bartonella and Rickettsia infections among intravenous drug users from Central and East Harlem, New York City. Am J Trop Med Hyg. 2001 Dec;65(6):855-60. PMID:11791987

Comer JA, Paddock CD, Childs JE. Urban zoonoses caused by Bartonella, Coxiella, Ehrlichia, and Rickettsia species. Vector Borne Zoonotic Dis. 2001 Summer;1(2):91-118. PMID:12653141

Commander NJ, Spencer SA, Wren BW, MacMillan AP. The identification of two protective DNA vaccines from a panel of five plasmid constructs encoding Brucella melitensis 16M genes. Vaccine. 2007 Jan 2;25(1):43-54. Epub 2006 Aug 4. PMID:17049676

Concannon R, Wynn-Owen K, Simpson VR, Birtles RJ. Molecular characterization of haemoparasites infecting bats (Microchiroptera) in Cornwall, UK. Parasitology. 2005 Oct;131(Pt 4):489-96. PMID:16174413

Conrad DA. Treatment of cat-scratch disease. Curr Opin Pediatr. 2001 Feb;13(1):56-9. PMID:11176245

Consigny S, Chosidow O. [Cutaneous infections in the homeless]. [Article in French]. Rev Prat. 2003 Nov 30;53(18):1977-81. PMID:15008208

Conyers GB, Wu G, Bessman MJ, Mildvan AS. Metal requirements of a diadenosine pyrophosphatase from Bartonella bacilliformis: magnetic resonance and kinetic studies of the role of Mn2+. Biochemistry. 2000 Mar 7;39(9):2347-54. PMID:10694402

Cooling MB. Pain in the neck. Pediatr Nurs. 2007 Jul-Aug;33(4):342-4. PMID:17907735

Cordeiro FN, Bruno CB, Paula CD, Motta Jde O. Familial occurrence of zoonotic sporotrichosis.[Article in English, Portuguese]. An Bras Dermatol. 2011 Jul-Aug;86(4 Suppl 1):S121-4. PMID:22068790

Corrain R, Drigo M, Fenati M, Menandro ML, Mondin A, Pasotto D, Martini M. Study on Ticks and Tick-Borne Zoonoses in Public Parks in Italy. Zoonoses Public Health. 2012 May 2. [Epub ahead of print]. PMID:22551055

Cortes EE, Saraceni V, Medeiros D, Ribeiro I. Bacillary angiomatosis and Kaposi's sarcoma in AIDS. AIDS Patient Care STDS. 2000 Apr;14(4):179-82. PMID:10806635

Corti M, Villafañe MF, Castello T, Méndez N, Gancedo E, Palmieri O. [Bacilar angiomatosis with hepatic peliosis in an AIDS patient].[Article in Spanish]. Medicina (B Aires). 2006;66(2):153. PMID:16715767

Costa V, Sommese L, Casamassimi A, Colicchio R, Angelini C, Marchesano V, Milone L, Farzati B, Giovane A, Fiorito C, Rienzo M, Picardi M, Avallone B, Marco Corsi M, Sarubbi B, Calabrò R, Salvatore P, Ciccodicola A, Napoli C. Impairment of circulating endothelial progenitors in Down syndrome. BMC Med Genomics. 2010 Sep 13;3:40. PMID:20836844

Cotar AI, Badescu D, Oprea M, Dinu S, Banu O, Dobreanu D, Dobreanu M, Ionac A, Flonta M, Straut M. Q Fever endocarditis in romania: the first cases confirmed by direct sequencing. Int J Mol Sci. 2011;12(12):9504-13. Epub 2011 Dec 20. PMID:22272146

Cotté V, Bonnet S, Cote M, Vayssier-Taussat M. Prevalence of five pathogenic agents in questing Ixodes ricinus ticks from western France. Vector Borne Zoonotic Dis. 2010 Oct;10(8):723-30. Epub 2009 Dec 18. PMID:20020814

Cotté V, Bonnet S, Le Rhun D, Le Naour E, Chauvin A, Boulouis HJ, Lecuelle B, Lilin T, Vayssier-Taussat M. Transmission of Bartonella henselae by Ixodes ricinus. Emerg Infect Dis. 2008 Jul;14(7):1074-80. PMID:18598628

Courtney JW, Kostelnik LM, Zeidner NS, Massung RF. Multiplex real-time PCR for detection of anaplasma phagocytophilum and Borrelia burgdorferi. J Clin Microbiol. 2004 Jul;42(7):3164-8. PMID:15243077

Cozzani E, Cinotti E, Ameri P, Sofia A, Murialdo G, Parodi A. Onset of cutaneous vasculitis and exacerbation of IgA nephropathy after Bartonella henselae infection. Clin Exp Dermatol. 2012 Apr;37(3):238-40. Epub 2011 Oct 10. PMID:21981612

Cramm KJ, Silverstein DM. Gross hematuria in a young child with axillary lymphadenopathy. Clin Pediatr (Phila). 2002 Jun;41(5):357-9. PMID:12086202

Crissiuma A, Favacho A, Gershony L, Mendes-de-Almeida F, Gomes R, Mares-Guia A, Rozental T, Barreira J, Lemos E, Labarthe N. Prevalence of Bartonella species DNA and antibodies in cats (Felis catus) submitted to a spay/neuter program in Rio de Janeiro, Brazil. J Feline Med Surg. 2011 Feb;13(2):149-51. Epub 2010 Nov 10. PMID:21071251

Cross JR, Rossmeisl JH, Maggi RG, Breitschwerdt EB, Duncan RB. Bartonella-associated meningoradiculoneuritis and dermatitis or panniculitis in 3 dogs. J Vet Intern Med. 2008 May-Jun;22(3):674-8. Epub 2008 May 2. PMID:18466250

Crossman L, Holden M, Pain A, Parkhill J. Genomes beyond compare. Nat Rev Microbiol. 2004 Aug;2(8):616-7. PMID:15303267

Cueto M. Nationalism, Carrión's disease and medical geography in the Peruvian Andes. Hist Philos Life Sci. 2003;25(3):319-35. PMID:15584200

Cunningham ET, Koehler JE. Ocular bartonellosis. Am J Ophthalmol. 2000 Sep;130(3):340-9. PMID:11020414

Curi AL, Campos WR, Barbosa L, Lana-Peixoto MA, Oréfice F. Unusual presentation of cat scratch disease in HIV+ patient. Br J Ophthalmol. 2003 Mar;87(3):371. PMID:12598467

Curi AL, Machado D, Heringer G, Campos WR, Lamas C, Rozental T, Gutierres A, Orefice F, Lemos E. Cat-scratch disease: ocular manifestations and visual outcome. Int Ophthalmol. 2010 Oct;30(5):553-8. Epub 2010 Jul 30. PMID:20668914

Curi AL, Machado DO, Heringer G, Campos WR, Orefice F. Ocular manifestation of cat-scratch disease in HIV-positive patients. Am J Ophthalmol. 2006 Feb;141(2):400-1. PMID:16458711

Cutler S, Abdissa A, Adamu H, Tolosa T, Gashaw A. Bartonella quintana in Ethiopian lice. Comp Immunol Microbiol Infect Dis. 2012 Jan;35(1):17-21.Epub 2011 Oct 21. PMID:22019400

da Costa PS, Brigatte ME, Greco DB. Antibodies to Rickettsia rickettsii, Rickettsia typhi, Coxiella burnetii, Bartonella henselae, Bartonella quintana, and Ehrlichia chaffeensis among healthy population in Minas Gerais, Brazil. Mem Inst Oswaldo Cruz. 2005 Dec;100(8):853-9. Epub 2006 Jan 20. PMID:16444416

Da Silva K, Chussid S. Cat scratch disease: clinical considerations for the pediatric dentist. Pediatr Dent. 2009 Jan-Feb;31(1):58-62. PMID:19320261

Dabo SM, Confer AW, Anderson BE, Gupta S. Bartonella henselae Pap31, an extracellular matrix adhesin, binds the fibronectin repeat III13 module. Infect Immun. 2006 May;74(5):2513-21. PMID:16622186

Dabo SM, Confer AW, Saliki JT, Anderson BE. Binding of Bartonella henselae to extracellular molecules: identification of potential adhesins. Microb Pathog. 2006 Jul;41(1):10-20. Epub 2006 May 24. PMID:16725305

Dabrowska-Bień J, Pietniczka-Załeska M, Rowicki T. [Cat scratch disease—a diagnostic problem, case report].[Article in Polish]. Otolaryngol Pol. 2009 Mar-Apr;63(2):154-7. PMID:19681487

Dai S, Best S, St John M. Bartonella henselae neuroretinitis in cat scratch disease. N Z Med J. 2001 Aug 10;114(1137):360-1. PMID:11587306

Daily JP, Waldron MA. Case records of the Massachusetts General Hospital. Weekly clinicopathological exercises. Case 22-2003. A 22-year-old man with chills and fever after a stay in South America. N Engl J Med. 2003 Jul 17;349(3):287-95. PMID:12867613

Danon O, Duval-Arnould M, Osman Z, Boukobza B, Kazerouni F, Cadranel JF, Neuenschwander S, Nocton F. Hepatic and splenic involvement in cat-scratch disease: imaging features. Abdom Imaging. 2000 Mar-Apr;25(2):182-3. PMID:10675462

Dardenne S, Coche E, Weynand B, Poncelet A, Zech F, De Meyer M. High suspicion of bacillary angiomatosis in a kidney transplant recipient: a difficult way to diagnose--case report. Transplant Proc. 2007 Jan-Feb;39(1):311-3. PMID:17275532

Das BB, Wasser E, Bryant KA, Woods CR, Yang SG, Zahn M. Culture negative endocarditis caused by Bartonella henselae in a child with congenital heart disease. Pediatr Infect Dis J. 2009 Oct;28(10):922-5. PMID:19738506

Das S, Paul S, Chatterjee S, Dutta C. Codon and amino acid usage in two major human pathogens of genus Bartonella--optimization between replicational-transcriptional selection, translational control and cost minimization. DNA Res. 2005;12(2):91-102. PMID:16303741

Day MJ. One health: the importance of companion animal vector-borne diseases. Parasit Vectors. 2011 Apr 13;4:49. PMID:21489237

Day MJ. The immunopathology of canine vector-borne diseases. Parasit Vectors. 2011 Apr 13;4:48. PMID:21489234

Daybell D, Paddock CD, Zaki SR, Comer JA, Woodruff D, Hansen KJ, Peacock JE Jr. Disseminated infection with Bartonella henselae as a cause of spontaneous splenic rupture. Clin Infect Dis. 2004 Aug 1;39(3):e21-4. Epub 2004 Jul 9. PMID:15307019

de Caprariis D, Dantas-Torres F, Capelli G, Mencke N, Stanneck D, Breitschwerdt EB, Otranto D. Evolution of clinical, haematological and biochemical findings in young dogs naturally infected by vector-borne pathogens. Vet Microbiol. 2011 Apr 21;149(1-2):206-12. Epub 2010 Oct 16. PMID:21106311

De Clerck KF, Van Offel JF, Vlieghe E, Van Marck E, Stevens WJ. Bartonella endocarditis mimicking adult Still's disease. Acta Clin Belg. 2008 May-Jun;63(3):190-2. PMID:18714850

de Kort JG, Robben SG, Schrander JJ, van Rhijn LW. Multifocal osteomyelitis in a child: a rare manifestation of cat scratch disease: a case report and systematic review of the literature. J Pediatr Orthop B. 2006 Jul;15(4):285-8. PMID:16751739

de La Blanchardière A, Fournier PE, Haustraete E, du Cheyron D, Lepage O, Verdon R. [Infective endocarditis due to Bartonella henselae following a rupture of a cerebral aneurysm].[Article in French]. Med Mal Infect. 2009 Jun;39(6):394-6. Epub 2008 Dec 18. PMID:19097835

De La Rosa GR, Barnett BJ, Ericsson CD, Turk JB. Native valve endocarditis due to Bartonella henselae in a middle-aged human immunodeficiency virus-negative woman. J Clin Microbiol. 2001 Sep;39(9):3417-9. PMID:11526194 de Paiva Diniz PP, Schwartz DS, de Morais HS, Breitschwerdt EB. Surveillance for zoonotic vector-borne infections using sick dogs from southeastern Brazil. Vector Borne Zoonotic Dis. 2007 Winter;7(4):689-97. PMID:18021025

de Paz HD, Larrea D, Zunzunegui S, Dehio C, de la Cruz F, Llosa M. Functional dissection of the conjugative coupling protein TrwB. J Bacteriol. 2010 Jun;192(11):2655-69. Epub 2010 Apr 2. PMID:20363945

de Paz HD, Sangari FJ, Bolland S, García-Lobo JM, Dehio C, de la Cruz F, Llosa M. Functional interactions between type IV secretion systems involved in DNA transfer and virulence. Microbiology. 2005 Nov;151(Pt 11):3505-16. PMID:16272374

De Schryver I, Stevens AM, Vereecke G, Kestelyn P. Cat scratch disease (CSD) in patients with stellate neuroretinitis: 3 cases. Bull Soc Belge Ophtalmol. 2002;(286):41-6. PMID:12564316

De Sousa R, Edouard-Fournier P, Santos-Silva M, Amaro F, Bacellar F, Raoult D. Molecular detection of Rickettsia felis, Rickettsia typhi and two genotypes closely related to Bartonella elizabethae. Am J Trop Med Hyg. 2006 Oct;75(4):727-31. PMID:17038702

de Souza Zanutto M, Mamizuka EM, Raiz R Jr, de Lima TM, Diogo CL, Okay TS, Hagiwara MK. Experimental infection and horizontal transmission of Bartonella henselae in domestic cats. Rev Inst Med Trop Sao Paulo. 2001 Sep-Oct;43(5):257-61. PMID:11696847

Dean RL, Eisenbeis JF. Neck abscess secondary to cat-scratch disease. Ear Nose Throat J. 2004 Nov;83(11):781-3. PMID:15628637

Degueldre F, Bonnet S. [Cause of unusual unilateral vitreous hemorrhage: neuroretinitis of Cat-Scratch disease. Presentation of a case].[Article in French]. Bull Soc Belge Ophtalmol. 2002;(285):37-40. PMID:12442341

Dehio C, Lanz C, Pohl R, Behrens P, Bermond D, Piémont Y, Pelz K, Sander A. Bartonella schoenbuchii sp. nov., isolated from the blood of wild roe deer. Int J Syst Evol Microbiol. 2001 Jul;51(Pt 4):1557-65. PMID:11491358

Dehio C, Sauder U, Hiestand R. Isolation of Bartonella schoenbuchensis from Lipoptena cervi, a blood-sucking arthropod causing deer ked dermatitis. J Clin Microbiol. 2004 Nov;42(11):5320-3. PMID:15528732

Dehio C. Bartonella interactions with endothelial cells and erythrocytes. Trends Microbiol. 2001 Jun;9(6):279-85. PMID:11390243

Dehio C. Bartonella-host-cell interactions and vascular tumour formation. Nat Rev Microbiol. 2005 Aug;3(8):621-31. PMID:16064054

Dehio C. Infection-associated type IV secretion systems of Bartonella and their diverse roles in host cell interaction. Cell Microbiol. 2008 Aug;10(8):1591-8. Epub 2008 Jul 30. PMID:18489724

Dehio C. Molecular and cellular basis of bartonella pathogenesis. Annu Rev Microbiol. 2004;58:365-90. PMID:15487942

Dehio C. Recent progress in understanding Bartonella-induced vascular proliferation. Curr Opin Microbiol. 2003 Feb;6(1):61-5. PMID:12615221

Dehio M, Québatte M, Foser S, Certa U. The transcriptional response of human endothelial cells to infection with Bartonella henselae is dominated by genes controlling innate immune responses, cell cycle, and vascular remodelling. Thromb Haemost. 2005 Aug;94(2):347-61. PMID:16113825

Dekkers MJ, Dees A, Weidema WF, Bartelsman M, Veeken H, Hart W. [Clinical thinking and decision making in practice. A man with abdominal pain, weight loss and fever].[Article in Dutch]. Ned Tijdschr Geneeskd. 2009 Jan 31;153(5):174-80. PMID:19256242

Del Prete R, Fumarola D, Fumarola L, Miragliotta G. Detection of Bartonella henselae and Afipia felis DNA by polymerase chain reaction in specimens from patients with cat scratch disease. Eur J Clin Microbiol Infect Dis. 2000 Dec;19(12):964-7. PMID:11205638

Del Prete R, Fumarola D, Ungari S, Fumarola L, Miragliotta G. Polymerase chain reaction detection of Bartonella henselae bacteraemia in an immunocompetent child with cat-scratch disease. Eur J Pediatr. 2000 May;159(5):356-9. PMID:10834521

Del Santo M, Malorgio C, Not T, Maranzana G, Cerasoli G, Facchini S, Zennaro F, Ventura A. Vertebral osteomyelitis in 2 children. Clin Pediatr (Phila). 2002 Nov-Dec;41(9):711-3. PMID:12462322

del Valle LJ, Flores L, Vargas M, García-de-la-Guarda R, Quispe RL, Ibañez ZB, Alvarado D, Ramírez P, Ruiz J. Bartonella bacilliformis, endemic pathogen of the Andean region, is intrinsically resistant to quinolones. Int J Infect Dis. 2010 Jun;14(6):e506-10. Epub 2009 Dec 6. PMID:19969497

Delahaye F, Hoen B, McFadden E, Roth O, de Gevigney G. Treatment and prevention of infective endocarditis. Expert Opin Pharmacother. 2002 Feb;3(2):131-45. PMID:11829727

Delpino MV, Cassataro J, Fossati CA, Goldbaum FA, Baldi PC. Brucella outer membrane protein Omp31 is a haemin-binding protein. Microbes Infect. 2006 Apr;8(5):1203-8. Epub 2006 Jan 19. PMID:16517201

Deng H, Le Rhun DC, Cotte V, Buffet JP, Read A, Birtles RJ, Vayssier-Taussat M. Strategies of exploitation of mammalian reservoirs by Bartonella species. Vet Res. 2012 Feb 27;43(1):15. [Epub ahead of print]. PMID:22369683

Deng HK, Le Rhun D, Lecuelle B, Le Naour E, Vayssier-Taussat M. Role of the spleen in Bartonella spp. infection. FEMS Immunol Med Microbiol. 2012 Feb;64(1):143-5. PMID:22098417

Depeyre C, Mancel E, Besson-Leaud L, Goursaud R. [Abrupt visual loss in children. Three case studies of ocular bartonellosis].[Article in French]. J Fr Ophtalmol. 2005 Nov;28(9):968-75. PMID:16395224

Derrick SC, Ihler GM. Deformin, a substance found in Bartonella bacilliformis culture supernatants, is a small, hydrophobic molecule with an affinity for albumin. Blood Cells Mol Dis. 2001 Nov-Dec;27(6):1013-9. PMID:11831868

Descamps V, Bouscarat F. [Bartonellosis].[Article in French]. Ann Dermatol Venereol. 2001 May;128(5):669-73. PMID:11427808

Desenclos JC, Laporte A, Brouqui P. [Louse-borne infections in humans].[Article in French]. Med Mal Infect. 2011 Jun;41(6):295-300. Epub 2011 Mar 30. PMID:21450425

Dharnidharka VR, Richard GA, Neiberger RE, Fennell RS 3rd. Cat scratch disease and acute rejection after pediatric renal transplantation. Pediatr Transplant. 2002 Aug;6(4):327-31. PMID:12234274

Di Francesco A, Sanguinetti V, Gallina L, Gavioli R, Piva S, Baldelli R. Prevalence of antibodies to Bartonella henselae in dogs in Italy. Vet Rec. 2007 Oct 6;161(14):489-90. PMID:17921442

Di Lorenzo G, Rizzo M, Mansueto P, Falci C, Mazzola G, Affronti M, Rini GB, Mansueto S. [Three cases of bartonellosis (cat scratch disease)].[Article in Italian]. Ann Ital Med Int. 2002 Oct-Dec;17(4):256-60. PMID:12532565

Diaz MH, Bai Y, Malania L, Winchell JM, Kosoy MY. Development of a novel genus-specific real-time PCR assay for detection and differentiation of bartonella species and genotypes. J Clin Microbiol. 2012 May;50(5):1645-9. Epub 2012 Feb 29. PMID:22378904

Díaz-Valle D, Toledano Fernández N, Arteaga Sánchez A, Miguélez Sánchez R, Pascual Allen D. [Severe retinal phlebitis in ocular bartonellosis].[Article in Spanish]. Arch Soc Esp Oftalmol. 2003 Apr;78(4):223-6. PMID:12743848

Diederen BM, Vermeulen MJ, Verbakel H, van der Zee A, Bergmans A, Peeters MF. Evaluation of an internally controlled real-time polymerase chain reaction assay targeting the groEL gene for the detection of Bartonella spp. DNA in patients with suspected cat-scratch disease. Eur J Clin Microbiol Infect Dis. 2007 Sep;26(9):629-33. PMID:17624560

Dietrich F, Schmidgen T, Maggi RG, Richter D, Matuschka FR, Vonthein R, Breitschwerdt EB, Kempf VA. Prevalence of Bartonella henselae and Borrelia burgdorferi sensu lato DNA in ixodes ricinus ticks in Europe. Appl Environ Microbiol. 2010 Mar;76(5):1395-8. Epub 2010 Jan 8. PMID:20061459

Dillon B, Cagney M, Manolios N, Iredell JR. Failure to detect Bartonella henselae infection in synovial fluid from sufferers of chronic arthritis. Rheumatol Int. 2000;19(6):219-22. PMID:11063291

Dillon B, Iredell J, Breitschwerdt EB, Maggi RG. Potential limitations of the 16S-23S rRNA intergenic region for molecular detection of Bartonella species. J Clin Microbiol. 2005 Sep;43(9):4921-2. PMID:16145180

Dillon B, Iredell J. DdeI RFLP for 16S rDNA typing in Bartonella henselae. J Med Microbiol. 2004 Dec;53(Pt 12):1263-5. PMID:15585508

Dillon B, Valenzuela J, Don R, Blanckenberg D, Wigney DI, Malik R, Morris AJ, Robson JM, Iredell J. Limited diversity among human isolates of Bartonella henselae. J Clin Microbiol. 2002 Dec;40(12):4691-9. PMID:12454174

Ding HJ. [Cat scrach disease].[Article in Chinese]. Zhonghua Bing Li Xue Za Zhi. 2004 Oct;33(5):475-7. PMID:15498227

Diniz PP, Beall MJ, Omark K, Chandrashekar R, Daniluk DA, Cyr KE, Koterski JF, Robbins RG, Lalo PG, Hegarty BC, Breitschwerdt EB. High prevalence of tick-borne pathogens in dogs from an Indian reservation in northeastern Arizona. Vector Borne Zoonotic Dis. 2010 Mar;10(2):117-23. PMID:19469667

Diniz PP, Billeter SA, Otranto D, De Caprariis D, Petanides T, Mylonakis ME, Koutinas AF, Breitschwerdt EB. Molecular documentation of Bartonella infection in dogs in Greece and Italy. J Clin Microbiol. 2009 May;47(5):1565-7. Epub 2009 Mar 4. PMID:19261798

Diniz PP, de Morais HS, Breitschwerdt EB, Schwartz DS. Serum cardiac troponin I concentration in dogs with ehrlichiosis. J Vet Intern Med. 2008 Sep-Oct;22(5):1136-43. Epub 2008 Jul 11. PMID:18638021

Diniz PP, Maggi RG, Schwartz DS, Cadenas MB, Bradley JM, Hegarty B, Breitschwerdt EB. Canine bartonellosis: serological and molecular prevalence in Brazil and evidence of co-infection with Bartonella henselae and Bartonella vinsonii subsp. berkhoffii. Vet Res. 2007 Sep-Oct;38(5):697-710. Epub 2007 Jun 23. PMID:17583666

Diniz PP, Wood M, Maggi RG, Sontakke S, Stepnik M, Breitschwerdt EB. Co-isolation of Bartonella henselae and Bartonella vinsonii subsp. Berkhoffii from blood, joint and subcutaneous seroma fluids from two naturally infected dogs. Vet Microbiol. 2009 Sep 18;138(3-4):368-72. Epub 2009 Feb 4. PMID:19560291

Dlova NC. Photo capsules. Bacillary angiomatosis. Skinmed. 2005 Jul-Aug;4(4):213. PMID:16015069

Dobler G, Pfeffer M. Fleas as parasites of the family Canidae. Parasit Vectors. 2011 Jul 18;4:139. PMID:21767354

Doern GV. Detection of selected fastidious bacteria. Clin Infect Dis. 2000 Jan;30(1):166-73. PMID:10619747

Dong J, Olano JP, McBride JW, Walker DH. Emerging pathogens: challenges and successes of molecular diagnostics. J Mol Diagn. 2008 May;10(3):185-97. Epub 2008 Apr 10. PMID:18403608

Donnio A, Buestel C, Ventura E, Merle H. [Cat-scratch disease neuroretinitis].[Article in French]. J Fr Ophtalmol. 2004 Mar;27(3):285-90. PMID:15039632

Donnio A, Jean-Charles A, Merle H. Macular hole following Bartonella henselae neuroretinitis. Eur J Ophthalmol. 2008 May-Jun;18(3):456-8. PMID:18465733

Dorado Moles MJ, López-Ibor B, Figueredo MA, González Laguillo A. [Atypical cat scratch disease in an immunocompetent school-aged child].[Article in Spanish]. An Pediatr (Barc). 2007 Apr;66(4):418-9. PMID:17430722

Dörbecker C, Sander A, Oberle K, Schülin-Casonato T. In vitro susceptibility of Bartonella species to 17 antimicrobial compounds: comparison of Etest and agar dilution. J Antimicrob Chemother. 2006 Oct;58(4):784-8. Epub 2006 Aug 17. PMID:16916864

dos Santos AP, dos Santos RP, Biondo AW, Dora JM, Goldani LZ, de Oliveira ST, de Sá Guimarães AM, Timenetsky J, de Morais HA, González FH, Messick JB. Hemoplasma infection in HIV-positive patient, Brazil. Emerg Infect Dis. 2008 Dec;14(12):1922-4. PMID:19046522

dos Santos RP, Cartell A, Goldani LZ. An HIV-positive patient with cervical lymphadenopathy and skin lesions. Clin Infect Dis. 2007 Mar 15;44(6):849, 884-5. PMID:17304465

Dowers KL, Hawley JR, Brewer MM, Morris AK, Radecki SV, Lappin MR. Association of Bartonella species, feline calicivirus, and feline herpesvirus 1 infection with gingivostomatitis in cats. J Feline Med Surg. 2010 Apr;12(4):314-21. Epub 2009 Dec 2. PMID:19959386

Drancourt M, Berger P, Terrada C, Bodaghi B, Conrath J, Raoult D, LeHoang P. High prevalence of fastidious bacteria in 1520 cases of uveitis of unknown etiology. Medicine (Baltimore). 2008 May;87(3):167-76. PMID:18520326

Drancourt M, Bodaghi B, Lepidi H, Le Hoang P, Raoult D. Intraocular detection of Bartonella henselae in a patient with HLA-B27 uveitis. J Clin Microbiol. 2004 Apr;42(4):1822-5. PMID:15071060

Drancourt M, Carrieri P, Gévaudan MJ, Raoult D. Blood agar and Mycobacterium tuberculosis: the end of a dogma. J Clin Microbiol. 2003 Apr;41(4):1710-1. PMID:12682165

Drancourt M, Tran-Hung L, Courtin J, Lumley H, Raoult D. Bartonella quintana in a 4000-year-old human tooth. J Infect Dis. 2005 Feb 15;191(4):607-11. Epub 2005 Jan 10. PMID:15655785

Drebber U, Kasper HU, Ratering J, Wedemeyer I, Schirmacher P, Dienes HP, Odenthal M. Hepatic granulomas: histological and molecular pathological approach to differential diagnosis--a study of 442 cases. Liver Int. 2008 Jul;28(6):828-34. PMID:18312287

Dreier J, Vollmer T, Freytag CC, Bäumer D, Körfer R, Kleesiek K. Culture-negative infectious endocarditis caused by Bartonella spp.: 2 case reports and a review of the literature. Diagn Microbiol Infect Dis. 2008 Aug;61(4):476-83. Epub 2008 May 1. PMID:18455348

Drummond MR, Gilioli R, Velho PE. Bartonellosis diagnosis requires careful evaluation. Braz J Infect Dis. 2010 May-Jun;14(3):217. PMID:20835501

Dubey JP, Bhatia CR, Lappin MR, Ferreira LR, Thorn A, Kwok OC. Seroprevalence of Toxoplasma gondii and Bartonella spp. antibodies in cats from Pennsylvania. J Parasitol. 2009 Jun;95(3):578-80. PMID:19061304

Dubey JP, Lappin MR, Kwok OC, Mofya S, Chikweto A, Baffa A, Doherty D, Shakeri J, Macpherson CN, Sharma RN. Seroprevalence of Toxoplasma gondii and concurrent Bartonella spp., feline immunodeficiency virus, and feline leukemia virus infections in cats from Grenada, West Indies. J Parasitol. 2009 Oct;95(5):1129-33. Epub 2009 Apr 22. PMID:19385716

Duchemin JB, Fournier PE, Parola P. [Fleas and diseases transmissible to man].[Article in French]. Med Trop (Mars). 2006 Feb;66(1):21-9. PMID:16615611

Duncan AW, Maggi RG, Breitschwerdt EB. A combined approach for the enhanced detection and isolation of Bartonella species in dog blood samples:pre-enrichment liquid culture followed by PCR and subculture onto agar plates. J Microbiol Methods. 2007 May;69(2):273-81. Epub 2007 Feb 2. PMID:17346836

Duncan AW, Maggi RG, Breitschwerdt EB. Bartonella DNA in dog saliva. Emerg Infect Dis. 2007 Dec;13(12):1948-50. PMID:18258056

Duncan AW, Marr HS, Birkenheuer AJ, Maggi RG, Williams LE, Correa MT, Breitschwerdt EB. Bartonella DNA in the blood and lymph nodes of Golden Retrievers with lymphoma and in healthy controls. J Vet Intern Med. 2008 Jan-Feb;22(1):89-95. PMID:18289294

Durá Travé T, Yoldi Petri ME, Lavilla Oiz A, Molins Castiella T. [Neuroretinitis in cat-scratch disease].[Article in Spanish]. An Pediatr (Barc). 2010 Apr;72(4):290-1. Epub 2010 Mar 2. PMID:20199895

Durá-Travé T, Yoldi-Petri ME, Gallinas-Victoriano F, Lavilla-Oiz A, Bove-Guri M. Neuroretinitis Caused by Bartonella henselae (Cat-Scratch Disease) in a 13-Year-Old Girl. Int J Pediatr. 2010;2010:763105. Epub 2010 Jun 15. PMID:20628521

Durden LA, Ellis BA, Banks CW, Crowe JD, Oliver JH Jr. Ectoparasites of gray squirrels in two different habitats and screening of selected ectoparasites for bartonellae. J Parasitol. 2004 Jun;90(3):485-9. PMID:15270090

Durupt F, Seve P, Roure C, Biron F, Raoult D, Broussolle C. Liver and spleen abscesses without endocarditis due to Bartonella quintana in an immunocompetent host. Eur J Clin Microbiol Infect Dis. 2004 Oct;23(10):790-1. PMID:15365873

Dutkiewicz J, Cisak E, Sroka J, Wójcik-Fatla A, Zając V. Biological agents as occupational hazards - selected issues. Ann Agric Environ Med. 2011 Dec;18(2):286-93. PMID:22216801

Dutta A, Schwarzwald HL, Edwards MS. Disseminated bartonellosis presenting as neuroretinitis in a young adult with human immunodeficiency virus infection. Pediatr Infect Dis J. 2010 Jul;29(7):675-7. PMID:20216243

Dyachenko P, Ziv M, Raz R, Chazan B, Lev A, Rozenman D. Cat scratch disease encephalopathy in an immunocompetent patient. Eur J Intern Med. 2005 Dec;16(8):610-1. PMID:16314249

Dzelalija B, Avsic-Zupanc T. [Bartonella henselae as the causative agent in cat-scratch disease: case report].[Article in Croatian]. Lijec Vjesn. 2001 Jan-Feb;123(1-2):14-5. PMID:11379192

Dzelalija B, Medić A, Rode OD, Mazzi A. [Rash and purulent lymphadenitis in cat scratch disease].[Article in Croatian]. Acta Med Croatica. 2006 Dec;60(5):483-6. PMID:17217106

Dzelalija B, Petrovec M, Avsic-Zupanc T. Probable atypical cat scratch disease presenting as isolated posterior pancreatic duodenal lymphadenitis and abdominal pain. Clin Infect Dis. 2001 Sep 15;33(6):912-4. Epub 2001 Aug 21. PMID:11512100

Earhart KC, Power MH. Images in clinical medicine. Bartonella neuroretinitis. N Engl J Med. 2000 Nov 16;343(20):1459. PMID:11078771

Easterbrook JD, Kaplan JB, Vanasco NB, Reeves WK, Purcell RH, Kosoy MY, Glass GE, Watson J, Klein SL. A survey of zoonotic pathogens carried by Norway rats in Baltimore, Maryland, USA. Epidemiol Infect. 2007 Oct;135(7):1192-9. Epub 2007 Jan 15. PMID:17224086

Ebani VV, Bertelloni F, Fratini F. Occurrence of Bartonella henselae types I and II in Central Italian domestic cats. Res Vet Sci. 2011 Aug 6. [Epub ahead of print]. PMID:21824634

Ebani VV, Cerri D, Andreani E. Cat scratch disease. Survey on the presence of Bartonella henselae among cats of Tuscany. New Microbiol. 2002 Jul;25(3):307-13. PMID:12173772

Eberhardt C, Engelmann S, Kusch H, Albrecht D, Hecker M, Autenrieth IB, Kempf VA. Proteomic analysis of the bacterial pathogen Bartonella henselae and identification of immunogenic proteins for serodiagnosis. Proteomics. 2009 Apr;9(7):1967-81. PMID:19333998

Eberhardt JM, Neal K, Shackelford T, Lappin MR. Prevalence of selected infectious disease agents in cats from Arizona. J Feline Med Surg. 2006 Jun;8(3):164-8. Epub 2006 Jan 27. PMID:16443383

Eckart P, Tournade G, Amiour M, Guillot M, Courthéoux P, Rousselot P. [Pseudotumoral presentation of cat scratch disease].[Article in French]. Arch Pediatr. 2001 Apr;8(4):393-6. PMID:11339132

Economou M, Lithoxopoulou M, Aivazis V, Tsakalidis C, Athanassiou-Metaxa M. Bartonella henselae: association with the development of transient lupus anticoagulant and asymptomatic prolongation of activated partial thromboplastin time. Scand J Infect Dis. 2003;35(2):149. PMID:12693573

Edlow JA. Erythema migrans. Med Clin North Am. 2002 Mar;86(2):239-60. PMID:11982300

Edmonson BC, Morris WR, Osborn FD. Bacillary angiomatosis with cytomegaloviral and mycobacterial infections of the palpebral conjunctiva in a patient with AIDS. Ophthal Plast Reconstr Surg. 2004 Mar;20(2):168-70. PMID:15083089

Edouard S, Gonin K, Turc Y, Angelakis E, Socolovschi C, Raoult D. Eschar and neck lymphadenopathy caused by Francisella tularensis after a tick bite: a case report. J Med Case Reports. 2011 Mar 19;5:108. PMID:21418587

Edouard S, Raoult D. [Bartonella henselae, an ubiquitous agent of proteiform zoonotic disease].[Article in French]. Med Mal Infect. 2010 Jun;40(6):319-30. Epub 2009 Dec 29. PMID:20042306

Eggenberger E. Cat scratch disease: posterior segment manifestations. Ophthalmology. 2000 May;107(5):817-8. PMID:10811065

Eglantin F, Hamdad F, El Samad Y, Monge AS, Sevestre H, Eb F, Schmit JL. [The diagnosis of cat-scratch-disease-associated adenitis: diagnostic value of serology and polymerase chain reaction].[Article in French]. Pathol Biol (Paris). 2008 Nov-Dec;56(7-8):461-6. Epub 2008 Oct 7. PMID:18842353

Egyed L, Elő P, Sréter-Lancz Z, Széll Z, Balogh Z, Sréter T. Seasonal activity and tick-borne pathogen infection rates of Ixodes ricinus ticks in Hungary. Ticks Tick Borne Dis. 2012 Apr;3(2):90-4. Epub 2012 Mar 23. PMID:22445929

Ehrenborg C, Byström R, Hjelm E, Friman G, Holmberg M. High Bartonella spp. seroprevalence in a Swedish homeless population but no evidence of trench fever. Scand J Infect Dis. 2008;40(3):208-15. Epub 2007 Sep 6. PMID:17852922

Ehrenborg C, Hagberg S, Alden J, Makitalo S, Myrdal G, Larsson E, Hjelm E, Friman G. First known case of Bartonella quintana endocarditis in Sweden. Scand J Infect Dis. 2009;41(1):73-5. PMID:18985544

Ehrenborg C, Handley S, Ellis B, Mills J, Holmberg M. Bartonella grahamii infecting rodents display high genetic diversity over short geographic distances. Ann N Y Acad Sci. 2003 Jun;990:233-5. PMID:12860632

Ehrenborg C, Wesslén L, Jakobson A, Friman G, Holmberg M. Sequence variation in the ftsZ gene of Bartonella henselae isolates and clinical samples. J Clin Microbiol. 2000 Feb;38(2):682-7. PMID:10655367

Eicher SC, Dehio C. Bartonella entry mechanisms into mammalian host cells. Cell Microbiol. 2012 Apr 23. [Epub ahead of print]. PMID:22519749

Eichhorn-Sens J, Bund T, Vogt PM. [Painful soft-tissue swelling of the upper arm].[Article in German]. Chirurg. 2008 Mar;79(3):249-51. PMID:17443304

Eidlitz-Markus T, Zeharia A. Images in clinical medicine. Cat scratch disease lymphadenopathy. N Engl J Med. 2006 Apr 27;354(17):e17. PMID:16641391

Eisen RJ, Gage KL. Transmission of flea-borne zoonotic agents. Annu Rev Entomol. 2012;57:61-82. Epub 2011 Aug 29. PMID:21888520

El-Atrouni W, Berbari E, Temesgen Z. HIV-associated opportunistic infections. Bacterial infections. J Med Liban. 2006 Apr-Jun;54(2):80-3. PMID:17086998

Elliott TS, Foweraker J, Gould FK, Perry JD, Sandoe JA; Working Party of the British Society for Antimicrobial Chemotherapy. Guidelines for the antibiotic treatment of endocarditis in adults: report of the Working Party of the British Society for Antimicrobial Chemotherapy. J Antimicrob Chemother. 2004 Dec;54(6):971-81. Epub 2004 Nov 16. PMID:15546974

Elston DM, Do H. What's eating you? Cat flea (Ctenocephalides felis), Part 1: Clinical features and role as a disease vector. Cutis. 2010 May;85(5):231-6. PMID:20540412

Endara SA, Roati AA, Alizzi AM, Boldery JO, Bidstrup BP. Aortic valve endocarditis caused by Bartonella henselae: a rare surgical entity. Heart Surg Forum. 2001;4(4):359-60; discussion 360. PMID:11803150

Ender PT, Phares J, Gerson G, Taylor SE, Regnery R, Challener RC, Dolan MJ. Association of Bartonella species and Coxiella burnetii infection with coronary artery disease. J Infect Dis. 2001 Mar 1;183(5):831-4. Epub 2001 Jan 24. PMID:11181164

Engbaek K, Lawson PA. Identification of Bartonella species in rodents, shrews and cats in Denmark: detection of two B. henselae variants, one in cats and the other in the long-tailed field mouse. APMIS. 2004 Jun;112(6):336-41. PMID:15511270

Engel P, Dehio C. Genomics of host-restricted pathogens of the genus bartonella. Genome Dyn. 2009;6:158-69. Epub 2009 Aug 19. PMID:19696500

Engel P, Goepfert A, Stanger FV, Harms A, Schmidt A, Schirmer T, Dehio C. Adenylylation control by intra- or intermolecular active-site obstruction in Fic proteins. Nature. 2012 Jan 22;482(7383):107-10. PMID:22266942

Engel P, Salzburger W, Liesch M, Chang CC, Maruyama S, Lanz C, Calteau A, Lajus A, Médigue C, Schuster SC, Dehio C. Parallel evolution of a type IV secretion system in radiating lineages of the host-restricted bacterial pathogen Bartonella. PLoS Genet. 2011 Feb 10;7(2):e1001296. PMID:21347280

English R. Cat-scratch disease. Pediatr Rev. 2006 Apr;27(4):123-8; quiz 128. PMID:16581952

Engvall EO, Brändström B, Fermér C, Blomqvist G, Englund L. Prevalence of Bartonella henselae in young, healthy cats in Sweden. Vet Rec. 2003 Mar 22;152(12):366-9. PMID:12678262

Enia F, Di Stefano G, Floresta AM, Matassa C. [New etiologies responsible for infective endocarditis with negative blood cultures]. [Article in Italian]. Ital Heart J Suppl. 2005 Mar;6(3):128-34. PMID:15875498

Erbe M, Lindenfelser R. [Solitary nontuberculous mycobacterial infection of a cervical lymph node caused by Bartonella henselae (cat scratch disease)].[Article in German]. Mund Kiefer Gesichtschir. 2004 Nov;8(6):381-6. Epub 2004 Sep 9. PMID:15365888

Eremeeva ME, Gerns HL, Lydy SL, Goo JS, Ryan ET, Mathew SS, Ferraro MJ, Holden JM, Nicholson WL, Dasch GA, Koehler JE. Bacteremia, fever, and splenomegaly caused by a newly recognized bartonella species. N Engl J Med. 2007 Jun 7;356(23):2381-7. PMID:17554119

Ergin C, Akkaya Y, Kiriş Satılmış O, Yılmaz C. [Comparison of the indirect immunofluorescence assay performance of Bartonella henselae antigens obtained by co-cultivation in Vero and HeLa cells].[Article in Turkish]. Mikrobiyol Bul. 2011 Jul;45(3):461-7. PMID:21935779

Eroğlu C, Candir N, Dervişoğlu A, Kefeli M. [A case of cat scratch disease].[Article in Turkish]. Mikrobiyol Bul. 2007 Oct;41(4):603-6. PMID:18173081

Escarmelle A, Delbrassine N, De Potter P. [Cat's cratch disease and Parinaud's oculoglandular syndrome].[Article in French]. J Fr Ophtalmol. 2004 Feb;27(2):179-83. PMID:15029049

Eskow E, Rao RV, Mordechai E. Concurrent infection of the central nervous system by Borrelia burgdorferi and Bartonella henselae: evidence for a novel tick-borne disease complex. Arch Neurol. 2001 Sep;58(9):1357-63. PMID:11559306

Estrella M, Cosgrove SE. Cases from the Osler Medical Service at Johns Hopkins University. Bartonella henselae infection of the liver and spleen. Am J Med. 2002 Sep;113(4):344-6. PMID:12361825

Evguenieva-Hackenberg E, Klug G. RNase III processing of intervening sequences found in helix 9 of 23S rRNA in the alpha subclass of Proteobacteria. J Bacteriol. 2000 Sep;182(17):4719-29. PMID:10940010

Eymin G, Zapata A, Andrade M, Aizman A, Rojas L, Rabagliati R. [Cat-scratch disease. Review of eight adult patients hospitalized for fever or adenopathy].[Article in Spanish]. Rev Med Chil. 2006 Oct;134(10):1243-8. Epub 2006 Dec 13. PMID:17186093

Fabbi M, De Giuli L, Tranquillo M, Bragoni R, Casiraghi M, Genchi C. Prevalence of Bartonella henselae in Italian stray cats: evaluation of serology to assess the risk of transmission of Bartonella to humans. J Clin Microbiol. 2004 Jan;42(1):264-8. PMID:14715763

Fabbi M, Vicari N, Tranquillo M, Pozzi C, Prati P, De Meneghi D, Bertoletti I, Lauzi S, Guiso P, Genchi C. [Prevalence of Bartonella henselae in stray and domestic cats in different Italian areas: evaluation of the potential risk of transmission of Bartonella to humans].[Article in Italian]. Parassitologia. 2004 Jun;46(1-2):127-9. PMID:15305701

Family-Pigné D, Mouchet B, Lousteau V, Borie MF, Deforges L, Lesprit P, Godeau B. [Hepatosplenic localization of cat scratch disease: two cases in immunocompetent adult patients].[Article in French]. Rev Med Interne. 2006 Oct;27(10):772-5. Epub 2006 Jul 7. PMID:16959382

Farooque P, Khurana DS, Melvin JJ. Persistent focal seizures after cat scratch encephalopathy. Pediatr Neurol. 2010 Mar;42(3):215-8. PMID:20159433

Fei S, Feng L, Hongzhong J. Bacillary angiomatosis after skin autografting in a patient without human immunodeficiency virus who was treated with interferon alfa. Arch Dermatol. 2010 Aug;146(8):928-30. PMID:20713840

Feliciangeli MD. Natural breeding places of phlebotomine sandflies. Med Vet Entomol. 2004 Mar;18(1):71-80. PMID:15009450

Feng S, Kasten RW, Werner JA, Hodzic E, Barthold SW, Chomel BB. Immunogenicity of Bartonella henselae P26 in cats. Vet Immunol Immunopathol. 2009 Dec 15;132(2-4):251-6. Epub 2009 May 18. PMID:19500857

Fenimore A, Varanat M, Maggi R, Schultheiss P, Breitschwerdt E, Lappin MR. Bartonella spp. DNA in cardiac tissues from dogs in Colorado and Wyoming. J Vet Intern Med. 2011 May-Jun;25(3):613-6. PMID:21539606

Fenollar F, Lepidi H, Raoult D. Whipple's endocarditis: review of the literature and comparisons with Q fever, Bartonella infection, and blood culture-positive endocarditis. Clin Infect Dis. 2001 Oct 15;33(8):1309-16. Epub 2001 Sep 14. PMID:11565070

Fenollar F, Raoult D. Molecular diagnosis of bloodstream infections caused by non-cultivable bacteria. Int J Antimicrob Agents. 2007 Nov;30 Suppl 1:S7-15. Epub 2007 Aug 17. PMID:17707613

Fenollar F, Raoult D. Molecular genetic methods for the diagnosis of fastidious microorganisms. APMIS. 2004 Nov-Dec;112(11-12):785-807. PMID:15638838

Fenollar F, Sire S, Raoult D. Bartonella vinsonii subsp. arupensis as an agent of blood culture-negative endocarditis in a human. J Clin Microbiol. 2005 Feb;43(2):945-7. PMID:15695714

Fernández-González E, de Paz HD, Alperi A, Agúndez L, Faustmann M, Sangari FJ, Dehio C, Llosa M. Transfer of R388 derivatives by a pathogenesis-associated type IV secretion system into both bacteria and human cells. J Bacteriol. 2011 Nov;193(22):6257-65. Epub 2011 Sep 9. PMID:21908662

Fernández-López R, Garcillán-Barcia MP, Revilla C, Lázaro M, Vielva L, de la Cruz F. Dynamics of the IncW genetic backbone imply general trends in conjugative plasmid evolution. FEMS Microbiol Rev. 2006 Nov;30(6):942-66. Epub 2006 Oct 6. PMID:17026718

Ferrés G M, Abarca V K, Prado D P, Montecinos P L, Navarrete C M, Vial C PA. [Prevalence of Bartonella henselae antibodies in Chilean children, adolescents and veterinary workers].[Article in Spanish]. Rev Med Chil. 2006 Jul;134(7):863-7. Epub 2006 Aug 29. PMID:17130969

Ferrés M, Abarca K, Godoy P, García P, Palavecino E, Méndez G, Valdés A, Ernst S, Thibaut J, Koberg J, Chanqueo L, Vial PA. [Presence of Bartonella henselae in cats: natural reservoir quantification and human exposition risk of this zoonoses in Chile].[Article in Spanish]. Rev Med Chil. 2005 Dec;133(12):1465-71. Epub 2006 Jan 27. PMID:16446874

Fichet-Calvet E, Jomâa I, Ben Ismail R, Ashford RW. Patterns of infection of haemoparasites in the fat sand rat, Psammomys obesus, in Tunisia, and effect on the host. Ann Trop Med Parasitol. 2000 Jan;94(1):55-68. PMID:10723524

Ficociello J, Bradbury C, Morris A, Lappin MR. Detection of Bartonella henselae IgM in serum of experimentally infected and naturally exposed cats. J Vet Intern Med. 2011 Nov-Dec;25(6):1264-9. Epub 2011 Nov 1. PMID:22092615

Filoni C, Catão-Dias JL, Bay G, Durigon EL, Jorge RS, Lutz H, Hofmann-Lehmann R. First evidence of feline herpesvirus, calicivirus, parvovirus, and Ehrlichia exposure in Brazilian free-ranging felids. J Wildl Dis. 2006 Apr;42(2):470-7. PMID:16870878

Filoni C, Catão-Dias JL, Cattori V, Willi B, Meli ML, Corrêa SH, Marques MC, Adania CH, Silva JC, Marvulo MF, Ferreira Neto JS, Durigon EL, de Carvalho VM, Coutinho SD, Lutz H, Hofmann-Lehmann R. Surveillance using serological and molecular methods for the detection of infectious agents in captive Brazilian neotropic and exotic felids. J Vet Diagn Invest. 2012 Jan;24(1):166-73. Epub 2011 Jul 21. PMID:21908268

Finkelstein JL, Brown TP, O'Reilly KL, Wedincamp J Jr, Foil LD. Studies on the growth of Bartonella henselae in the cat flea (Siphonaptera: Pulicidae). J Med Entomol. 2002 Nov;39(6):915-9. PMID:12495192

Fischer D, Moeller P, Thomas SM, Naucke TJ, Beierkuhnlein C. Combining climatic projections and dispersal ability: a method for estimating the responses of sandfly vector species to climate change. PLoS Negl Trop Dis. 2011 Nov;5(11):e1407. Epub 2011 Nov 29. PMID:22140590

Fisher W. Images in emergency medicine. Bartonella henselae lymphadenitis. Ann Emerg Med. 2007 Jul;50(1):90, 97. PMID:17572294

Fiskus W, Padmalayam I, Kelly T, Guibao C, Baumstark BR. Identification and characterization of the DdlB, FtsQ and FtsA genes upstream of FtsZ in Bartonella bacilliformis and Bartonella henselae. DNA Cell Biol. 2003 Nov;22(11):743-52. PMID:14659047

Fleury RN, Taborda PR, Gupta AK, Fujita MS, Rosa PS, Weckwerth AC, Negrão MS, Bastazini I. Zoonotic sporotrichosis. Transmission to humans by infected domestic cat scratching: report of four cases in São Paulo, Brazil. Int J Dermatol. 2001 May;40(5):318-22. PMID:11575308

Flodr P. [What is your diagnosis? 1. Lymphadenopathy in sarcoidosis. 2. Toxoplasmic lymphadenitis (Piringer-Kuchinkov). 3. Reactive (paraneoplastic) granulomatous lymphadenopathy. 4. Granulomatous cat-scratch lymphadenitis].[Article in Czech]. Cesk Patol. 2011 Jul;47(3):122-4. PMID:21887930

Florin TA, Zaoutis TE, Zaoutis LB. Beyond cat scratch disease: widening spectrum of Bartonella henselae infection. Pediatrics. 2008 May;121(5):e1413-25. Epub 2008 Apr 28. PMID:18443019

Fohlman J, Blomberg J, Fröman G, Engstrand L, Johansson A, Friman G. [Microbial diagnosis with PCR will become clinically beneficial with a faster analysis].[Article in Swedish]. Lakartidningen. 2004 Apr 22;101(17):1488-92. PMID:15150950

Foley JE, Brown RN, Gabriel MW, Henn J, Drazenovich N, Kasten R, Green SL, Chomel BB. Spatial analysis of the exposure of dogs in rural north-coastal California to vectorborne pathogens. Vet Rec. 2007 Nov 10;161(19):653-7. PMID:17993656

Fonollosa A, Galdos M, Artaraz J, Perez-Irezabal J, Martinez-Alday N. Occlusive vasculitis and optic disk neovascularization associated with neuroretinitis. Ocul Immunol Inflamm. 2011 Feb;19(1):62-4. Epub 2010 Oct 31. PMID:21034304

Font RL, Del Valle M, Mitchell BM, Boniuk M. Cat-scratch uveitis confirmed by histological, serological, and molecular diagnoses. Cornea. 2011 Apr;30(4):468-71. PMID:21099401

Fontenelle JP, Powell CC, Hill AE, Radecki SV, Lappin MR. Prevalence of serum antibodies against Bartonella species in the serum of cats with or without uveitis. J Feline Med Surg. 2008 Feb;10(1):41-6. Epub 2007 Aug 23. PMID:17719256

Foongladda S, Inthawong D, Kositanont U, Gaywee J. Rickettsia, Ehrlichia, Anaplasma, and Bartonella in ticks and fleas from dogs and cats in Bangkok. Vector Borne Zoonotic Dis. 2011 Oct;11(10):1335-41. Epub 2011 May 25. PMID:21612535

Forbes SH, Robert SC, Martin JE, Rajakariar R. Quiz page January 2012 – Acute kidney injury with hematuria, a positive ANCA test, and low levels of complement. Am J Kidney Dis. 2012 Jan;59(1):A28-31. PMID:22177451

Foroozan R. Cat scratch disease in two brothers. J Neuroophthalmol. 2004 Jun;24(2):186-7. PMID:15179075

Fortune SM, Kaelin CM, Gulizia JM, Daily JP. Cat scratch disease presenting as a breast mass. Obstet Gynecol. 2000 Jun;95(6 Pt 2):1027. PMID:10808015

Foucault C, Barrau K, Brouqui P, Raoult D. Bartonella quintana Bacteremia among Homeless People. Clin Infect Dis. 2002 Sep 15;35(6):684-9. Epub 2002 Aug 20. PMID:12203165

Foucault C, Brouqui P, Raoult D. Bartonella quintana characteristics and clinical management. Emerg Infect Dis. 2006 Feb;12(2):217-23. PMID:16494745

Foucault C, La Scola B, Lindroos H, Andersson SG, Raoult D. Multispacer typing technique for sequence-based typing of Bartonella quintana. J Clin Microbiol. 2005 Jan;43(1):41-8. PMID:15634949

Foucault C, Raoult D, Brouqui P. Randomized open trial of gentamicin and doxycycline for eradication of Bartonella quintana from blood in patients with chronic bacteremia. Antimicrob Agents Chemother. 2003 Jul;47(7):2204-7. PMID:12821469

Foucault C, Rolain JM, Raoult D, Brouqui P. Detection of Bartonella quintana by direct immunofluorescence examination of blood smears of a patient with acute trench fever. J Clin Microbiol. 2004 Oct;42(10):4904-6. PMID:15472378

Fouch B, Coventry S. A case of fatal disseminated Bartonella henselae infection (cat-scratch disease) with encephalitis. Arch Pathol Lab Med. 2007 Oct;131(10):1591-4. PMID:17922599

Fournier PE, Couderc C, Buffet S, Flaudrops C, Raoult D. Rapid and cost-effective identification of Bartonella species using mass spectrometry. J Med Microbiol. 2009 Sep;58(Pt 9):1154-9. Epub 2009 Jun 15. PMID:19528172

Fournier PE, Lelievre H, Eykyn SJ, Mainardi JL, Marrie TJ, Bruneel F, Roure C, Nash J, Clave D, James E, Benoit-Lemercier C, Deforges L, Tissot-Dupont H, Raoult D. Epidemiologic and clinical characteristics of Bartonella quintana and Bartonella henselae endocarditis: a study of 48 patients. Medicine (Baltimore). 2001 Jul;80(4):245-51. PMID:11470985

Fournier PE, Mainardi JL, Raoult D. Value of microimmunofluorescence for diagnosis and follow-up of Bartonella endocarditis. Clin Diagn Lab Immunol. 2002 Jul;9(4):795-801. PMID:12093675

Fournier PE, Minnick MF, Lepidi H, Salvo E, Raoult D. Experimental model of human body louse infection using green fluorescent protein-expressing Bartonella quintana. Infect Immun. 2001 Mar;69(3):1876-9. PMID:11179366

Fournier PE, Ndihokubwayo JB, Guidran J, Kelly PJ, Raoult D. Human pathogens in body and head lice. Emerg Infect Dis. 2002 Dec;8(12):1515-8. PMID:12498677

Fournier PE, Robson J, Zeaiter Z, McDougall R, Byrne S, Raoult D. Improved culture from lymph nodes of patients with cat scratch disease and genotypic characterization of Bartonella henselae isolates in Australia. J Clin Microbiol. 2002 Oct;40(10):3620-4. PMID:12354855

Fournier PE, Taylor C, Rolain JM, Barrassi L, Smith G, Raoult D. Bartonella australis sp. nov. from kangaroos, Australia. Emerg Infect Dis. 2007 Dec;13(12):1961-2. PMID:18258063

Fournier PE, Thuny F, Richet H, Lepidi H, Casalta JP, Arzouni JP, Maurin M, Célard M, Mainardi JL, Caus T, Collart F, Habib G, Raoult D. Comprehensive diagnostic strategy for blood culture-negative endocarditis: a prospective study of 819 new cases. Clin Infect Dis. 2010 Jul 15;51(2):131-40. PMID:20540619

Fox JW, Studley JK, Cohen DM. Recurrent expressive aphasia as a presentation of cat-scratch encephalopathy. Pediatrics. 2007 Mar;119(3):e760-3. PMID:17332191

Franz B, Kempf VA. Adhesion and host cell modulation: critical pathogenicity determinants of Bartonella henselae. Parasit Vectors. 2011 Apr 13;4:54. PMID:21489243

Frean J, Arndt S, Spencer D. High rate of Bartonella henselae infection in HIV-positive outpatients in Johannesburg, South Africa. Trans R Soc Trop Med Hyg. 2002 Sep-Oct;96(5):549-50. PMID:12474487

Fretzayas A, Papadopoulos NG, Moustaki M, Bossios A, Koukoutsakis P, Karpathios T. Unsuspected extralymphocutaneous dissemination in febrile cat scratch disease. Scand J Infect Dis. 2001;33(8):599-603. PMID:11525355

From the Centers for Disease Control and Prevention. Cat-Scratch Disease in children--Texas, September 2000-August 2001. JAMA. 2002 May 22-29;287(20):2647-9. PMID:12035788

Fu J, Muttaiyah S, Pandey S, Thomas M. Two cases of endocarditis due to Bartonella henselae. N Z Med J. 2007 Jun 1;120(1255):U2558. PMID:17546106

Fuchs M, Kondracka E. [Cat-scratch disease in a 17-year old patient—case report].[Article in Polish]. Otolaryngol Pol. 2001;55(1):105-6. PMID:11355467

Fuentes-Páez G, Martínez-Osorio H, Herreras JM, Calonge M. Subretinal fibrosis and uveitis syndrome associated with ulcerative colitis. Int J Colorectal Dis. 2007 Mar;22(3):333-4. Epub 2006 May 24. PMID:16721489

Fuhrmann O, Arvand M, Göhler A, Schmid M, Krüll M, Hippenstiel S, Seybold J, Dehio C, Suttorp N. Bartonella henselae induces NF-kappaB-dependent upregulation of adhesion molecules in cultured human endothelial cells: possible role of outer membrane proteins as pathogenic factors. Infect Immun. 2001 Aug;69(8):5088-97. PMID:11447190

Fukuchi T, Morisawa Y. [A case of cat-scratch-induced Pasteurella multocida infection presenting with disseminated intravascular coagulation and acute renal failure].[Article in Japanese]. Kansenshogaku Zasshi. 2009 Sep;83(5):557-60. PMID:19860260

Fukushima A, Yasuoka M, Tsukahara M, Ueno H. A case of cat scratch disease neuroretinitis confirmed by polymerase chain reaction. Jpn J Ophthalmol. 2003 Jul-Aug;47(4):405-8. PMID:12842212

Fukushima H, Numaga J, Yoshimoto M, Kato S, Kawashima H. An ocular cat-scratch disease patient positive for cytoplasmic anti-neutrophil cytoplasmic antibody. Graefes Arch Clin Exp Ophthalmol. 2001 Nov;239(11):882-5. PMID:11789871

Gabler B, Linde HJ, Reischl U, Lohmann CP. [Disciform keratatis caused by Bartonella henselae infection: detection of a rare ocular complication of cat-scratch disease with PCR].[Article in German]. Klin Monbl Augenheilkd. 2000 Nov;217(5):299-302. PMID:11146830

Gabriel MW, Henn J, Foley JE, Brown RN, Kasten RW, Foley P, Chomel BB. Zoonotic Bartonella species in fleas collected on gray foxes (Urocyon cinereoargenteus). Vector Borne Zoonotic Dis. 2009 Dec;9(6):597-602. PMID:19125660

Gamblin TC, Nobles-James C, Bradley RA, Katner HP, Dale PS. Cat scratch disease presenting as breast mastitis. Can J Surg. 2005 Jun;48(3):254-5. PMID:16013636

Gan JJ, Mandell AM, Otis JA, Holmuhamedova M, Perloff MD. Suspecting optic neuritis, diagnosing Bartonella cat scratch disease. Arch Neurol. 2011 Jan;68(1):122-6. PMID:21220684

Ganesan K, Mizen K. Cat scratch disease: an unusual cause of facial palsy and partial ptosis: case report. J Oral Maxillofac Surg. 2005 Jun;63(6):869-72. PMID:15944991

García CJ, Varela C, Abarca K, Ferrés M, Prado P, Vial PA. Regional lymphadenopathy in cat-scratch disease: ultrasonographic findings. Pediatr Radiol. 2000 Sep;30(9):640-3. PMID:11009305

García Puga JM, Ramos Ramos MV, Muwaqued Rodríguez F, Santos Pérez JL, Vega Pérez S. [Submandibular tumor].[Article in Spanish]. An Pediatr (Barc). 2006 May;64(5):503-4. PMID:16756901

García-Esteban C, Gil H, Rodríguez-Vargas M, Gerrikagoitia X, Barandika J, Escudero R, Jado I, García-Amil C, Barral M, García-Pérez AL, Bhide M, Anda P. Molecular method for Bartonella species identification in clinical and environmental samples. J Clin Microbiol. 2008 Feb;46(2):776-9. Epub 2007 Dec 19. PMID:18094134

García-García JA, Baquerizo R, Vargas J, Mira JA, Merchante N, Macías J, Pineda JA. [Prevalence of serum antibodies against Bartonella ssp. in a health population from the south area of the Seville province].[Article in Spanish]. Rev Clin Esp. 2005 Nov;205(11):541-4. PMID:16381097

García-García JA, Vargas J, Mira JA, Vergara-López S, Macías J, Pineda JA. [Kinetics of Bartonella spp. IgG antibodies in cat-scratch disease and in asymptomatic HIV-infected patients].[Article in Spanish]. Med Clin (Barc). 2003 Apr 12;120(13):494-5. PMID:12716542

Gardberg A, Abendroth J, Bhandari J, Sankaran B, Staker B. Structure of fructose bisphosphate aldolase from Bartonella henselae bound to fructose 1,6-bisphosphate. Acta Crystallogr Sect F Struct Biol Cryst Commun. 2011 Sep 1;67(Pt 9):1051-4. Epub 2011 Aug 13. PMID:21904049

Gardner MB, Luciw PA. Macaque models of human infectious disease. ILAR J. 2008;49(2):220-55. PMID:18323583

Garré L, Guaraglia W, Cuatz D, Kaufman S, Gil H, De Rosa AF. [Infective endocarditis due to Bartonella quintana].[Article in Spanish]. Medicina (B Aires). 2008;68(2):144-6. PMID:18499964

Garvey J, Joyce MR, Khan F, Ammar A, Connolly CE, Cormican MR, McAnena O. Axillary lymphadenopathy secondary to cat-scratch disease. Ir Med J. 2005 Sep;98(8):243-4. PMID:16255119

Gary AT, Webb JA, Hegarty BC, Breitschwerdt EB. The low seroprevalence of tick-transmitted agents of disease in dogs from southern Ontario and Quebec. Can Vet J. 2006 Dec;47(12):1194-200. PMID:17217089

Gaskin AA, Schantz P, Jackson J, Birkenheuer A, Tomlinson L, Gramiccia M, Levy M, Steurer F, Kollmar E, Hegarty BC, Ahn A, Breitschwerdt EB. Visceral leishmaniasis in a New York foxhound kennel. J Vet Intern Med. 2002 Jan-Feb;16(1):34-44. PMID:11822802

Gaubitz M, Herrmann M, Shahin M, Schotte H, Willeke P, Domschke W. Cat scratch disease (bartonellosis) mimicking an SLE flare. Lupus. 2001;10(12):883-5. PMID:11787880

Gauduchon V, Chalabreysse L, Etienne J, Célard M, Benito Y, Lepidi H, Thivolet-Béjui F, Vandenesch F. Molecular diagnosis of infective endocarditis by PCR amplification and direct sequencing of DNA from valve tissue. J Clin Microbiol. 2003 Feb;41(2):763-6. PMID:12574279

Gazineo JL, Trope BM, Maceira JP, May SB, Coelho JM, Lambert JS, Nogueira SA. Bacillary angiomatosis: description of 13 cases reported in five reference centers for AIDS treatment in Rio de Janeiro, Brazil. Rev Inst Med Trop Sao Paulo. 2001 Jan-Feb;43(1):1-6. PMID:11246275

Geffray L, Poynard JP, Collet T, Armand P, Verdon R. [A "diagnosis of goldsmith"].[Article in French]. Rev Med Interne. 2000 Jun;21 Suppl 3:326s-329s. PMID:10916845

Geissdörfer W, Moos V, Moter A, Loddenkemper C, Jansen A, Tandler R, Morguet AJ, Fenollar F, Raoult D, Bogdan C, Schneider T. High frequency of Tropheryma whipplei in culture-negative endocarditis. J Clin Microbiol. 2012 Feb;50(2):216-22. Epub 2011 Nov 30. PMID:22135251

Genizi J, Kasis I, Schif A, Shahar E. Effect of high-dose methyl-prednisolone on brainstem encephalopathy and basal ganglia impairment complicating cat scratch disease. Brain Dev. 2007 Jul;29(6):377-9. Epub 2006 Dec 15. PMID:17174500

George JG, Bradley JC, Kimbrough RC 3rd, Shami MJ. Bartonella quintana associated neuroretinitis. Scand J Infect Dis. 2006;38(2):127-8. PMID:16449005

Gerber JE, Johnson JE, Scott MA, Madhusudhan KT. Fatal meningitis and encephalitis due to Bartonella henselae bacteria. J Forensic Sci. 2002 May;47(3):640-4. PMID:12051353

Gerrikagoitia X, Gil H, García-Esteban C, Anda P, Juste RA, Barral M. Presence of Bartonella species in wild carnivores of northern Spain. Appl Environ Microbiol. 2012 Feb;78(3):885-8. Epub 2011 Dec 2. PMID:22138983

Gerrits JA, Wolfs TF, Geelen SP. [Three toddlers with a swelling in the neck].[Article in Dutch]. Ned Tijdschr Geneeskd. 2003 Feb 8;147(6):225-9. PMID:12621974

Gescher DM, Mallmann C, Kovacevic D, Schmiedel D, Borges AC, Schweickert B, Göbel UB, Moter A. A view on Bartonella quintana endocarditis--confirming the molecular diagnosis by specific fluorescence in situ hybridization. Diagn Microbiol Infect Dis. 2008 Jan;60(1):99-103. Epub 2007 Sep 21. PMID:17889492

Ghez D, Bernard L, Bayou E, Bani-Sadr F, Vallée C, Perronne C. Bartonella henselae infection mimicking a splenic lymphoma. Scand J Infect Dis. 2001;33(12):935-6. PMID:11868771

Ghidoni JJ. Role of Bartonella henselae endocarditis in the nucleation of aortic valvular calcification. Ann Thorac Surg. 2004 Feb;77(2):704-6. PMID:14759468

Gielen J, Wang XL, Vanhoenacker F, De Schepper H, De Beuckeleer L, Vandevenne J, De Schepper A. Lymphadenopathy at the medial epitrochlear region in cat-scratch disease. Eur Radiol. 2003 Jun;13(6):1363-9. Epub 2002 Oct 2. PMID:12764654

Gil H, García-Esteban C, Barandika JF, Peig J, Toledo A, Escudero R, Jado I, Rodríguez-Vargas M, García-Amil C, Lobo B, Roales P, Rodríguez-Moreno I, Olmeda AS, García-Pérez AL, Anda P. Variability of Bartonella genotypes among small mammals in Spain. Appl Environ Microbiol. 2010 Dec;76(24):8062-70. Epub 2010 Oct 8. PMID:20935117

Gilad J, Wolak A, Borer A, Benharroch D, Avidor B, Giladi M, Schlaeffer F. Isolated splenic cat scratch disease in an immunocompetent adult woman. Clin Infect Dis. 2003 Jan 1;36(1):e10-3. Epub 2002 Dec 10. PMID:12491224

Giladi M, Kletter Y, Avidor B, Metzkor-Cotter E, Varon M, Golan Y, Weinberg M, Riklis I, Ephros M, Slater L. Enzyme immunoassay for the diagnosis of cat-scratch disease defined by polymerase chain reaction. Clin Infect Dis. 2001 Dec 1;33(11):1852-8. Epub 2001 Oct 23. PMID:11692296

Giladi M, Maman E, Paran D, Bickels J, Comaneshter D, Avidor B, Varon-Graidy M, Ephros M, Wientroub S. Cat-scratch disease-associated arthropathy. Arthritis Rheum. 2005 Nov;52(11):3611-7. PMID:16255053

Gillaspie D, Perkins I, Larsen K, McCord A, Pangonis S, Sweger D, Seleem MN, Sriranganathan N, Anderson BE. Plasmid-based system for high-level gene expression and antisense gene knockdown in Bartonella henselae. Appl Environ Microbiol. 2009 Aug;75(16):5434-6. Epub 2009 Jun 19. PMID:19542333

Gillespie TN, Washabau RJ, Goldschmidt MH, Cullen JM, Rogala AR, Breitschwerdt EB. Detection of Bartonella henselae and Bartonella clarridgeiae DNA in hepatic specimens from two dogs with hepatic disease. J Am Vet Med Assoc. 2003 Jan 1;222(1):47-51, 35. PMID:12523479

Gilmore RD Jr, Bellville TM, Sviat SL, Frace M. The Bartonella vinsonii subsp. arupensis immunodominant surface antigen BrpA gene, encoding a 382-kilodalton protein composed of repetitive sequences, is a member of a multigene family conserved among bartonella species. Infect Immun. 2005 May;73(5):3128-36. PMID:15845521

Gilmore RD Jr, Carpio AM, Kosoy MY, Gage KL. Molecular characterization of the sucB gene encoding the immunogenic dihydrolipoamide succinyltransferase protein of Bartonella vinsonii subsp. berkhoffii and Bartonella quintana. Infect Immun. 2003 Aug;71(8):4818-22. PMID:12874367

Girardeau B, Boursier J, Pilette C. [Common bile duct obstruction by lymph node enlargment due to cat scratch disease].[Article in French]. Gastroenterol Clin Biol. 2005 Oct;29(10):1061-3. PMID:16435519

Glaser C, Lewis P, Wong S. Pet-, animal-, and vector-borne infections. Pediatr Rev. 2000 Jul;21(7):219-32. PMID:10878184

Glaser CA, Gilliam S, Schnurr D, Forghani B, Honarmand S, Khetsuriani N, Fischer M, Cossen CK, Anderson LJ; California Encephalitis Project, 1998-2000. In search of encephalitis etiologies: diagnostic challenges in the California Encephalitis Project, 1998-2000. Clin Infect Dis. 2003 Mar 15;36(6):731-42. Epub 2003 Mar 3. PMID:12627357

Godet C, Roblot F, Le Moal G, Roblot P, Frat JP, Becq-Giraudon B. Cat-scratch disease presenting as a breast mass. Scand J Infect Dis. 2004;36(6-7):494-5. PMID:15307578

Goldstein DA, Mouritsen L, Friedlander S, Tessler HH, Edward DP. Acute endogenous endophthalmitis due to Bartonella henselae. Clin Infect Dis. 2001 Sep 1;33(5):718-21. Epub 2001 Jul 30. PMID:11486295

Goldstein LH, Saliba WR, Elias M, Zlotnik A, Raz R, Giladi M. Bartonella quintana endocarditis in east Africa. Eur J Intern Med. 2005 Nov;16(7):518-9. PMID:16275550

Gonzalez BE, Correa AG, Kaplan SL. Cat-scratch disease occurring in three siblings simultaneously. Pediatr Infect Dis J. 2003 May;22(5):467-8. PMID:12797315

Goodman RA, Breitschwerdt EB. Clinicopathologic findings in dogs seroreactive to Bartonella henselae antigens. Am J Vet Res. 2005 Dec;66(12):2060-4. PMID:16379647

Goodrich JM, Quigley KS, Lewis JC, Astafiev AA, Slabi EV, Miquelle DG, Smirnov EN, Kerley LL, Armstrong DL, Quigley HB, Hornocker MG. Serosurvey of free-ranging Amur tigers in the Russian Far East. J Wildl Dis. 2012 Jan;48(1):186-9. PMID:22247389

Gouriet F, Fenollar F, Patrice JY, Drancourt M, Raoult D. Use of shell-vial cell culture assay for isolation of bacteria from clinical specimens: 13 years of experience. J Clin Microbiol. 2005 Oct;43(10):4993-5002. PMID:16207953

Gouriet F, Lepidi H, Habib G, Collart F, Raoult D. From cat scratch disease to endocarditis, the possible natural history of Bartonella henselae infection. BMC Infect Dis. 2007 Apr 18;7:30. PMID:17442105

Gouriet F, Samson L, Delaage M, Mainardi JL, Meconi S, Drancourt M, Raoult D. Multiplexed whole bacterial antigen microarray, a new format for the automation of serodiagnosis: the culture-negative endocarditis paradigm. Clin Microbiol Infect. 2008 Dec;14(12):1112-8. PMID:19076842

Graffin B, Genty I, Crétel E, Jean R, Drancourt M, Durand JM. [Erythema nodosum in cat scratch disease].[Article in French]. Presse Med. 2000 Jun 10;29(20):1125. PMID:10901791

Grand A, Celard M, el Belghiti R, Ghadban W, De Gevigney G, Dabboura A, Besnard C, Ouanes K, Huret JF, Fichter P. [Subacute infectious endocarditis due to the agent of cat scratch fever: Bartonella henselae].[Article in French]. Arch Mal Coeur Vaiss. 2001 Feb;94(2):157-61. PMID:11265556

Granowitz EV, Tabor KJ, Kirchhoffer JB. Potentially fatal interaction between azithromycin and disopyramide. Pacing Clin Electrophysiol. 2000 Sep;23(9):1433-5. PMID:11025903

Graveleau J, Grossi O, Lefebvre M, Redon H, Caignon JM, Pallardy A, Bodet-Milin C, Néel A, Hamidou MA. Vertebral osteomyelitis: an unusual presentation of Bartonella henselae infection. Semin Arthritis Rheum. 2011 Dec;41(3):511-6. Epub 2011 Aug 15. PMID:21840042

Gray AV, Michels KS, Lauer AK, Samples JR. Bartonella henselae infection associated with neuroretinitis, central retinal artery and vein occlusion, neovascular glaucoma, and severe vision loss. Am J Ophthalmol. 2004 Jan;137(1):187-9. PMID:14700670

Greco AJ, Baluarte JH, Meyers KE, Sellers MT, Suchi M, Biegel JA, Kaplan BS. Chromophobe renal cell carcinoma in a pediatric living-related kidney transplant recipient. Am J Kidney Dis. 2005 Jun;45(6):e105-8. PMID:15957121

Greub G, Raoult D. Bartonella: new explanations for old diseases. J Med Microbiol. 2002 Nov;51(11):915-23. PMID:12448674

Grilo N, Modi D, Barrow P. Cutaneous bacillary angiomatosis: a marker of systemic disease in HIV. S Afr Med J. 2009 Apr;99(4):220-1. PMID:19588770

Grumbkow PV, Zipp A, Seidenberg V, Fehren-Schmitz L, Kempf VA, Gross U, Hummel S. Brief communication: evidence of Bartonella quintana infections in skeletons of a historical mass grave in Kassel, Germany. Am J Phys Anthropol. 2011 Sep;146(1):134-7. PMID:21710687

Grzeszczuk A, Stańczak J, Pogorzelska J, Prokopowicz D. [Diagnostics of human granulocytic anaplasmosis].[Article in Polish]. Wiad Parazytol. 2005;51(2):109-14. PMID:16838619

Grzeszczuk A, Ziarko S, Kovalchuk O, Stańczak J. Etiology of tick-borne febrile illnesses in adult residents of North-Eastern Poland: report from a prospective clinical study. Int J Med Microbiol. 2006 May;296 Suppl 40:242-9. Epub 2006 Mar 10. PMID:16530481

Guay DR. Pet-assisted therapy in the nursing home setting: potential for zoonosis. Am J Infect Control. 2001 Jun;29(3):178-86. PMID:11391280

Guibal F, de La Salmonière P, Rybojad M, Hadjrabia S, Dehen L, Arlet G. High seroprevalence to Bartonella quintana in homeless patients with cutaneous parasitic infestations in downtown Paris. J Am Acad Dermatol. 2001 Feb;44(2):219-23. PMID:11174378

Guillén Martín S, Jensen J, Prieto Tato LM, Ramos Amador JT, García-Esteban C, García-Bermejo I, Sánchez-Pina C, Anda P. [A presentation of two female siblings with a disease caused by a cat scratch].[Article in Spanish]. An Pediatr (Barc). 2009 Jan;70(1):101-3. Epub 2008 Nov 17. PMID:19174134

Guimaraes AM, Brandão PE, Moraes W, Kiihl S, Santos LC, Filoni C, Cubas ZS, Robes RR, Marques LM, Neto RL, Yamaguti M, Oliveira RC, Catão-Dias JL, Richtzenhain LJ, Messick JB, Biondo AW, Timenetsky J. Detection of Bartonella spp. in neotropical felids and evaluation of risk factors and hematological abnormalities associated with infection. Vet Microbiol. 2010 May 19;142(3-4):346-51. Epub 2009 Oct 20. PMID:19913372

Guittet V, Ménager C, Missotte I, Duparc B, Verhaegen F, Duhamel JF. [Hepatic abscesses in childhood: retrospective study about 33 cases observed in New-Caledonia between 1985 and 2003].[Article in French]. Arch Pediatr. 2004 Sep;11(9):1046-53. PMID:15350993

Gulati A, Yalamanchili S, Golnik KC, Lee AG. Cat Scratch Neuroretinitis: The Role of Acute and Convalescent Titers for Diagnosis. J Neuroophthalmol. 2011 Sep 21. [Epub ahead of print]. PMID:21941214

Gundi VA, Billeter SA, Rood MP, Kosoy MY. Bartonella spp. in Rats and Zoonoses, Los Angeles, California, USA. Emerg Infect Dis. 2012 Apr;18(4):631-3. PMID:22469313

Gundi VA, Bourry O, Davous B, Raoult D, La Scola B. Bartonella clarridgeiae and B. henselae in dogs, Gabon. Emerg Infect Dis. 2004 Dec;10(12):2261-2. PMID:15672535

Gundi VA, Davoust B, Khamis A, Boni M, Raoult D, La Scola B. Isolation of Bartonella rattimassiliensis sp. nov. and Bartonella phoceensis sp. nov. from European Rattus norvegicus. J Clin Microbiol. 2004 Aug;42(8):3816-8. PMID:15297537

Gundi VA, Kosoy MY, Myint KS, Shrestha SK, Shrestha MP, Pavlin JA, Gibbons RV. Prevalence and genetic diversity of bartonella species detected in different tissues of small mammals in Nepal. Appl Environ Microbiol. 2010 Dec;76(24):8247-54. Epub 2010 Oct 29. PMID:21037303

Gundi VA, Taylor C, Raoult D, La Scola B. Bartonella rattaustraliani sp. nov., Bartonella queenslandensis sp. nov. and Bartonella coopersplainsensis sp. nov., identified in Australian rats. Int J Syst Evol Microbiol. 2009 Dec;59(Pt 12):2956-61. Epub 2009 Jul 23. PMID:19628592

Gunson TH, Oliver GF. Osler's nodes and Janeway lesions. Australas J Dermatol. 2007 Nov;48(4):251-5. PMID:17956487

Gupta D, Green J, Franco-Paredes C, Lerakis S. Challenges in the clinical management of blood-culture negative endocarditis: case of Bartonella henselae infection. Am J Med. 2011 Mar;124(3):e1-2. PMID:21396492

Gupta PK, Patel R, Bhatti MT. Neuroretinitis secondary to concurrent infection with cat scratch disease and lyme disease. Eye (Lond). 2009 Jul;23(7):1607. Epub 2008 Sep 12. PMID:18791545

Guptill L, Wu CC, Glickman L, Turek J, Slater L, HogenEsch H. Extracellular Bartonella henselae and artifactual intraerythrocytic pseudoinclusions in experimentally infected cats. Vet Microbiol. 2000 Oct 1;76(3):283-90. PMID:10973702

Guptill L, Wu CC, HogenEsch H, Slater LN, Glickman N, Dunham A, Syme H, Glickman L. Prevalence, risk factors, and genetic diversity of Bartonella henselae infections in pet cats in four regions of the United States. J Clin Microbiol. 2004 Feb;42(2):652-9. PMID:14766832

Guptill L. Bartonellosis. Vet Clin North Am Small Anim Pract. 2003 Jul;33(4):809-25. PMID:12910745

Guptill L. Bartonellosis. Vet Microbiol. 2010 Jan 27;140(3-4):347-59. Epub 2009 Nov 18. PMID:20018462

Guptill L. Feline bartonellosis. Vet Clin North Am Small Anim Pract. 2010 Nov;40(6):1073-90. PMID:20933137

Guranowski A. Specific and nonspecific enzymes involved in the catabolism of mononucleoside and dinucleoside polyphosphates. Pharmacol Ther. 2000 Aug-Sep;87(2-3):117-39. PMID:11007995

Gurfield AN, Boulouis HJ, Chomel BB, Kasten RW, Heller R, Bouillin C, Gandoin C, Thibault D, Chang CC, Barrat F, Piemont Y. Epidemiology of Bartonella infection in domestic cats in France. Vet Microbiol. 2001 May 21;80(2):185-98. PMID:11295338

Guzel M, Celebi B, Yalcin E, Koenhemsi L, Mamak N, Pasa S, Aslan O. A serological investigation of Bartonella henselae infection in cats in Turkey. J Vet Med Sci. 2011 Nov;73(11):1513-6. Epub 2011 Jul 7. PMID:21737965

Gyémánt N, Molnár A, Spengler G, Mándi Y, Szabó M, Molnár J. Bacterial models for tumor development. Mini-Acta Microbiol Immunol Hung. 2004;51(3):321-32. PMID:15571072

H Fischer A, van der Loo B, M Shär G, Zbinden R, Duru F, Brunckhorst C, Rousson V, Delacrétaz Y E, Stuber T, Oechslin EN, Follath F, Jenni R. Serological evidence for the association of Bartonella henselae infection with arrhythmogenic right ventricular cardiomyopathy. Clin Cardiol. 2008 Oct;31(10):469-71. PMID:18666174

Haberl R, Wenisch C. Case 33-2002: a 28-year-old woman with ocular inflammation, fever, and headache. N Engl J Med. 2003 Jan 30;348(5):474-6; author reply 474-6. PMID:12556554

Habot-Wilner Z, Zur D, Goldstein M, Goldenberg D, Shulman S, Kesler A, Giladi M, Neudorfer M. Macular findings on optical coherence tomography in cat-scratch disease neuroretinitis. Eye (Lond). 2011 Aug;25(8):1064-8. Epub 2011 Jun 10. PMID:21660065

Hackett TB, Jensen WA, Lehman TL, Hohenhaus AE, Crawford PC, Giger U, Lappin MR. Prevalence of DNA of Mycoplasma haemofelis, 'Candidatus Mycoplasma haemominutum,' Anaplasma phagocytophilum, and species of Bartonella, Neorickettsia, and Ehrlichia in cats used as blood donors in the United States. J Am Vet Med Assoc. 2006 Sep 1;229(5):700-5. PMID:16948578

Hagen K. [Risk of infections among orienteers].[Article in Norwegian]. Tidsskr Nor Laegeforen. 2009 Jun 25;129(13):1326-8. PMID:19561657

Hajjaji N, Hocqueloux L, Kerdraon R, Bret L. Bone infection in cat-scratch disease: a review of the literature. J Infect. 2007 May;54(5):417-21. Epub 2006 Nov 29. PMID:17140668

Hajj-Chahine J, Houmaida H, Plouzeau C, Tomasi J, Corbi P. Bartonella as a cause of mechanical prosthetic aortic root endocarditis. Ann Thorac Surg. 2012 Apr;93(4):e93-5. PMID:22450112

Halos L, Jamal T, Maillard R, Beugnet F, Le Menach A, Boulouis HJ, Vayssier-Taussat M. Evidence of Bartonella sp. in questing adult and nymphal Ixodes ricinus ticks from France and co-infection with Borrelia burgdorferi sensu lato and Babesia sp. Vet Res. 2005 Jan-Feb;36(1):79-87. PMID:15610725

Halos L, Jamal T, Maillard R, Girard B, Guillot J, Chomel B, Vayssier-Taussat M, Boulouis HJ. Role of Hippoboscidae flies as potential vectors of Bartonella spp. infecting wild and domestic ruminants. Appl Environ Microbiol. 2004 Oct;70(10):6302-5. PMID:15466580

Halperin JJ, Wormser GP. Of fleas and ticks on cats and mice... Arch Neurol. 2001 Sep;58(9):1345-7. PMID:11559304

Hambuch TM, Handley SA, Ellis B, Chamberlin J, Romero S, Regnery R. Population genetic analysis of Bartonella bacilliformis isolates from areas of peru where Carrion's disease is endemic and epidemic. J Clin Microbiol. 2004 Aug;42(8):3675-80. PMID:15297516

Hamel D, Silaghi C, Knaus M, Visser M, Kusi I, Rapti D, Rehbein S, Pfister K. Detection of Babesia canis subspecies and other arthropod-borne diseases in dogs from Tirana, Albania. Wien Klin Wochenschr. 2009 Oct;121 Suppl 3:42-5. PMID:19915816

Handley SA, Regnery RL. Differentiation of pathogenic Bartonella species by infrequent restriction site PCR. J Clin Microbiol. 2000 Aug;38(8):3010-5. PMID:10921969

Hansmann Y, DeMartino S, Piémont Y, Meyer N, Mariet P, Heller R, Christmann D, Jaulhac B. Diagnosis of cat scratch disease with detection of Bartonella henselae by PCR: a study of patients with lymph node enlargement. J Clin Microbiol. 2005 Aug;43(8):3800-6. PMID:16081914

Hara H, Ito K, Akimoto M, Suzuki H, Asai S, Maruyama S. Detection of Bartonella henselae DNA using polymerase chain reaction assay in patient with cat scratch disease. Acta Derm Venereol. 2003;83(1):67-8. PMID:12636034

Harada T. [Newly emerging infections: Catscratch disease].[Article in Japanese]. Nihon Jibiinkoka Gakkai Kaiho. 2004 Nov;107(11):1016-9. PMID:15700401

Harms A, Dehio C. Intruders below the radar: molecular pathogenesis of Bartonella spp. Clin Microbiol Rev. 2012 Jan;25(1):42-78. PMID:22232371

Harms CA, Maggi RG, Breitschwerdt EB, Clemons-Chevis CL, Solangi M, Rotstein DS, Fair PA, Hansen LJ, Hohn AA, Lovewell GN, McLellan WA, Pabst DA, Rowles TK, Schwacke LH, Townsend FI, Wells RS. Bartonella species detection in captive, stranded and free-ranging cetaceans. Vet Res. 2008 Nov-Dec;39(6):59. Epub 2008 Aug 23. PMID:18721502

Harrison A, Bown KJ, Montgomery WI, Birtles RJ. Ixodes ricinus Is Not an Epidemiologically Relevant Vector of Bartonella Species in the Wood Mouse (Apodemus sylvaticus). Vector Borne Zoonotic Dis. 2012 Jan 4. [Epub ahead of print]. PMID:22217173

Harrus S, Bar-Gal GK, Golan A, Elazari-Volcani R, Kosoy MY, Morick D, Avidor B, Baneth G. Isolation and genetic characterization of a Bartonella strain closely related to Bartonella tribocorum and Bartonella elizabethae in Israeli commensal rats. Am J Trop Med Hyg. 2009 Jul;81(1):55-8. PMID:19556567

Harrus S, Perlman-Avrahami A, Mumcuoglu KY, Morick D, Eyal O, Baneth G. Molecular detection of Ehrlichia canis, Anaplasma bovis, Anaplasma platys, Candidatus Midichloria mitochondrii and Babesia canis vogeli in ticks from Israel. Clin Microbiol Infect. 2011 Mar;17(3):459-63. PMID:20636417

Harsch IA, Schahin SP, Schmelzer A, Hahn EG, Konturek PC. Cat-scratch disease in an immunocompromised host. Med Sci Monit. 2002 Mar;8(3):CS26-9. PMID:11887039

Hartung JS, Shao J, Kuykendall LD. Comparison of the 'Ca. Liberibacter asiaticus' genome adapted for an intracellular lifestyle with other members of the Rhizobiales. PLoS One. 2011;6(8):e23289. Epub 2011 Aug 18. PMID:21876745

Hawkins EC, Johnson LR, Guptill L, Marr HS, Breitschwerdt EB, Birkenheuer AJ. Failure to identify an association between serologic or molecular evidence of Bartonella infection and idiopathic rhinitis in dogs. J Am Vet Med Assoc. 2008 Aug 15;233(4):597-9. PMID:18710315

Hemsworth S, Pizer B. Pet ownership in immunocompromised children--a review of the literature and survey of existing guidelines. Eur J Oncol Nurs. 2006 Apr;10(2):117-27. Epub 2006 Apr 3. PMID:16581294

Hendrix LR, Kiss K. Studies on the identification of deforming factor from Bartonella bacilliformis. Ann N Y Acad Sci. 2003 Jun;990:596-604. PMID:12860696

Hendrix LR. Contact-dependent hemolytic activity distinct from deforming activity of Bartonella bacilliformis. FEMS Microbiol Lett. 2000 Jan 1;182(1):119-24. PMID:10612742

Henn JB, Chomel BB, Boulouis HJ, Kasten RW, Murray WJ, Bar-Gal GK, King R, Courreau JF, Baneth G. Bartonella rochalimae in raccoons, coyotes, and red foxes. Emerg Infect Dis. 2009 Dec;15(12):1984-7. PMID:19961681

Henn JB, Gabriel MW, Kasten RW, Brown RN, Koehler JE, MacDonald KA, Kittleson MD, Thomas WP, Chomel BB. Infective endocarditis in a dog and the phylogenetic relationship of the associated "Bartonella rochalimae" strain with isolates from dogs, gray foxes, and a human. J Clin Microbiol. 2009 Mar;47(3):787-90. Epub 2008 Dec 24. PMID:19109472

Henn JB, Gabriel MW, Kasten RW, Brown RN, Theis JH, Foley JE, Chomel BB. Gray foxes (Urocyon cinereoargenteus) as a potential reservoir of a Bartonella clarridgeiae-like bacterium and domestic dogs as part of a sentinel system for surveillance of zoonotic arthropod-borne pathogens in northern California. J Clin Microbiol. 2007 Aug;45(8):2411-8. Epub 2007 Jun 6. PMID:17553970

Henn JB, Liu CH, Kasten RW, VanHorn BA, Beckett LA, Kass PH, Chomel BB. Seroprevalence of antibodies against Bartonella species and evaluation of risk factors and clinical signs associated with seropositivity in dogs. Am J Vet Res. 2005 Apr;66(4):688-94. PMID:15900951

Henn JB, Vanhorn BA, Kasten RW, Kachani M, Chomel BB. Antibodies to Bartonella vinsonii subsp. Berkhoffii in Moroccan dogs. Am J Trop Med Hyg. 2006 Feb;74(2):222-3. PMID:16474074

Henríquez C, Hinojosa JC, Ventosilla P, Infante B, Merello J, Mallqui V, Verastegui M, Maguiña C. Report of an unusual case of persistent bacteremia by Bartonella bacilliformis in a splenectomized patient. Am J Trop Med Hyg. 2004 Jul;71(1):53-5. PMID:15238689

Hercík K, Hásová V, Janecek J, Branny P. Molecular evidence of Bartonella DNA in ixodid ticks in Czechia. Folia Microbiol (Praha). 2007;52(5):503-9. PMID:18298048

Hercík K, Melter O, Janecek J, Branny P. In situ detection of Bartonella henselae cells. Mol Cell Probes. 2002 Feb;16(1):49-56. PMID:12005447

Hermans SM, Schouten WE, Faber TE, Hoepelman IM, Andriesse GI. [Subcutaneous nodules with malignant presentation, but caused by infection].[Article in Dutch]. Ned Tijdschr Geneeskd. 2004 Aug 14;148(33):1636-41. PMID:15455512

Hernandez-Da-Mota S, Escalante-Razo F. Bartonellosis causing bilateral Leber neuroretinitis: a case report. Eur J Ophthalmol. 2009 Mar-Apr;19(2):307-9. PMID:19253255

Herremans M, Bakker J, Vermeulen MJ, Schellekens JF, Koopmans MP. Evaluation of an in-house cat scratch disease IgM ELISA to detect Bartonella henselae in a routine laboratory setting. Eur J Clin Microbiol Infect Dis. 2009 Feb;28(2):147-52. Epub 2008 Aug 5. PMID:18679728

Herremans M, Vermeulen MJ, Van de Kassteele J, Bakker J, Schellekens JF, Koopmans MP. The use of Bartonella henselae-specific age dependent IgG and IgM in diagnostic models to discriminate diseased from non-diseased in Cat Scratch Disease serology. J Microbiol Methods. 2007 Nov;71(2):107-13. Epub 2007 Sep 15. PMID:17916395

Herz AM, Lahey JM. Images in clinical medicine. Optic neuritis due to Bartonella henselae infection. N Engl J Med. 2004 Jan 8;350(2):e1. PMID:14711929

Heye S, Matthijs P, Wallon J, van Campenhoudt M. Cat-scratch disease osteomyelitis. Skeletal Radiol. 2003 Jan;32(1):49-51. Epub 2002 Oct 23. PMID:12525945

Higgins R. Emerging or re-emerging bacterial zoonotic diseases: bartonellosis, leptospirosis, Lyme borreliosis, plague. Rev Sci Tech. 2004 Aug;23(2):569-81. PMID:15702720

Hinrichsen VL, Whitworth UG, Breitschwerdt EB, Hegarty BC, Mather TN. Assessing the association between the geographic distribution of deer ticks and seropositivity rates to various tick-transmitted disease organisms in dogs. J Am Vet Med Assoc. 2001 Apr 1;218(7):1092-7. PMID:11318358

Hipp SJ, O'Shields A, Fordham LA, Blatt J, Hamrick HJ, Henderson FW. Multifocal bone marrow involvement in cat-scratch disease. Pediatr Infect Dis J. 2005 May;24(5):472-4. PMID:15876956

Hippenstiel S, Suttorp N. Interaction of pathogens with the endothelium. Thromb Haemost. 2003 Jan;89(1):18-24. PMID:12540949

Hjelle JT, Miller-Hjelle MA, Poxton IR, Kajander EO, Ciftcioglu N, Jones ML, Caughey RC, Brown R, Millikin PD, Darras FS. Endotoxin and nanobacteria in polycystic kidney disease. Kidney Int. 2000 Jun;57(6):2360-74. PMID:10844606

Hjelm E, McGill S, Blomqvist G. Prevalence of antibodies to Bartonella henselae, B. elizabethae and B. quintana in Swedish domestic cats. Scand J Infect Dis. 2002;34(3):192-6. PMID:12030392

Hmaimess G, Kadhim H, Saint Martin C, Abu Serieh B, Mousny M, Sébire G. Cat scratch disease presenting as meningomyeloradiculopathy. Arch Dis Child. 2004 Jul;89(7):691-2. PMID:15210515

Hoar BR, Chomel BB, Rolfe DL, Chang CC, Fritz CL, Sacks BN, Carpenter TE. Spatial analysis of Yersinia pestis and Bartonella vinsonii subsp. berkhoffii seroprevalence in California coyotes (Canis latrans). Prev Vet Med. 2003 Jan 15;56(4):299-311. PMID:12507856

Hoey JG, Valois-Cruz F, Goldenberg H, Voskoboynik Y, Pfiffner J, Tilton RC, Mordechai E, Adelson ME. Development of an immunoglobulin M capture-based enzyme-linked immunosorbent assay for diagnosis of acute infections with Bartonella henselae. Clin Vaccine Immunol. 2009 Feb;16(2):282-4. Epub 2008 Dec 3. PMID:19052161

Hoffman CF, Papadopoulos D, Palmer DM, Austin C, Gropper CA. A case report of bacillary angiomatosis in a patient infected with human immunodeficiency virus. Cutis. 2002 Mar;69(3):175-8. PMID:11926335

Hoffman RM, AboulHosn J, Child JS, Pegues DA. Bartonella endocarditis in complex congenital heart disease. Congenit Heart Dis. 2007 Jan-Feb;2(1):79-84. PMID:18377522

Holden K, Boothby JT, Kasten RW, Chomel BB. Co-detection of Bartonella henselae, Borrelia burgdorferi, and Anaplasma phagocytophilum in Ixodes pacificus ticks from California, USA. Vector Borne Zoonotic Dis. 2006 Spring;6(1):99-102. PMID:16584332

Holmberg M, Mills JN, McGill S, Benjamin G, Ellis BA. Bartonella infection in sylvatic small mammals of central Sweden. Epidemiol Infect. 2003 Feb;130(1):149-57. PMID:12613756

Holmes NE, Opat S, Kelman A, Korman TM. Refractory Bartonella quintana bacillary angiomatosis following chemotherapy for chronic lymphocytic leukaemia. J Med Microbiol. 2011 Jan;60(Pt 1):142-6. Epub 2010 Oct 14. PMID:20947664

Honadel TE, Chomel BB, Yamamoto K, Chang C, Farver TB. Seroepidemiology of Bartonella vinsonii subsp berkhoffii exposure among healthy dogs. J Am Vet Med Assoc. 2001 Aug 15;219(4):480-4. PMID:11518174

Hopp L, Eppes SC. Development of IgA nephritis following cat scratch disease in a 13-year-old boy. Pediatr Nephrol. 2004 Jun;19(6):682-4. Epub 2004 Mar 11. PMID:15015065

Houhamdi L, Parola P, Raoult D. [Lice and lice-borne diseases in humans].[Article in French]. Med Trop (Mars). 2005;65(1):13-23. PMID:15903070

Houhamdi L, Raoult D. Experimental infection of human body lice with Acinetobacter baumannii. Am J Trop Med Hyg. 2006 Apr;74(4):526-31. PMID:16606978

Houpikian P, Fournier PE, Raoult D. Phylogenetic position of Bartonella vinsonii subsp. arupensis based on 16S rDNA and gltA gene sequences. Int J Syst Evol Microbiol. 2001 Jan;51(Pt 1):179-82. PMID:11211257

Houpikian P, Raoult D. 16S/23S rRNA intergenic spacer regions for phylogenetic analysis, identification, and subtyping of Bartonella species. J Clin Microbiol. 2001 Aug;39(8):2768-78. PMID:11473990

Houpikian P, Raoult D. Blood culture-negative endocarditis in a reference center: etiologic diagnosis of 348 cases. Medicine (Baltimore). 2005 May;84(3):162-73. PMID:15879906

Houpikian P, Raoult D. Diagnostic methods current best practices and guidelines for identification of difficult-to-culture pathogens in infective endocarditis. Infect Dis Clin North Am. 2002 Jun;16(2):377-92, x. PMID:12092478

Houpikian P, Raoult D. Diagnostic methods. Current best practices and guidelines for identification of difficult-to-culture pathogens in infective endocarditis. Cardiol Clin. 2003 May;21(2):207-17. PMID:12874894

Houpikian P, Raoult D. Molecular phylogeny of the genus Bartonella: what is the current knowledge? FEMS Microbiol Lett. 2001 Jun 12;200(1):1-7. PMID:11410341

Houpikian P, Raoult D. Western immunoblotting for Bartonella endocarditis. Clin Diagn Lab Immunol. 2003 Jan;10(1):95-102. PMID:12522046

Houston G. Oral pathology. Case of the quarter. J Okla Dent Assoc. 2000 Autumn;91(2):24-7. PMID:11314170

Hsieh JW, Tung KC, Chen WC, Lin JW, Chien LJ, Hsu YM, Wang HC, Chomel BB, Chang CC. Epidemiology of Bartonella infection in rodents and shrews in Taiwan. Zoonoses Public Health. 2010 Sep;57(6):439-46. PMID:19538457

Hu V, Dong B, MacFarlane A. Visual loss after cat scratch. J R Soc Med. 2005 Jan;98(1):28-9. PMID:15632237

Huang J, Dai L, Lei S, Liao DY, Wang XQ, Luo TY, Chen Y, Hang ZB, Li GD, Dong DD, Xu G, Gu ZC, Hao JL, Hua P, He L, Duan FL. [Application of Warthin-Starry stain, immunohistochemistry and transmission electron microscopy in diagnosis of cat scratch disease].[Article in Chinese]. Zhonghua Bing Li Xue Za Zhi. 2010 Apr;39(4):225-9. PMID:20654119

Huang R, Liu Q, Li G, Li D, Song X, Birtles RJ, Zhao F. Bartonella quintana infections in captive monkeys, China. Emerg Infect Dis. 2011 Sep;17(9):1707-9. PMID:21888799

Huarcaya E, Best I, Rodriguez-Tafur J, Maguiña C, Solórzano N, Menacho J, Lopez De Guimaraes D, Chauca J, Ventosilla P. Cytokines and T-Lymphocute count in patients in the acute and chronic phases of Bartonella bacilliformis infection in an endemic area in peru: a pilot study. Rev Inst Med Trop Sao Paulo. 2011 May-Jun;53(3):149-54. PMID:21755237

Huarcaya E, Maguina C, Best I, Solorzano N, Leeman L. Immunological response in cases of complicated and uncomplicated bartonellosis during pregnancy. Rev Inst Med Trop Sao Paulo. 2007 Sep-Oct;49(5):335-7. PMID:18026643

Huarcaya E, Maguiña C, Merello J, Cok J, Birtles R, Infante B, Vidal J, Tello A, Ventosilla P. A prospective study of Cat-Scratch Disease in Lima-Peru. Rev Inst Med Trop Sao Paulo. 2002 Nov-Dec;44(6):325-30. PMID:12532216

Huarcaya E, Maguiña C, Torres R, Rupay J, Fuentes L. Bartonelosis (Carrion's Disease) in the pediatric population of Peru: an overview and update. Braz J Infect Dis. 2004 Oct;8(5):331-9. Epub 2005 Mar 17. PMID:15798808

Hubert J, Kopecký J, Perotti MA, Nesvorná M, Braig HR, Ságová-Marečková M, Macovei L, Zurek L. Detection and Identification of Species-Specific Bacteria Associated with Synanthropic Mites. Microb Ecol. 2011 Nov 5. [Epub ahead of print]. PMID:22057398

Hulinska D, Votypka J, Plch J, Vlcek E, Valesová M, Bojar M, Hulinsky V, Smetana K. Molecular and microscopical evidence of Ehrlichia spp. and Borrelia burgdorferi sensu lato in patients, animals and ticks in the Czech Republic. New Microbiol. 2002 Oct;25(4):437-48. PMID:12437223

Husain S, Singh N. Pyomyositis associated with bacillary angiomatosis in a patient with HIV infection. Infection. 2002 Jan;30(1):50-3. PMID:11876519

Hussain S, Rathore MH. Cat scratch disease with epidural extension while on antimicrobial treatment. Pediatr Neurosurg. 2007;43(2):164-6. PMID:17337934

Hutton TA, Goldstein RE, Njaa BL, Atwater DZ, Chang YF, Simpson KW. Search for Borrelia burgdorferi in kidneys of dogs with suspected "Lyme nephritis". J Vet Intern Med. 2008 Jul-Aug;22(4):860-5. PMID:18564223

Ide F, Tanaka A, Kusama K. Two unusual vascular lesions: epithelioid angiomatous nodule and spindle cell hemangiomatosis. J Oral Pathol Med. 2008 Apr;37(4):252-4. Epub 2008 Jan 15. PMID:18205744

Idrees J, Albacker TB, Gordon SM, Shin J, Menon V, Roselli EE. Bartonella infective endocarditis of a prosthetic aortic valve with a subvalvular abscess. J Card Surg. 2011 Sep;26(5):483-5. Epub 2011 Aug 17. PMID:21848606

Ignatovich VF, Lukin EP, Umnova NS, Penkina GA, Vorob'ev AA. [Seroimmunologic monitoring of microorganisms of Rickettsia and Bartonella species microorganisms in the Moscow region].[Article in Russian]. Zh Mikrobiol Epidemiol Immunobiol. 2001 Jan-Feb;(1):14-7. PMID:11236493

Il'ina TS, Bashkirov VN. [Interaction of bacteria of the genus Bartonella with the host: inhibition of apoptosis, induction of proliferation, and formation of tumors].[Article in Russian]. Mol Gen Mikrobiol Virusol. 2008;(3):3-11. PMID:18763333

Il'ina TS, Irkhin AI. [Bacteria of Bartonella genus: characteristics, pathogenicity factors and methods of molecular-genetic investigation]. [Article in Russian]. Mol Gen Mikrobiol Virusol. 2004;(2):3-10. PMID:15164714

Imperiale A, Blondet C, Ben-Sellem D, Forestier E, Mohseni M, Piemont Y, Ojeda M, Christmann D, Constantinesco A, Hansmann Y. Unusual abdominal localization of cat scratch disease mimicking malignancy on F-18 FDG PET/CT examination. Clin Nucl Med. 2008 Sep;33(9):621-3. PMID:18716512

Incandela S, Raoult D, Vitale G, Micalizzi A, Mansueto P. Hepatosplenic cat-scratch fever with seropositivity for Bartonella quintana? Lancet Infect Dis. 2008 Nov;8(11):663. PMID:18992392

Infante B, Villar S, Palma S, Merello J, Valencia R, Torres L, Cok J, Ventosilla P, Manguiña C, Guerra H, Henriquez C. BALB/c Mice resist infection with Bartonella bacilliformis. BMC Res Notes. 2008 Oct 28;1:103. PMID:18957122

Inoue K, Kabeya H, Hagiya K, Kosoy MY, Une Y, Yoshikawa Y, Maruyama S. Multi-locus sequence analysis reveals host specific association between Bartonella washoensis and squirrels. Vet Microbiol. 2011 Feb 24;148(1):60-5. Epub 2010 Aug 22. PMID:20884133

Inoue K, Kabeya H, Kosoy MY, Bai Y, Smirnov G, McColl D, Artsob H, Maruyama S. Evolutional and geographical relationships of Bartonella grahamii isolates from wild rodents by multi-locus sequencing analysis. Microb Ecol. 2009 Apr;57(3):534-41. Epub 2009 Feb 14. PMID:19219487

Inoue K, Kabeya H, Shiratori H, Ueda K, Kosoy MY, Chomel BB, Boulouis HJ, Maruyama S. Bartonella japonica sp. nov. and Bartonella silvatica sp. nov., isolated from Apodemus mice. Int J Syst Evol Microbiol. 2010 Apr;60(Pt 4):759-63. Epub 2009 Aug 5. PMID:19656930

Inoue K, Maruyama S, Kabeya H, Hagiya K, Izumi Y, Une Y, Yoshikawa Y. Exotic small mammals as potential reservoirs of zoonotic Bartonella spp. Emerg Infect Dis. 2009 Apr;15(4):526-32. PMID:19331727

Inoue K, Maruyama S, Kabeya H, Kawanami K, Yanai K, Jitchum S, Jittaparapong S. Prevalence of Bartonella infection in cats and dogs in a metropolitan area, Thailand. Epidemiol Infect. 2009 Nov;137(11):1568-73. Epub 2009 Apr 20. PMID:19379541

Inoue K, Maruyama S, Kabeya H, Yamada N, Ohashi N, Sato Y, Yukawa M, Masuzawa T, Kawamori F, Kadosaka T, Takada N, Fujita H, Kawabata H. Prevalence and genetic diversity of Bartonella species isolated from wild rodents in Japan. Appl Environ Microbiol. 2008 Aug;74(16):5086-92. Epub 2008 Jul 7. PMID:18606803

Iralu J, Bai Y, Crook L, Tempest B, Simpson G, Mckenzie T, Koster F. Rodent-associated Bartonella febrile illness, Southwestern United States. Emerg Infect Dis. 2006 Jul;12(7):1081-6. PMID:16836824

Iredell J, Blanckenberg D, Arvand M, Grauling S, Feil EJ, Birtles RJ. Characterization of the natural population of Bartonella henselae by multilocus sequence typing. J Clin Microbiol. 2003 Nov;41(11):5071-9. PMID:14605141

Iredell J, McHattan J, Kyme P, Dillon B, Blanckenberg D. Antigenic and genotypic relationships between Bartonella henselae strains. J Clin Microbiol. 2002 Nov;40(11):4397-8. PMID:12409443

Irshad FA, Gordon RA. Bartonella henselae neuroretinitis in a 15-year-old girl with chronic myelogenous leukemia. J AAPOS. 2009 Dec;13(6):602-4. PMID:20006827

Ishak AM, Radecki S, Lappin MR. Prevalence of Mycoplasma haemofelis, 'Candidatus Mycoplasma haemominutum', Bartonella species, Ehrlichia species, and Anaplasma phagocytophilum DNA in the blood of cats with anemia. J Feline Med Surg. 2007 Feb;9(1):1-7. Epub 2006 Jul 17. PMID:16846745

Ishida C, Tsuneoka H, Iino H, Murakami K, Inokuma H, Ohnishi T, Tsukahara M. [Bartonella henselae infection in domestic cat and dog fleas].[Article in Japanese]. Kansenshogaku Zasshi. 2001 Feb;75(2):133-6. PMID:11260879

Ishikawa T, Suzuki T, Shinoda M, Takashi H, Yamaguchi H, Suzuki T, Miyake N, Kamiya T. [A case of hepatosplenic cat scratch disease]. [Article in Japanese]. Nihon Shokakibyo Gakkai Zasshi. 2006 Sep;103(9):1050-4. PMID:16953102

Ives TJ, Marston EL, Regnery RL, Butts JD, Majerus TC. In vitro susceptibilities of Rickettsia and Bartonella spp. to 14-hydroxy-clarithromycin as determined by immunofluorescent antibody analysis of infected vero cell monolayers. J Antimicrob Chemother. 2000 Mar;45(3):305-10. PMID:10702548

Ives TJ, Marston EL, Regnery RL, Butts JD. In vitro susceptibilities of Bartonella and Rickettsia spp. to fluoroquinolone antibiotics as determined by immunofluorescent antibody analysis of infected Vero cell monolayers. Int J Antimicrob Agents. 2001 Sep;18(3):217-22. PMID:11673033

Izri A, Depaquit J, Parola P. [Phlebotomine sandflies and transmission of disease agents around the Mediterranean basin].[Article in French]. Med Trop (Mars). 2006 Oct;66(5):429-35. PMID:17201284

Izzedine H, Launay-Vacher V, Mercadal L, Vernant JP, Deray G. Doxycycline, gastrointestinal bleeding, and thrombotic microangiopathy. Am J Hematol. 2004 Nov;77(3):319. PMID:15495239

Jäckel MC, Glock T, Künster A. [Parinaud's oculoglandular syndrome. A rare differential diagnosis of "red eye"].[Article in German]. HNO. 2006 Jan;54(1):37-40. PMID:15702352

Jacobs DJ, Scott ML, Slusher MM. Localised retinal vasculitis in cat scratch disease. BMJ Case Rep. 2009;2009. pii: bcr09.2008.0904. Epub 2009 Mar 17. PMID:21686569

Jacomo V, Kelly PJ, Raoult D. Natural history of Bartonella infections (an exception to Koch's postulate). Clin Diagn Lab Immunol. 2002 Jan;9(1):8-18. PMID:11777823

James EA, Hill J, Uppal R, Prentice MB. Bartonella infection: a significant cause of native valve endocarditis necessitating surgical management. J Thorac Cardiovasc Surg. 2000 Jan;119(1):171-2. PMID:10612779

Jardine C, Appleyard G, Kosoy MY, McColl D, Chirino-Trejo M, Wobeser G, Leighton FA. Rodent-associated Bartonella in Saskatchewan, Canada. Vector Borne Zoonotic Dis. 2005 Winter;5(4):402-9. PMID:16417436

Jardine C, McColl D, Wobeser G, Leighton FA. Diversity of Bartonella genotypes in Richardson's ground squirrel populations. Vector Borne Zoonotic Dis. 2006 Winter;6(4):395-403. PMID:17187575

Jardine C, Waldner C, Wobeser G, Leighton FA. Demographic features of Bartonella infections in Richardson's ground squirrels (Spermophilus richardsonii). J Wildl Dis. 2006 Oct;42(4):739-49. PMID:17255440

Jardine C, Waldner C, Wobeser G, Leighton FA. Effect of experimental ectoparasite control on bartonella infections in wild Richardson's ground squirrels. J Wildl Dis. 2006 Oct;42(4):750-8. PMID:17255441

Jeanclaude D, Godmer P, Leveiller D, Pouedras P, Fournier PE, Raoult D, Rolain JM. Bartonella alsatica endocarditis in a French patient in close contact with rabbits. Clin Microbiol Infect. 2009 Dec;15 Suppl 2:110-1. Epub 2009 Apr 30. PMID:19438633

Jenkins NE, Ferguson DJ, Alp NJ, Harrison TG, Bowler IC. Urban trench fever presenting as culture-negative endocarditis. QJM. 2009 Jan;102(1):63-5. Epub 2008 Oct 3. PMID:18835881

Jensen WA, Fall MZ, Rooney J, Kordick DL, Breitschwerdt EB. Rapid identification and differentiation of Bartonella species using a single-step PCR assay. J Clin Microbiol. 2000 May;38(5):1717-22. PMID:10790087

Jensenius M, Davis X, von Sonnenburg F, Schwartz E, Keystone JS, Leder K, Lopéz-Véléz R, Caumes E, Cramer JP, Chen L, Parola P; GeoSentinel Surveillance Network. Multicenter GeoSentinel analysis of rickettsial diseases in international travelers, 1996-2008. Emerg Infect Dis. 2009 Nov;15(11):1791-8. PMID:19891867

Jeong W, Seiter K, Strauchen J, Rafael T, Lau HC, Breakstone B, Ahmed T, Liu D. PET scan-positive cat scratch disease in a patient with T cell lymphoblastic lymphoma. Leuk Res. 2005 May;29(5):591-4. PMID:15755513

Jeyaprakash A, Hoy MA, Allsopp MH. Bacterial diversity in worker adults of Apis mellifera capensis and Apis mellifera scutellata (Insecta: Hymenoptera) assessed using 16S rRNA sequences. J Invertebr Pathol. 2003 Oct;84(2):96-103. PMID:14615218

Jiang G, Guo M, Wen Z. [Cat-scratch disease].[Article in Chinese]. Lin Chuang Er Bi Yan Hou Ke Za Zhi. 2005 Sep;19(18):820-2. PMID:16375109

Jiang J, Temenak JJ, Richards AL. Real-time PCR duplex assay for Rickettsia prowazekii and Borrelia recurrentis. Ann N Y Acad Sci. 2003 Jun;990:302-10. PMID:12860643

Johnson G, Ayers M, McClure SC, Richardson SE, Tellier R. Detection and identification of Bartonella species pathogenic for humans by PCR amplification targeting the riboflavin synthase gene (ribC). J Clin Microbiol. 2003 Mar;41(3):1069-72. PMID:12624031

Johnson R, Ramos-Vara J, Vemulapalli R. Identification of Bartonella henselae in an aborted equine fetus. Vet Pathol. 2009 Mar;46(2):277-81. PMID:19261640

Johnston AW, Todd JD, Curson AR, Lei S, Nikolaidou-Katsaridou N, Gelfand MS, Rodionov DA. Living without Fur: the subtlety and complexity of iron-responsive gene regulation in the symbiotic bacterium Rhizobium and other alpha-proteobacteria. Biometals. 2007 Jun;20(3-4):501-11. Epub 2007 Feb 20. PMID:17310401

Jöhrens K, Anagnostopoulos I, Dürkop H, Stein H. Different T-bet expression patterns characterize particular reactive lymphoid tissue lesions. Histopathology. 2006 Mar;48(4):343-52. PMID:16487356

Jones RT, McCormick KF, Martin AP. Bacterial communities of Bartonella-positive fleas: diversity and community assembly patterns. Appl Environ Microbiol. 2008 Mar;74(5):1667-70. Epub 2008 Jan 18. PMID:18203862

Jones SL, Maggi R, Shuler J, Alward A, Breitschwerdt EB. Detection of Bartonella henselae in the blood of 2 adult horses. J Vet Intern Med. 2008 Mar-Apr;22(2):495-8. Epub 2008 Mar 10. PMID:18346149

Jovanović J, Lalosević V. [Treatment of bite wounds and cat-scratch disease].[Article in Croatian]. Med Pregl. 2001;54 Suppl 1:39-42. PMID:12078126

Juncker-Voss M, Prosl H, Lussy H, Enzenberg U, Auer H, Lassnig H, Müller M, Nowotny N. [Screening for antibodies against zoonotic agents among employees of the Zoological Garden of Vienna, Schönbrunn, Austria].[Article in German]. Berl Munch Tierarztl Wochenschr. 2004 Sep-Oct;117(9-10):404-9. PMID:15495931

Juskevicius R, Vnencak-Jones C. Pathologic quiz case: a 17-year-old renal transplant patient with persistent fever, pancytopenia, and axillary lymphadenopathy. Bacillary angiomatosis of the lymph node in the renal transplant recipient. Arch Pathol Lab Med. 2004 Jan;128(1):e12-4. PMID:14692837

Just FT, Gilles J, Pradel I, Pfalzer S, Lengauer H, Hellmann K, Pfister K. Molecular evidence for Bartonella spp. in cat and dog fleas from Germany and France. Zoonoses Public Health. 2008 Oct;55(8-10):514-20. Epub 2008 May 16. PMID:18489542

Justa RF, Carneiro AB, Rodrigues JL, Cavalcante A, Girão ES, Silva PS, Valença Júnior JT, de Menezes DB, Leitão Tdo M. Bacillary angiomatosis in HIV-positive patient from Northeastern Brazil: a case report. Rev Soc Bras Med Trop. 2011 Oct;44(5):641-3. PMID:22031085

Juvet F, Lappin MR, Brennan S, Mooney CT. Prevalence of selected infectious agents in cats in Ireland. J Feline Med Surg. 2010 Jun;12(6):476-82. Epub 2010 May 15. PMID:20472484

Kabeya H, Colborn JM, Bai Y, Lerdthusnee K, Richardson JH, Maruyama S, Kosoy MY. Detection of Bartonella tamiae DNA in ectoparasites from rodents in Thailand and their sequence similarity with bacterial cultures from Thai patients. Vector Borne Zoonotic Dis. 2010 Jun;10(5):429-34. PMID:20017718

Kabeya H, Inoue K, Izumi Y, Morita T, Imai S, Maruyama S. Bartonella species in wild rodents and fleas from them in Japan. J Vet Med Sci. 2011 Dec;73(12):1561-7. Epub 2011 Jul 27. PMID:21791887

Kabeya H, Maruyama S, Hirano K, Mikami T. Cloning and expression of Bartonella henselae sucB gene encoding an immunogenic dihydrolipoamide succinyltransferase homologous protein. Microbiol Immunol. 2003;47(8):571-6. PMID:14524617

Kabeya H, Maruyama S, Irei M, Takahashi R, Yamashita M, Mikami T. Genomic variations among Bartonella henselae isolates derived from naturally infected cats. Vet Microbiol. 2002 Oct 22;89(2-3):211-21. PMID:12243898

Kabeya H, Sase M, Yamashita M, Maruyama S. Predominant T helper 2 immune responses against Bartonella henselae in naturally infected cats. Microbiol Immunol. 2006;50(3):171-8. PMID:16547414

Kabeya H, Tsunoda E, Maruyama S, Mikami T. Immune responses of immunocompetent and immunocompromised mice experimentally infected with Bartonella henselae. J Vet Med Sci. 2003 Apr;65(4):479-84. PMID:12736430

Kabeya H, Umehara T, Okanishi H, Tasaki I, Kamiya M, Misawa A, Mikami T, Maruyama S. Experimental infection of cats with Bartonella henselae resulted in rapid clearance associated with T helper 1 immune responses. Microbes Infect. 2009 May-Jun;11(6-7):716-20. Epub 2009 Apr 5. PMID:19348961

Kabeya H, Yamasaki A, Ikariya M, Negishi R, Chomel BB, Maruyama S. Characterization of Th1 activation by Bartonella henselae stimulation in BALB/c mice: Inhibitory activities of interleukin-10 for the production of interferon-gamma in spleen cells. Vet Microbiol. 2007 Jan 31;119(2-4):290-6. Epub 2006 Aug 14. PMID:17005337

Kaçar N, Taşli L, Demirkan N, Ergin C, Ergin S. HIV-negative case of bacillary angiomatosis with chronic hepatitis B. J Dermatol. 2010 Aug;37(8):722-5. PMID:20649715

Kacker A, Kuhel WI, Hoda RS. Quiz case 2. Cat-scratch disease (CSD). Arch Otolaryngol Head Neck Surg. 2000 May;126(5):677, 681-2. PMID:10807342

Kaewmongkol G, Kaewmongkol S, Burmej H, Bennett MD, Fleming PA, Adams PJ, Wayne AF, Ryan U, Irwin PJ, Fenwick SG. Diversity of Bartonella species detected in arthropod vectors from animals in Australia. Comp Immunol Microbiol Infect Dis. 2011 Sep;34(5):411-7. Epub 2011 Aug 20. PMID:21862131

Kaewmongkol G, Kaewmongkol S, Fleming PA, Adams PJ, Ryan U, Irwin PJ, Fenwick SG. Zoonotic Bartonella species in fleas and blood from red foxes in Australia. Vector Borne Zoonotic Dis. 2011 Dec;11(12):1549-53. Epub 2011 Sep 15. PMID:21919728

Kaewmongkol G, Kaewmongkol S, McInnes LM, Burmej H, Bennett MD, Adams PJ, Ryan U, Irwin PJ, Fenwick SG. Genetic characterization of flea-derived Bartonella species from native animals in Australia suggests host-parasite co-evolution. Infect Genet Evol. 2011 Dec;11(8):1868-72. Epub 2011 Aug 12. PMID:21856444

Kaewmongkol G, Kaewmongkol S, Owen H, Fleming PA, Adams PJ, Ryan U, Irwin PJ, Fenwick SG. Candidatus Bartonella antechini: a novel Bartonella species detected in fleas and ticks from the yellow-footed antechinus (Antechinus flavipes), an Australian marsupial. Vet Microbiol. 2011 May 5;149(3-4):517-21. Epub 2010 Dec 8. PMID:21215534

Kahr A, Kerbl R, Gschwandtner K, Heinzl B, Lackner H, Schwinger W, Stünzner D, Lindbichler F, Urban EC. Visceral manifestation of cat scratch disease in children. A consequence of altered immunological state? Infection. 2000 Mar-Apr;28(2):116-8. PMID:10782400

Kainth P, Gupta RS. Signature proteins that are distinctive of alpha proteobacteria. BMC Genomics. 2005 Jun 16;6:94. PMID:15960851

Kaiser PO, Linke D, Schwarz H, Leo JC, Kempf VA. Analysis of the BadA stalk from Bartonella henselae reveals domain-specific and domain-overlapping functions in the host cell infection process. Cell Microbiol. 2012 Feb;14(2):198-209. Epub 2011 Nov 10. PMID:21981119

Kaiser PO, Riess T, O'Rourke F, Linke D, Kempf VA. Bartonella spp.: throwing light on uncommon human infections. Int J Med Microbiol. 2011 Jan;301(1):7-15. Epub 2010 Sep 15. PMID:20833105

Kaiser PO, Riess T, Wagner CL, Linke D, Lupas AN, Schwarz H, Raddatz G, Schäfer A, Kempf VA. The head of Bartonella adhesin A is crucial for host cell interaction of Bartonella henselae. Cell Microbiol. 2008 Nov;10(11):2223-34. Epub 2008 Jul 7. PMID:18627378

Kalogeropoulos C, Koumpoulis I, Mentis A, Pappa C, Zafeiropoulos P, Aspiotis M. Bartonella and intraocular inflammation: a series of cases and review of literature. Clin Ophthalmol. 2011;5:817-29. Epub 2011 Jun 16. PMID:21750616

Kamoi K, Yoshida T, Takase H, Yokota M, Kawaguchi T, Mochizuki M. Seroprevalence of Bartonella henselae in patients with uveitis and healthy individuals in Tokyo. Jpn J Ophthalmol. 2009 Sep;53(5):490-3. Epub 2009 Oct 22. PMID:19847604

Kämpfer P, Rosselló-Mora R, Scholz HC, Welinder-Olsson C, Falsen E, Busse HJ. Description of Pseudochrobactrum gen. nov., with the two species Pseudochrobactrum asaccharolyticum sp. nov. and Pseudochrobactrum saccharolyticum sp. nov. Int J Syst Evol Microbiol. 2006 Aug;56(Pt 8):1823-9. PMID:16902015

Kamrani A, Parreira VR, Greenwood J, Prescott JF. The prevalence of Bartonella, hemoplasma, and Rickettsia felis infections in domestic cats and in cat fleas in Ontario. Can J Vet Res. 2008 Oct;72(5):411-9. PMID:19086373

Kantas I, Katotomichelakis M, Vafiadis M, Kaloutsa ZV, Papadakis CE. Serous labyrinthitis as a manifestation of cat scratch disease: a case report. J Med Case Reports. 2009 Sep 15;3:7405. PMID:20519021

Kaplan JE, Masur H, Holmes KK; USPHS; Infectious Disease Society of America. Guidelines for preventing opportunistic infections among HIV-infected persons--2002. Recommendations of the U.S. Public Health Service and the Infectious Diseases Society of America. MMWR Recomm Rep. 2002 Jun 14;51(RR-8):1-52. PMID:12081007

Karakaş M, Baba M, Aksungur VL, Homan S, Memisoğlu HR, Uğuz A. Bacillary angiomatosis on a region of burned skin in a immunocompetent patient. Br J Dermatol. 2000 Sep;143(3):609-11. PMID:10971338

Karakaş M, Baba M, Homan S, Akman A, Acar MA, Memişoğlu HR, Gümürdülü D. A case of bacillary angiomatosis presenting as leg ulcers. J Eur Acad Dermatol Venereol. 2003 Jan;17(1):65-7. PMID:12602974

Karbowiak G, Fricová J, Stanko M, Hapunik J, Várfalvyová D. Blood parasites of mound-building mouse, Mus spicilegus Petényi, 1882 (Mammalia, Rodentia). Wiad Parazytol. 2010;56(1):63-6. PMID:20450010

Karem KL, Paddock CD, Regnery RL. Bartonella henselae, B. quintana, and B. bacilliformis: historical pathogens of emerging significance. Microbes Infect. 2000 Aug;2(10):1193-205. PMID:11008109

Karem KL. Immune aspects of Bartonella. Crit Rev Microbiol. 2000;26(3):133-45. PMID:11052646

Karolak J, Gotz-Wipckowska A. [Neuroretinitis in cat scratch disease]. [Article in Polish]. Klin Oczna. 2010;112(4-6):131-4. PMID:20825068

Karras A, Thervet E, Legendre C; Groupe Coopératif de transplantation d'Ile de France. Hemophagocytic syndrome in renal transplant recipients: report of 17 cases and review of literature. Transplantation. 2004 Jan 27;77(2):238-43. PMID:14742988

Karris MY, Litwin CM, Dong HS, Vinetz J. Bartonella henselae infection of prosthetic aortic valve associated with colitis. Vector Borne Zoonotic Dis. 2011 Nov;11(11):1503-5. Epub 2011 Jun 24. PMID:21702667

Katsinelos P, Kountouras J, Chatzimavroudis G, Zavos C, Paroutoglou G. "Cat scratch" colon: an impressive but innocent endoscopic finding. Endoscopy. 2007 Nov;39(11):1026; author reply 1026. PMID:18008212

Kawasaki A, Wilson DL. Mass lesions of the posterior segment associated with Bartonella henselae. Br J Ophthalmol. 2003 Feb;87(2):248-9. PMID:12543767

Kayaselçuk F, Ceken I, Bircan S, Tuncer I. Bacillary angiomatosis of the scalp in a human immunodeficiency virus-negative patient. J Eur Acad Dermatol Venereol. 2002 Nov;16(6):612-4. PMID:12482046

Kelly P, Roberts S, Fournier PE. A review of emerging flea-borne bacterial pathogens in New Zealand. N Z Med J. 2005 Jan 28;118(1208):U1257. PMID:15682209

Kelly P, Rolain JM, Maggi R, Sontakke S, Keene B, Hunter S, Lepidi H, Breitschwerdt KT, Breitschwerdt EB. Bartonella quintana endocarditis in dogs. Emerg Infect Dis. 2006 Dec;12(12):1869-72. PMID:17326937

Kelly P, Rolain JM, Raoult D. Prevalence of human pathogens in cat and dog fleas in New Zealand. N Z Med J. 2005 Nov 25;118(1226):U1754. PMID:16311612

Kelly PJ, Eoghain GN, Raoult D. Antibodies reactive with Bartonella henselae and Ehrlichia canis in dogs from the communal lands of Zimbabwe. J S Afr Vet Assoc. 2004 Sep;75(3):116-20. PMID:15628802

Kelly PJ, Meads N, Theobald A, Fournier PE, Raoult D. Rickettsia felis, Bartonella henselae, and B. clarridgeiae, New Zealand. Emerg Infect Dis. 2004 May;10(5):967-8. PMID:15216855

Kelly PJ, Midwinter A, Rolain JM, Raoult D. Polymerase chain reaction (PCR) survey for rickettsias and bartonellas in ticks from New Zealand. N Z Vet J. 2005 Dec;53(6):468-9. PMID:16317451

Kelly PJ, Moura L, Miller T, Thurk J, Perreault N, Weil A, Maggio R, Lucas H, Breitschwerdt E. Feline immunodeficiency virus, feline leukemia virus and Bartonella species in stray cats on St Kitts, West Indies. J Feline Med Surg. 2010 Jun;12(6):447-50. Epub 2010 Feb 6. PMID:20138558

Kelly PJ. A review of bacterial pathogens in Ctenocephalides felis in New Zealand. N Z Vet J. 2004 Dec;52(6):352-7. PMID:15768135

Kempf VA, Hitziger N, Riess T, Autenrieth IB. Do plant and human pathogens have a common pathogenicity strategy? Trends Microbiol. 2002 Jun;10(6):269-75. PMID:12088662

Kempf VA, Lebiedziejewski M, Alitalo K, Wälzlein JH, Ehehalt U, Fiebig J, Huber S, Schütt B, Sander CA, Müller S, Grassl G, Yazdi AS, Brehm B, Autenrieth IB. Activation of hypoxia-inducible factor-1 in bacillary angiomatosis: evidence for a role of hypoxia-inducible factor-1 in bacterial infections. Circulation. 2005 Mar 1;111(8):1054-62. Epub 2005 Feb 21. PMID:15723970

Kempf VA, Petzold H, Autenrieth IB. Cat scratch disease due to Bartonella henselae infection mimicking parotid malignancy. Eur J Clin Microbiol Infect Dis. 2001 Oct;20(10):732-3. PMID:11757975

Kempf VA, Schairer A, Neumann D, Grassl GA, Lauber K, Lebiedziejewski M, Schaller M, Kyme P, Wesselborg S, Autenrieth IB. Bartonella henselae inhibits apoptosis in Mono Mac 6 cells. Cell Microbiol. 2005 Jan;7(1):91-104. PMID:15617526

Kempf VA, Schaller M, Behrendt S, Volkmann B, Aepfelbacher M, Cakman I, Autenrieth IB. Interaction of Bartonella henselae with endothelial cells results in rapid bacterial rRNA synthesis and replication. Cell Microbiol. 2000 Oct;2(5):431-41. PMID:11207598

Kempf VA, Volkmann B, Schaller M, Sander CA, Alitalo K, Riess T, Autenrieth IB. Evidence of a leading role for VEGF in Bartonella henselae-induced endothelial cell proliferations. Cell Microbiol. 2001 Sep;3(9):623-32. PMID:11553014

Kerkhoff FT, Rothova A. Bartonella henselae associated uveitis and HLA-B27. Br J Ophthalmol. 2000 Oct;84(10):1125-9. PMID:11004097

Kernif T, Aissi M, Doumandji SE, Chomel BB, Raoult D, Bitam I. Molecular evidence of Bartonella infection in domestic dogs from Algeria, North Africa, by polymerase chain reaction (PCR). Am J Trop Med Hyg. 2010 Aug;83(2):298-300. PMID:20682871

Kernif T, Parola P, Davoust B, Plaire L, Cabre O, Raoult D, Rolain JM. Bartonella clarridgeiae in fleas, Tahiti, French Polynesia. Emerg Infect Dis. 2011 Sep;17(9):1773-5. PMID:21888825

Kernif T, Parola P, Ricci JC, Raoult D, Rolain JM. Molecular detection of Bartonella alsatica in rabbit fleas, France. Emerg Infect Dis. 2010 Dec;16(12):2013-4. PMID:21122251

Kernif T, Socolovschi C, Wells K, Lakim MB, Inthalad S, Slesak G, Boudebouch N, Beaucournu JC, Newton PN, Raoult D, Parola P. Bartonella and Rickettsia in arthropods from the Lao PDR and from Borneo, Malaysia. Comp Immunol Microbiol Infect Dis. 2012 Jan;35(1):51-7. Epub 2011 Dec 5. PMID:22153360

Ketring KL, Zuckerman EE, Hardy WD Jr. Bartonella: a new etiological agent of feline ocular disease. J Am Anim Hosp Assoc. 2004 Jan-Feb;40(1):6-12. PMID:14736899

Keynan Y, Yakirevitch E, Shusterman T, Alter-Migdal E, Avidor B, Weber G, Giladi M. Bone marrow and skin granulomatosis in a patient with Bartonella infection. J Med Microbiol. 2007 Jan;56(Pt 1):133-5. PMID:17172528

Khairallah M, Chee SP, Rathinam SR, Attia S, Nadella V. Novel infectious agents causing uveitis. Int Ophthalmol. 2010 Oct;30(5):465-83. Epub 2009 Aug 27. PMID:19711015

Khairallah M, Jelliti B, Jenzeri S. Emergent infectious uveitis. Middle East Afr J Ophthalmol. 2009 Oct;16(4):225-38. PMID:20404989

Khoudri I, Frémont G, Flageul B, Brière J, Dubertret L, Viguier M. [Bilateral inguinal lymphadenopathy and erythema nodosum: an uncommon presentation of cat scratch disease].[Article in French]. Rev Med Interne. 2011 Mar;32(3):e34-6. Epub 2010 Jun 19. PMID:20646798

Khurana RN, Albini T, Green RL, Rao NA, Lim JI. Bartonella henselae infection presenting as a unilateral panuveitis simulating Vogt-Koyanagi-Harada syndrome. Am J Ophthalmol. 2004 Dec;138(6):1063-5. PMID:15629311

Kikuchi E, Maruyama S, Sakai T, Tanaka S, Yamaguchi F, Hagiwara T, Katsube Y, Mikami T. Serological investigation of Bartonella henselae infections in clinically cat-scratch disease-suspected patients, patients with cardiovascular diseases, and healthy veterinary students in Japan. Microbiol Immunol. 2002;46(5):313-6. PMID:12139390

Kim CM, Kim JY, Yi YH, Lee MJ, Cho MR, Shah DH, Klein TA, Kim HC, Song JW, Chong ST, O'Guinn ML, Lee JS, Lee IY, Park JH, Chae JS. Detection of Bartonella species from ticks, mites and small mammals in Korea. J Vet Sci. 2005 Dec;6(4):327-34. PMID:16293997

Kim DM, Yu KD, Lee JH, Kim HK, Lee SH. Controlled trial of a 5-day course of telithromycin versus doxycycline for treatment of mild to moderate scrub typhus. Antimicrob Agents Chemother. 2007 Jun;51(6):2011-5. Epub 2007 Apr 2. PMID:17404000

Kim YS, Seo KW, Lee JH, Choi EW, Lee HW, Hwang CY, Shin NS, Youn HJ, Youn HY. Prevalence of Bartonella henselae and Bartonella clarridgeiae in cats and dogs in Korea. J Vet Sci. 2009 Mar;10(1):85-7. PMID:19255530

Kirby JE, Nekorchuk DM. Bartonella-associated endothelial proliferation depends on inhibition of apoptosis. Proc Natl Acad Sci U S A. 2002 Apr 2;99(7):4656-61. Epub 2002 Mar 19. PMID:11904386

Kirby JE. In vitro model of Bartonella henselae-induced angiogenesis. Infect Immun. 2004 Dec;72(12):7315-7. PMID:15557658

Kirillov MIu, Markov AP, Lopyrev IV, Pankratova VN, Levitskiĭ SA, Bashkirov VN, Smirnov GB, Kruglov AN, Osadchaia VA, Frolova GP, Barmina GV, Morozova OA, Kosoy MY. [Molecular genetic methods of typing of the Bartonellae].[Article in Russian]. Mol Gen Mikrobiol Virusol. 2007;(1):8-15. PMID:17354603

Kiss A, Moodley N, Sheldon J, Tun M. Misdiagnosed bacillary angiomatosis. S Afr Med J. 2007 Nov;97(11):1050. PMID:18254198

Kitchell BE, Fan TM, Kordick D, Breitschwerdt EB, Wollenberg G, Lichtensteiger CA. Peliosis hepatis in a dog infected with Bartonella henselae. J Am Vet Med Assoc. 2000 Feb 15;216(4):519-23, 517. PMID:10687006

Klein JL, Nair SK, Harrison TG, Hunt I, Fry NK, Friedland JS. Prosthetic valve endocarditis caused by Bartonella quintana. Emerg Infect Dis. 2002 Feb;8(2):202-3. PMID:11897074

Klose TC, MacPhail CM, Schultheiss PC, Rosychuk RA, Hawley JR, Lappin MR. Prevalence of select infectious agents in inflammatory aural and nasopharyngeal polyps from client-owned cats. J Feline Med Surg. 2010 Oct;12(10):769-74. PMID:20850367

Klotz SA, Ianas V, Elliott SP. Cat-scratch Disease. Am Fam Physician. 2011 Jan 15;83(2):152-5. PMID:21243990

Knap N, Duh D, Birtles R, Trilar T, Petrovec M, Avsic-Zupanc T. Molecular detection of Bartonella species infecting rodents in Slovenia. FEMS Immunol Med Microbiol. 2007 Jun;50(1):45-50. Epub 2007 Mar 21. PMID:17374132

Knopper LD, Mineau P. Organismal effects of pesticide exposure on meadow voles (Microtus pennsylvanicus) living in golf course ecosystems: developmental instability, clinical hematology, body condition, and blood parasitology. Environ Toxicol Chem. 2004 Jun;23(6):1512-9. PMID:15376537

Kobayashi K, Koga T, Oki T, Iwao K, Okumura A, Okinami S. [Cat scratch disease with posterior segment involvement].[Article in Japanese]. Nihon Ganka Gakkai Zasshi. 2003 Feb;107(2):99-104. PMID:12647335

Kodama T, Masuda H, Ohira A. Neuroretinitis associated with cat-scratch disease in Japanese patients. Acta Ophthalmol Scand. 2003 Dec;81(6):653-7. PMID:14641271

Kodama Y, Maeno N, Nishi J, Imuta N, Oda H, Tanaka S, Kono Y, Kawano Y. Multifocal osteomyelitis due to Bartonella henselae in a child without focal pain. J Infect Chemother. 2007 Oct;13(5):350-2. Epub 2007 Oct 30. PMID:17982727

Koehler JE, Duncan LM. Case records of the Massachusetts General Hospital. Case 30-2005. A 56-year-old man with fever and axillary lymphadenopathy. N Engl J Med. 2005 Sep 29;353(13):1387-94. PMID:16192484

Koehler JE, Sanchez MA, Tye S, Garrido-Rowland CS, Chen FM, Maurer T, Cooper JL, Olson JG, Reingold AL, Hadley WK, Regnery RR, Tappero JW. Prevalence of Bartonella infection among human immunodeficiency virus-infected patients with fever. Clin Infect Dis. 2003 Aug 15;37(4):559-66. Epub 2003 Jul 31. PMID:12905141

Koesling J, Aebischer T, Falch C, Schülein R, Dehio C. Cutting edge: antibody-mediated cessation of hemotropic infection by the intraerythrocytic mouse pathogen Bartonella grahamii. J Immunol. 2001 Jul 1;167(1):11-4. PMID:11418625

Koga T, Taguchi J, Suzuki M, Higa Y, Kamimura T, Nishimura M, Arakawa M. Cat scratch disease presenting with a retroperitoneal abscess in a patient without animal contacts. J Infect Chemother. 2009 Dec;15(6):414-6. PMID:20012734

Köhler W. Killed in action: microbiologists and clinicians as victims of their occupation. Part 2: Yellow fever and bartonellosis. Int J Med Microbiol. 2005 Aug;295(4):193-200. PMID:16128394

Kojima M, Morita Y, Shimizu K, Itoh H, Masawa N, Nakamura S. Plasmacytoid monocytes in cat scratch disease with special reference to the histological diversity of suppurative lesions. Pathol Res Pract. 2006;202(1):17-22. Epub 2005 Dec 13. PMID:16352403

Komitova R, Bosheva M, Sander A, Spasova M, Atanasova M. First case in Bulgaria of Parinaud's oculoglandular syndrome associated with Bartonella henselae. Scand J Infect Dis. 2003;35(5):358-9. PMID:12875532

Koo M, Manalili S, Bankowski MJ, Sampath R, Hofstadler SA, Koo J. A "silent culture-negative" abdominal aortic mycotic aneurysm: Rapid detection of Bartonella species using PCR and high-throughput mass spectrometry. Hawaii Med J. 2010 Mar;69(3):68-9. PMID:20397506

Koretke KK, Szczesny P, Gruber M, Lupas AN. Model structure of the prototypical non-fimbrial adhesin YadA of Yersinia enterocolitica. J Struct Biol. 2006 Aug;155(2):154-61. Epub 2006 Apr 3. PMID:16675268

Kornreich BG, Craven M, McDonough SP, Nydam DV, Scorza V, Assarasakorn S, Lappin M, Simpson KW. Fluorescence In-situ Hybridization for the Identification of Bacterial Species in Archival Heart Valve Sections of Canine Bacterial Endocarditis. J Comp Pathol. 2012 May;146(4):298-307. Epub 2011 Oct 24. PMID:22030263

Koryzna K, Skomro P, Leśniewski S, Szych Z. [Oral cavity health condition of HIV carriers].[Article in Polish]. Ann Acad Med Stetin. 2008;54(3):77-80. PMID:19839516

Kosek M, Lavarello R, Gilman RH, Delgado J, Maguiña C, Verástegui M, Lescano AG, Mallqui V, Kosek JC, Recavarren S, Cabrera L. Natural history of infection with Bartonella bacilliformis in a nonendemic population. J Infect Dis. 2000 Sep;182(3):865-72. Epub 2000 Aug 17. PMID:10950782

Kosoy M, Bai Y, Lynch T, Kuzmin IV, Niezgoda M, Franka R, Agwanda B, Breiman RF, Rupprecht CE. Bartonella spp. in bats, Kenya. Emerg Infect Dis. 2010 Dec;16(12):1875-81. PMID:21122216

Kosoy M, Bai Y, Sheff K, Morway C, Baggett H, Maloney SA, Boonmar S, Bhengsri S, Dowell SF, Sitdhirasdr A, Lerdthusnee K, Richardson J, Peruski LF. Identification of Bartonella infections in febrile human patients from Thailand and their potential animal reservoirs. Am J Trop Med Hyg. 2010 Jun;82(6):1140-5. PMID:20519614

Kosoy M, Hayman DT, Chan KS. Bartonella bacteria in nature: Where does population variability end and a species start? Infect Genet Evol. 2012 Jul;12(5):894-904. Epub 2012 Mar 23. PMID:22449771

Kosoy M, Mandel E, Green D, Marston E, Childs J. Prospective studies of Bartonella of rodents. Part I. Demographic and temporal patterns in population dynamics. Vector Borne Zoonotic Dis. 2004 Winter;4(4):285-95. PMID:15671735

Kosoy M, Mandel E, Green D, Marston E, Jones D, Childs J. Prospective studies of Bartonella of rodents. Part II. Diverse infections in a single rodent community. Vector Borne Zoonotic Dis. 2004 Winter;4(4):296-305. PMID:15671736

Kosoy M, Morway C, Sheff KW, Bai Y, Colborn J, Chalcraft L, Dowell SF, Peruski LF, Maloney SA, Baggett H, Sutthirattana S, Sidhirat A, Maruyama S, Kabeya H, Chomel BB, Kasten R, Popov V, Robinson J, Kruglov A, Petersen LR. Bartonella tamiae sp. nov., a newly recognized pathogen isolated from three human patients from Thailand. J Clin Microbiol. 2008 Feb;46(2):772-5. Epub 2007 Dec 12. PMID:18077632

Kosoy M, Murray M, Gilmore RD Jr, Bai Y, Gage KL. Bartonella strains from ground squirrels are identical to Bartonella washoensis isolated from a human patient. J Clin Microbiol. 2003 Feb;41(2):645-50. PMID:12574261

Kosoy MY, Saito EK, Green D, Marston EL, Jones DC, Childs JE. Experimental evidence of host specificity of Bartonella infection in rodents. Comp Immunol Microbiol Infect Dis. 2000 Oct;23(4):221-38. PMID:11038125

Kossiva L, Vakaki M, Pasparakis D, Kallergi K, Karavanaki K, Garoufi A. Hip monoarthritis in a child with cat-scratch disease: Rare manifestation. Pediatr Int. 2010 Aug;52(4):680-1. PMID:20958885

Kotake S. [Zoonosis and ocular diseases].[Article in Japanese]. Nihon Ganka Gakkai Zasshi. 2003 Feb;107(2):69-70. PMID:12647329

Kotilainen P, Heiro M, Jalava J, Rantakokko V, Nikoskelainen J, Nikkari S, Rantakokko-Jalava K. Aetiological diagnosis of infective endocarditis by direct amplification of rRNA genes from surgically removed valve tissue. An 11-year experience in a Finnish teaching hospital. Ann Med. 2006;38(4):263-73. PMID:16754257

Krause R, Auner HW, Daxböck F, Mulabecirovic A, Krejs GJ, Wenisch C, Reisinger EC. Monoclonal and biclonal gammopathy in two patients infected with Bartonella henselae. Ann Hematol. 2003 Jul;82(7):455-7. Epub 2003 May 23. PMID:12764550

Krause R, Piswanger-Soelkner C, Lipp RW, Daxböck F, Schnedl WJ, Hoier S, Reisinger EC. Somatostatin receptor scintigraphy in patients with cat-scratch disease. Nuklearmedizin. 2006;45(4):160-2. PMID:16964341

Krause R, Wenisch C, Fladerer P, Daxböck F, Krejs GJ, Reisinger EC. Osteomyelitis of the hip joint associated with systemic cat-scratch disease in an adult. Eur J Clin Microbiol Infect Dis. 2000 Oct;19(10):781-3. PMID:11117643

Krause R, Wenisch C, Reisinger EC. Primary lesion of cat-scratch disease and inguinal cat-scratch disease. Wien Klin Wochenschr. 2003 Feb 28;115(3-4):88. PMID:12674683

Kreisel D, Pasque MK, Damiano RJ Jr, Medoff G, Kates A, Kreisel FH, Lawton JS. Bartonella species-induced prosthetic valve endocarditis associated with rapid progression of valvular stenosis. J Thorac Cardiovasc Surg. 2005 Aug;130(2):567-8. PMID:16077432

Kreitzer T, Saoud A. Bacillary angiomatosis following the use of long-term methotrexate therapy: a case report. W V Med J. 2006 Jan-Feb;102(1):317-8. PMID:16706324

Kumar T, Epstein M, Markovskaya Y, Narasimhan M, Rosen M, Talwar A. Bronchoscopy and endobronchial disease in patients with human immunodeficiency virus infection. Indian J Chest Dis Allied Sci. 2011 Apr-Jun;53(2):99-105. PMID:21545071

Kumasaka K, Arashima Y, Yanai M, Hosokawa N, Kawano K. Survey of veterinary professionals for antibodies to Bartonella henselae in Japan. Rinsho Byori. 2001 Sep;49(9):906-10. PMID:11685779

Kunz S, Oberle K, Sander A, Bogdan C, Schleicher U. Lymphadenopathy in a novel mouse model of Bartonella-induced cat scratch disease results from lymphocyte immigration and proliferation and is regulated by interferon-alpha/beta. Am J Pathol. 2008 Apr;172(4):1005-18. Epub 2008 Feb 21. PMID:18292236

Kusaba N, Yoshida H, Sumino M, Sata M. [Longitudinal study of serological response to Bartonella henselae by indirect fluorescence assay in cat scratch disease].[Article in Japanese]. Kansenshogaku Zasshi. 2001 Jul;75(7):557-61. PMID:11521278

Kusuhara K, Nakao F, Saito M, Nakamura K, Ieiri S, Taguchi T, Hara T. Pyogenic splenic abscess in an infant with serological evidence of cat scratch disease. Eur J Pediatr. 2007 Dec;166(12):1289-91. Epub 2006 Dec 22. PMID:17186270

Kuykendall LD, Shao JY, Hartung JS. Conservation of Gene Order and Content in the Circular Chromosomes of 'Candidatus Liberibacter asiaticus' and Other Rhizobiales. PLoS One. 2012;7(4):e34673. Epub 2012 Apr 4. PMID:22496839

Kyme P, Dillon B, Iredell J. Phase variation in Bartonella henselae. Microbiology. 2003 Mar;149(Pt 3):621-9. PMID:12634331

Kyme PA, Haas A, Schaller M, Peschel A, Iredell J, Kempf VA. Unusual trafficking pattern of Bartonella henselae -containing vacuoles in macrophages and endothelial cells. Cell Microbiol. 2005 Jul;7(7):1019-34. PMID:15953033

Kymionis GD, Siganos CS, Pallikaris IG. Late onset of serologic positive titers in a patient with Parinaud's oculoglandular syndrome. Semin Ophthalmol. 2004 Sep-Dec;19(3-4):125-6. PMID:15590554

La Scola B, Davoust B, Boni M, Raoult D. Lack of correlation between Bartonella DNA detection within fleas, serological results, and results of blood culture in a Bartonella-infected stray cat population. Clin Microbiol Infect. 2002 Jun;8(6):345-51. PMID:12084102

La Scola B, Fournier PE, Brouqui P, Raoult D. Detection and culture of Bartonella quintana, Serratia marcescens, and Acinetobacter spp. from decontaminated human body lice. J Clin Microbiol. 2001 May;39(5):1707-9. PMID:11325978

La Scola B, Holmberg M, Raoult D. Lack of Bartonella sp. in 167 Ixodes ricinus ticks collected in central Sweden. Scand J Infect Dis. 2004;36(4):305-6. PMID:15198190

La Scola B, Liang Z, Zeaiter Z, Houpikian P, Grimont PA, Raoult D. Genotypic characteristics of two serotypes of Bartonella henselae. J Clin Microbiol. 2002 Jun;40(6):2002-8. PMID:12037055

La Scola B, Raoult D. Acinetobacter baumannii in human body louse. Emerg Infect Dis. 2004 Sep;10(9):1671-3. PMID:15498175

La Scola B, Zeaiter Z, Khamis A, Raoult D. Gene-sequence-based criteria for species definition in bacteriology: the Bartonella paradigm. Trends Microbiol. 2003 Jul;11(7):318-21. PMID:12875815

La VD, Clavel B, Lepetz S, Aboudharam G, Raoult D, Drancourt M. Molecular detection of Bartonella henselae DNA in the dental pulp of 800-year-old French cats. Clin Infect Dis. 2004 Nov 1;39(9):1391-4. Epub 2004 Oct 12. PMID:15494918

La VD, Tran-Hung L, Aboudharam G, Raoult D, Drancourt M. Bartonella quintana in domestic cat. Emerg Infect Dis. 2005 Aug;11(8):1287-9. PMID:16102321

La Via WV. Urban trench fever and cat scratch disease. Clin Infect Dis. 2003 Apr 15;36(8):1089. PMID:12684929

Labalette P, Bermond D, Dedes V, Savage C. Cat-scratch disease neuroretinitis diagnosed by a polymerase chain reaction approach. Am J Ophthalmol. 2001 Oct;132(4):575-6. PMID:11589885

Lafferty KD. Microbiology. Interacting parasites. Science. 2010 Oct 8;330(6001):187-8. PMID:20929765

Laham FR, Kaplan SL. Hepatosplenic cat-scratch fever. Lancet Infect Dis. 2008 Feb;8(2):140. PMID:18222165

Lamas C, Curi A, Bóia M, Lemos E. Human bartonellosis: seroepidemiological and clinical features with an emphasis on data from Brazil - a review. Mem Inst Oswaldo Cruz. 2008 May;103(3):221-35. PMID:18592096

Lamas C, Favacho A, Ramos RG, Santos MS, Ferravoli GI, Weksler C, Rozental T, Bóia MN, Lemos ER. Bartonella native valve endocarditis: the first Brazilian case alive and well. Braz J Infect Dis. 2007 Dec;11(6):591-4. PMID:18327472

Lamas CC, Eykyn SJ. Blood culture negative endocarditis: analysis of 63 cases presenting over 25 years. Heart. 2003 Mar;89(3):258-62. PMID:12591823

Lamas CC, Mares-Guia MA, Rozental T, Moreira N, Favacho AR, Barreira J, Guterres A, Bóia MN, de Lemos ER. Bartonella spp. infection in HIV positive individuals, their pets and ectoparasites in Rio de Janeiro, Brazil: serological and molecular study. Acta Trop. 2010 Jul-Aug;115(1-2):137-41. Epub 2010 Mar 3. PMID:20206113

Lamps LW, Scott MA. Cat-scratch disease: historic, clinical, and pathologic perspectives. Am J Clin Pathol. 2004 Jun;121 Suppl:S71-80. PMID:15298152

Lange D, Oeder C, Waltermann K, Mueller A, Oehme A, Rohrberg R, Marsch W, Fischer M. Bacillary angiomatosis.[Article in English, German]. J Dtsch Dermatol Ges. 2009 Sep;7(9):767-69. PMID:19298547

Lappin MR, Breitschwerdt E, Brewer M, Hawley J, Hegarty B, Radecki S. Prevalence of Bartonella species antibodies and Bartonella species DNA in the blood of cats with and without fever. J Feline Med Surg. 2009 Feb;11(2):141-8. Epub 2008 Aug 29. PMID:18760647

Lappin MR, Griffin B, Brunt J, Riley A, Burney D, Hawley J, Brewer MM, Jensen WA. Prevalence of Bartonella species, haemoplasma species, Ehrlichia species, Anaplasma phagocytophilum, and Neorickettsia risticii DNA in the blood of cats and their fleas in the United States. J Feline Med Surg. 2006 Apr;8(2):85-90. Epub 2005 Nov 14. PMID:16290092

Lappin MR, Hawley J. Presence of Bartonella species and Rickettsia species DNA in the blood, oral cavity, skin and claw beds of cats in the United States. Vet Dermatol. 2009 Oct;20(5-6):509-14. PMID:20178489

Lappin MR, Kordick DL, Breitschwerdt EB. Bartonella spp antibodies and DNA in aqueous humour of cats. J Feline Med Surg. 2000 Mar;2(1):61-8. PMID:11716593

Larrey D. [Bacterial hepatitis].[Article in French]. Gastroenterol Clin Biol. 2003 May;27(5 Suppl):B27-31. PMID:12843934

Laudisoit A, Iverson J, Neerinckx S, Shako JC, Nsabimana JM, Kersh G, Kosoy M, Zeidner N. Human seroreactivity against Bartonella species in the Democratic Republic of Congo. Asian Pac J Trop Med. 2011 Apr;4(4):320-2. Epub 2011 May 29. PMID:21771478

Laumbacher B, Fellerhoff B, Herzberger B, Wank R. Do dogs harbour risk factors for human breast cancer? Med Hypotheses. 2006;67(1):21-6. Epub 2006 Mar 3. PMID:16516398

Lawes R. Cat scratch disease. Nursing. 2009 Mar;39(3):72. PMID:19247139

Lax AJ, Thomas W. How bacteria could cause cancer: one step at a time. Trends Microbiol. 2002 Jun;10(6):293-9. PMID:12088666

Laycock GM, Day MJ, Birtles RJ. Prevalence of Bartonella henselae in cats in the UK. Vet Rec. 2001 Feb 17;148(7):219. PMID:11266008

Le Rhun D, Malou N, Labed S, Le Naour E, Vayssier-Taussat M. In vitro effect of Bartonella birtlesii on mouse red cell viability. Clin Microbiol Infect. 2009 Dec;15 Suppl 2:112-3. Epub 2009 Apr 30. PMID:19438632

Le Tallec V, Abgueguen P, Pichard E, Chennebault JM, Bellec V, Delbos V, Rousselet MC, Dib N, Boyer J. [Hepatosplenic localization of cat scratch disease in immunocompetent adults. Two cases]. [Article in French]. Gastroenterol Clin Biol. 2003 Feb;27(2):225-9. PMID:12658133

Ledina D, Rincić J, Ivić I, Marasović D, Ledina D. A child with Bartonella henselae osteomyelitis of the right humerus. Acta Dermatovenerol Croat. 2004;12(2):92-5. PMID:15075043

Lee J, Fernandes R. Neck masses: evaluation and diagnostic approach. Oral Maxillofac Surg Clin North Am. 2008 Aug;20(3):321-37. PMID:18603194

Lee J, Lynde C. Pyogenic granuloma: pyogenic again? Association between pyogenic granuloma and Bartonella. J Cutan Med Surg. 2001 Nov-Dec;5(6):467-70. PMID:11907853

Lee J, Michael AJ, Martynowski D, Goldsmith EJ, Phillips MA. Phylogenetic diversity and the structural basis of substrate specificity in the beta/alpha-barrel fold basic amino acid decarboxylases. J Biol Chem. 2007 Sep 14;282(37):27115-25. Epub 2007 Jul 11. PMID:17626020

Lee KN, Padmalayam I, Baumstark B, Baker SL, Massung RF. Characterization of the ftsZ gene from Ehrlichia chaffeensis, Anaplasma phagocytophilum, and Rickettsia rickettsii, and use as a differential PCR target. DNA Cell Biol. 2003 Mar;22(3):179-86. PMID:12804116

Leeper T, Zhang S, Van Voorhis WC, Myler PJ, Varani G. Comparative analysis of glutaredoxin domains from bacterial opportunistic pathogens. Acta Crystallogr Sect F Struct Biol Cryst Commun. 2011 Sep 1;67(Pt 9):1141-7. Epub 2011 Aug 16. PMID:21904064

Leibovitz K, Pearce L, Brewer M, Lappin MR. Bartonella species antibodies and DNA in cerebral spinal fluid of cats with central nervous system disease. J Feline Med Surg. 2008 Aug;10(4):332-7. Epub 2008 Apr 8. PMID:18400536

Leidholm MD. Encountering cat-scratch disease. Nurse Pract. 2002 Feb;27(2):14, 60. PMID:11858582

Leighton FA, Artsob HA, Chu MC, Olson JG. A serological survey of rural dogs and cats on the southwestern Canadian prairie for zoonotic pathogens. Can J Public Health. 2001 Jan-Feb;92(1):67-71. PMID:11257996

Lejko-Zupanc T, Slemenik-Pusnik C, Kozelj M, Klokocovnik T, Avsic-Zupanc T, Dolenc-Strazar Z, Benko D, Duh D, Rojko T. Native valve endocarditis due to Bartonella henselae in an immunocompetent man. Wien Klin Wochenschr. 2008;120(7-8):246-9. PMID:18500601

Lemme KA, Seupaul RA. Images in emergency medicine. Parinaud's oculoglandular syndrome. Ann Emerg Med. 2005 Nov;46(5):406, 423. Epub 2005 Jul 22. PMID:16271667

Lemos ER, Mares-Guia MA, Almeida DN, Silva RG, Silva CM, Britto C, Lamas CC. [Traveler's fever associated with cervical adenomegaly and antibodies for Bartonella sp in a Brazilian patient returning from South Africa].[Article in Portuguese]. Rev Soc Bras Med Trop. 2010 Jul-Aug;43(4):472-3. PMID:20802956

Lepidi H, Coulibaly B, Casalta JP, Raoult D. Autoimmunohistochemistry: a new method for the histologic diagnosis of infective endocarditis. J Infect Dis. 2006 Jun 15;193(12):1711-7. Epub 2006 May 12. PMID:16703515

Lepidi H, Fournier PE, Raoult D. Quantitative analysis of valvular lesions during Bartonella endocarditis. Am J Clin Pathol. 2000 Dec;114(6):880-9. PMID:11338477

Lerdluedeeporn P, Krogstad P, Roberts RL, Stiehm ER. Oral corticosteroids in cat-scratch disease. Clin Pediatr (Phila). 2003 Jan-Feb;42(1):71-3. PMID:12635985

Lerdthusnee K, Nigro J, Monkanna T, Leepitakrat W, Leepitakrat S, Insuan S, Charoensongsermkit W, Khlaimanee N, Akkagraisee W, Chayapum K, Jones JW. Surveys of rodent-borne disease in Thailand with a focus on scrub typhus assessment. Integr Zool. 2008 Dec;3(4):267-73. PMID:21396076

Lesprit P, Noël V, Chazouillères P, Brun-Buisson C, Deforges L. Cure of bartonella endocarditis of a prosthetic aortic valve without surgery: value of serologic follow-up. Clin Microbiol Infect. 2003 Mar;9(3):239-41. PMID:12667258

Lester JL, Buccolo LS, McAdams CA. Breast swelling and erythema in a teen. J Fam Pract. 2011 Nov;60(11):675-7. PMID:22049351

Letranchant L, Ruivard M, Dauphin C, Chanet V, Philippe P. [Non infectious endocarditis: retrospective study (6 cases)].[Article in French]. Rev Med Interne. 2005 Mar;26(3):189-95. Epub 2005 Jan 5. PMID:15777581

Levy I, Rolain JM, Lepidi H, Raoult D, Feinmesser M, Lapidoth M, Ben-Amitai D. Is pyogenic granuloma associated with Bartonella infection? J Am Acad Dermatol. 2005 Dec;53(6):1065-6. PMID:16310070

Levy JK, Crawford PC, Lappin MR, Dubovi EJ, Levy MG, Alleman R, Tucker SJ, Clifford EL. Infectious diseases of dogs and cats on Isabela Island, Galapagos. J Vet Intern Med. 2008 Jan-Feb;22(1):60-5. PMID:18289290

Levy JK, Lappin MR, Glaser AL, Birkenheuer AJ, Anderson TC, Edinboro CH. Prevalence of infectious diseases in cats and dogs rescued following Hurricane Katrina. J Am Vet Med Assoc. 2011 Feb 1;238(3):311-7. PMID:21281213

Levy PY, Corey R, Berger P, Habib G, Bonnet JL, Levy S, Messana T, Djiane P, Frances Y, Botta C, DeMicco P, Dumon H, Mundler O, Chomel JJ, Raoult D. Etiologic diagnosis of 204 pericardial effusions. Medicine (Baltimore). 2003 Nov;82(6):385-91. PMID:14663288

Levy PY, Fournier PE, Carta M, Raoult D. Pericardial effusion in a homeless man due to Bartonella quintana. J Clin Microbiol. 2003 Nov;41(11):5291-3. PMID:14605187

Lewis P, Glaser CA. Encephalitis. Pediatr Rev. 2005 Oct;26(10):353-63. PMID:16199589

Li CW, Yin J, Zhang XL. [Cat scratch disease: report of a case]. [Article in Chinese]. Zhonghua Er Ke Za Zhi. 2007 Aug;45(8):573. PMID:18021527

Li D, Liu Q, Song X, Zhang J, Xu C, Yang X. [Biological and molecular characteristics of a cat-borne Bartonella clarridgeiae]. [Article in Chinese]. Wei Sheng Wu Xue Bao. 2009 Apr;49(4):429-37. PMID:19621628

Li DM, Liu QY, Yu DZ, Zhang JZ, Gong ZD, Song XP. Phylogenetic analysis of Bartonella detected in rodent fleas in Yunnan, China. J Wildl Dis. 2007 Oct;43(4):609-17. PMID:17984255

Li DM, Liu QY, Zhao F, Hu Y, Xiao D, Gu YX, Song XP, Zhang JZ. Proteomic and bioinformatic analysis of outer membrane proteins of the protobacterium Bartonella henselae (Bartonellaceae). Genet Mol Res. 2011 Aug 26;10(3):1789-818. PMID:21948745

Li DM, Meng FX, Song XP, Qin ZJ, Yang XR, Wu HX, Ren DS, Liu QY. [Study on Bartonella vinsonii berkhoffii isolated from blood of native dogs in China].[Article in Chinese]. Zhonghua Liu Xing Bing Xue Za Zhi. 2006 Apr;27(4):333-8. PMID:16875539

Li DM, Yu DZ, Liu QY, Gong ZD. [Study on the prevalence of Bartonella species in rodent hosts from different environmental areas in Yunnan].[Article in Chinese]. Zhonghua Liu Xing Bing Xue Za Zhi. 2004 Nov;25(11):934-7. PMID:15769319

Li DM, Yu DZ, Liu QY, Hai R, Guo BH. [Study on Bartonella infection using molecular biological diagnostic techniques from China].[Article in Chinese]. Zhonghua Liu Xing Bing Xue Za Zhi. 2004 Jul;25(7):602-6. PMID:15308042

Li W, Chomel BB, Maruyama S, Guptil L, Sander A, Raoult D, Fournier PE. Multispacer typing to study the genotypic distribution of Bartonella henselae populations. J Clin Microbiol. 2006 Jul;44(7):2499-506. PMID:16825371

Li W, Raoult D, Fournier PE. Genetic diversity of Bartonella henselae in human infection detected with multispacer typing. Emerg Infect Dis. 2007 Aug;13(8):1178-83. PMID:17953088

Liang Z, La Scola B, Lepidi H, Raoult D. Production of Bartonella genus-specific monoclonal antibodies. Clin Diagn Lab Immunol. 2001 Jul;8(4):847-9. PMID:11427441

Liang Z, Raoult D. Differentiation of Bartonella species by a microimmunofluorescence assay, sodium dodecyl sulfate-polyacrylamide gel electrophoresis, and Western immunoblotting. Clin Diagn Lab Immunol. 2000 Jul;7(4):617-24. PMID:10882662

Liang Z, Raoult D. Species-specific monoclonal antibodies for rapid identification of Bartonella quintana. Clin Diagn Lab Immunol. 2000 Jan;7(1):21-4. PMID:10618271

Liao HM, Huang FY, Chi H, Wang NL, Chen BF. Systemic cat scratch disease. J Formos Med Assoc. 2006 Aug;105(8):674-9. PMID:16935770

Liapi-Adamidou G, Tsolia M, Magiakou AM, Zeis PM, Theodoropoulos V, Karpathios T. Cat scratch disease in 2 siblings presenting as acute gastroenteritis. Scand J Infect Dis. 2000;32(3):317-9. PMID:10879606

Liberto MC, Lamberti AG, Marascio N, Matera G, Quirino A, Barreca GS, Baudi F, Focà A. Molecular identification of Bartonella quintana infection using species-specific real-time PCR targeting transcriptional regulatory protein (bqtR) gene. Mol Cell Probes. 2011 Oct-Dec;25(5-6):238-42. Epub 2011 Jul 28. PMID:21816218

Liberto MC, Matera G, Lamberti AG, Barreca GS, Focà D, Quirino A, Soria MR, Focà A. Bartonella quintana-induced apoptosis inhibition of human endothelial cells is associated with p38 and SAPK/JNK modulation and with stimulation of mitosis. Diagn Microbiol Infect Dis. 2004 Nov;50(3):159-66. PMID:15541600

Liberto MC, Matera G, Lamberti AG, Barreca GS, Quirino A, Focà A. In vitro Bartonella quintana infection modulates the programmed cell death and inflammatory reaction of endothelial cells. Diagn Microbiol Infect Dis. 2003 Feb;45(2):107-15. PMID:12614981

Liberto MC, Matera G. Pathogenic mechanisms of Bartonella quintana. New Microbiol. 2000 Oct;23(4):449-56. PMID:11061635

Lieberman JM. North American zoonoses. Pediatr Ann. 2009 Apr;38(4):193-8. PMID:19455948

Lien SH, Lo WT, Lee CM, Cheng SN, Chu ML, Wang CC. Cat-scratch disease in children at a medical center. Acta Paediatr Taiwan. 2004 Sep-Oct;45(5):282-6. PMID:15868811

Lienhardt B, Irani S, Gaspert A, Weishaupt D, Boehler A. Disseminated infection with Bartonella henselae in a lung transplant recipient. J Heart Lung Transplant. 2009 Jul;28(7):736-9. PMID:19560704

Lin EY, Tsigrelis C, Baddour LM, Lepidi H, Rolain JM, Patel R, Raoult D. Candidatus Bartonella mayotimonensis and endocarditis. Emerg Infect Dis. 2010 Mar;16(3):500-3. PMID:20202430

Lin JW, Chen CM, Chang CC. Unknown fever and back pain caused by Bartonella henselae in a veterinarian after a needle puncture: a case report and literature. Vector Borne Zoonotic Dis. 2011 May;11(5):589-91. Epub 2010 Jun 23. PMID:20569013

Lin JW, Chen CY, Chen WC, Chomel BB, Chang CC. Isolation of Bartonella species from rodents in Taiwan including a strain closely related to 'Bartonella rochalimae' from Rattus norvegicus. J Med Microbiol. 2008 Dec;57(Pt 12):1496-501. PMID:19018019

Lin JW, Hsu YM, Chomel BB, Lin LK, Pei JC, Wu SH, Chang CC. Identification of novel Bartonella spp. in bats and evidence of Asian gray shrew as a new potential reservoir of Bartonella. Vet Microbiol. 2012 Apr 23;156(1-2):119-26. Epub 2011 Oct 2. PMID:22005177

Lin YY, Hsiao CH, Hsu YH, Lee CC, Tsai HJ, Pan MJ. Immunohistochemical study of lymph nodes in patients with cat scratch disease. J Formos Med Assoc. 2006 Nov;105(11):911-7. PMID:17098692

Lindroos H, Vinnere O, Mira A, Repsilber D, Näslund K, Andersson SG. Genome rearrangements, deletions, and amplifications in the natural population of Bartonella henselae. J Bacteriol. 2006 Nov;188(21):7426-39. Epub 2006 Aug 25. PMID:16936024

Lindroos HL, Mira A, Repsilber D, Vinnere O, Näslund K, Dehio M, Dehio C, Andersson SG. Characterization of the genome composition of Bartonella koehlerae by microarray comparative genomic hybridization profiling. J Bacteriol. 2005 Sep;187(17):6155-65. PMID:16109957

Lindsey J, Patel S. PCR for bacterial 16S ribosomal DNA in multiple sclerosis cerebrospinal fluid. Mult Scler. 2008 Mar;14(2):147-52. Epub 2007 Nov 6. PMID:17986505

Listernick R. A 14-month-old boy with prolonged fever and splenomegaly. Pediatr Ann. 2004 Oct;33(10):637-8, 640-2. PMID:15515351

Littman MP. Canine borreliosis. Vet Clin North Am Small Anim Pract. 2003 Jul;33(4):827-62. PMID:12910746

Litwin CM, Johnson JM, Martins TB. The Bartonella henselae sucB gene encodes a dihydrolipoamide succinyltransferase protein reactive with sera from patients with cat-scratch disease. J Med Microbiol. 2004 Dec;53(Pt 12):1221-7. PMID:15585501

Litwin CM, Johnson JM. Identification, cloning, and expression of the CAMP-like factor autotransporter gene (cfa) of Bartonella henselae. Infect Immun. 2005 Jul;73(7):4205-13. PMID:15972511

Litwin CM, Rawlins ML, Swenson EM. Characterization of an immunogenic outer membrane autotransporter protein, Arp, of Bartonella henselae. Infect Immun. 2007 Nov;75(11):5255-63. Epub 2007 Sep 4. PMID:17785470

Liu MF, Cescau S, Mechold U, Wang J, Cohen D, Danchin A, Boulouis HJ, Biville F. Identification of a novel nanoRNase in Bartonella. Microbiology. 2012 Apr;158(Pt 4):886-95. Epub 2012 Jan 19. PMID:22262096

Liu Q, Eremeeva ME, Li D. Bartonella and Bartonella infections in China: from the clinic to the laboratory. Comp Immunol Microbiol Infect Dis. 2012 Mar;35(2):93-102. Epub 2012 Feb 2. PMID:22304899

Liu Q, Sun J, Lu L, Fu G, Ding G, Song X, Meng F, Wu H, Yang T, Ren Z, Chen E, Lin J, Lv H, Chai C. Detection of bartonella species in small mammals from Zhejiang Province, China. J Wildl Dis. 2010 Jan;46(1):179-85. PMID:20090031

Loa CC, Adelson ME, Mordechai E, Raphaelli I, Tilton RC. Serological diagnosis of human babesiosis by IgG enzyme-linked immunosorbent assay. Curr Microbiol. 2004 Dec;49(6):385-9. PMID:15696612

Loa CC, Mordechai E, Tilton RC, Adelson ME. Production of recombinant Bartonella henselae 17-kDa protein for antibody-capture enzyme-linked immunosorbent assay. Diagn Microbiol Infect Dis. 2006 May;55(1):1-7. Epub 2006 Feb 20. PMID:16490335

Lobanov VA, Gajadhar AA, Al-Adhami B, Schwantje HM. Molecular Study of Free-ranging Mule Deer and White-tailed Deer from British Columbia, Canada, for Evidence of Anaplasma spp. and Ehrlichia spp. Transbound Emerg Dis. 2012 Jun;59(3):233-43. Epub 2011 Sep 20. PMID:21933360

Loeckx I, Tuerlinckx D, Jespers S, Marchant AS, Bodart E. [A clinical case of spontaneous involution of systemic cat scratch disease].[Article in French]. Rev Med Liege. 2010 Feb;65(2):78-80. PMID:20344917

Loftis AD, Gill JS, Schriefer ME, Levin ML, Eremeeva ME, Gilchrist MJ, Dasch GA. Detection of Rickettsia, Borrelia, and Bartonella in Carios kelleyi (Acari: Argasidae). J Med Entomol. 2005 May;42(3):473-80. PMID:15962801

Loftis AD, Reeves WK, Szumlas DE, Abbassy MM, Helmy IM, Moriarity JR, Dasch GA. Population survey of Egyptian arthropods for rickettsial agents. Ann N Y Acad Sci. 2006 Oct;1078:364-7. PMID:17114742

Loftis AD, Reeves WK, Szumlas DE, Abbassy MM, Helmy IM, Moriarity JR, Dasch GA. Rickettsial agents in Egyptian ticks collected from domestic animals. Exp Appl Acarol. 2006;40(1):67-81. Epub 2006 Sep 27. PMID:17004028

Loftis AD, Reeves WK, Szumlas DE, Abbassy MM, Helmy IM, Moriarity JR, Dasch GA. Surveillance of Egyptian fleas for agents of public health significance: Anaplasma, Bartonella, Coxiella, Ehrlichia, Rickettsia, and Yersinia pestis. Am J Trop Med Hyg. 2006 Jul;75(1):41-8. PMID:16837707

Lohmann CP, Gabler B, Kroher G, Spiegel D, Linde HJ, Reischl U. Disciforme keratitis caused by Bartonella henselae: an unusual ocular complication in cat scratch disease. Eur J Ophthalmol. 2000 Jul-Sep;10(3):257-8. PMID:11071035

Lohmann CP, Winkler von Mohrenfels C, Gabler B, Reischl U, Kochanowski B. [Polymerase chain reaction (PCR) for microbiological diagnosis in refractory infectious keratitis: a clinical study in 16 patients].[Article in German]. Klin Monbl Augenheilkd. 2000 Jul;217(1):37-42. PMID:10949815

López de Blanc S, Sambuelli R, Femopase F, Luna N, Gravotta M, David D, Bistoni A, Criscuolo MI. Bacillary angiomatosis affecting the oral cavity. Report of two cases and review. J Oral Pathol Med. 2000 Feb;29(2):91-6. PMID:10718405

López-Goñi I, Guzmán-Verri C, Manterola L, Sola-Landa A, Moriyón I, Moreno E. Regulation of Brucella virulence by the two-component system BvrR/BvrS. Vet Microbiol. 2002 Dec 20;90(1-4):329-39. PMID:12414153

Lortholary O, Mainardi JL, La Scola B, Gallais V, Frenaux P, Casassus P. Consecutive bacillary angiomatosis and Rhodococcus equi bacteremia during acute leukemia: zoonoses may cause fever in neutropenic patients. Clin Microbiol Infect. 2000 Jun;6(6):334-6. PMID:11168145

Losanoff JE, Sauter ER, Rider KD. Cat scratch disease presenting with abdominal pain and retroperitoneal lymphadenopathy. J Clin Gastroenterol. 2004 Mar;38(3):300-1. PMID:15128085

Lukin EP, Vorob'ev AA, Bykov AS. [Taxonomy and classification of Rickettsiae].[Article in Russian]. Zh Mikrobiol Epidemiol Immunobiol. 2001 Mar-Apr;(2):105-10. PMID:11548242

Luong A, McClay JE, Jafri HS, Brown O. Antibiotic therapy for nontuberculous mycobacterial cervicofacial lymphadenitis. Laryngoscope. 2005 Oct;115(10):1746-51. PMID:16222188

Lupi O, Madkan V, Tyring SK. Tropical dermatology: bacterial tropical diseases. J Am Acad Dermatol. 2006 Apr;54(4):559-78; quiz 578-80. PMID:16546577

Luria BJ, Levy JK, Lappin MR, Breitschwerdt EB, Legendre AM, Hernandez JA, Gorman SP, Lee IT. Prevalence of infectious diseases in feral cats in Northern Florida. J Feline Med Surg. 2004 Oct;6(5):287-96. PMID:15363760

Luther TT, Roters S, Diestelhorst M. [Papillary swelling and macular edema].[Article in German]. Ophthalmologe. 2003 Jul;100(7):558-60. Epub 2003 Jun 26. PMID:12920558

Lydy SL, Eremeeva ME, Asnis D, Paddock CD, Nicholson WL, Silverman DJ, Dasch GA. Isolation and characterization of Bartonella bacilliformis from an expatriate Ecuadorian. J Clin Microbiol. 2008 Feb;46(2):627-37. Epub 2007 Dec 19. PMID:18094131

Lynch T, Iverson J, Kosoy M. Combining culture techniques for Bartonella: the best of both worlds. J Clin Microbiol. 2011 Apr;49(4):1363-8. Epub 2011 Feb 2. PMID:21289156

Macdonald K. Infective endocarditis in dogs: diagnosis and therapy. Vet Clin North Am Small Anim Pract. 2010 Jul;40(4):665-84. PMID:20610018

MacDonald KA, Chomel BB, Kittleson MD, Kasten RW, Thomas WP, Pesavento P. A prospective study of canine infective endocarditis in northern California (1999-2001): emergence of Bartonella as a prevalent etiologic agent. J Vet Intern Med. 2004 Jan-Feb;18(1):56-64. PMID:14765733

Machi T. [Cat scratch disease showing clinical picture resembling tuberculous lymphadenitis: a case report].[Article in Japanese]. Kekkaku. 2001 Jul;76(7):545-8. PMID:11517562

MacKichan JK, Gerns HL, Chen YT, Zhang P, Koehler JE. A SacB mutagenesis strategy reveals that the Bartonella quintana variably expressed outer membrane proteins are required for bloodstream infection of the host. Infect Immun. 2008 Feb;76(2):788-95. Epub 2007 Dec 10. PMID:18070893

Maco V, Maguiña C, Tirado A, Maco V, Vidal JE. Carrion's disease (Bartonellosis bacilliformis) confirmed by histopathology in the High Forest of Peru. Rev Inst Med Trop Sao Paulo. 2004 May-Jun;46(3):171-4. Epub 2004 Jul 20. PMID:15286824

Maczka I, Chmielewski T, Walczak E, Rózański J, Religa G, Tylewska-Wierzbanowska S. Tick-borne infections as a cause of heart transplantation. Pol J Microbiol. 2011;60(4):341-3. PMID:22390070

Maeno N, Yoshiie K, Matayoshi S, Fujimura T, Mao S, Wahid MR, Oda H. A heat-stable component of Bartonella henselae upregulates intercellular adhesion molecule-1 expression on vascular endothelial cells. Scand J Immunol. 2002 Apr;55(4):366-72. PMID:11967118

Mafee MF. Ocular manifestations of cat-scratch disease: role of MR imaging. AJNR Am J Neuroradiol. 2005 Jun-Jul;26(6):1303-4. PMID:15956483

Magalhães RF, Cintra ML, Barjas-Castro ML, Del Negro GM, Okay TS, Velho PE. Blood donor infected with Bartonella henselae. Transfus Med. 2010 Aug 1;20(4):280-2. Epub 2010 Mar 24. PMID:20345384

Magalhães RF, Pitassi LH, Salvadego M, de Moraes AM, Barjas-Castro ML, Velho PE. Bartonella henselae survives after the storage period of red blood cell units: is it transmissible by transfusion? Transfus Med. 2008 Oct;18(5):287-91. PMID:18937735

Magalhães RF, Urso Pitassi LH, Lania BG, Barjas-Castro ML, Neves Ferreira Velho PE. Bartonellosis as cause of death after red blood cell unit transfusion. Ultrastruct Pathol. 2009 Jul-Aug;33(4):151-4. PMID:19728230

Magand F, Frésard A, Manoli P, Cazorla C, Lucht F. [Stellar neuroretinitis and Bartonella henselae infection. A case report without exposure to cats].[Article in French]. Med Mal Infect. 2008 May;38(5):275-7. Epub 2008 Jan 9. PMID:18187281

Maggi RG, Breitschwerdt EB. Isolation of bacteriophages from Bartonella vinsonii subsp. berkhoffii and the characterization of Pap31 gene sequences from bacterial and phage DNA. J Mol Microbiol Biotechnol. 2005;9(1):44-51. PMID:16254445

Maggi RG, Breitschwerdt EB. Potential limitations of the 16S-23S rRNA intergenic region for molecular detection of Bartonella species. J Clin Microbiol. 2005 Mar;43(3):1171-6. PMID:15750079

Maggi RG, Chomel B, Hegarty BC, Henn J, Breitschwerdt EB. A Bartonella vinsonii berkhoffii typing scheme based upon 16S-23S ITS and Pap31 sequences from dog, coyote, gray fox, and human isolates. Mol Cell Probes. 2006 Apr;20(2):128-34. Epub 2006 Feb 7. PMID:16460911

Maggi RG, Duncan AW, Breitschwerdt EB. Novel chemically modified liquid medium that will support the growth of seven bartonella species. J Clin Microbiol. 2005 Jun;43(6):2651-5. PMID:15956379

Maggi RG, Harms CA, Hohn AA, Pabst DA, McLellan WA, Walton WJ, Rotstein DS, Breitschwerdt EB. Bartonella henselae in porpoise blood. Emerg Infect Dis. 2005 Dec;11(12):1894-8. PMID:16485476

Maggi RG, Kosoy M, Mintzer M, Breitschwerdt EB. Isolation of Candidatus Bartonella melophagi from human blood. Emerg Infect Dis. 2009 Jan;15(1):66-8. PMID:19116054

Maggi RG, Mascarelli PE, Pultorak EL, Hegarty BC, Bradley JM, Mozayeni BR, Breitschwerdt EB. Bartonella spp. bacteremia in high-risk immunocompetent patients. Diagn Microbiol Infect Dis. 2011 Dec;71(4):430-7. Epub 2011 Oct 13. PMID:21996096

Maggi RG, Mozayeni BR, Pultorak EL, Hegarty BC, Bradley JM, Correa M, Breitschwerdt EB. Bartonella spp. Bacteremia and Rheumatic Symptoms in Patients from Lyme Disease-endemic Region. Emerg Infect Dis. 2012 May;18(5):783-91. PMID:22516098

Maggi RG, Raverty SA, Lester SJ, Huff DG, Haulena M, Ford SL, Nielsen O, Robinson JH, Breitschwerdt EB. Bartonella henselae in captive and hunter-harvested beluga (Delphinapterus leucas). J Wildl Dis. 2008 Oct;44(4):871-7. PMID:18957643

Maggi RG, Reichelt S, Toliver M, Engber B. Borrelia species in Ixodes affinis and Ixodes scapularis ticks collected from the coastal plain of North Carolina. Ticks Tick Borne Dis. 2010 Dec;1(4):168-71. Epub 2010 Oct 20. PMID:21771524

Maguina C, Garcia PJ, Gotuzzo E, Cordero L, Spach DH. Bartonellosis (Carrión's disease) in the modern era. Clin Infect Dis. 2001 Sep 15;33(6):772-9. Epub 2001 Aug 10. PMID:11512081

Maguiña C, Gotuzzo E. Bartonellosis. New and old. Infect Dis Clin North Am. 2000 Mar;14(1):1-22, vii. PMID:10738670

Maguiña C, Guerra H, Ventosilla P. Bartonellosis. Clin Dermatol. 2009 May-Jun;27(3):271-80. PMID:19362689

Mahler M, Kessenbrock K, Raats J, Williams R, Fritzler MJ, Blüthner M. Characterization of the human autoimmune response to the major C-terminal epitope of the ribosomal P proteins. J Mol Med (Berl). 2003 Mar;81(3):194-204. Epub 2003 Mar 14. PMID:12682728

Maillard R, Grimard B, Chastant-Maillard S, Chomel B, Delcroix T, Gandoin C, Bouillin C, Halos L, Vayssier-Taussat M, Boulouis HJ. Effects of cow age and pregnancy on Bartonella infection in a herd of dairy cattle. J Clin Microbiol. 2006 Jan;44(1):42-6. PMID:16390945

Maillard R, Petit E, Chomel B, Lacroux C, Schelcher F, Vayssier-Taussat M, Haddad N, Boulouis HJ. Endocarditis in cattle caused by Bartonella bovis. Emerg Infect Dis. 2007 Sep;13(9):1383-5. PMID:18252116

Maillard R, Riegel P, Barrat F, Bouillin C, Thibault D, Gandoin C, Halos L, Demanche C, Alliot A, Guillot J, Piémont Y, Boulouis HJ, Vayssier-Taussat M. Bartonella chomelii sp. nov., isolated from French domestic cattle (Bos taurus). Int J Syst Evol Microbiol. 2004 Jan;54(Pt 1):215-20. PMID:14742483

Maillard R, Vayssier-Taussat M, Bouillin C, Gandoin C, Halos L, Chomel B, Piémont Y, Boulouis HJ. Identification of Bartonella strains isolated from wild and domestic ruminants by a single-step PCR analysis of the 16S-23S intergenic spacer region. Vet Microbiol. 2004 Jan 14;98(1):63-9. PMID:14738783

Malatskey S, Fradis M, Ben-David J, Podoshin L. Cat-scratch disease of the parotid gland: an often-misdiagnosed entity. Ann Otol Rhinol Laryngol. 2000 Jul;109(7):679-82. PMID:10903051

Mallqui V, Speelmon EC, Verástegui M, Maguiña-Vargas C, Pinell-Salles P, Lavarello R, Delgado J, Kosek M, Romero S, Arana Y, Gilman RH. Sonicated diagnostic immunoblot for bartonellosis. Clin Diagn Lab Immunol. 2000 Jan;7(1):1-5. PMID:10618267

Maman E, Bickels J, Ephros M, Paran D, Comaneshter D, Metzkor-Cotter E, Avidor B, Varon-Graidy M, Wientroub S, Giladi M. Musculoskeletal manifestations of cat scratch disease. Clin Infect Dis. 2007 Dec 15;45(12):1535-40. PMID:18190312

Mancino P, Ucciferri C, Falasca K, Racciatti D, Di Girolamo A, Vecchiet J, Pizzigallo E. Inguinal lymphadenopathy due to Bartonella henselae. Infez Med. 2008 Jun;16(2):91-3. PMID:18622149

Mandel L, Surattanont F, Miremadi R. Cat-scratch disease: considerations for dentistry. J Am Dent Assoc. 2001 Jul;132(7):911-4. PMID:11480644

Mändle T, Einsele H, Schaller M, Neumann D, Vogel W, Autenrieth IB, Kempf VA. Infection of human CD34+ progenitor cells with Bartonella henselae results in intraerythrocytic presence of B. henselae. Blood. 2005 Aug 15;106(4):1215-22. Epub 2005 Apr 28. PMID:15860668

Manfredi R, Sabbatani S, Chiodo F. Bartonellosis: light and shadows in diagnostic and therapeutic issues. Clin Microbiol Infect. 2005 Mar;11(3):167-9. PMID:15715712

Manfredi R, Sabbatani S. Bartonellosis: suggestive case reports in adult and pediatric patients and therapeutic issues. Braz J Infect Dis. 2006 Dec;10(6):411-5. PMID:17420917

Mann P, Nye F, Williams G, Walker A, Amadi A. From trench fever to endocarditis. Postgrad Med J. 2003 Nov;79(937):655-6. PMID:14654579

Mansueto P, Di Lorenzo G, Rizzo M, Mazzola G, Affronti M, Battista Rini G, Mansueto S. [Bartonellosis].[Article in Italian]. Recenti Prog Med. 2003 Apr;94(4):177-85. PMID:12677790

Mansueto P, Pepe I, Cillari E, Arcoleo F, Micalizzi A, Bonura F, Seidita A, Palillo L, Di Gregorio MF, Affronti M, Di Rosa S, Rini G, Vitale G. Prevalence of antibodies anti-bartonella henselae in Western sicily: children, blood donors, and cats. J Immunoassay Immunochem. 2012 Jan;33(1):18-25. PMID:22181817

Mantadakis E, Spanaki AM, Psaroulaki A, Fitrolaki D, Minadakis G, Michaeloudi E, Tselentis Y, Briassoulis G. Encephalopathy complicated by Guillain-Barre syndrome and hydrocephalus and associated with acute Bartonella quintana infection. Pediatr Infect Dis J. 2007 Sep;26(9):860-2. PMID:17721391

Marano N, Rupprecht C, Regnery R. Vaccines for emerging infections. Rev Sci Tech. 2007 Apr;26(1):203-15. PMID:17633303

Marchant DJ. Inflammation of the breast. Obstet Gynecol Clin North Am. 2002 Mar;29(1):89-102. PMID:11892876

Margileth AM. Recent Advances in Diagnosis and Treatment of Cat Scratch Disease. Curr Infect Dis Rep. 2000 Apr;2(2):141-146. PMID:11095849

Margolis B, Kuzu I, Herrmann M, Raible MD, Hsi E, Alkan S. Rapid polymerase chain reaction-based confirmation of cat scratch disease and Bartonella henselae infection. Arch Pathol Lab Med. 2003 Jun;127(6):706-10. PMID:12741894

Marié JL, Davoust B, Socolovschi C, Mediannikov O, Roqueplo C, Beaucournu JC, Raoult D, Parola P. Rickettsiae in arthropods collected from red foxes (Vulpes vulpes) in France. Comp Immunol Microbiol Infect Dis. 2012 Jan;35(1):59-62. Epub 2011 Nov 25. PMID:22118782

Marié JL, Fournier PE, Rolain JM, Briolant S, Davoust B, Raoult D. Molecular detection of Bartonella quintana, B. Elizabethae, B. Koehlerae, B. Doshiae, B. Taylorii, and Rickettsia felis in rodent fleas collected in Kabul, Afghanistan. Am J Trop Med Hyg. 2006 Mar;74(3):436-9. PMID:16525103

Marienfeld CB, Dicapua DB, Sze GK, Goldstein JM. Expressive aphasia as a presentation of encephalitis with Bartonella henselae infection in an immunocompetent adult. Yale J Biol Med. 2010 Jun;83(2):67-71. PMID:20589186

Marignac G, Barrat F, Chomel B, Vayssier-Taussat M, Gandoin C, Bouillin C, Boulouis HJ. Murine model for Bartonella birtlesii infection: New aspects. Comp Immunol Microbiol Infect Dis. 2010 Mar;33(2):95-107. Epub 2010 Jan 25. PMID:20097421

Marín M, Muñoz P, Sánchez M, del Rosal M, Alcalá L, Rodríguez-Créixems M, Bouza E; Group for the Management of Infective Endocarditis of the Gregorio Marañón Hospital. Molecular diagnosis of infective endocarditis by real-time broad-range polymerase chain reaction (PCR) and sequencing directly from heart valve tissue. Medicine (Baltimore). 2007 Jul;86(4):195-202. PMID:17632260

Markaki S, Sotiropoulou M, Papaspirou P, Lazaris D. Cat-scratch disease presenting as a solitary tumour in the breast: report of three cases. Eur J Obstet Gynecol Reprod Biol. 2003 Feb 10;106(2):175-8. PMID:12551788

Markov AP, Lopyrev IV, Irkhin AI, Khliap LA, Levitskiĭ SA, Kirillov MIu, Manuvera VA, Il'ina TS, Pokrovskaia MS, Aleshkin GI, Bashkirov VN, Smirnov GB, Kosoĭ M. [Wild small mammals are the reservoir hosts of the Bartonella genus bacteria in the south of Moscow region]. [Article in Russian]. Mol Gen Mikrobiol Virusol. 2006;(4):8-13. PMID:17094651

Márquez FJ, Millán J, Rodríguez-Liébana JJ, García-Egea I, Muniain MA. Detection and identification of Bartonella sp. in fleas from carnivorous mammals in Andalusia, Spain. Med Vet Entomol. 2009 Dec;23(4):393-8. PMID:19941605

Márquez FJ, Rodríguez-Liébana JJ, Pachón-Ibáñez ME, Docobo-Pérez F, Hidalgo-Fontiveros A, Bernabeu-Wittel M, Muniain MA, Pachón J. Molecular screening of Bartonella species in rodents from south western Spain. Vector Borne Zoonotic Dis. 2008 Oct;8(5):695-700. PMID:18620508

Márquez FJ. Molecular detection of Bartonella alsatica in European wild rabbits (Oryctolagus cuniculus) in Andalusia (Spain). Vector Borne Zoonotic Dis. 2010 Oct;10(8):731-4. Epub 2010 Jan 8. PMID:20059317

Marr BP, Shields CL, Shields JA, Eagle RC Jr. Conjunctival cat-scratch disease simulating rhabdomyosarcoma. J Pediatr Ophthalmol Strabismus. 2003 Sep-Oct;40(5):302-3. PMID:14560840

Marseglia GL, Monafo V, Marone P, Meloni F, Martini A, Burgio GR. Asymptomatic persistent pulmonary infiltrates in an immunocompetent boy with cat-scratch disease. Eur J Pediatr. 2001 Apr;160(4):260-1. PMID:11317652

Marsilia GM, La Mura A, Galdiero R, Galdiero E, Aloj G, Ragozzino A. Isolated hepatic involvement of cat scratch disease in immunocompetent adults: Enhanced magnetic resonance imaging, pathological findings, and molecular analysis--two cases. Int J Surg Pathol. 2006 Oct;14(4):349-54. PMID:17041206

Martín Díaz MA, Rubio Flores C, Corral de la Calle M, De Lucas Laguna R. [Cat scratch disease].[Article in Spanish]. An Pediatr (Barc). 2006 Nov;65(5):506-8. PMID:17184616

Martín L, Vidal L, Campins A, Salvá F, Riera M, Carrillo A, Sáez de Ibarra JI. Bartonella as a cause of blood culture-negative endocarditis. Description of five cases.[Article in English, Spanish]. Rev Esp Cardiol. 2009 Jun;62(6):694-7. PMID:19480767

Martinez-Diaz GJ, Kim J, Bruckner AL. A toddler with facial nodules: a case of idiopathic facial aseptic granuloma. Dermatol Online J. 2010 Jan 15;16(1):9. PMID:20137751

Martínez-Osorio H, Calonge M, Torres J, González F. Cat-scratch disease (ocular bartonellosis) presenting as bilateral recurrent iridocyclitis. Clin Infect Dis. 2005 Mar 1;40(5):e43-5. Epub 2005 Feb 1. PMID:15714406

Martini M, Menandro ML, Mondin A, Pasotto D, Mazzariol S, Lauzi S, Stelletta C. Detection of Bartonella bovis in a cattle herd in Italy. Vet Rec. 2008 Jan 12;162(2):58-9. PMID:18192660

Maruyama S, Boonmar S, Morita Y, Sakai T, Tanaka S, Yamaguchi F, Kabeya H, Katsube Y. Seroprevalence of Bartonella henselae and Toxoplasma gondii among healthy individuals in Thailand. J Vet Med Sci. 2000 Jun;62(6):635-7. PMID:10907691

Maruyama S, Izumikawa K, Miyashita M, Kabeya H, Mikami T, Yamanouchi H, Sasaki E, Yoshida H, Izumikawa K. First isolation of Bartonella henselae type I from a cat-scratch disease patient in Japan and its molecular analysis. Microbiol Immunol. 2004;48(2):103-9. PMID:14978335

Maruyama S, Kabeya H, Nakao R, Tanaka S, Sakai T, Xuan X, Katsube Y, Mikami T. Seroprevalence of Bartonella henselae, Toxoplasma gondii, FIV and FeLV infections in domestic cats in Japan. Microbiol Immunol. 2003;47(2):147-53. PMID:12680718

Maruyama S, Kabeya H, Nogami S, Sakai H, Suzuki J, Suzuki H, Sugita H, Katsube Y. Three cases of cat scratch disease diagnosed by indirect immunofluorescence antibody assay and/or polymerase chain reaction of 16S rRNA gene of Bartonella henselae. J Vet Med Sci. 2000 Dec;62(12):1321-4. PMID:11193351

Maruyama S, Kasten RW, Boulouis HJ, Gurfield NA, Katsube Y, Chomel BB. Genomic diversity of Bartonella henselae isolates from domestic cats from Japan, the USA and France by pulsed-field gel electrophoresis. Vet Microbiol. 2001 Apr 19;79(4):337-49. PMID:11267793

Maruyama S, Nakamura Y, Kabeya H, Tanaka S, Sakai T, Katsube Y. Prevalence of Bartonella henselae, Bartonella clarridgeiae and the 16S rRNA gene types of Bartonella henselae among pet cats in Japan. J Vet Med Sci. 2000 Mar;62(3):273-9. PMID:10770599

Maruyama S, Sakai T, Morita Y, Tanaka S, Kabeya H, Boonmar S, Poapolathep A, Chalarmchaikit T, Chang CC, Kasten RW, Chomel BB, Katsube Y. Prevalence of Bartonella species and 16s rRNA gene types of Bartonella henselae from domestic cats in Thailand. Am J Trop Med Hyg. 2001 Dec;65(6):783-7. PMID:11791975

Maruyama S. [Cat-scratch disease].[Article in Japanese]. Nihon Rinsho. 2010 Jun;68 Suppl 6:244-7. PMID:20942049

Maruyama S. [Diagnostic tests: Cat-scratch disease].[Article in Japanese]. Nihon Rinsho. 2005 Jul;63 Suppl 7:237-40. PMID:16111236

Mascarelli PE, Iredell JR, Maggi RG, Weinberg G, Breitschwerdt EB. Bartonella species bacteremia in two patients with epithelioid hemangioendothelioma. J Clin Microbiol. 2011 Nov;49(11):4006-12. Epub 2011 Sep 14. PMID:21918021

Mason JO 3rd. Retinal and optic nerve neovascularization associated with cat scratch neuroretinitis. Retina. 2004 Feb;24(1):176-8. PMID:15076968

Massei F, Gori L, Macchia P, Maggiore G. The expanded spectrum of bartonellosis in children. Infect Dis Clin North Am. 2005 Sep;19(3):691-711. PMID:16102656

Massei F, Gori L, Taddeucci G, Macchia P, Maggiore G. Bartonella henselae infection associated with Guillain-Barre syndrome. Pediatr Infect Dis J. 2006 Jan;25(1):90-1. PMID:16395116

Massei F, Massimetti M, Messina F, Macchia P, Maggiore G. Bartonella henselae and inflammatory bowel disease. Lancet. 2000 Oct 7;356(9237):1245-6. PMID:11072951

Massei F, Messina F, Gori L, Macchia P, Maggiore G. High prevalence of antibodies to Bartonella henselae among Italian children without evidence of cat scratch disease. Clin Infect Dis. 2004 Jan 1;38(1):145-8. Epub 2003 Dec 5. PMID:14679462

Massei F, Messina F, Massimetti M, Macchia P, Maggiore G. Pseudoinfectious mononucleosis: a presentation of Bartonella henselae infection. Arch Dis Child. 2000 Nov;83(5):443-4. PMID:11040157

Massei F, Messina F, Talini I, Massimetti M, Palla G, Macchia P, Maggiore G. Widening of the clinical spectrum of Bartonella henselae infection as recognized through serodiagnostics. Eur J Pediatr. 2000 Jun;159(6):416-9. PMID:10867845

Massung RF, Slater KG. Comparison of PCR assays for detection of the agent of human granulocytic ehrlichiosis, Anaplasma phagocytophilum. J Clin Microbiol. 2003 Feb;41(2):717-22. PMID:12574272

Mastrandrea S, Simonetta Taras M, Capitta P, Tola S, Marras V, Strusi G, Masala G. Detection of Bartonella henselae--DNA in macronodular hepatic lesions of an immunocompetent woman. Clin Microbiol Infect. 2009 Dec;15 Suppl 2:116-7. Epub 2009 Sep 28. PMID:19793123

Masur H, Kaplan JE, Holmes KK; U.S. Public Health Service; Infectious Diseases Society of America. Guidelines for preventing opportunistic infections among HIV-infected persons--2002. Recommendations of the U.S. Public Health Service and the Infectious Diseases Society of America. Ann Intern Med. 2002 Sep 3;137(5 Pt 2):435-78. PMID:12617574

Mateen FJ, Newstead JC, McClean KL. Bacillary angiomatosis in an HIV-positive man with multiple risk factors: A clinical and epidemiological puzzle. Can J Infect Dis Med Microbiol. 2005 Jul;16(4):249-52. PMID:18159553

Matera G, Liberto MC, Joosten LA, Vinci M, Quirino A, Pulicari MC, Kullberg BJ, Van der Meer JW, Netea MG, Focà A. The Janus face of Bartonella quintana recognition by Toll-like receptors (TLRs): a review. Eur Cytokine Netw. 2008 Sep;19(3):113-8. Epub 2008 Sep 8. PMID:18775802

Matera G, Liberto MC, Quirino A, Barreca GS, Lamberti AG, Iannone M, Mancuso E, Palma E, Cufari FA, Rotiroti D, Focà A. Bartonella quintana lipopolysaccharide effects on leukocytes, CXC chemokines and apoptosis: a study on the human whole blood and a rat model. Int Immunopharmacol. 2003 Jun;3(6):853-64. PMID:12781702

Matera G, Muto V, Vinci M, Zicca E, Abdollahi-Roodsaz S, van de Veerdonk FL, Kullberg BJ, Liberto MC, van der Meer JW, Focà A, Netea MG, Joosten LA. Receptor recognition of and immune intracellular pathways for Veillonella parvula lipopolysaccharide. Clin Vaccine Immunol. 2009 Dec;16(12):1804-9. Epub 2009 Oct 14. PMID:19828771

Mathieu S, Vellin JF, Poujol D, Ristori JM, Soubrier M. Cat scratch disease during etanercept therapy. Joint Bone Spine. 2007 Mar;74(2):184-6. Epub 2007 Feb 5. PMID:17337229

Matsumoto K, Berrada ZL, Klinger E, Goethert HK, Telford SR 3rd. Molecular detection of Bartonella schoenbuchensis from ectoparasites of deer in Massachusetts. Vector Borne Zoonotic Dis. 2008 Aug;8(4):549-54. PMID:18454595

Matsumoto K, Cook JA, Goethert HK, Telford SR 3rd. Bartonella sp. Infection of voles trapped from an interior Alaskan site where ticks are absent. J Wildl Dis. 2010 Jan;46(1):173-8. PMID:20090030

Matsuo T, Kato M. Submacular exudates with serous retinal detachment caused by cat scratch disease. Ocul Immunol Inflamm. 2002 Jun;10(2):147-50. PMID:12778351

Matsuo T, Notohara K. Bartonella henselae bacilli detected in vitrectomy aspirates in a patient with massive vitreous opacity with total retinal detachment. Ocul Immunol Inflamm. 2006 Feb;14(1):47-9. PMID:16507491

Matsuo T, Yamaoka A, Shiraga F, Takasu I, Okanouchi T, Nagayama M, Baba T, Hayashi M, Sarada K. Clinical and angiographic characteristics of retinal manifestations in cat scratch disease. Jpn J Ophthalmol. 2000 Mar-Apr;44(2):182-6. PMID:10715390

Maurin M, Raoult D. Isolation in endothelial cell cultures of chlamydia trachomatis LGV (Serovar L2) from a lymph node of a patient with suspected cat scratch disease. J Clin Microbiol. 2000 Jun;38(6):2062-4. PMID:10834954

Maurin M, Rolain JM, Raoult D. Comparison of in-house and commercial slides for detection by immunofluorescence of immunoglobulins G and M against Bartonella henselae and Bartonella quintana. Clin Diagn Lab Immunol. 2002 Sep;9(5):1004-9. PMID:12204950

Mavris M, Saenz H, Monteil M, Boulouis HJ, Dehio C, Vayssier-Taussat M. Characterization of genes involved in long-term bacteremia in mice by Bartonella birtlesii. Ann N Y Acad Sci. 2005 Dec;1063:312-4. PMID:16481533

Mayne PJ. Emerging incidence of Lyme borreliosis, babesiosis, bartonellosis, and granulocytic ehrlichiosis in Australia. Int J Gen Med. 2011;4:845-52. Epub 2011 Dec 16. PMID:22267937

Mba PA, Marié JL, Rolain JM, Davoust B, Beaucournu JC, Raoult D, Parola P. Rickettsia felis and Bartonella henselae in fleas from Lebanon. Vector Borne Zoonotic Dis. 2011 Jul;11(7):991-2. Epub 2011 Feb 1. PMID:21284512

McAvoy CE, Best J, Sharkey JA. Extensive peripapillary exudation secondary to cat-scratch disease. Eye (Lond). 2004 Mar;18(3):331-2. PMID:15004593

McCool TL, Hoey JG, Montileone F, Goldenberg HB, Mordechai E, Adelson ME. Discovery and analysis of Bartonella henselae antigens for use in clinical serologic assays. Diagn Microbiol Infect Dis. 2008 Jan;60(1):17-23. Epub 2007 Sep 21. PMID:17889484

McCord AM, Burgess AW, Whaley MJ, Anderson BE. Interaction of Bartonella henselae with endothelial cells promotes monocyte/macrophage chemoattractant protein 1 gene expression and protein production and triggers monocyte migration. Infect Immun. 2005 Sep;73(9):5735-42. PMID:16113290

McCord AM, Cuevas J, Anderson BE. Bartonella-induced endothelial cell proliferation is mediated by release of calcium from intracellular stores. DNA Cell Biol. 2007 Sep;26(9):657-63. PMID:17678436

McCord AM, Resto-Ruiz SI, Anderson BE. Autocrine role for interleukin-8 in Bartonella henselae-induced angiogenesis. Infect Immun. 2006 Sep;74(9):5185-90. PMID:16926411

McDonald RA, Day MJ, Birtles RJ. Histological evidence of disease in wild stoats (Mustela erminea) in England. Vet Rec. 2001 Dec 1;149(22):671-5. PMID:11765324

McElroy KM, Blagburn BL, Breitschwerdt EB, Mead PS, McQuiston JH. Flea-associated zoonotic diseases of cats in the USA: bartonellosis, flea-borne rickettsioses, and plague. Trends Parasitol. 2010 Apr;26(4):197-204. Epub 2010 Feb 23. PMID:20185369

McEwan J, Basha S, Rogers S, Harkness P. An unusual presentation of cat-scratch disease. J Laryngol Otol. 2001 Oct;115(10):826-8. PMID:11667999

McGill S, Hjelm E, Rajs J, Lindquist O, Friman G. Bartonella spp. antibodies in forensic samples from Swedish heroin addicts. Ann N Y Acad Sci. 2003 Jun;990:409-13. PMID:12860665

McGill S, Rajs J, Hjelm E, Lindquist O, Friman G. A study on forensic samples of Bartonella spp antibodies in Swedish intravenous heroin addicts. APMIS. 2003 Apr;111(4):507-13. PMID:12780526

McGill S, Wesslén L, Hjelm E, Holmberg M, Auvinen MK, Berggren K, Grandin-Jarl B, Johnson U, Wikström S, Friman G. Bartonella spp. Seroprevalence in healthy Swedish blood donors. Scand J Infect Dis. 2005;37(10):723-30. PMID:16191889

McGill S, Wesslen L, Hjelm E, Holmberg M, Rolf C, Friman G. Serological and epidemiological analysis of the prevalence of Bartonella spp. antibodies in Swedish elite orienteers 1992-93. Scand J Infect Dis. 2001;33(6):423-8. PMID:11450861

McLean CR, Hargrove R, Behn E. The first fatal case of capnocytophaga canimorsus sepsis caused by a cat scratch. J R Nav Med Serv. 2004;90(1):13-5. PMID:15457651

McLemore MS, Huo L, Deavers MT, Curry JL, Torres-Cabala CA, Wang WL, Prieto VG. Cutaneous epithelioid angiomatous nodule of the chest wall with expression of estrogen receptor: a mimic of carcinoma and a potential diagnostic pitfall. J Cutan Pathol. 2011 Oct;38(10):818-22. Epub 2011 Jul 14. PMID:21752053

McNeill PM, Verrips A, Mullaart R, Gabreëls FJ, Gabreëls-Festen AW, Knibbeler JG. Chronic inflammatory demyelinating polyneuropathy as a complication of cat scratch disease. J Neurol Neurosurg Psychiatry. 2000 Jun;68(6):797. PMID:10877628

Mediannikov O, Cabre O, Qu F, Socolovschi C, Davoust B, Marié JL, Parola P, Raoult D. Rickettsia felis and Bartonella clarridgeiae in fleas from New Caledonia. Vector Borne Zoonotic Dis. 2011 Feb;11(2):181-3. Epub 2010 Jun 23. PMID:20569017

Mediannikov O, Davoust B, Cabre O, Rolain JM, Raoult D. Bartonellae in animals and vectors in New Caledonia. Comp Immunol Microbiol Infect Dis. 2011 Dec;34(6):497-501. Epub 2011 Oct 20. PMID:22018646

Mediannikov O, Ivanov L, Zdanovskaya N, Vysochina N, Fournier PE, Tarasevich I, Raoult D. Molecular screening of Bartonella species in rodents from the Russian Far East. Ann N Y Acad Sci. 2005 Dec;1063:308-11. PMID:16481532

Mediannikov OIu, Likhoded LIa, Penkina GA, Manzeniuk OIu, Fatalieva SF, Tarasevich IV. [Bartonella and bartonellosis--emerging and re-emerging infections: epidemiology, clinical course, diagnosis]. [Article in Russian]. Zh Mikrobiol Epidemiol Immunobiol. 2005 Jan-Feb;(1):83-9. PMID:15773411

Mediannikov OIu, Likhoded LIa, Penkina GA, Manzeniuk OIu, Fatalieva SF, Tarasevich IV. [Bartonella and bartonellosis--emerging and re-emerging infections. Taxonomy, bacteriology, pathogenesis and genetics].[Article in Russian]. Zh Mikrobiol Epidemiol Immunobiol. 2004 Nov-Dec;(6):113-21. PMID:15636157

Mediannikov OIu, Melikian AL. [A case of cat scratch disease in a patient with diabetes mellitus and chronic renal failure].[Article in Russian]. Klin Med (Mosk). 2006;84(7):61-3. PMID:16924805

Medici Olaso C, García Gariglio L, Ferreira García MI, Giachetto Larraz G, Gutierrez Bottino MC, Pírez García MC. [Cat scratch disease: clinical characteristics in hospitalised children].[Article in Spanish]. An Pediatr (Barc). 2011 Jan;74(1):42-6. PMID:20870475

Medková Z. [Bartonelloses].[Article in Czech]. Klin Mikrobiol Infekc Lek. 2004 Oct;10(5):207-13. PMID:15558448

Meghari S, Rolain JM, Grau GE, Platt E, Barrassi L, Mege JL, Raoult D. Antiangiogenic effect of erythromycin: an in vitro model of Bartonella quintana infection. J Infect Dis. 2006 Feb 1;193(3):380-6. Epub 2005 Dec 27. PMID:16388485

Mehanna D, Peck N, Arnot R, Solano T, Sheldon D. Cat scratch disease presenting as splenic abscess. Aust N Z J Surg. 2000 Aug;70(8):622-4. PMID:10945561

Mehmi M, Lim SP, Tan CY. An unusual cutaneous presentation of cat-scratch disease. Clin Exp Dermatol. 2007 Mar;32(2):219-20. Epub 2006 Dec 14. PMID:17176268

Meininger GR, Nadasdy T, Hruban RH, Bollinger RC, Baughman KL, Hare JM. Chronic active myocarditis following acute Bartonella henselae infection (cat scratch disease). Am J Surg Pathol. 2001 Sep;25(9):1211-4. PMID:11688584

Melikian AL, Mediannikov OIu, Kaplanskaia IB, Komarova AI, Tarasevich IV. [Bartonella infection in hematological practice].[Article in Russian]. Ter Arkh. 2007;79(4):58-62. PMID:17564022

Mellor PJ, Fetz K, Maggi RG, Haugland S, Dunning M, Villiers EJ, Mellanby RJ, Williams D, Breitschwerdt E, Herrtage ME. Alpha1-proteinase inhibitor deficiency and Bartonella infection in association with panniculitis, polyarthritis, and meningitis in a dog. J Vet Intern Med. 2006 Jul-Aug;20(4):1023-8. PMID:16955834

Melter O, Arvand M, Votýpka J, Hulínská D. Bartonella quintana transmission from mite to family with high socioeconomic status. Emerg Infect Dis. 2012 Jan;18(1):163-5. PMID:22257438

Melter O, Hercík K, Weyant RS, Janecek J, Nemec A, Mecera J, Gonzorová L, Branny P. Detection and characterization of feline Bartonella henselae in the Czech Republic. Vet Microbiol. 2003 May 29;93(3):261-73. PMID:12695049

Mennel S, Meyer CH, Schroeder FM. [Multifocal chorioretinitis, papillitis, and recurrent optic neuritis in cat-scratch disease].[Article in French]. J Fr Ophtalmol. 2005 Dec;28(10):e10. PMID:16395190

Merle De Boever C, Mura F, Brun M, Reynes J. [Ocular bartonellosis in an HIV-HVC coinfected patient].[Article in French]. Med Mal Infect. 2008 Sep;38(9):504-6. Epub 2008 Aug 15. PMID:18706780

Merrell DS, Falkow S. Frontal and stealth attack strategies in microbial pathogenesis. Nature. 2004 Jul 8;430(6996):250-6. PMID:15241423

Messam LL, Kasten RW, Ritchie MJ, Chomel BB. Bartonella henselae and domestic cats, Jamaica. Emerg Infect Dis. 2005 Jul;11(7):1146-7. PMID:16032793

Messina F, Doria R, Gabriellini G, Sartini MS, Tascini C, Menichetti F. Bartonella henselae neuroretinitis. Clin Microbiol Infect. 2001 Jul;7(7):387-8. PMID:11531989

Metola Sacristán L, Acha Arrieta V, Merino Rubio C, García de Lucas MD, Casas Fernández de Tejerina JM. [Maxillary osteolysis, bacillary angiomatosis in HIV infection].[Article in Spanish]. An Med Interna. 2001 Mar;18(3):162-3. PMID:11594185

Metz CH, Buer J, Bornfeld N, Lipski A. Bilateral Bartonella henselae neuroretinitis with stellate maculopathy in a 6-year-old boy. Infection. 2012 Apr;40(2):191-4. Epub 2011 Aug 9. PMID:21826435

Metzkor-Cotter E, Kletter Y, Avidor B, Varon M, Golan Y, Ephros M, Giladi M. Long-term serological analysis and clinical follow-up of patients with cat scratch disease. Clin Infect Dis. 2003 Nov 1;37(9):1149-54. Epub 2003 Oct 7. PMID:14557957

Mexas AM, Hancock SI, Breitschwerdt EB. Bartonella henselae and Bartonella elizabethae as potential canine pathogens. J Clin Microbiol. 2002 Dec;40(12):4670-4. PMID:12454170

Meyniel C, Wiertlewski S. [Optic neuritis].[Article in French]. Rev Med Interne. 2010 Jul;31(7):481-5. PMID:20434241

Michau TM, Breitschwerdt EB, Gilger BC, Davidson MG. Bartonella vinsonii subspecies berkhoffi as a possible cause of anterior uveitis and choroiditis in a dog. Vet Ophthalmol. 2003 Dec;6(4):299-304. PMID:14641826

Michos A, Dessypris N, Pourtsidis A, Moschovi M, Polychronopoulou S, Athanasiadou-Piperopoulou F, Kalmanti M, Syriopoulou VP, Mavrouli MD, Petridou ET. Delayed exposure to infections and childhood lymphomas: a case-control study. Cancer Causes Control. 2009 Jul;20(5):795-802. Epub 2009 Jan 25. PMID:19169895

Mietze A, Morick D, Köhler H, Harrus S, Dehio C, Nolte I, Goethe R. Combined MLST and AFLP typing of Bartonella henselae isolated from cats reveals new sequence types and suggests clonal evolution. Vet Microbiol. 2011 Mar 24;148(2-4):238-45. Epub 2010 Sep 21. PMID:20863631

Mietze A, Strube C, Beyerbach M, Schnieder T, Goethe R. Occurrence of Bartonella henselae and Borrelia burgdorferi sensu lato co-infections in ticks collected from humans in Germany. Clin Microbiol Infect. 2011 Jun;17(6):918-20. Epub 2010 Nov 10. PMID:21682805

Miftode E, Luca V. [Bartonella infection].[Article in Romanian]. Rev Med Chir Soc Med Nat Iasi. 2001 Jul-Sep;105(3):486-9. PMID:12092178

Mikolajczyk MG, O'Reilly KL. Clinical disease in kittens inoculated with a pathogenic strain of Bartonella henselae. Am J Vet Res. 2000 Apr;61(4):375-9. PMID:10772100

Mikula I, Vrtiak OJ, Novak M, Sokol J. [The niches and pathways of animal pathogens].[Article in Slovak]. Bratisl Lek Listy. 2000;101(6):340-7. PMID:11039207

Millán J. Comments on the manuscript by Bitam et al., 'Fleas and flea-borne diseases'. Int J Infect Dis. 2011 Mar;15(3):e219. Epub 2010 Dec 28. PMID:21193340

Millar B, Moore J, Mallon P, Xu J, Crowe M, Mcclurg R, Raoult D, Earle J, Hone R, Murphy P. Molecular diagnosis of infective endocarditis--a new Duke's criterion. Scand J Infect Dis. 2001;33(9):673-80. PMID:11669225

Millar BC, Moore JE. Emerging issues in infective endocarditis. Emerg Infect Dis. 2004 Jun;10(6):1110-6. PMID:15207065

Miller DS, Sauther ML, Hunter-Ishikawa M, Fish K, Culbertson H, Cuozzo PF, Campbell TW, Andrews GA, Chavey PS, Nachreiner R, Rumbeiha W, Stacewicz-Sapuntzakis M, Lappin MR. Biomedical evaluation of free-ranging ring-tailed lemurs (Lemur catta) in three habitats at the Beza Mahafaly Special Reserve, Madagascar. J Zoo Wildl Med. 2007 Jun;38(2):201-16. PMID:17679503

Minadakis G, Chochlakis D, Kokkini S, Gikas A, Tselentis Y, Psaroulaki A. Seroprevalence of Bartonella henselae antibodies in blood donors in Crete. Scand J Infect Dis. 2008;40(10):846-7. PMID:18609206

Minga KA, Gberi I, Boka MB, Gourvellec G, Abo Y, Dohoun L, Abe H, Ekra D, Bonard D, Danel C, Huet C, Salamon R, Bondurand A, N'Dri-Yoman T, Anglaret X. [Bacillary angiomatosis in an adult infected with HIV-1 at an early stage of immunodepression in Abidjan, Côte d'Ivoire].[Article in French]. Bull Soc Pathol Exot. 2002 Mar;95(1):34-6. PMID:12012962

Minnick MF, Anderson BE. Bartonella interactions with host cells. Subcell Biochem. 2000;33:97-123. PMID:10804853

Minnick MF, Battisti JM. Pestilence, persistence and pathogenicity: infection strategies of Bartonella. Future Microbiol. 2009 Aug;4(6):743-58. PMID:19659429

Minnick MF, Sappington KN, Smitherman LS, Andersson SG, Karlberg O, Carroll JA. Five-member gene family of Bartonella quintana. Infect Immun. 2003 Feb;71(2):814-21. PMID:12540561

Minnick MF, Smitherman LS, Samuels DS. Mitogenic effect of Bartonella bacilliformis on human vascular endothelial cells and involvement of GroEL. Infect Immun. 2003 Dec;71(12):6933-42. PMID:14638782

Minnick MF, Wilson ZR, Smitherman LS, Samuels DS. gyrA mutations in ciprofloxacin-resistant Bartonella bacilliformis strains obtained in vitro. Antimicrob Agents Chemother. 2003 Jan;47(1):383-6. PMID:12499219

Mirakhur B, Shah SS, Ratner AJ, Goldstein SM, Bell LM, Kim JO. Cat scratch disease presenting as orbital abscess and osteomyelitis. J Clin Microbiol. 2003 Aug;41(8):3991-3. PMID:12904438

Mitchell BM, Font RL. Molecular detection of Bartonella henselae for the diagnosis of cat scratch disease and bacillary angiomatosis of the conjunctiva. Cornea. 2011 Jul;30(7):807-14. PMID:21282991

Miyatake C, Asano T, Mishina-Ikegami K, Takeuchi H, Koizumi S, Hatori T, Fujino O. Cat scratch disease confirmed by immunological and polymerase-chain-reaction-based diagnosis using serum. Pediatr Int. 2010 Apr;52(2):e98-e100. PMID:20500473

Mnif H, Kallel R, Ghorbel R, Znazen A, Gouiaa N, Ellouze S, Makni S, Sellami Boudawara T. [Bacillary angiomatosis].[Article in French]. Ann Dermatol Venereol. 2010 Mar;137(3):248-50. Epub 2010 Feb 1. PMID:20227575

Modi SP, Eppes SC, Klein JD. Cat-scratch disease presenting as multifocal osteomyelitis with thoracic abscess. Pediatr Infect Dis J. 2001 Oct;20(10):1006-7. PMID:11642619

Mofenson LM, Brady MT, Danner SP, Dominguez KL, Hazra R, Handelsman E, Havens P, Nesheim S, Read JS, Serchuck L, Van Dyke R; Centers for Disease Control and Prevention; National Institutes of Health; HIV Medicine Association of the Infectious Diseases Society of America; Pediatric Infectious Diseases Society; American Academy of Pediatrics. Guidelines for the Prevention and Treatment of Opportunistic Infections among HIV-exposed and HIV-infected children: recommendations from CDC, the National Institutes of Health, the HIV Medicine Association of the Infectious Diseases Society of America, the Pediatric Infectious Diseases Society, and the American Academy of Pediatrics. MMWR Recomm Rep. 2009 Sep 4;58(RR-11):1-166. PMID:19730409

Mogollon-Pasapera E, Otvos L Jr, Giordano A, Cassone M. Bartonella: emerging pathogen or emerging awareness? Int J Infect Dis. 2009 Jan;13(1):3-8. Epub 2008 Jul 14. PMID:18621561

Mokhtar AS, Tay ST. Molecular detection of Rickettsia felis, Bartonella henselae, and B. clarridgeiae in fleas from domestic dogs and cats in Malaysia. Am J Trop Med Hyg. 2011 Nov;85(5):931-3. PMID:22049052

Molia S, Chomel BB, Kasten RW, Leutenegger CM, Steele BR, Marker L, Martenson JS, Keet DF, Bengis RG, Peterson RP, Munson L, O'Brien SJ. Prevalence of Bartonella infection in wild African lions (Panthera leo) and cheetahs (Acinonyx jubatus). Vet Microbiol. 2004 May 20;100(1-2):31-41. PMID:15135511

Monks D, Fisher M, Forbes NA. Ixodes frontalis and avian tick-related syndrome in the United Kingdom. J Small Anim Pract. 2006 Aug;47(8):451-5. PMID:16911113

Montcriol A, Benard F, Fenollar F, Ribeiri A, Bonnet M, Collart F, Guidon C. Fatal myocarditis-associated Bartonella quintana endocarditis: a case report. J Med Case Reports. 2009 Jul 17;3:7325. PMID:19830188

Monteil M, Durand B, Bouchouicha R, Petit E, Chomel B, Arvand M, Boulouis HJ, Haddad N. Development of discriminatory multiple-locus variable number tandem repeat analysis for Bartonella henselae. Microbiology. 2007 Apr;153(Pt 4):1141-8. PMID:17379723

Morales SC, Breitschwerdt EB, Washabau RJ, Matise I, Maggi RG, Duncan AW. Detection of Bartonella henselae DNA in two dogs with pyogranulomatous lymphadenitis. J Am Vet Med Assoc. 2007 Mar 1;230(5):681-5. PMID:17331050

Moreillon P, Que YA. Infective endocarditis. Lancet. 2004 Jan 10;363(9403):139-49. PMID:14726169

Morick D, Baneth G, Avidor B, Kosoy MY, Mumcuoglu KY, Mintz D, Eyal O, Goethe R, Mietze A, Shpigel N, Harrus S. Detection of Bartonella spp. in wild rodents in Israel using HRM real-time PCR. Vet Microbiol. 2009 Nov 18;139(3-4):293-7. Epub 2009 Jun 21. PMID:19595521

Morick D, Krasnov BR, Khokhlova IS, Gottlieb Y, Harrus S. Investigation of Bartonella acquisition and transmission in Xenopsylla ramesis fleas (Siphonaptera: Pulicidae). Mol Ecol. 2011 Jul;20(13):2864-70. Epub 2011 Feb 24. PMID:21692752

Morick D, Krasnov BR, Khokhlova IS, Shenbrot GI, Kosoy MY, Harrus S. Bartonella genotypes in fleas (insecta: siphonaptera) collected from rodents in the negev desert, Israel. Appl Environ Microbiol. 2010 Oct;76(20):6864-9. Epub 2010 Aug 27. PMID:20802081

Morick D, Osinga N, Gruys E, Harrus S. Identification of a Bartonella species in the harbor seal (Phoca vitulina) and in seal lice (Echinophtirius horridus). Vector Borne Zoonotic Dis. 2009 Dec;9(6):751-3. PMID:19402763

Morozova OV, Cabello FC, Dobrotvorsky AK. Semi-nested PCR detection of Bartonella henselae in Ixodes persulcatus ticks from Western Siberia, Russia. Vector Borne Zoonotic Dis. 2004 Winter;4(4):306-9. PMID:15671737

Morozova OV, Chernousova NIa, Morozov IV. [Detection of the Bartonella DNA by the method of nested PCR in patients after tick bites in Novosibirsk region].[Article in Russian]. Mol Gen Mikrobiol Virusol. 2005;(4):14-7. PMID:16334219

Mortelé KJ, Segatto E, Ros PR. The infected liver: radiologic-pathologic correlation. Radiographics. 2004 Jul-Aug;24(4):937-55. PMID:15256619

Morway C, Kosoy M, Eisen R, Montenieri J, Sheff K, Reynolds PJ, Powers N. A longitudinal study of Bartonella infection in populations of woodrats and their fleas. J Vector Ecol. 2008 Dec;33(2):353-64. PMID:19263856

Mosbacher M, Elliott SP, Shehab Z, Pinnas JL, Klotz JH, Klotz SA. Cat scratch disease and arthropod vectors: more to it than a scratch? J Am Board Fam Med. 2010 Sep-Oct;23(5):685-6. PMID:20823366

Mosbacher ME, Klotz S, Klotz J, Pinnas JL. Bartonella henselae and the potential for arthropod vector-borne transmission. Vector Borne Zoonotic Dis. 2011 May;11(5):471-7. Epub 2010 Oct 25. PMID:20973657

Mosepele M, Mazo D, Cohn J. Bartonella infection in immunocompromised hosts: immunology of vascular infection and vasoproliferation. Clin Dev Immunol. 2012;2012:612809. Epub 2011 Nov 17. PMID:22162717

Moulin C, Kanitakis J, Ranchin B, Chauvet C, Gillet Y, Morelon E, Euvrard S. Cutaneous bacillary angiomatosis in renal transplant recipients: report of three new cases and literature review. Transpl Infect Dis. 2012 Feb 9. [Epub ahead of print]. PMID:22316326

Müller NF, Kaiser PO, Linke D, Schwarz H, Riess T, Schäfer A, Eble JA, Kempf VA. Trimeric autotransporter adhesin-dependent adherence of Bartonella henselae, Bartonella quintana, and Yersinia enterocolitica to matrix components and endothelial cells under static and dynamic flow conditions. Infect Immun. 2011 Jul;79(7):2544-53. Epub 2011 May 2. PMID:21536788

Muenzel D, Duetsch S, Fauser C, Slotta-Huspenina J, Gaa J, Rummeny EJ, Holzapfel K. Diffusion-weighted magnetic resonance imaging in cervical lymphadenopathy: report of three cases of patients with Bartonella henselae infection mimicking malignant disease. Acta Radiol. 2009 Oct;50(8):914-6. PMID:19636985

Muñana KR, Vitek SM, Hegarty BC, Kordick DL, Breitschwerdt EB. Infection of fetal feline brain cells in culture with Bartonella henselae. Infect Immun. 2001 Jan;69(1):564-9. PMID:11119554

Munson PD, Boyce TG, Salomao DR, Orvidas LJ. Cat-scratch disease of the head and neck in a pediatric population: surgical indications and outcomes. Otolaryngol Head Neck Surg. 2008 Sep;139(3):358-63. PMID:18722212

Murakami K, Tsukahara M, Tsuneoka H, Iino H, Ishida C, Tsujino K, Umeda A, Furuya T, Kawauchi S, Sasaki K. Cat scratch disease: analysis of 130 seropositive cases. J Infect Chemother. 2002 Dec;8(4):349-52. PMID:12525897

Murano I, Tsuneoka H, Iino H, Kamei T, Nakamura I, Tsukahara M. [Two patients with Bartonella henselae infection from a dog]. [Article in Japanese]. Kansenshogaku Zasshi. 2001 Sep;75(9):808-11. PMID:11605190

Murano I, Yoshii H, Kurashige H, Sugio Y, Tsukahara M. Giant hepatic granuloma caused by Bartonella henselae. Pediatr Infect Dis J. 2001 Mar;20(3):319-20. PMID:11303841

Murillo O, Mimbrera D, Petit A, Gil H, Anda P, Carrera M, Podzamczer D. Fatal bacillary angiomatosis mimicking an infiltrative vascular tumour in the immune restoration phase of an HIV-infected patient. Antivir Ther. 2012;17(2):405-7. Epub 2011 Oct 21. PMID:22293094

Murphy M, Ball CA, Gross S. Comparative in vivo adulticidal activity of a topical dinotefuran versus an imidacloprid-based formulation against cat fleas (Ctenocephalides felis) on cats. Vet Ther. 2009 Spring-Summer;10(1-2):9-16. PMID:19742443

Murray MA, Zamecki KJ, Paskowski J, Lelli GJ Jr. Ocular bacillary angiomatosis in an immunocompromised man. Ophthal Plast Reconstr Surg. 2010 Sep-Oct;26(5):371-2. PMID:20683276

Murthy SN, Faden HS, Cohen ME, Bakshi R. Acute disseminated encephalomyelitis in children. Pediatrics. 2002 Aug;110(2 Pt 1):e21. PMID:12165620

Musso T, Badolato R, Ravarino D, Stornello S, Panzanelli P, Merlino C, Savoia D, Cavallo R, Ponzi AN, Zucca M. Interaction of Bartonella henselae with the murine macrophage cell line J774: infection and proinflammatory response. Infect Immun. 2001 Oct;69(10):5974-80. PMID:11553533

Myint KS, Gibbons RV, Iverson J, Shrestha SK, Pavlin JA, Mongkolsirichaikul D, Kosoy MY. Serological response to Bartonella species in febrile patients from Nepal. Trans R Soc Trop Med Hyg. 2011 Dec;105(12):740-2. Epub 2011 Sep 28. PMID:21955739

Mylonakis ME, Koutinas AF, Breitschwerdt EB, Hegarty BC, Billinis CD, Leontides LS, Kontos VS. Chronic canine ehrlichiosis (Ehrlichia canis): a retrospective study of 19 natural cases. J Am Anim Hosp Assoc. 2004 May-Jun;40(3):174-84. PMID:15131097

Naber CK, Erbel R. Infective endocarditis with negative blood cultures. Int J Antimicrob Agents. 2007 Nov;30 Suppl 1:S32-6. Epub 2007 Sep 24. PMID:17890062

Nakamura RK, Zimmerman SA, Lesser MB. Suspected Bartonella-associated myocarditis and supraventricular tachycardia in a cat. J Vet Cardiol. 2011 Dec;13(4):277-81. Epub 2011 Nov 3. PMID:22051527

Namekata DY, Kasten RW, Boman DA, Straub MH, Siperstein-Cook L, Couvelaire K, Chomel BB. Oral shedding of Bartonella in cats: correlation with bacteremia and seropositivity. Vet Microbiol. 2010 Dec 15;146(3-4):371-5. Epub 2010 Jun 1. PMID:20646879

Namekata MS, Clifford DL, Kasten RW, Henn JB, Garcelon DK, Coonan TJ, Chomel BB. Seroprevalence of Bartonella spp. in the endangered island fox (Urocyon littoralis). Vet Microbiol. 2009 Apr 14;136(1-2):184-7. Epub 2008 Oct 28. PMID:19058928

Nelder MP, Reeves WK, Adler PH, Wozniak A, Wills W. Ectoparasites and associated pathogens of free-roaming and captive animals in zoos of South Carolina. Vector Borne Zoonotic Dis. 2009 Oct;9(5):469-77. PMID:18973443

Nghiem PP, Schatzberg SJ. Conventional and molecular diagnostic testing for the acute neurologic patient. J Vet Emerg Crit Care (San Antonio). 2010 Feb;20(1):46-61. PMID:20230434

Niedzielska G, Kotowski M, Niedzielski A, Dybiec E, Wieczorek P. Cervical lymphadenopathy in children--incidence and diagnostic management. Int J Pediatr Otorhinolaryngol. 2007 Jan;71(1):51-6. Epub 2006 Nov 9. PMID:17097154

Nijssen E, Cescau S, Vayssier-Taussat M, Wang J, Biville F. Identification of mechanisms involved in iron and haem uptake in Bartonella birtlesii: in silico and in vivo approaches. Clin Microbiol Infect. 2009 Dec;15 Suppl 2:118-9. Epub 2009 Apr 30. PMID:19438629

Nilsson K, Liu A, Påhlson C, Lindquist O. Demonstration of intracellular microorganisms (Rickettsia spp., Chlamydia pneumoniae, Bartonella spp.) in pathological human aortic valves by PCR. J Infect. 2005 Jan;50(1):46-52. PMID:15603840

Nishio N, Kubota T, Nakao Y, Hidaka H. Cat scratch disease with encephalopathy in a 9-year-old girl. Pediatr Int. 2008 Dec;50(6):823-4. PMID:19067901

No authors listed. Cat-scratch disease in children--Texas, September 2000 to August 2001. Can Commun Dis Rep. 2002 Apr 15;28(8):64-7. [Article in English, French]. PMID:11974428

Nowakowski GS, Katz A. Epilepsia partialis continua as an atypical presentation of cat scratch disease in a young adult. Neurology. 2002 Dec 10;59(11):1815-6. PMID:12473786

Nowicki M. Persistent abdominal pain: commentary. Clin Pediatr (Phila). 2005 Jul-Aug;44(6):554-5. PMID:16015407

Nthumba PM. Giant pyogenic granuloma of the thigh: a case report. J Med Case Reports. 2008 Mar 31;2:95. PMID:18377654

Numazaki K, Chiba S, Ueno H. Bartonella hensela in inflammatory bowel disease. Lancet. 2001 Jun 16;357(9272):1974-5. PMID:11430386

Numazaki K, Ueno H, Yokoo K, Muramatsu Y, Chiba S, Morita C. Detection of serum antibodies to Bartonella henselae and Coxiella burnetii from Japanese children and pregnant women. Microbes Infect. 2000 Oct;2(12):1431-4. PMID:11099929

Nutter FB, Dubey JP, Levine JF, Breitschwerdt EB, Ford RB, Stoskopf MK. Seroprevalences of antibodies against Bartonella henselae and Toxoplasma gondii and fecal shedding of Cryptosporidium spp, Giardia spp, and Toxocara cati in feral and pet domestic cats. J Am Vet Med Assoc. 2004 Nov 1;225(9):1394-8. PMID:15552314

Nystedt B, Frank AC, Thollesson M, Andersson SG. Diversifying selection and concerted evolution of a type IV secretion system in Bartonella. Mol Biol Evol. 2008 Feb;25(2):287-300. Epub 2007 Dec 7. PMID:18065487

Odenthal M, Koenig S, Farbrother P, Drebber U, Bury Y, Dienes HP, Eichinger L. Detection of opportunistic infections by low-density microarrays: a diagnostic approach for granulomatous lymphadenitis. Diagn Mol Pathol. 2007 Mar;16(1):18-26. PMID:17471154

Ogura K, Hara Y, Tsukahara H, Maeda M, Tsukahara M, Mayumi M. MR signal changes in a child with cat scratch disease encephalopathy and status epilepticus. Eur Neurol. 2004;51(2):109-10. Epub 2004 Feb 11. PMID:14963382

Ohad DG, Morick D, Avidor B, Harrus S. Molecular detection of Bartonella henselae and Bartonella koehlerae from aortic valves of Boxer dogs with infective endocarditis. Vet Microbiol. 2010 Feb 24;141(1-2):182-5. Epub 2009 Aug 8. PMID:19716241

Ohl ME, Spach DH. Bartonella quintana and urban trench fever. Clin Infect Dis. 2000 Jul;31(1):131-5. Epub 2000 Jul 25. PMID:10913410

Ohnishi H, Mizunoe Y, Takade A, Tanaka Y, Miyamoto H, Harada M, Yoshida S. Legionella dumoffii DjlA, a member of the DnaJ family, is required for intracellular growth. Infect Immun. 2004 Jun;72(6):3592-603. PMID:15155669

Okamoto M, Murai K, Okayama A, Sekiya R, Kataoka H, Iino H, Tsuneoka H, Tsukahara M, Tsubouchi H. [An adult case of systemic cat-scratch disease with hepatosplenic involvement].[Article in Japanese]. Kansenshogaku Zasshi. 2001 Jun;75(6):499-503. PMID:11494569

Olarte L, Ampofo K, Thorell EA, Sanderson S, Doby E, Pavia AT, Rosado H, Raoult D, Socolovschi C, Hersh AL. Bartonella vinsonii Endocarditis in an Adolescent With Congenital Heart Disease. Pediatr Infect Dis J. 2012 May;31(5):531-4. PMID:22301474

Oldrini G, Denny P, Becker S, Alexandre JL, Thomas D. [Systemic cat scratch disease in an immunocompetent adult].[Article in French]. J Radiol. 2009 Mar;90(3 Pt 1):318-21. PMID:19421118

Oliveira AM, Maggi RG, Woods CW, Breitschwerdt EB. Suspected needle stick transmission of Bartonella vinsonii subspecies berkhoffii to a veterinarian. J Vet Intern Med. 2010 Sep-Oct;24(5):1229-32. Epub 2010 Jul 28. PMID:20695992

Oliver MK, Telfer S, Piertney SB. Major histocompatibility complex (MHC) heterozygote superiority to natural multi-parasite infections in the water vole (Arvicola terrestris). Proc Biol Sci. 2009 Mar 22;276(1659):1119-28. PMID:19129114

Oman K, Norton R, Gunawardane K. Bartonella henselae infective endocarditis in north Queensland. Intern Med J. 2003 Jan-Feb;33(1-2):55-6. PMID:12534881

O'Reilly KL, Parr KA, Brown TP, Tedder-Ferguson B, Scholl DT. Passive antibody to Bartonella henselae protects against clinical disease following homologous challenge but does not prevent bacteremia in cats. Infect Immun. 2001 Mar;69(3):1880-2. PMID:11179367

O'Rourke F, Schmidgen T, Kaiser PO, Linke D, Kempf VA. Adhesins of Bartonella spp. Adv Exp Med Biol. 2011;715:51-70. PMID:21557057

O'Rourke K. Zoonotic risks of pets: how to handle questions. J Am Vet Med Assoc. 2002 May 15;220(10):1439, 1442. PMID:12018364

O'Rourke LG, Pitulle C, Hegarty BC, Kraycirik S, Killary KA, Grosenstein P, Brown JW, Breitschwerdt EB. Bartonella quintana in cynomolgus monkey (Macaca fascicularis). Emerg Infect Dis. 2005 Dec;11(12):1931-4. PMID:16485482

Ortiz-Santamaría V, Tural Llacher C, Pérez Andrés R, Olivé Marqués A. [Bacillary angiomatosis or Kaposi's sarcoma].[Article in Spanish]. Rev Clin Esp. 2004 Aug;204(8):440. PMID:15274773

Oskouizadeh K, Zahraei-Salehi T, Aledavood S. Detection of Bartonella henselae in domestic cats' saliva. Iran J Microbiol. 2010 Jun;2(2):80-4. PMID:22347553

Oteo JA, Castilla A, Arosey A, Blanco JR, Ibarra V, Morano LE. [Endocarditis due to Bartonella spp. Three new clinical cases and Spanish literature review].[Article in Spanish]. Enferm Infecc Microbiol Clin. 2006 May;24(5):297-301. PMID:16762254

Otranto D, de Caprariis D, Lia RP, Tarallo V, Lorusso V, Testini G, Dantas-Torres F, Latrofa S, Diniz PP, Mencke N, Maggi RG, Breitschwerdt E, Capelli G, Stanneck D. Prevention of endemic canine vector-borne diseases using imidacloprid 10% and permethrin 50% in young dogs: a longitudinal field study. Vet Parasitol. 2010 Sep 20;172(3-4):323-32. Epub 2010 May 25. PMID:20591573

Padmalayam I, Fiskus W, Massung RF, Baumstark BR. Molecular cloning and analysis of a region of the Bartonella bacilliformis genome encoding NlpD, L-isoaspartyl methyltransferase and YajC homologs. DNA Cell Biol. 2003 May;22(5):347-53. PMID:12941162

Padmalayam I, Karem K, Baumstark B, Massung R. The gene encoding the 17-kDa antigen of Bartonella henselae is located within a cluster of genes homologous to the virB virulence operon. DNA Cell Biol. 2000 Jun;19(6):377-82. PMID:10882236

Padmalayam I, Kelly T, Baumstark B, Massung R. Molecular cloning, sequencing, expression, and characterization of an immunogenic 43-kilodalton lipoprotein of Bartonella bacilliformis that has homology to NlpD/LppB. Infect Immun. 2000 Sep;68(9):4972-9. PMID:10948113

Paitoonpong L, Chitsomkasem A, Chantrakooptungool S, Kanjanahareutai S, Tribuddharat C, Srifuengfung S. Bartonella henselae: first reported isolate in a human in Thailand. Southeast Asian J Trop Med Public Health. 2008 Jan;39(1):123-9. PMID:18567451

Palanivelu DV, Goepfert A, Meury M, Guye P, Dehio C, Schirmer T. Fic domain-catalyzed adenylylation: insight provided by the structural analysis of the type IV secretion system effector BepA. Protein Sci. 2011 Mar;20(3):492-9. Epub 2011 Feb 17. PMID:21213248

Palmero J, Pusterla N, Cherry NA, Kasten RW, Mapes S, Boulouis HJ, Breitschwerdt EB, Chomel BB. Experimental infection of horses with Bartonella henselae and Bartonella bovis. J Vet Intern Med. 2012 Mar-Apr;26(2):377-83. Epub 2012 Feb 22. PMID:22356473

Palumbo E, Sodini F, Boscarelli G, Nasca G, Branchi M, Pellegrini G. Immune thrombocytopenic purpura as a complication of Bartonella henselae infection. Infez Med. 2008 Jun;16(2):99-102. PMID:18622151

Pamo OG. Daniel Carrion's experiment: the use of self-infection in the advance of medicine. J R Coll Physicians Edinb. 2012 Mar;42(1):81-6. PMID:22441071

Pandak N, Daković-Rode O, Cabraja I, Kristof Z, Kotarac S. Prevalence of Bartonella henselae antibodies in children and blood donors in Croatia. Infection. 2009 Apr;37(2):166-7. Epub 2009 Mar 9. PMID:19274430

Papadopouli E, Michailidi E, Papadopoulou E, Paspalaki P, Vlahakis I, Kalmanti M. Cervical lymphadenopathy in childhood epidemiology and management. Pediatr Hematol Oncol. 2009 Sep;26(6):454-60. PMID:19657996

Papadopoulos NG, Gourgiotis D, Bossios A, Fretzayas A, Moustaki M, Karpathios T. Circulating cytokines in patients with cat scratch disease. Clin Infect Dis. 2001 Sep 15;33(6):e54-6. Epub 2001 Aug 13. PMID:11512109

Papagrigorakis MJ, Yapijakis C, Synodinos PN, Baziotopoulou-Valavani E. DNA examination of ancient dental pulp incriminates typhoid fever as a probable cause of the Plague of Athens. Int J Infect Dis. 2006 May;10(3):206-14. Epub 2006 Jan 18. PMID:16412683

Papakonstantinou O, Bakantaki A, Paspalaki P, Charoulakis N, Gourtsoyiannis N. High-resolution and color Doppler ultrasonography of cervical lymphadenopathy in children. Acta Radiol. 2001 Sep;42(5):470-6. PMID:11552884

Pape M, Kollaras P, Mandraveli K, Tsona A, Metallidis S, Nikolaidis P, Alexiou-Daniel S. Occurrence of Bartonella henselae and Bartonella quintana among human immunodeficiency virus-infected patients. Ann N Y Acad Sci. 2005 Dec;1063:299-301. PMID:16481530

Pape M, Mandraveli K, Alexiou-Daniel S. Clinical aspects of Bartonella infection in northern Greece. Clin Microbiol Infect. 2009 Dec;15 Suppl 2:91-2. Epub 2009 May 18. PMID:19456804

Pappalardo BL, Brown T, Gebhardt D, Sontakke S, Breitschwerdt EB. Cyclic CD8+ lymphopenia in dogs experimentally infected with Bartonella vinsonii subsp. berkhoffii. Vet Immunol Immunopathol. 2000 Jun 30;75(1-2):43-57. PMID:10889298

Pappalardo BL, Brown T, Gookin JL, Morrill CL, Breitschwerdt EB. Granulomatous disease associated with Bartonella infection in 2 dogs. J Vet Intern Med. 2000 Jan-Feb;14(1):37-42. PMID:10668815

Pappalardo BL, Brown TT, Tompkins M, Breitschwerdt EB. Immunopathology of Bartonella vinsonii (berkhoffii) in experimentally infected dogs. Vet Immunol Immunopathol. 2001 Dec;83(3-4):125-47. PMID:11730925

Parisi E, Glick M. Cervical lymphadenopathy in the dental patient: a review of clinical approach. Quintessence Int. 2005 Jun;36(6):423-36. PMID:15954248

Park SY, Kelminson KL, Lee AK, Zhang P, Warner RE, Rehkopf DH, Calderwood SB, Koehler JE. Identification, characterization, and functional analysis of a gene encoding the ferric uptake regulation protein in Bartonella species. J Bacteriol. 2001 Oct;183(19):5751-5. PMID:11544240

Parola P, Fournier PE, Raoult D. Bartonella quintana, lice, and molecular tools. J Med Entomol. 2006 Sep;43(5):787; author reply 788. PMID:17017209

Parola P, Sanogo OY, Lerdthusnee K, Zeaiter Z, Chauvancy G, Gonzalez JP, Miller RS, Telford SR 3rd, Wongsrichanalai C, Raoult D. Identification of Rickettsia spp. and Bartonella spp. in ffrom the Thai-Myanmar border. Ann N Y Acad Sci. 2003 Jun;990:173-81. PMID:12860622

Parola P, Shpynov S, Montoya M, Lopez M, Houpikian P, Zeaiter Z, Guerra H, Raoult D. First molecular evidence of new Bartonella spp. in fleas and a tick from Peru. Am J Trop Med Hyg. 2002 Aug;67(2):135-6. PMID:12389935

Parrow NL, Abbott J, Lockwood AR, Battisti JM, Minnick MF. Function, regulation, and transcriptional organization of the hemin utilization locus of Bartonella quintana. Infect Immun. 2009 Jan;77(1):307-16. Epub 2008 Nov 3. PMID:18981245

Pasticci MB, Di Candilo F, Egidi MA, Lapalorcia LM, Marroni M, Tinca E, Sfara C, Stagni G. Bartonella henselae lymphadenitis progressing to hepatosplenic disease with slow clinical response despite early diagnosis and treatment. Int J Clin Pract. 2008 Dec;62(12):1956-7. Epub 2007 Mar 1. PMID:17343673

Patel SJ, Petrarca R, Shah SM, Zimmer-Galler I, Janjua KA, Do DV, Nguyen QD. Atypical Bartonella hensalae chorioretinitis in an immunocompromised patient. Ocul Immunol Inflamm. 2008 Jan-Feb;16(1):45-9. PMID:18379943

Patel UD, Hollander H, Saint S. Clinical problem-solving. Index of suspicion. N Engl J Med. 2004 May 6;350(19):1990-5. PMID:15128900

Pavlidakey PG, Burroughs C, Karrs T, Somach SC. Cutaneous epithelioid angiomatous nodule: a case with metachronous lesions. Am J Dermatopathol. 2011 Dec;33(8):831-4. PMID:21931284

Pawelczyk A, Bajer A, Behnke JM, Gilbert FS, Sinski E. Factors affecting the component community structure of haemoparasites in common voles (Microtus arvalis) from the Mazury Lake District region of Poland. Parasitol Res. 2004 Mar;92(4):270-84. Epub 2004 Jan 9. PMID:14714180

Paziewska A, Harris PD, Zwolińska L, Bajer A, Siński E. Differences in the ecology of Bartonella infections of Apodemus flavicollis and Myodes glareolus in a boreal forest. Parasitology. 2012 Feb 16:1-13. [Epub ahead of print]. PMID:22336264

Paziewska A, Harris PD, Zwolińska L, Bajer A, Siński E. Recombination within and between species of the alpha proteobacterium Bartonella infecting rodents. Microb Ecol. 2011 Jan;61(1):134-45. Epub 2010 Aug 26. PMID:20740281

Paziewska A, Siński E, Harris PD. Recombination, Diversity and Allele Sharing of Infectivity Proteins Between Bartonella Species from Rodents. Microb Ecol. 2012 Mar 15. [Epub ahead of print]. PMID:22419104

Paziewska A. [Diversity of blood parasites of genus Bartonella in wild rodents in Mazury Lakes District].[Article in Polish]. Wiad Parazytol. 2011;57(1):53-4. PMID:21638804

Peacock A, Pearson W. The Peacock versus the louse (pediculus humanus corporis): one soldier's contribution to combating trench fever in the First World War. J R Coll Physicians Edinb. 2010 Sep;40(3):256-62. PMID:20973437

Pearce LK, Radecki SV, Brewer M, Lappin MR. Prevalence of Bartonella henselae antibodies in serum of cats with and without clinical signs of central nervous system disease. J Feline Med Surg. 2006 Oct;8(5):315-20. Epub 2006 Sep 1. PMID:16949848

Pedersen BK. [Bartonella bacterium is suspected as the cause of sudden death among Swedish cross-country runners].[Article in Danish]. Ugeskr Laeger. 2001 May 21;163(21):2951. PMID:11402978

Pedersen BK. Sudden cardiac death in Swedish orienteers--a mystery solved? Scand J Med Sci Sports. 2001 Oct;11(5):259. PMID:11696208

Pelton SI, Kim JY, Kradin RL. Case records of the Massachusetts General Hospital. Case 27-2006. A 17-year-old boy with fever and lesions in the liver and spleen. N Engl J Med. 2006 Aug 31;355(9):941-8. PMID:16943407

Pendle S, Ginn A, Iredell J. Antimicrobial susceptibility of Bartonella henselae using Etest methodology. J Antimicrob Chemother. 2006 Apr;57(4):761-3. Epub 2006 Feb 7. PMID:16464897

Pennisi MG, La Camera E, Giacobbe L, Orlandella BM, Lentini V, Zummo S, Fera MT. Molecular detection of Bartonella henselae and Bartonella clarridgeiae in clinical samples of pet cats from Southern Italy. Res Vet Sci. 2010 Jun;88(3):379-84. Epub 2009 Dec 5. PMID:19963231

Perez C, Hummel JB, Keene BW, Maggi RG, Diniz PP, Breitschwerdt EB. Successful treatment of Bartonella henselae endocarditis in a cat. J Feline Med Surg. 2010 Jun;12(6):483-6. Epub 2010 Feb 6. PMID:20138559

Pérez C, Maggi RG, Diniz PP, Breitschwerdt EB. Molecular and serological diagnosis of Bartonella infection in 61 dogs from the United States. J Vet Intern Med. 2011 Jul-Aug;25(4):805-10. Epub 2011 May 25. PMID:21615498

Pérez G J, Munita S JM, Araos B R, López G JP, Stevenson A R, González A P, Pérez C D, Noriega R LM. [Cat scratch disease associated neuroretinitis: clinical report and review of the literature]. [Article in Spanish]. Rev Chilena Infectol. 2010 Oct;27(5):417-22. PMID:21186508

Pérez-Gil J, Calisto BM, Behrendt C, Kurz T, Fita I, Rodríguez-Concepción M. Crystal Structure of Brucella abortus Deoxyxylulose-5-phosphate Reductoisomerase-like (DRL) Enzyme Involved in Isoprenoid Biosynthesis. J Biol Chem. 2012 May 4;287(19):15803-9. Epub 2012 Mar 22. PMID:22442144

Pérez-Irezábal J, Aguirrebengoa K, Cilla G. [Endocarditis due to Bartonella spp. Three new clinical cases and Spanish literature review].[Article in Spanish]. Enferm Infecc Microbiol Clin. 2006 Nov;24(9):597. PMID:17125688

Pérez-Martínez L, Blanco JR, Oteo JA. [Treatment of human infections caused by Bartonella spp].[Article in Spanish]. Rev Esp Quimioter. 2010 Sep;23(3):109-14. PMID:20844840

Pérez-Martínez L, Venzal JM, González-Acuña D, Portillo A, Blanco JR, Oteo JA. Bartonella rochalimae and other Bartonella spp. in fleas, Chile. Emerg Infect Dis. 2009 Jul;15(7):1150-2. PMID:19624952

Pérez-Salcedo L, Herrera D, Esteban-Saltiveri D, León R, Jeusette I, Torre C, O'Connor A, González I, Sanz M. Comparison of two sampling methods for microbiological evaluation of periodontal disease in cats. Vet Microbiol. 2011 May 5;149(3-4):500-3. Epub 2010 Nov 21. PMID:21168288

Perry A, Ramdass MJ, Maharaj D, Naraynsingh V. Cat-scratch disease of the upper limb with ulnar nerve involvement. Am J Orthop (Belle Mead NJ). 2004 Jul;33(7):349-50. PMID:15344577

Pesavento PA, Chomel BB, Kasten RW, McDonald KA, Mohr FC. Pathology of bartonella endocarditis in six dogs. Vet Pathol. 2005 May;42(3):370-3. PMID:15872387

Petanides TA, Koutinas AF, Mylonakis ME, Day MJ, Saridomichelakis MN, Leontides LS, Mischke R, Diniz P, Breitschwerdt EB, Kritsepi M, Garipidou VA, Koutinas CK, Lekkas S. Factors associated with the occurrence of epistaxis in natural canine leishmaniasis (Leishmania infantum). J Vet Intern Med. 2008 Jul-Aug;22(4):866-72. PMID:18564224

Petersen K, Earhart KC, Wallace MR. Bacillary angiomatosis in a patient with chronic lymphocytic leukemia. Infection. 2008 Oct;36(5):480-4. Epub 2007 Dec 28. PMID:18165862

Petrogiannopoulos C, Valla K, Mikelis A, Kalogeropoulos SG, Karachalios G, Karachaliou I, Skandami I. Parotid mass due to cat scratch disease. Int J Clin Pract. 2006 Dec;60(12):1679-80. Epub 2006 Mar 27. PMID:16669837

Pfrommer S, Maier M, Mayer C, Erben A, Engelmann V, Lohmann CP. [Vasoproliferative retinal tumours].[Article in German]. Ophthalmologe. 2011 Mar;108(3):265-8. PMID:21153829

Philip J, Bhatia S, Sugar A, Berry N, Ruddy M. Mycobacterium lentiflavum--a cause of infections in the head and neck: case report and literature review. J Oral Maxillofac Surg. 2011 Apr;69(4):1114-6. Epub 2010 Jul 31. PMID:20674119

Philippon A. [Bacterial zoonoses: emerging concepts].[Article in French]. Bull Acad Natl Med. 2006 Mar;190(3):579-94; discussion 595, 625-7. PMID:17140097

Pieh C, Ness T, Lagrèze WA. [Cotton wool spots in a 16-year-old girl].[Article in German]. Ophthalmologe. 2005 May;102(5):524-6. PMID:15095109

Piémont Y, Bermond D. [Infections caused by Bartonella spp].[Article in French]. Ann Biol Clin (Paris). 2001 Sep-Oct;59(5):593-604. PMID:11602390

Piérard-Franchimont C, Quatresooz P, Piérard GE. Skin diseases associated with Bartonella infection: facts and controversies. Clin Dermatol. 2010 Sep-Oct;28(5):483-8. PMID:20797506

Pignataro L, Torretta S, Capaccio P, Esposito S, Marchisio P. Unusual otolaryngological manifestations of certain systemic bacterial and fungal infections in children. Int J Pediatr Otorhinolaryngol. 2009 Dec;73 Suppl 1:S33-7. PMID:20114153

Pinilla Moraza J, Labarga Echevarría P, Cachorro San Pedro I. [Inguinal mass as presentation of cat-scratch disease].[Article in Spanish]. An Med Interna. 2005 Aug;22(8):400-1. PMID:16358433

Pinna A, Puglia E, Dore S. Unusual retinal manifestations of cat scratch disease. Int Ophthalmol. 2011 Apr;31(2):125-8. Epub 2011 Jan 26. PMID:21267628

Pinna Parpaglia ML, Masu G, Masala G, Porcu R, Zobba R, Pintori G, Cocco R. Seroprevalence of Bartonella henselae in dogs and cats in Sassari. Vet Res Commun. 2007 Aug;31 Suppl 1:317-20. PMID:17682904

Pinto Jr VL, Curi AL, Pinto Ada S, Nunes EP, Teixeira Mde L, Rozental T, Favacho AR, Castro EL, Bóia MN. Cat scratch disease complicated with aseptic meningitis and neuroretinitis. Braz J Infect Dis. 2008 Apr;12(2):158-60. PMID:18641856

Pipili C, Katsogridakis K, Cholongitas E. Myocarditis due to Bartonella henselae. South Med J. 2008 Nov;101(11):1186. PMID:19088543

Pitassi LH, Cintra ML, Ferreira MR, Magalhães RF, Velho PE. Blood cell findings resembling Bartonella spp. Ultrastruct Pathol. 2010 Feb;34(1):2-6. PMID:20070147

Pitassi LH, Magalhães RF, Barjas-Castro ML, de Paula EV, Ferreira MR, Velho PE. Bartonella henselae infects human erythrocytes. Ultrastruct Pathol. 2007 Nov-Dec;31(6):369-72. PMID:18098053

Pitchford CW, Creech CB 2nd, Peters TR, Vnencak-Jones CL. Bartonella henselae endocarditis in a child. Pediatr Cardiol. 2006 Nov-Dec;27(6):769-71. Epub 2006 Nov 16. PMID:17111290

Pitulle C, Strehse C, Brown JW, Breitschwerdt EB. Investigation of the phylogenetic relationships within the genus Bartonella based on comparative sequence analysis of the rnpB gene, 16S rDNA and 23S rDNA. Int J Syst Evol Microbiol. 2002 Nov;52(Pt 6):2075-80. PMID:12508871

Plettenberg A, Lorenzen T, Burtsche BT, Rasokat H, Kaliebe T, Albrecht H, Mertensközter T, Bogner JR, Stoehr A, Schöfer H. Bacillary angiomatosis in HIV-infected patients--an epidemiological and clinical study. Dermatology. 2000;201(4):326-31. PMID:11146343

Pocheville I, Morteruel E, Alvarez J, Pérez-Irezabal J. [Vertebral osteomyelitis associated with cat scratch disease].[Article in Spanish]. Enferm Infecc Microbiol Clin. 2002 Dec;20(10):538-9. PMID:12433360

Podglajen I, Bellery F, Poyart C, Coudol P, Buu-Hoï A, Bruneval P, Mainardi JL. Comparative molecular and microbiologic diagnosis of bacterial endocarditis. Emerg Infect Dis. 2003 Dec;9(12):1543-7. PMID:14720393

Podsiadły E, Chmielewski T, Karbowiak G, Kędra E, Tylewska-Wierzbanowska S. The occurrence of spotted fever rickettsioses and other tick-borne infections in forest workers in Poland. Vector Borne Zoonotic Dis. 2011 Jul;11(7):985-9. Epub 2010 Nov 17. PMID:21083370

Podsiadly E, Chmielewski T, Marczak R, Sochon E, Tylewska-Wierzbanowska S. Bartonella henselae in the human environment in Poland. Scand J Infect Dis. 2007;39(11-12):956-62. Epub 2007 Jun 1. PMID:17852890

Podsiadly E, Chmielewski T, Sochon E, Tylewska-Wierzbanowska S. Bartonella henselae in Ixodes ricinus ticks removed from dogs. Vector Borne Zoonotic Dis. 2007 Summer;7(2):189-92. PMID:17627437

Podsiadły E, Chmielewski T, Tylewska-Wierzbanowska S. Bartonella henselae and Borrelia burgdorferi infections of the central nervous system. Ann N Y Acad Sci. 2003 Jun;990:404-6. PMID:12860663

Podsiadly E, Karbowiak G, Tylewska-Wierzbanowska S. Presence of Bartonella spp. in Ixodidae ticks. Clin Microbiol Infect. 2009 Dec;15 Suppl 2:120-1. Epub 2009 Mar 26. PMID:19416286

Podsiadły E, Sapiejka E, Dabrowska-Bień J, Majkowski J, Tylewska-Wierzbanowska S. [Diagnostics of cat scratch disease and present methods of bartonellosis recognition--a case report].[Article in Polish]. Pol Merkur Lekarski. 2009 Feb;26(152):131-5. PMID:19388519

Podsiadły E, Sokołowska E, Tylewska-Wierzbanowska S. [Seroprevalence of Bartonella henselae and Bartonella quintana infections in Poland in 1998-2001].[Article in Polish]. Przegl Epidemiol. 2002;56(3):399-407. PMID:12608089

Podsiadły E, Sokolowska E, Tylewska-Wierzbanowska S. Seroprevalence of Bartonella henselae and Bartonella quintana infections in Poland in 1998-2001. Ann N Y Acad Sci. 2003 Jun;990:407-8. PMID:12860664

Pons I, Sanfeliu I, Cardeñosa N, Nogueras MM, Font B, Segura F. Serological evidence of Bartonella henselae infection in healthy people in Catalonia, Spain. Epidemiol Infect. 2008 Dec;136(12):1712-6. Epub 2008 Feb 25. PMID:18294428

Pons I, Sanfeliu I, Nogueras MM, Sala M, Cervantes M, Amengual MJ, Segura F. Seroprevalence of Bartonella spp. infection in HIV patients in Catalonia, Spain. BMC Infect Dis. 2008 May 1;8:58. PMID:18452613

Pons I, Sanfeliu I, Quesada M, Anton E, Sampere M, Font B, Pla J, Segura F. Prevalence of Bartonella henselae in cats in Catalonia, Spain. Am J Trop Med Hyg. 2005 Apr;72(4):453-7. PMID:15827285

Pont M, Delaporte E, Patenotre P, Piette F. [A cat scratch and finger swelling].[Article in French]. Ann Dermatol Venereol. 2000 Dec;127(12):1103-4. PMID:11173693

Popa C, Abdollahi-Roodsaz S, Joosten LA, Takahashi N, Sprong T, Matera G, Liberto MC, Foca A, van Deuren M, Kullberg BJ, van den Berg WB, van der Meer JW, Netea MG. Bartonella quintana lipopolysaccharide is a natural antagonist of Toll-like receptor 4. Infect Immun. 2007 Oct;75(10):4831-7. Epub 2007 Jul 2. PMID:17606598

Popov A, Abdullah Z, Wickenhauser C, Saric T, Driesen J, Hanisch FG, Domann E, Raven EL, Dehus O, Hermann C, Eggle D, Debey S, Chakraborty T, Krönke M, Utermöhlen O, Schultze JL. Indoleamine 2,3-dioxygenase-expressing dendritic cells form suppurative granulomas following Listeria monocytogenes infection. J Clin Invest. 2006 Dec;116(12):3160-70. Epub 2006 Nov 16. PMID:17111046

Posfay Barbe K, Jaeggi E, Ninet B, Liassine N, Donatiello C, Gervaix A, Suter S. Bartonella quintana endocarditis in a child. N Engl J Med. 2000 Jun 15;342(24):1841-2. PMID:10866564

Povoski SP, Spigos DG, Marsh WL. An unusual case of cat-scratch disease from Bartonella quintana mimicking inflammatory breast cancer in a 50-year-old woman. Breast J. 2003 Nov-Dec;9(6):497-500. PMID:14616946

Powell CC, Kordick DL, Lappin MR. Inoculation with Bartonella henselae followed by feline herpesvirus 1 fails to activate ocular toxoplasmosis in chronically infected cats. J Feline Med Surg. 2002 Jun;4(2):107-10. PMID:12027509

Powell CC, McInnis CL, Fontenelle JP, Lappin MR. Bartonella species, feline herpesvirus-1, and Toxoplasma gondii PCR assay results from blood and aqueous humor samples from 104 cats with naturally occurring endogenous uveitis. J Feline Med Surg. 2010 Dec;12(12):923-8. PMID:20817587

Prasher P, Di Pascuale M, Cavanagh HD. Bilateral chronic peripheral ulcerative keratitis secondary to cat-scratch disease. Eye Contact Lens. 2008 May;34(3):191-3. PMID:18463489

Pretorius AM, Beati L, Birtles RJ. Diversity of bartonellae associated with small mammals inhabiting Free State province, South Africa. Int J Syst Evol Microbiol. 2004 Nov;54(Pt 6):1959-67. PMID:15545418

Pretorius AM, Kelly PJ, Birtles RJ, Raoult D. Are Bartonella emerging and re-emerging pathogens in southern Africa? S Afr Med J. 2000 Jun;90(6):566. PMID:10918880

Pretorius AM, Kelly PJ, Birtles RJ, Raoult D. Are Bartonella emerging and re-emerging pathogens in southern Africa? S Afr Med J. 2000 Jan;90(1):12. PMID:10721382

Pretorius AM, Kelly PJ. An update on human bartonelloses. Cent Afr J Med. 2000 Jul;46(7):194-200. PMID:11317589

Pretorius AM, Kuyl JM, Isherwood DR, Birtles RJ. Bartonella henselae in African lion, South Africa. Emerg Infect Dis. 2004 Dec;10(12):2257-8. PMID:15672532

Probert W, Louie JK, Tucker JR, Longoria R, Hogue R, Moler S, Graves M, Palmer HJ, Cassady J, Fritz CL. Meningitis due to a "Bartonella washoensis"-like human pathogen. J Clin Microbiol. 2009 Jul;47(7):2332-5. Epub 2009 May 13. PMID:19439538

Prybis BG, Eady JL, Kotchmar GS Jr. Chronic osteomyelitis associated with cat-scratch disease. J South Orthop Assoc. 2002 Summer;11(2):119-23. PMID:12741593

Psaroulaki A, Antoniou M, Toumazos P, Mazeris A, Ioannou I, Chochlakis D, Christophi N, Loukaides P, Patsias A, Moschandrea I, Tselentis Y. Rats as indicators of the presence and dispersal of six zoonotic microbial agents in Cyprus, an island ecosystem: a seroepidemiological study. Trans R Soc Trop Med Hyg. 2010 Nov;104(11):733-9. Epub 2010 Sep 25. PMID:20870259

Psarros G, Riddell J 4th, Gandhi T, Kauffman CA, Cinti SK. Bartonella henselae infections in solid organ transplant recipients: report of 5 cases and review of the literature. Medicine (Baltimore). 2012 Mar;91(2):111-21. PMID:22391473

Puligheddu M, Giagheddu A, Genugu F, Giagheddu M, Marrosu F. Epilepsia partialis continua in cat scratch disease. Seizure. 2004 Apr;13(3):191-5. PMID:15010059

Pulliainen AT, Dehio C. Bartonella henselae: subversion of vascular endothelial cell functions by translocated bacterial effector proteins. Int J Biochem Cell Biol. 2009 Mar;41(3):507-10. Epub 2008 Oct 25. PMID:19010441

Pulliainen AT, Dehio C. Persistence of Bartonella spp. stealth pathogens: from subclinical infections to vasoproliferative tumor formation. FEMS Microbiol Rev. 2012 May;36(3):563-99. Epub 2012 Feb 7. PMID:22229763

Qian X, Jin L, Hayden RT, Macon WR, Lloyd RV. Diagnosis of cat scratch disease with Bartonella henselae infection in formalin-fixed paraffin-embedded tissues by two different PCR assays. Diagn Mol Pathol. 2005 Sep;14(3):146-51. PMID:16106195

Qin X, Urdahl KB. PCR and sequencing of independent genetic targets for the diagnosis of culture negative bacterial endocarditis. Diagn Microbiol Infect Dis. 2001 Aug;40(4):145-9. PMID:11576785

Qiu J, Ma Y, Wen Y, Chen L, Wu L, Liu W. Functional identification of two novel genes from Pseudomonas sp. strain HZN6 involved in the catabolism of nicotine. Appl Environ Microbiol. 2012 Apr;78(7):2154-60. Epub 2012 Jan 20. PMID:22267672

Que YA, Moreillon P. Infective endocarditis. Nat Rev Cardiol. 2011 Jun;8(6):322-36. Epub 2011 Apr 12. PMID:21487430

Quebatte M, Dehio M, Tropel D, Basler A, Toller I, Raddatz G, Engel P, Huser S, Schein H, Lindroos HL, Andersson SG, Dehio C. The BatR/BatS two-component regulatory system controls the adaptive response of Bartonella henselae during human endothelial cell infection. J Bacteriol. 2010 Jul;192(13):3352-67. Epub 2010 Apr 23. PMID:20418395

Quimby JM, Elston T, Hawley J, Brewer M, Miller A, Lappin MR. Evaluation of the association of Bartonella species, feline herpesvirus 1, feline calicivirus, feline leukemia virus and feline immunodeficiency virus with chronic feline gingivostomatitis. J Feline Med Surg. 2008 Feb;10(1):66-72. Epub 2007 Sep 4. PMID:17766156

Quinn JH, Girard YA, Gilardi K, Hernandez Y, Poppenga R, Chomel BB, Foley JE, Johnson CK. Pathogen and Rodenticide Exposure in American Badgers (Taxidea taxus) in California. J Wildl Dis. 2012 Apr;48(2):467-72. PMID:22493124

Rahimian J, Raoult D, Tang YW, Hanna BA. Bartonella quintana endocarditis with positive serology for Coxiella burnetii. J Infect. 2006 Sep;53(3):e151-3. Epub 2005 Dec 27. PMID:16386308

Ramharter A, Kremser B. [Bilateral panuveitis with serous retinal detachment].[Article in German]. Ophthalmologe. 2009 Apr;106(4):351-5. PMID:18696078

Ramos AJ, Vargas J, Fernández-Rivera J, Macías J, Mira JA, Pineda JA. [Prevalence of Bartonella spp. seropositivity in human immunodeficiency virus-infected and non infected intravenous drug abusers].[Article in Spanish]. Med Clin (Barc). 2002 Nov 2;119(15):565-7. PMID:12421507

Rampersad JN, Watkins JD, Samlal MS, Deonanan R, Ramsubeik S, Ammons DR. A nested-PCR with an Internal Amplification Control for the detection and differentiation of Bartonella henselae and B. clarridgeiae: an examination of cats in Trinidad. BMC Infect Dis. 2005 Aug 12;5:63. PMID:16098227

Raoult D, Casalta JP, Richet H, Khan M, Bernit E, Rovery C, Branger S, Gouriet F, Imbert G, Bothello E, Collart F, Habib G. Contribution of systematic serological testing in diagnosis of infective endocarditis. J Clin Microbiol. 2005 Oct;43(10):5238-42. PMID:16207989

Raoult D, Dutour O, Houhamdi L, Jankauskas R, Fournier PE, Ardagna Y, Drancourt M, Signoli M, La VD, Macia Y, Aboudharam G. Evidence for louse-transmitted diseases in soldiers of Napoleon's Grand Army in Vilnius. J Infect Dis. 2006 Jan 1;193(1):112-20. Epub 2005 Nov 18. PMID:16323139

Raoult D, Foucault C, Brouqui P. Infections in the homeless. Lancet Infect Dis. 2001 Sep;1(2):77-84. PMID:11871479

Raoult D, Fournier PE, Vandenesch F, Mainardi JL, Eykyn SJ, Nash J, James E, Benoit-Lemercier C, Marrie TJ. Outcome and treatment of Bartonella endocarditis. Arch Intern Med. 2003 Jan 27;163(2):226-30. PMID:12546614

Raoult D, La Scola B, Kelly PJ, Davoust B, Gomez J. Bartonella bovis in cattle in Africa. Vet Microbiol. 2005 Jan 31;105(2):155-6. Epub 2004 Dec 15. PMID:15627528

Raoult D, Roblot F, Rolain JM, Besnier JM, Loulergue J, Bastides F, Choutet P. First isolation of Bartonella alsatica from a valve of a patient with endocarditis. J Clin Microbiol. 2006 Jan;44(1):278-9. PMID:16390990

Raoult D. Etiological diagnosis of blood-culture-negative endocarditis. Enferm Infecc Microbiol Clin. 2006 May;24(5):295-6. PMID:16762253

Raoult D. From Cat scratch disease to Bartonella henselae infection. Clin Infect Dis. 2007 Dec 15;45(12):1541-2. PMID:18190313

Rar VA, Fomenko NV, Dobrotvorsky AK, Livanova NN, Rudakova SA, Fedorov EG, Astanin VB, Morozova OV. Tickborne pathogen detection, Western Siberia, Russia. Emerg Infect Dis. 2005 Nov;11(11):1708-15. PMID:16318722

Rawlins ML, Gerstner C, Hill HR, Litwin CM. Evaluation of a western blot method for the detection of Yersinia antibodies: evidence of serological cross-reactivity between Yersinia outer membrane proteins and Borrelia burgdorferi. Clin Diagn Lab Immunol. 2005 Nov;12(11):1269-74. PMID:16275939

Razaq M, Godkar D, Mankan N, Sridhar S, Hussain S, Ohri A. Cat scratch disease mimicking Richter's Syndrome in a patient with chronic lymphocytic leukemia. Leuk Lymphoma. 2005 Mar;46(3):443-5. PMID:15621836

Rebolleda G, Muñoz-Negrete FJ. [Neuroretinitis in an HIV-infected patient].[Article in Spanish]. Arch Soc Esp Oftalmol. 2001 Aug;76(8):511-4. PMID:11484147

Reddy AK, Morriss MC, Ostrow GI, Stass-Isern M, Olitsky SE, Lowe LH. Utility of MR imaging in cat-scratch neuroretinitis. Pediatr Radiol. 2007 Aug;37(8):840-3. Epub 2007 Jun 22. PMID:17583805

Reeves WK, Dowling AP, Dasch GA. Rickettsial agents from parasitic dermanyssoidea (Acari: Mesostigmata). Exp Appl Acarol. 2006;38(2-3):181-8. PMID:16596351

Reeves WK, Kato CY, Gilchriest T. Pathogen screening and bionomics of Lutzomyia apache (Diptera: Psychodidae) in Wyoming, USA. J Am Mosq Control Assoc. 2008 Sep;24(3):444-7. PMID:18939699

Reeves WK, Loftis AD, Gore JA, Dasch GA. Molecular evidence for novel bartonella species in Trichobius major (Diptera: Streblidae) and Cimex adjunctus (Hemiptera: Cimicidae) from two southeastern bat caves, U.S.A. J Vector Ecol. 2005 Dec;30(2):339-41. PMID:16599175

Reeves WK, Loftis AD, Sanders F, Spinks MD, Wills W, Denison AM, Dasch GA. Borrelia, Coxiella, and Rickettsia in Carios capensis (Acari: Argasidae) from a brown pelican (Pelecanus occidentalis) rookery in South Carolina, USA. Exp Appl Acarol. 2006;39(3-4):321-9. Epub 2006 Jul 5. PMID:16821092

Reeves WK, Loftis AD, Szumlas DE, Abbassy MM, Helmy IM, Hanafi HA, Dasch GA. Rickettsial pathogens in the tropical rat mite Ornithonyssus bacoti (Acari: Macronyssidae) from Egyptian rats (Rattus spp.). Exp Appl Acarol. 2007;41(1-2):101-7. Epub 2007 Jan 16. PMID:17225079

Reeves WK, Nelder MP, Cobb KD, Dasch GA. Bartonella spp. in deer keds, Lipoptena mazamae (Diptera: Hippoboscidae), from Georgia and South Carolina, USA. J Wildl Dis. 2006 Apr;42(2):391-6. PMID:16870863

Reeves WK, Nelder MP, Korecki JA. Bartonella and Rickettsia in fleas and lice from mammals in South Carolina, U.S.A. J Vector Ecol. 2005 Dec;30(2):310-5. PMID:16599169

Reeves WK, Rogers TE, Dasch GA. Bartonella and Rickettsia from fleas (Siphonaptera: Ceratophyllidae) of prairie dogs (Cynomys spp.) from the western United States. J Parasitol. 2007 Aug;93(4):953-5. PMID:17918386

Reeves WK, Rogers TE, Durden LA, Dasch GA. Association of Bartonella with the fleas (Siphonaptera) of rodents and bats using molecular techniques. J Vector Ecol. 2007 Jun;32(1):118-22. PMID:17633432

Reeves WK, Streicker DG, Loftis AD, Dasch GA. Serologic survey of Eptesicus fuscus from Georgia, U.S.A. for Rickettsia and Borrelia and laboratory transmission of a Rickettsia by bat ticks. J Vector Ecol. 2006 Dec;31(2):386-9. PMID:17249357

Reeves WK, Szumlas DE, Moriarity JR, Loftis AD, Abbassy MM, Helmy IM, Dasch GA. Louse-borne bacterial pathogens in lice (Phthiraptera) of rodents and cattle from Egypt. J Parasitol. 2006 Apr;92(2):313-8. PMID:16729688

Reine NJ. Infection and blood transfusion: a guide to donor screening. Clin Tech Small Anim Pract. 2004 May;19(2):68-74. PMID:15179926

Reis C, Cote M, Le Rhun D, Lecuelle B, Levin ML, Vayssier-Taussat M, Bonnet SI. Vector competence of the tick Ixodes ricinus for transmission of Bartonella birtlesii. PLoS Negl Trop Dis. 2011;5(5):e1186. Epub 2011 May 31. PMID:21655306

Reis C, Cote M, Paul RE, Bonnet S. Questing ticks in suburban forest are infected by at least six tick-borne pathogens. Vector Borne Zoonotic Dis. 2011 Jul;11(7):907-16. Epub 2010 Dec 15. PMID:21158500

Renesto P, Gautheret D, Drancourt M, Raoult D. Determination of the rpoB gene sequences of Bartonella henselae and Bartonella quintana for phylogenic analysis. Res Microbiol. 2000 Dec;151(10):831-6. PMID:11191808

Renesto P, Gouvernet J, Drancourt M, Roux V, Raoult D. Use of rpoB gene analysis for detection and identification of Bartonella species. J Clin Microbiol. 2001 Feb;39(2):430-7. PMID:11158086

Renou F, Raffray L, Gerber A, Moiton MP, Ferrandiz D, Yvin JL. [Hepatic localization of cat scratch disease in an immunocompetent patient].[Article in French]. Med Mal Infect. 2010 Mar;40(3):172-4. Epub 2009 Jul 17. PMID:19616394

Requena Caballero C, Nicolau MJ, Haro R, Martorell A, Sanmartín O, Llombart B, Botella R, Guillén C, Requena L. [Proliferative cutaneous epithelioid angiomatous nodule].[Article in Spanish]. Actas Dermosifiliogr. 2009 Mar;100(2):137-41. PMID:19445879

Resto-Ruiz S, Burgess A, Anderson BE. The role of the host immune response in pathogenesis of Bartonella henselae. DNA Cell Biol. 2003 Jun;22(6):431-40. PMID:12906736

Resto-Ruiz SI, Schmiederer M, Sweger D, Newton C, Klein TW, Friedman H, Anderson BE. Induction of a potential paracrine angiogenic loop between human THP-1 macrophages and human microvascular endothelial cells during Bartonella henselae infection. Infect Immun. 2002 Aug;70(8):4564-70. PMID:12117969

Resto-Ruiz SI, Sweger D, Widen RH, Valkov N, Anderson BE. Transcriptional activation of the htrA (High-temperature requirement A) gene from Bartonella henselae. Infect Immun. 2000 Oct;68(10):5970-8. PMID:10992509

Reye AL, Hübschen JM, Sausy A, Muller CP. Prevalence and seasonality of tick-borne pathogens in questing Ixodes ricinus ticks from Luxembourg. Appl Environ Microbiol. 2010 May;76(9):2923-31. Epub 2010 Mar 12. PMID:20228110

Reynolds MG, Holman RC, Curns AT, O'Reilly M, McQuiston JH, Steiner CA. Epidemiology of cat-scratch disease hospitalizations among children in the United States. Pediatr Infect Dis J. 2005 Aug;24(8):700-4. PMID:16094224

Rheault MN, van Burik JA, Mauer M, Ingulli E, Ferrieri P, Jessurun J, Chavers BM. Cat-scratch disease relapse in a kidney transplant recipient. Pediatr Transplant. 2007 Feb;11(1):105-9. PMID:17239132

Rhomberg TA, Karlberg O, Mini T, Zimny-Arndt U, Wickenberg U, Röttgen M, Jungblut PR, Jenö P, Andersson SG, Dehio C. Proteomic analysis of the sarcosine-insoluble outer membrane fraction of the bacterial pathogen Bartonella henselae. Proteomics. 2004 Oct;4(10):3021-33. PMID:15378747

Rhomberg TA, Truttmann MC, Guye P, Ellner Y, Dehio C. A translocated protein of Bartonella henselae interferes with endocytic uptake of individual bacteria and triggers uptake of large bacterial aggregates via the invasome. Cell Microbiol. 2009 Jun;11(6):927-45. Epub 2009 Feb 27. PMID:19302579

Ricart JJ. [Infective endocarditis due to Bartonella quintana].[Article in Spanish]. Medicina (B Aires). 2008;68(6):478. PMID:19147434

Ridder GJ, Boedeker CC, Lee TK, Sander A. B-mode sonographic criteria for differential diagnosis of cervicofacial lymphadenopathy in cat-scratch disease and toxoplasmosis. Head Neck. 2003 Apr;25(4):306-12. PMID:12658735

Ridder GJ, Boedeker CC, Technau-Ihling K, Grunow R, Sander A. Role of cat-scratch disease in lymphadenopathy in the head and neck. Clin Infect Dis. 2002 Sep 15;35(6):643-9. Epub 2002 Aug 14. PMID:12203159

Ridder GJ, Boedeker CC, Technau-Ihling K, Sander A. Cat-scratch disease: Otolaryngologic manifestations and management. Otolaryngol Head Neck Surg. 2005 Mar;132(3):353-8. PMID:15746844

Ridder GJ, Eglinger CF, Sander A, Technau-Ihling K. [Neck abscess as primary manifestation of head and neck carcinoma: implications for diagnostic management].[Article in German]. Laryngorhinootologie. 2000 Oct;79(10):604-8. PMID:11089210

Ridder GJ, Richter B, Disko U, Sander A. Gray-scale sonographic evaluation of cervical lymphadenopathy in cat-scratch disease. J Clin Ultrasound. 2001 Mar-Apr;29(3):140-5. PMID:11329156

Ridder GJ, Richter B, Laszig R, Sander A. [Parotid involvement in cat scratch disease: a differential diagnosis with increased significance]. [Article in German]. Laryngorhinootologie. 2000 Aug;79(8):471-7. PMID:11006911

Ridder-Schröter R, Marx A, Beer M, Tappe D, Kreth HW, Girschick HJ. Abscess-forming lymphadenopathy and osteomyelitis in children with Bartonella henselae infection. J Med Microbiol. 2008 Apr;57(Pt 4):519-24. PMID:18349375

Riess T, Anderson B, Fackelmayer A, Autenrieth IB, Kempf VA. Rapid and efficient transposon mutagenesis of Bartonella henselae by transposome technology. Gene. 2003 Aug 14;313:103-9. PMID:12957381

Riess T, Andersson SG, Lupas A, Schaller M, Schäfer A, Kyme P, Martin J, Wälzlein JH, Ehehalt U, Lindroos H, Schirle M, Nordheim A, Autenrieth IB, Kempf VA. Bartonella adhesin a mediates a proangiogenic host cell response. J Exp Med. 2004 Nov 15;200(10):1267-78. Epub 2004 Nov 8. PMID:15534369

Riess T, Dietrich F, Schmidt KV, Kaiser PO, Schwarz H, Schäfer A, Kempf VA. Analysis of a novel insect cell culture medium-based growth medium for Bartonella species. Appl Environ Microbiol. 2008 Aug;74(16):5224-7. Epub 2008 Jun 20. PMID:18567689

Riess T, Raddatz G, Linke D, Schäfer A, Kempf VA. Analysis of Bartonella adhesin A expression reveals differences between various B. henselae strains. Infect Immun. 2007 Jan;75(1):35-43. Epub 2006 Oct 23. PMID:17060468

Rigopoulos D, Paparizos V, Katsambas A. Cutaneous markers of HIV infection. Clin Dermatol. 2004 Nov-Dec;22(6):487-98. PMID:15596320

Riley SP, Foley J, Chomel B. Exposure to feline and canine pathogens in bobcats and gray foxes in urban and rural zones of a national park in California. J Wildl Dis. 2004 Jan;40(1):11-22. PMID:15137484

Roberts DR. DDT risk assessments. Environ Health Perspect. 2001 Jul;109(7):A302-3. PMID:11485878

Robinson JL, Spady DW, Prasad E, McColl D, Artsob H. Bartonella seropositivity in children with Henoch-Schonlein purpura. BMC Infect Dis. 2005 Apr 5;5:21. PMID:15807903

Robinson MT, Hillman T, Langton DA, Shaw SE. Bartonella clarridgeiae in a cat in the UK. Vet Rec. 2009 Jan 10;164(2):58-9. PMID:19136687

Robinson MT, Morgan ER, Woods D, Shaw SE. Real-time and multiplex real-time polymerase chain reactions for the detection of Bartonella henselae within cat flea, Ctenocephalides felis, samples. Med Vet Entomol. 2010 Dec;24(4):449-55. PMID:20704655

Roblot F. [Cat-scratch disease].[Article in French]. Med Mal Infect. 2005 Jan;35(1):46-7. PMID:15695034

Robson CD. Imaging of granulomatous lesions of the neck in children. Radiol Clin North Am. 2000 Sep;38(5):969-77. PMID:11054963

Rocha JL, Pellegrino LN, Riella LV, Martins LT. Acute hemiplegia associated with cat-scratch disease. Braz J Infect Dis. 2004 Jun;8(3):263-6. Epub 2004 Sep 29. PMID:15476060

Roden JA, Wells DH, Chomel BB, Kasten RW, Koehler JE. Hemin binding protein C is found in outer membrane vesicles and protects Bartonella henselae against toxic concentrations of hemin. Infect Immun. 2012 Mar;80(3):929-42. Epub 2012 Jan 9. PMID:22232189

Rodrick D, Dillon B, Dexter M, Nicholson I, Marcel S, Dickeson D, Iredell J. Culture-negative endocarditis due to Houston Complex Bartonella henselae acquired in Noumea, New Caledonia. J Clin Microbiol. 2004 Apr;42(4):1846-8. PMID:15071067

Rodríguez C M, Giachetto L G, Cuneo E A, Gutiérrez B Mdel C, Shimchack R M, Pírez G MC. [Cat-scratch disease with bone compromise: atypical manifestation].[Article in Spanish]. Rev Chilena Infectol. 2009 Aug;26(4):363-9. Epub 2009 Sep 23. PMID:19802407

Rodríguez G, Torres BE, Motta A. [Bacillary angiomatosis].[Article in Spanish]. Biomedica. 2002 Jun;22(2):141-54. PMID:12152480

Roe RH, Michael Jumper J, Fu AD, Johnson RN, Richard McDonald H, Cunningham ET. Ocular bartonella infections. Int Ophthalmol Clin. 2008 Summer;48(3):93-105. PMID:18645403

Rogers LF. Magnetic resonance images of reactive lymphadenitis. Lymphology. 2006 Mar;39(1):53-4. PMID:16724511

Rolain JM, Arnoux D, Parzy D, Sampol J, Raoult D. Experimental infection of human erythrocytes from alcoholic patients with Bartonella quintana. Ann N Y Acad Sci. 2003 Jun;990:605-11. PMID:12860697

Rolain JM, Boureau-Voultoury A, Raoult D. Serological evidence of Bartonella vinsonii lymphadenopathies in a child bitten by a dog. Clin Microbiol Infect. 2009 Dec;15 Suppl 2:122-3. Epub 2009 Apr 3. PMID:19374641

Rolain JM, Bourry O, Davoust B, Raoult D. Bartonella quintana and Rickettsia felis in Gabon. Emerg Infect Dis. 2005 Nov;11(11):1742-4. PMID:16318727

Rolain JM, Brouqui P, Koehler JE, Maguina C, Dolan MJ, Raoult D. Recommendations for treatment of human infections caused by Bartonella species. Antimicrob Agents Chemother. 2004 Jun;48(6):1921-33. PMID:15155180

Rolain JM, Chanet V, Laurichesse H, Lepidi H, Beytout J, Raoult D. Cat scratch disease with lymphadenitis, vertebral osteomyelitis, and spleen abscesses. Ann N Y Acad Sci. 2003 Jun;990:397-403. PMID:12860662

Rolain JM, Foucault C, Brouqui P, Raoult D. Erythroblast cells as a target for Bartonella quintana in homeless people. Ann N Y Acad Sci. 2003 Jun;990:485-7. PMID:12860677

Rolain JM, Foucault C, Guieu R, La Scola B, Brouqui P, Raoult D. Bartonella quintana in human erythrocytes. Lancet. 2002 Jul 20;360(9328):226-8. PMID:12133660

Rolain JM, Fournier PE, Raoult D, Bonerandi JJ. First isolation and detection by immunofluorescence assay of Bartonella koehlerae in erythrocytes from a French cat. J Clin Microbiol. 2003 Aug;41(8):4001-2. PMID:12904442

Rolain JM, Franc M, Davoust B, Raoult D. Molecular detection of Bartonella quintana, B. koehlerae, B. henselae, B. clarridgeiae, Rickettsia felis, and Wolbachia pipientis in cat fleas, France. Emerg Infect Dis. 2003 Mar;9(3):338-42. PMID:12643829

Rolain JM, Gouriet F, Enea M, Aboud M, Raoult D. Detection by immunofluorescence assay of Bartonella henselae in lymph nodes from patients with cat scratch disease. Clin Diagn Lab Immunol. 2003 Jul;10(4):686-91. PMID:12853405

Rolain JM, La Scola B, Liang Z, Davoust B, Raoult D. Immunofluorescent detection of intraerythrocytic Bartonella henselae in naturally infected cats. J Clin Microbiol. 2001 Aug;39(8):2978-80. PMID:11474027

Rolain JM, Lecam C, Raoult D. Simplified serological diagnosis of endocarditis due to Coxiella burnetii and Bartonella. Clin Diagn Lab Immunol. 2003 Nov;10(6):1147-8. PMID:14607881

Rolain JM, Lepidi H, Zanaret M, Triglia JM, Michel G, Thomas PA, Texereau M, Stein A, Romaru A, Eb F, Raoult D. Lymph node biopsy specimens and diagnosis of cat-scratch disease. Emerg Infect Dis. 2006 Sep;12(9):1338-44. PMID:17073081

Rolain JM, Locatelli C, Chabanne L, Davoust B, Raoult D. Prevalence of Bartonella clarridgeiae and Bartonella henselae in domestic cats from France and detection of the organisms in erythrocytes by immunofluorescence. Clin Diagn Lab Immunol. 2004 Mar;11(2):423-5. PMID:15013998

Rolain JM, Maurin M, Bryskier A, Raoult D. In vitro activities of telithromycin (HMR 3647) against Rickettsia rickettsii, Rickettsia conorii, Rickettsia africae, Rickettsia typhi, Rickettsia prowazekii, Coxiella burnetii, Bartonella henselae, Bartonella quintana, Bartonella bacilliformis, and Ehrlichia chaffeensis. Antimicrob Agents Chemother. 2000 May;44(5):1391-3. PMID:10770788

Rolain JM, Maurin M, Mallet MN, Parzy D, Raoult D. Culture and antibiotic susceptibility of Bartonella quintana in human erythrocytes. Antimicrob Agents Chemother. 2003 Feb;47(2):614-9. PMID:12543668

Rolain JM, Maurin M, Raoult D. Bactericidal effect of antibiotics on Bartonella and Brucella spp.: clinical implications. J Antimicrob Chemother. 2000 Nov;46(5):811-4. PMID:11062204

Rolain JM, Novelli S, Ventosilla P, Maguina C, Guerra H, Raoult D. Immunofluorescence detection of Bartonella bacilliformis flagella in vitro and in vivo in human red blood cells as viewed by laser confocal microscopy. Ann N Y Acad Sci. 2003 Jun;990:581-4. PMID:12860693

Rolain JM, Rousset E, La Scola B, Duquesnel R, Raoult D. Bartonella schoenbuchensis isolated from the blood of a French cow. Ann N Y Acad Sci. 2003 Jun;990:236-8. PMID:12860633

Rombaux P, M'Bilo T, Badr-el-Din A, Theate I, Bigaignon G, Hamoir M. Cervical lymphadenitis and cat scratch disease (CSD): an overlooked disease? Acta Otorhinolaryngol Belg. 2000;54(4):491-6. PMID:11205454

Romero Ramírez DS, Ortigosa del Castillo L, Gaspar Guardado MA, Quintero Quintero M, Marrero García AR, Marrero Pérez CL. [Cat scratch disease with hepatosplenic involvement].[Article in Spanish]. An Pediatr (Barc). 2004 Nov;61(5):450-1. PMID:15530333

Rooks YL, Corwell B. Common urgent musculoskeletal injuries in primary care. Prim Care. 2006 Sep;33(3):751-77, viii. PMID:17088159

Rosado FG, Stratton CW, Mosse CA. Clinicopathologic correlation of epidemiologic and histopathologic features of pediatric bacterial lymphadenitis. Arch Pathol Lab Med. 2011 Nov;135(11):1490-3. PMID:22032579

Rosales CM, McLaughlin MD, Sata T, Katano H, Veno PA, de Las Casas LE, Miranda RN. AIDS presenting with cutaneous Kaposi's sarcoma and bacillary angiomatosis in the bone marrow mimicking Kaposi's sarcoma. AIDS Patient Care STDS. 2002 Dec;16(12):573-7. PMID:12542930

Rost Monahan S. Neuroretinitis: a clinical syndrome of cat-scratch disease. Clin Eye Vis Care. 2000 Dec;12(3-4):155-159. PMID:11137430

Rotstein DS, Taylor SK, Bradley J, Breitschwerdt EB. Prevalence of Bartonella henselae antibody in Florida panthers. J Wildl Dis. 2000 Jan;36(1):157-60. PMID:10682759

Roubaud-Baudron C, Fortineau N, Goujard C, Le Bras P, Lambotte O. [Cat scratch disease with bone involvement: a case report and literature review].[Article in French]. Rev Med Interne. 2009 Jul;30(7):602-8. Epub 2009 Mar 19. PMID:19303175

Roucher C, Mediannikov O, Diatta G, Trape JF, Raoult D. A New Rickettsia Species Found in Fleas Collected from Human Dwellings and from Domestic Cats and Dogs in Senegal. Vector Borne Zoonotic Dis. 2012 Jan 3. [Epub ahead of print]. PMID:22214272

Roux V, Eykyn SJ, Wyllie S, Raoult D. Bartonella vinsonii subsp. berkhoffii as an agent of afebrile blood culture-negative endocarditis in a human. J Clin Microbiol. 2000 Apr;38(4):1698-700. PMID:10747175

Rovery C, Greub G, Lepidi H, Casalta JP, Habib G, Collart F, Raoult D. PCR detection of bacteria on cardiac valves of patients with treated bacterial endocarditis. J Clin Microbiol. 2005 Jan;43(1):163-7. PMID:15634966

Rovery C, Rolain JM, Lepidi H, Zandotti C, Moreau J, Brouqui P. Bartonella quintana coinfection with Mycobacterium avium complex and CMV in an AIDS patient: case presentation. BMC Infect Dis. 2006 May 29;6:89. PMID:16732891

Roy AF, Corstvet RE, Tapp RA, Oreilly KL, Cox HU. Evaluation and use of a nested polymerase chain reaction assay in cats experimentally infected with Bartonella henselae genotype I and Bartonella henselae genotype II. J Vet Diagn Invest. 2001 Jul;13(4):312-22. PMID:11478603

Rozmanic V, Banac S, Miletic D, Manestar K, Kamber S, Paparic S. Role of magnetic resonance imaging and scintigraphy in the diagnosis and follow-up of osteomyelitis in cat-scratch disease. J Paediatr Child Health. 2007 Jul-Aug;43(7-8):568-70. PMID:17635689

Ruess M, Sander A, Brandis M, Berner R. Portal vein and bone involvement in disseminated cat-scratch disease: report of 2 cases. Clin Infect Dis. 2000 Sep;31(3):818-21. PMID:11017839

Ruiz J, Silva W, Pons MJ, Del Valle LJ, Tinco CR, Casabona VD, Gomes C, Bazan J, Zavaleta V, Cornejo H, Champin D, Del Valle J. Long time survival of Bartonella bacilliformis in blood stored at 4 °C. A risk for blood transfusions. Blood Transfus. 2012 Mar 29:1-2. [Epub ahead of print]. PMID:22507863

Rydzewski B, Lemańska-Kwiatkowska K, Lipińska M. [Cat scratch disease--diagnostic problems].[Article in Polish]. Otolaryngol Pol. 2002;56(6):727-31. PMID:12577490

Rymaszewska A, Adamska M. Molecular evidence of vector-borne pathogens coinfecting dogs from Poland. Acta Vet Hung. 2011 Jun;59(2):215-23. PMID:21665575

Saatci AO, Oner FH, Kargi A, Kavukcu S. Unilateral neuroretinitis and periparillary serous retinal detachment in cat-scratch disease. Korean J Ophthalmol. 2002 Jun;16(1):43-6. PMID:12162517

Sackal C, Laudisoit A, Kosoy M, Massung R, Eremeeva ME, Karpathy SE, Van Wyk K, Gabitzsch E, Zeidner NS. Bartonella spp. and Rickettsia felis in fleas, Democratic Republic of Congo. Emerg Infect Dis. 2008 Dec;14(12):1972-4. PMID:19046544

Saenz HL, Engel P, Stoeckli MC, Lanz C, Raddatz G, Vayssier-Taussat M, Birtles R, Schuster SC, Dehio C. Genomic analysis of Bartonella identifies type IV secretion systems as host adaptability factors. Nat Genet. 2007 Dec;39(12):1469-76. Epub 2007 Nov 25. PMID:18037886

Safdar A, McEvoy PL, Burns RG, Perfect JR. Clinical microbiological case: severe relapsing septal panniculitis in a healthy man from the south-eastern USA. Clin Microbiol Infect. 2002 Dec;8(12):801-2; 830-2. PMID:12519353

Safdar A. Urban trench fever in a healthy man from the southeastern United States. Clin Infect Dis. 2002 Dec 15;35(12):1577. PMID:12471587

Saisongkorh W, Barrassi L, Davoust B, de Broucker CA, Raoult D, Rolain JM. First isolation of Bartonella bovis from animals in French Guyana, South America. Clin Microbiol Infect. 2009 Dec;15 Suppl 2:124-6. Epub 2009 May 18. PMID:19456818

Saisongkorh W, Kowalczewska M, Azza S, Decloquement P, Rolain JM, Raoult D. Identification of candidate proteins for the diagnosis of Bartonella henselae infections using an immunoproteomic approach. FEMS Microbiol Lett. 2010 Sep 1;310(2):158-67. Epub 2010 Jul 9. PMID:20695898

Saisongkorh W, Robert C, La Scola B, Raoult D, Rolain JM. Evidence of transfer by conjugation of type IV secretion system genes between Bartonella species and Rhizobium radiobacter in amoeba. PLoS One. 2010 Sep 13;5(9):e12666. PMID:20856925

Saisongkorh W, Rolain JM, Suputtamongkol Y, Raoult D. Emerging Bartonella in humans and animals in Asia and Australia. J Med Assoc Thai. 2009 May;92(5):707-31. PMID:19459536

Saisongkorh W, Wootta W, Sawanpanyalert P, Raoult D, Rolain JM. "Candidatus Bartonella thailandensis": a new genotype of Bartonella identified from rodents. Vet Microbiol. 2009 Oct 20;139(1-2):197-201. Epub 2009 Jun 6. PMID:19574002

Sakellaris G, Kampitakis E, Karamitopoulou E, Scoulica E, Psaroulaki A, Mihailidou E, Charissis G. Cat scratch disease simulating a malignant process of the chest wall with coexistent osteomyelitis. Scand J Infect Dis. 2003;35(6-7):433-5. PMID:12953967

Sala E, Lipiec A, Zygmunt A, Burdzel Z, Ogórek M, Chyla M. [Cat scratch disease--course, diagnosis].[Article in Polish]. Przegl Epidemiol. 2006;60(2):307-13. PMID:16964683

Sala M, Font B, Sanfeliu I, Quesada M, Ponts I, Segura F. Bacillary angiomatosis caused by Bartonella quintana. Ann N Y Acad Sci. 2005 Dec;1063:302-7. PMID:16481531

Salehi N, Custodio H, Rathore MH. Renal microabscesses due to Bartonella infection. Pediatr Infect Dis J. 2010 May;29(5):472-3. PMID:20072078

Salgado CD, Weisse ME. Transverse myelitis associated with probable cat-scratch disease in a previously healthy pediatric patient. Clin Infect Dis. 2000 Aug;31(2):609-11. PMID:10987731

Salhi I, Boigegrain RA, Machold J, Weise C, Cloeckaert A, Rouot B. Characterization of new members of the group 3 outer membrane protein family of Brucella spp. Infect Immun. 2003 Aug;71(8):4326-32. PMID:12874309

Sällström B, Andersson SG. Genome reduction in the alpha-Proteobacteria. Curr Opin Microbiol. 2005 Oct;8(5):579-85. PMID:16099701

Salvatore P, Casamassimi A, Sommese L, Fiorito C, Ciccodicola A, Rossiello R, Avallone B, Grimaldi V, Costa V, Rienzo M, Colicchio R, Williams-Ignarro S, Pagliarulo C, Prudente ME, Abbondanza C, Lamberti F, Baroni A, Buommino E, Farzati B, Tufano MA, Ignarro LJ, Napoli C. Detrimental effects of Bartonella henselae are counteracted by L-arginine and nitric oxide in human endothelial progenitor cells. Proc Natl Acad Sci U S A. 2008 Jul 8;105(27):9427-32. Epub 2008 Jun 30. PMID:18595894

Salzberger B, Franzen C, Fätkenheuer G. [Update in infectious diseases. Part I: epidemiology].[Article in German]. Med Klin (Munich). 2000 Jun 15;95(6):314-20. PMID:10935415

Samson L, Drancourt M, Casalta JP, Raoult D. Corpuscular antigenic microarray for the serodiagnosis of blood culture-negative endocarditis. Ann N Y Acad Sci. 2006 Oct;1078:595-6. PMID:17114786

Sander A, Berner R, Ruess M. Serodiagnosis of cat scratch disease: response to Bartonella henselae in children and a review of diagnostic methods. Eur J Clin Microbiol Infect Dis. 2001 Jun;20(6):392-401. PMID:11476439

Sander A, Kretzer S, Bredt W, Oberle K, Bereswill S. Hemin-dependent growth and hemin binding of Bartonella henselae. FEMS Microbiol Lett. 2000 Aug 1;189(1):55-9. PMID:10913865

Sander A, Zagrosek A, Bredt W, Schiltz E, Piémont Y, Lanz C, Dehio C. Characterization of Bartonella clarridgeiae flagellin (FlaA) and detection of antiflagellin antibodies in patients with lymphadenopathy. J Clin Microbiol. 2000 Aug;38(8):2943-8. PMID:10921956

Sandrasegaran K, Hawes DR, Matthew G. Hepatic peliosis (bacillary angiomatosis) in AIDS: CT findings. Abdom Imaging. 2005 Nov-Dec;30(6):738-40. PMID:16245016

Sanfeliu I, Antón E, Pineda V, Pons I, Perez J, Font B, Segura F. Description of Bartonella spp. infections in a general hospital of Catalonia, Spain. Clin Microbiol Infect. 2009 Dec;15 Suppl 2:130-1. Epub 2009 May 18. PMID:19456816

Sanguinetti-Morelli D, Angelakis E, Richet H, Davoust B, Rolain JM, Raoult D. Seasonality of cat-scratch disease, France, 1999-2009. Emerg Infect Dis. 2011 Apr;17(4):705-7. PMID:21470466

Sankatsing SU, Kolader ME, Bouma BJ, Bennink RJ, Verberne HJ, Ansink TM, Visser CE, van der Meer JT. 18F-fluoro-2-deoxyglucose positron emission tomography-negative endocarditis lenta caused by Bartonella henselae. J Heart Valve Dis. 2011 Jan;20(1):100-2. PMID:21404906

Sanogo YO, Zeaiter Z, Caruso G, Merola F, Shpynov S, Brouqui P, Raoult D. Bartonella henselae in Ixodes ricinus ticks (Acari: Ixodida) removed from humans, Belluno province, Italy. Emerg Infect Dis. 2003 Mar;9(3):329-32. PMID:12643827

Santos R, Cardoso O, Rodrigues P, Cardoso J, Machado J, Afonso A, Bacellar F, Marston E, Proença R. Bacillary angiomatosis by Bartonella quintana in an HIV-infected patient. J Am Acad Dermatol. 2000 Feb;42(2 Pt 1):299-301. PMID:10642694

Saracević E, Sabanović S, Selimović A. [Cat-scratch disease].[Article in Croatian]. Med Arh. 2000;54(5-6):321-2. PMID:11219917

Sarret C, Barbier C, Faucher R, Lacombe P, Meyer M, Labbé A. [Erythema nodosum and adenopathy in a 15-year-old boy: uncommon signs of cat scratch disease].[Article in French]. Arch Pediatr. 2005 Mar;12(3):295-7. PMID:15734128

Sasaki T, Kobayashi M, Agui N. Detection of Bartonella quintana from body lice (Anoplura: Pediculidae) infesting homeless people in Tokyo by molecular technique. J Med Entomol. 2002 May;39(3):427-9. PMID:12061434

Sasaki T, Poudel SK, Isawa H, Hayashi T, Seki N, Tomita T, Sawabe K, Kobayashi M. First molecular evidence of Bartonella quintana in Pediculus humanus capitis (Phthiraptera: Pediculidae), collected from Nepalese children. J Med Entomol. 2006 Jan;43(1):110-2. PMID:16506456

Sasseigne G, Herbert A, Larvol L, Damade R, Cartry O. [Fever and abdominal pain in a 56-year-old woman].[Article in French]. Rev Med Interne. 2009 Dec;30(12):1049-53. Epub 2009 Oct 7. PMID:19815317

Satake K, Ohsawa I, Kobayashi N, Osaki K, Toyoda H, Horikoshi S, Tomino Y. Three cases of PR3-ANCA positive subacute endocarditis caused by attenuated bacteria (Propionibacterium, Gemella, and Bartonella) complicated with kidney injury. Mod Rheumatol. 2011 Oct;21(5):536-41. Epub 2011 Mar 15. PMID:21400245

Satta G, Chisu V, Cabras P, Fois F, Masala G. Pathogens and symbionts in ticks: a survey on tick species distribution and presence of tick-transmitted micro-organisms in Sardinia, Italy. J Med Microbiol. 2011 Jan;60(Pt 1):63-8. Epub 2010 Sep 30. PMID:20884769

Saunders GK, Monroe WE. Systemic granulomatous disease and sialometaplasia in a dog with Bartonella infection. Vet Pathol. 2006 May;43(3):391-2. PMID:16672593

Sayin-Kutlu S, Ergin C, Kutlu M, Akkaya Y, Akalin S. Bartonella henselae Seroprevalence in Cattle Breeders and Veterinarians in the Rural Areas of Aydin and Denizli, Turkey. Zoonoses Public Health. 2012 Apr 11. [Epub ahead of print]. PMID:22489645

Schabereiter-Gurtner C, Lubitz W, Rölleke S. Application of broad-range 16S rRNA PCR amplification and DGGE fingerprinting for detection of tick-infecting bacteria. J Microbiol Methods. 2003 Feb;52(2):251-60. PMID:12459246

Schad K, Kreyden OP, Trüeb RM. [When cats scratch].[Article in German]. Schweiz Med Wochenschr. 2000 Sep 30;130(39):1382. PMID:11059029

Schaefer HE. Introduction into pathology of ocular Zoonoses. Int J Med Sci. 2009;6(3):120-2. Epub 2009 Mar 19. PMID:19319226

Schaefer JD, Kasten RW, Coonan TJ, Clifford DL, Chomel BB. Isolation or detection of Bartonella vinsonii subspecies berkhoffii and Bartonella rochalimae in the endangered island foxes (Urocyon littoralis). Vet Microbiol. 2011 Dec 29;154(1-2):135-9. Epub 2011 Jul 2. PMID:21802869

Schaefer JD, Moore GM, Namekata MS, Kasten RW, Chomel BB. Seroepidemiology of Bartonella Infection in Gray Foxes from Texas. Vector Borne Zoonotic Dis. 2012 Jan 4. [Epub ahead of print]. PMID:22217178

Schaller JL, Burkland GA, Langhoff PJ. Do bartonella infections cause agitation, panic disorder, and treatment-resistant depression? MedGenMed. 2007 Sep 13;9(3):54. PMID:18092060

Schattner A, Zimhony O, Avidor B, Giladi M. Asking the right question. Lancet. 2003 May 24;361(9371):1786. PMID:12781538

Scheidegger F, Ellner Y, Guye P, Rhomberg TA, Weber H, Augustin HG, Dehio C. Distinct activities of Bartonella henselae type IV secretion effector proteins modulate capillary-like sprout formation. Cell Microbiol. 2009 Jul;11(7):1088-101. Epub 2009 Mar 12. PMID:19416269

Scheidegger F, Quebatte M, Mistl C, Dehio C. The Bartonella henselae VirB/Bep system interferes with vascular endothelial growth factor (VEGF) signalling in human vascular endothelial cells. Cell Microbiol. 2011 Mar;13(3):419-31. Epub 2010 Dec 3. PMID:21044238

Schiellerup P, Dyhr T, Rolain JM, Christensen M, Damsgaard R, Ethelberg S, Fisker N, Frost Andersen N, Raoult D, Krogfelt KA. Low seroprevalence of bartonella species in danish elite orienteers. Scand J Infect Dis. 2004;36(8):604-6. PMID:15370673

Schiellerup P, Krogfelt KA, Andersen AB. Bartonella henselae causing severe and protracted illness in an otherwise healthy person. Scand J Infect Dis. 2004;36(4):316-8. PMID:15198195

Schiettecatte A, Shahabpour M, Vanhoenacker FM, Goossens A, Pouliart N, Machiels F, de Mey J. An unusual case of cat-scratch disease of the knee: case report and differential diagnosis. JBR-BTR. 2007 Sep-Oct;90(5):391-4. PMID:18085195

Schiffmann A, Pers YM, Lukas C, Combe B, Morel J. Mesenteric and splenic cat-scratch disease during etanercept therapy. Rheumatology (Oxford). 2009 Nov;48(11):1461-2. Epub 2009 Aug 18. PMID:19690129

Schmalfuss IM, Dean CW, Sistrom C, Bhatti MT. Optic neuropathy secondary to cat scratch disease: distinguishing MR imaging features from other types of optic neuropathies. AJNR Am J Neuroradiol. 2005 Jun-Jul;26(6):1310-6. PMID:15956488

Schmid MC, Scheidegger F, Dehio M, Balmelle-Devaux N, Schulein R, Guye P, Chennakesava CS, Biedermann B, Dehio C. A translocated bacterial protein protects vascular endothelial cells from apoptosis. PLoS Pathog. 2006 Nov;2(11):e115. PMID:17121462

Schmid MC, Schulein R, Dehio M, Denecker G, Carena I, Dehio C. The VirB type IV secretion system of Bartonella henselae mediates invasion, proinflammatory activation and antiapoptotic protection of endothelial cells. Mol Microbiol. 2004 Apr;52(1):81-92. PMID:15049812

Schmiederer M, Anderson B. Cloning, sequencing, and expression of three Bartonella henselae genes homologous to the Agrobacterium tumefaciens VirB region. DNA Cell Biol. 2000 Mar;19(3):141-7. PMID:10749166

Schmiederer M, Arcenas R, Widen R, Valkov N, Anderson B. Intracellular induction of the Bartonella henselae virB operon by human endothelial cells. Infect Immun. 2001 Oct;69(10):6495-502. PMID:11553594

Schneer S, Marcoviciu D, Beilin V, Goffman M, Dicker D. [Stroke as a manifestation of acute Bartonella henselae endocarditis].[Article in Hebrew]. Harefuah. 2007 Nov;146(11):902-4, 908. PMID:18087840

Scholz HC, Al Dahouk S, Tomaso H, Neubauer H, Witte A, Schloter M, Kämpfer P, Falsen E, Pfeffer M, Engel M. Genetic diversity and phylogenetic relationships of bacteria belonging to the Ochrobactrum-Brucella group by recA and 16S rRNA gene-based comparative sequence analysis. Syst Appl Microbiol. 2008 Mar;31(1):1-16. Epub 2008 Jan 28. PMID:18222618

Schorn S, Pfister K, Reulen H, Mahling M, Silaghi C. Occurrence of Babesia spp., Rickettsia spp. and Bartonella spp. in Ixodes ricinus in Bavarian public parks, Germany. Parasit Vectors. 2011 Jul 15;4:135. PMID:21762494

Schröder G, Dehio C. Virulence-associated type IV secretion systems of Bartonella. Trends Microbiol. 2005 Jul;13(7):336-42. PMID:15935675

Schröder G, Schuelein R, Quebatte M, Dehio C. Conjugative DNA transfer into human cells by the VirB/VirD4 type IV secretion system of the bacterial pathogen Bartonella henselae. Proc Natl Acad Sci U S A. 2011 Aug 30;108(35):14643-8. Epub 2011 Aug 15. PMID:21844337

Schroff S. Update on emerging infections: news from the Centers for Disease Control and Prevention. Bartonella quintana in body lice and head lice from homeless persons, San Francisco, California, USA. Ann Emerg Med. 2010 Mar;55(3):280-2; discussion 282-3. PMID:20201124

Schülein R, Seubert A, Gille C, Lanz C, Hansmann Y, Piémont Y, Dehio C. Invasion and persistent intracellular colonization of erythrocytes. A unique parasitic strategy of the emerging pathogen Bartonella. J Exp Med. 2001 May 7;193(9):1077-86. PMID:11342592

Schulein R, Dehio C. The VirB/VirD4 type IV secretion system of Bartonella is essential for establishing intraerythrocytic infection. Mol Microbiol. 2002 Nov;46(4):1053-67. PMID:12421311

Schulein R, Guye P, Rhomberg TA, Schmid MC, Schröder G, Vergunst AC, Carena I, Dehio C. A bipartite signal mediates the transfer of type IV secretion substrates of Bartonella henselae into human cells. Proc Natl Acad Sci U S A. 2005 Jan 18;102(3):856-61. Epub 2005 Jan 10. PMID:15642951

Schulte B, Linke D, Klumpp S, Schaller M, Riess T, Autenrieth IB, Kempf VA. Bartonella quintana variably expressed outer membrane proteins mediate vascular endothelial growth factor secretion but not host cell adherence. Infect Immun. 2006 Sep;74(9):5003-13. PMID:16926391

Schultz MG. Who is this man? Emerg Infect Dis. 2010 Jun;16(6):1025-7. PMID:20507765

Schutze GE. Diagnosis and treatment of Bartonella henselae infections. Pediatr Infect Dis J. 2000 Dec;19(12):1185-7. PMID:11144381

Schweyer S, Fayyazi A. Activation and apoptosis of macrophages in cat scratch disease. J Pathol. 2002 Dec;198(4):534-40. PMID:12434424

Scolfaro C, Leunga GG, Bezzio S, Chiapello N, Riva C, Balbo L, Bertaina C, Tovo PA. Prolonged follow up of seven patients affected by hepatosplenic granulomata due to cat-scratch disease. Eur J Pediatr. 2008 Apr;167(4):471-3. Epub 2007 Jun 1. PMID:17541640

Scolfaro C, Mignone F, Gennari F, Alfarano A, Veltri A, Romagnoli R, Salizzoni M. Possible donor-recipient bartonellosis transmission in a pediatric liver transplant. Transpl Infect Dis. 2008 Dec;10(6):431-3. Epub 2008 Jul 22. PMID:18651873

Scott C, Azwa A, Cohen C, McIntyre M, Desmond N. Cat scratch disease: a diagnostic conundrum. Int J STD AIDS. 2009 Aug;20(8):585-6. PMID:19625597

Seah AB, Azran MS, Newman NJ. Cat-scratch encephalopathy. Arch Neurol. 2004 Jan;61(1):145-7. PMID:14732635

Seah AB, Azran MS, Rucker JC, Biousse V, Martin DF, Newman NJ. Magnetic resonance imaging abnormalities in cat-scratch disease encephalopathy. J Neuroophthalmol. 2003 Mar;23(1):16-21. PMID:12616083

Seas C, Villaverde H, Maguiña C. A 60-year-old man from the highlands of Peru with fever and hemolysis. Am J Trop Med Hyg. 2012 Mar;86(3):381. PMID:22403303

Sedlácková L, Bartosová D, Vydrzalová P, Crhová K, Zarosská E, Holcíková A, Habanec T, Janecek D. [Abscessing lymphadenitis in a 1.5-year-old boy].[Article in Czech]. Klin Mikrobiol Infekc Lek. 2007 Jun;13(3):119-21. PMID:17703405

Sekeyova Z, Subramanian G, Mediannikov O, Diaz MQ, Nyitray A, Blaskovicova H, Raoult D. Evaluation of clinical specimens for Rickettsia, Bartonella, Borrelia, Coxiella, Anaplasma, Franciscella and Diplorickettsia positivity using serological and molecular biology methods. FEMS Immunol Med Microbiol. 2012 Feb;64(1):82-91. Epub 2011 Dec 13. PMID:22098390

Seki N, Kasai S, Saito N, Komagata O, Mihara M, Sasaki T, Tomita T, Sasaki T, Kobayashi M. Quantitative analysis of proliferation and excretion of Bartonella quintana in body lice, Pediculus humanus L. Am J Trop Med Hyg. 2007 Sep;77(3):562-6. PMID:17827380

Seki N, Sasaki T, Sawabe K, Sasaki T, Matsuoka M, Arakawa Y, Marui E, Kobayashi M. Epidemiological studies on Bartonella quintana infections among homeless people in Tokyo, Japan. Jpn J Infect Dis. 2006 Feb;59(1):31-5. PMID:16495631

Serratrice J, Rolain JM, Granel B, Ene N, Conrath J, Avierinos JF, Disdier P, Raoult D, Weiller PJ. [Bilateral retinal artery branch occlusions revealing Bartonella grahamii infection].[Article in French]. Rev Med Interne. 2003 Sep;24(9):629-30. PMID:12951187

Seubert A, Falch C, Birtles RJ, Schulein R, Dehio C. Characterization of the cryptic plasmid pBGR1 from Bartonella grahamii and construction of a versatile Escherichia coli-Bartonella spp. shuttle cloning vector. Plasmid. 2003 Jan;49(1):44-52. PMID:12584000

Seubert A, Hiestand R, de la Cruz F, Dehio C. A bacterial conjugation machinery recruited for pathogenesis. Mol Microbiol. 2003 Sep;49(5):1253-66. PMID:12940985

Seubert A, Schulein R, Dehio C. Bacterial persistence within erythrocytes: a unique pathogenic strategy of Bartonella spp. Int J Med Microbiol. 2002 Feb;291(6-7):555-60. PMID:11890558

Sevall JS. Rapid allelic discrimination from real-time DNA amplification. Methods. 2001 Dec;25(4):452-5. PMID:11846614

Sève P, Turner R, Stankovic K, Perard L, Broussolle C. Transient monoclonal gammopathy in a patient with Bartonella quintana endocarditis. Am J Hematol. 2006 Feb;81(2):115-7. PMID:16432867

Shah SS, McGowan JP. Rickettsial, ehrlichial and Bartonella infections of the myocardium and pericardium. Front Biosci. 2003 Jan 1;8:e197-201. PMID:12456377

Shamaei-Tousi A, Cahill R, Frankel G. Interaction between protein subunits of the type IV secretion system of Bartonella henselae. J Bacteriol. 2004 Jul;186(14):4796-801. PMID:15231811

Shapira N, Merin O, Rosenmann E, Dzigivker I, Bitran D, Yinnon AM, Silberman S. Latent infective endocarditis: epidemiology and clinical characteristics of patients with unsuspected endocarditis detected after elective valve replacement. Ann Thorac Surg. 2004 Nov;78(5):1623-9. PMID:15511445

Shaw SE, Birtles RJ, Day MJ. Arthropod-transmitted infectious diseases of cats. J Feline Med Surg. 2001 Dec;3(4):193-209. PMID:11795958

Shaw SE, Kenny MJ, Tasker S, Birtles RJ. Pathogen carriage by the cat flea Ctenocephalides felis (Bouché) in the United Kingdom. Vet Microbiol. 2004 Sep 8;102(3-4):183-8. PMID:15327793

Shoham N, Miron D, Raz R, Garzozi HJ. [Familial parinaud oculo-glandular syndrome in cat-scratch disease].[Article in Hebrew]. Harefuah. 2000 Jun 15;138(12):1034-6, 1086. PMID:10979428

Short BH. Carrión's disease: an altitude-associated infectious disease. Intern Med J. 2003 Nov;33(11):545. PMID:14656265

Shulman ST. Attention: attention-deficit/ hyperactivity disorder. Pediatr Ann. 2008 Jan;37(1):5-6. PMID:18240846

Siciliano RF, Strabelli TM, Zeigler R, Rodrigues C, Castelli JB, Grinberg M, Colombo S, da Silva LJ, Mendes do Nascimento EM, Pereira dos Santos FC, Uip DE. Infective endocarditis due to Bartonella spp. and Coxiella burnetii: experience at a cardiology hospital in Sao Paulo, Brazil. Ann N Y Acad Sci. 2006 Oct;1078:215-22. PMID:17114712

Signorini L, Simeone F, Tonegatti L, Colombini P, Cadeo B, Cristini F, Matteeli A, Viale P. Co-infection with Esptein-Barr virus and Bartonella henselae resulting in systemic bartonellosis. J Infect. 2002 Oct;45(3):206-7. PMID:12387781

Silaghi C, Knaus M, Rapti D, Shukullari E, Pfister K, Rehbein S. Rickettsia felis and Bartonella spp. in fleas from cats in Albania. Vector Borne Zoonotic Dis. 2012 Jan;12(1):76-7. Epub 2011 Oct 13. PMID:21995262

Silva DF, Freitas RA, Franco AM. [Diversity and abundance of phlebotomine of the genus Lutzomyia (Diptera: Psychodidae) in areas of forest in the northeast of Manacapuru, Amazonas State, Brazil]. [Article in Portuguese]. Neotrop Entomol. 2007 Jan-Feb;36(1):138-44. PMID:17420872

Silveira Cancela M, Valdés Tascón F, Pita Carretero J, Montes Fontao M, Rico Bouza M. [Neonatal papular acrodermatitis (Gianotti-Crosti) and Bartonella henselae infection].[Article in Spanish]. An Esp Pediatr. 2000 Mar;52(3):299-300. PMID:11003916

Silveira Cancela M. [Cat scratch disease].[Article in Spanish]. An Pediatr (Barc). 2007 Apr;66(4):419-20. PMID:17569180

Singhal AB, Newstein MC, Budzik R, Cha JH, Rordorf G, Buonanno FS, Panzara MA. Diffusion-weighted magnetic resonance imaging abnormalities in Bartonella encephalopathy. J Neuroimaging. 2003 Jan;13(1):79-82. PMID:12593136

Skarphédinsson S, Jensen PM, Kristiansen K. Survey of tickborne infections in Denmark. Emerg Infect Dis. 2005 Jul;11(7):1055-61. PMID:16022780

Skerget M, Wenisch C, Daxboeck F, Krause R, Haberl R, Stuenzner D. Cat or dog ownership and seroprevalence of ehrlichiosis, Q fever, and cat-scratch disease. Emerg Infect Dis. 2003 Oct;9(10):1337-40. PMID:14609477

Smajlovic F, Ibralic M. Color Doppler pseudolymphomatous manifestations of the cat scratch disease. Med Arh. 2009;63(5):297-9. PMID:20380135

Smith BE, Tompkins MB, Breitschwerdt EB. Antinuclear antibodies can be detected in dog sera reactive to Bartonella vinsonii subsp. berkhoffii, Ehrlichia canis, or Leishmania infantum antigens. J Vet Intern Med. 2004 Jan-Feb;18(1):47-51. PMID:14765731

Smith DR. Cat scratch disease. Transmission and treatment. Answers still unfolding. Adv Nurse Pract. 2002 Sep;10(9):55-6. PMID:12400315

Smith HM, Reporter R, Rood MP, Linscott AJ, Mascola LM, Hogrefe W, Purcell RH. Prevalence study of antibody to ratborne pathogens and other agents among patients using a free clinic in downtown Los Angeles. J Infect Dis. 2002 Dec 1;186(11):1673-6. Epub 2002 Nov 1. PMID:12447746

Smith RA, Scott B, Beverley DW, Lyon F, Taylor R. Encephalopathy with retinitis due to cat-scratch disease. Dev Med Child Neurol. 2007 Dec;49(12):931-4. PMID:18039241

Smitherman LS, Minnick MF. Bartonella bacilliformis GroEL: effect on growth of human vascular endothelial cells in infected cocultures. Ann N Y Acad Sci. 2005 Dec;1063:286-98. PMID:16481529

Smoller BR, Madhusudhan KT, Scott MA, Horn TD. Granuloma annulare: another manifestation of Bartonella infection? Am J Dermatopathol. 2001 Dec;23(6):510-3. PMID:11801791

Sobha S, Reck AC, Evans A. Neuroretinitis associated with cat scratch disease in a child. Clin Experiment Ophthalmol. 2000 Apr;28(2):127-8. PMID:10933777

Solano-Gallego L, Bradley J, Hegarty B, Sigmon B, Breitschwerdt E. Bartonella henselae IgG antibodies are prevalent in dogs from southeastern USA. Vet Res. 2004 Sep-Oct;35(5):585-95. PMID:15369661

Solano-Gallego L, Hegarty B, Espada Y, Llull J, Breitschwerdt E. Serological and molecular evidence of exposure to arthropod-borne organisms in cats from northeastern Spain. Vet Microbiol. 2006 Dec 20;118(3-4):274-7. Epub 2006 Aug 17. PMID:16919405

Solano-Gallego L, Llull J, Osso M, Hegarty B, Breitschwerdt E. A serological study of exposure to arthropod-borne pathogens in dogs from northeastern Spain. Vet Res. 2006 Mar-Apr;37(2):231-44. PMID:16472522

Somech R, Spirer Z. Uncommon presentation of some common pediatric diseases. Adv Pediatr. 2003;50:269-304. PMID:14626491

Sondermeijer HP, Claas EC, Orendi JM, Tamsma JT. Bartonella quintana prosthetic valve endocarditis detected by blood culture incubation beyond 10 days. Eur J Intern Med. 2006 Oct;17(6):441-3. PMID:16962956

Song AT, Gory M, Roussi J, Salomon J, Cremieux AC, Perronne C, Bernard L. Familial occurrence of cat-scratch disease, with varying clinical expression. Scand J Infect Dis. 2007;39(8):728-30. PMID:17654352

Soós Z, Bakos M, Kovács G, Baranyai L, Jakab F, Winkler G. [Multiple hepatic abscesses due to actinomycosis: difficulties of diagnosis]. [Article in Hungarian]. Orv Hetil. 2011 Feb 13;152(7):268-72. PMID:21296736

Spitalská E, Boldis V, Kostanová Z, Kocianová E, Stefanidesová K. Incidence of various tick-borne microorganisms in rodents and ticks of central Slovakia. Acta Virol. 2008;52(3):175-9. PMID:18999892

Sréter-Lancz Z, Tornyai K, Széll Z, Sréter T, Márialigeti K. Bartonella infections in fleas (Siphonaptera: Pulicidae) and lack of bartonellae in ticks (Acari: Ixodidae) from Hungary. Folia Parasitol (Praha). 2006 Dec;53(4):313-6. PMID:17252927

Staggemeier R, Venker CA, Klein DH, Petry M, Spilki FR, Cantarelli VV. Prevalence of Bartonella henselae and Bartonella clarridgeiae in cats in the south of Brazil: a molecular study. Mem Inst Oswaldo Cruz. 2010 Nov;105(7):873-8. PMID:21120356

Stanek G. [Pandora's Box: pathogens in Ixodes ricinus ticks in Central Europe].[Article in German]. Wien Klin Wochenschr. 2009;121(21-22):673-83. PMID:19998007

Starck T, Madsen BW. Positive polymerase chain reaction and histology with borderline serology in Parinaud's oculoglandular syndrome. Cornea. 2002 Aug;21(6):625-7. PMID:12131048

Stek CJ, van Eijk JJ, Jacobs BC, Enting RH, Sprenger HG, van Alfen N, van Assen S. Neuralgic amyotrophy associated with Bartonella henselae infection. J Neurol Neurosurg Psychiatry. 2011 Jun;82(6):707-8. Epub 2010 Aug 14. PMID:20710009

Stevenson HL, Bai Y, Kosoy MY, Montenieri JA, Lowell JL, Chu MC, Gage KL. Detection of novel Bartonella strains and Yersinia pestis in prairie dogs and their fleas (Siphonaptera: Ceratophyllidae and Pulicidae) using multiplex polymerase chain reaction. J Med Entomol. 2003 May;40(3):329-37. PMID:12943112

Stiles J. Bartonellosis in cats: a role in uveitis? Vet Ophthalmol. 2011 Sep;14 Suppl 1:9-14. PMID:21923819

Stockmeyer B, Schoerner C, Frangou P, Moriabadi T, Heuss D, Harrer T. Chronic vasculitis and polyneuropathy due to infection with Bartonella henselae. Infection. 2007 Apr;35(2):107-9. PMID:17401716

Stojanovic V, Foley P. Infectious disease prevalence in a feral cat population on Prince Edward Island, Canada. Can Vet J. 2011 Sep;52(9):979-82. PMID:22379197

Stöllberger C, Mölzer G, Finsterer J. Seroprevalence of antibodies to microorganisms known to cause arterial and myocardial damage in patients with or without coronary stenosis. Clin Diagn Lab Immunol. 2001 Sep;8(5):997-1002. PMID:11527817

Stoob K, Beer G, Weishaupt D. [Adult, afebrile patient with rapidly growing tumor of the upper arm: Bartonella henselae as the etiology]. [Article in German]. Rofo. 2002 Mar;174(3):363-4. PMID:11885017

Stricker RB, Brewer JH, Burrascano JJ, Horowitz R, Johnson L, Phillips SE, Savely VR, Sherr VT. Possible role of tick-borne infection in "cat-scratch disease": comment on the article by Giladi et al. Arthritis Rheum. 2006 Jul;54(7):2347-8. PMID:16802385

Stricker RB, Johnson L. Lyme disease: the next decade. Infect Drug Resist. 2011;4:1-9. Epub 2011 Jan 7. PMID:21694904

Stricker RB, Lautin A, Burrascano JJ. Lyme disease: point/counterpoint. Expert Rev Anti Infect Ther. 2005 Apr;3(2):155-65. PMID:15918774

Stricker RB, Lautin A. The Lyme Wars: time to listen. Expert Opin Investig Drugs. 2003 Oct;12(10):1609-14. PMID:14519082

Stricker RB. Counterpoint: long-term antibiotic therapy improves persistent symptoms associated with lyme disease. Clin Infect Dis. 2007 Jul 15;45(2):149-57. Epub 2007 Jun 5. PMID:17578772

Struk DW, Munk PL, Lee MJ, Ho SG, Worsley DF. Imaging of soft tissue infections. Radiol Clin North Am. 2001 Mar;39(2):277-303. PMID:11316360

Sugiyama H, Sahara M, Imai Y, Ono M, Okamoto K, Kikuchi K, Nagai R. Infective endocarditis by Bartonella quintana masquerading as antineutrophil cytoplasmic antibody-associated small vessel vasculitis. Cardiology. 2009;114(3):208-11. Epub 2009 Jul 15. PMID:19602882

Suh B, Chun JK, Yong D, Lee YS, Jeong SH, Yang WI, Kim DS. A report of cat scratch disease in Korea confirmed by PCR amplification of the 16S-23S rRNA intergenic region of Bartonella henselae. Korean J Lab Med. 2010 Feb;30(1):34-7. PMID:20197720

Suhler EB, Lauer AK, Rosenbaum JT. Prevalence of serologic evidence of cat scratch disease in patients with neuroretinitis. Ophthalmology. 2000 May;107(5):871-6. PMID:10811077

Suksawat J, Xuejie Y, Hancock SI, Hegarty BC, Nilkumhang P, Breitschwerdt EB. Serologic and molecular evidence of coinfection with multiple vector-borne pathogens in dogs from Thailand. J Vet Intern Med. 2001 Sep-Oct;15(5):453-62. PMID:11596732

Sun J, Fu G, Lin J, Song X, Lu L, Liu Q. Seroprevalence of Bartonella in Eastern China and analysis of risk factors. BMC Infect Dis. 2010 May 20;10:121. PMID:20482887

Sun J, Liu Q, Lu L, Ding G, Guo J, Fu G, Zhang J, Meng F, Wu H, Song X, Ren D, Li D, Guo Y, Wang J, Li G, Liu J, Lin H. Coinfection with four genera of bacteria (Borrelia, Bartonella, Anaplasma, and Ehrlichia) in Haemaphysalis longicornis and Ixodes sinensis ticks from China. Vector Borne Zoonotic Dis. 2008 Dec;8(6):791-5. PMID:18637722

Sureda A, García D, Loma-Osorio P. [Embolic stroke as the first manifestation of Bartonella henselae endocarditis in an immunocompetent patient].[Article in Spanish]. Enferm Infecc Microbiol Clin. 2010 Jan;28(1):64-5. Epub 2009 May 1. PMID:19409676

Swanson KI, Norris DE. Co-circulating microorganisms in questing Ixodes scapularis nymphs in Maryland. J Vector Ecol. 2007 Dec;32(2):243-51. PMID:18260514

Swanson SJ, Neitzel D, Reed KD, Belongia EA. Coinfections acquired from ixodes ticks. Clin Microbiol Rev. 2006 Oct;19(4):708-27. PMID:17041141

Sweger D, Resto-Ruiz S, Johnson DP, Schmiederer M, Hawke N, Anderson B. Conservation of the 17-kilodalton antigen gene within the genus Bartonella. Clin Diagn Lab Immunol. 2000 Mar;7(2):251-7. PMID:10702501

Swick BL, Walling HW, Stone MS. Solitary erythematous nodule on the back. Arch Dermatol. 2010 Apr;146(4):439-44. PMID:20404237

Sykes JE, Henn JB, Kasten RW, Allen C, Chomel BB. Bartonella henselae infection in splenectomized domestic cats previously infected with hemotropic Mycoplasma species. Vet Immunol Immunopathol. 2007 Mar 15;116(1-2):104-8. Epub 2006 Dec 22. PMID:17254639

Sykes JE, Kittleson MD, Pesavento PA, Byrne BA, MacDonald KA, Chomel BB. Evaluation of the relationship between causative organisms and clinical characteristics of infective endocarditis in dogs: 71 cases (1992-2005). J Am Vet Med Assoc. 2006 Jun 1;228(11):1723-34. PMID:16740074

Sykes JE, Lindsay LL, Maggi RG, Breitschwerdt EB. Human coinfection with Bartonella henselae and two hemotropic mycoplasma variants resembling Mycoplasma ovis. J Clin Microbiol. 2010 Oct;48(10):3782-5. Epub 2010 Aug 11. PMID:20702675

Sykes JE, Westropp JL, Kasten RW, Chomel BB. Association between Bartonella species infection and disease in pet cats as determined using serology and culture. J Feline Med Surg. 2010 Aug;12(8):631-6. Epub 2010 May 31. PMID:20570199

Sykes JE. Feline hemotropic mycoplasmas. J Vet Emerg Crit Care (San Antonio). 2010 Feb;20(1):62-9. PMID:20230435

Szaleniec J, Oleś K, Składzień J, Strek P. [Cat scratch disease—an underestimated diagnosis].[Article in Polish]. Otolaryngol Pol. 2009 May-Jun;63(3):271-3. PMID:19886535

Szczesny P, Linke D, Ursinus A, Bär K, Schwarz H, Riess TM, Kempf VA, Lupas AN, Martin J, Zeth K. Structure of the head of the Bartonella adhesin BadA. PLoS Pathog. 2008 Aug 8;4(8):e1000119. PMID:18688279

Szczesny P, Lupas A. Domain annotation of trimeric autotransporter adhesins--daTAA. Bioinformatics. 2008 May 15;24(10):1251-6. Epub 2008 Apr 8. PMID:18397894

Szymański M, Siwiec H, Gołabek W. [Cat-scratch disease of the parotid gland].[Article in Polish]. Wiad Lek. 2004;57(11-12):704-6. PMID:15865254

Tabar MD, Altet L, Francino O, Sánchez A, Ferrer L, Roura X. Vector-borne infections in cats: molecular study in Barcelona area (Spain). Vet Parasitol. 2008 Feb 14;151(2-4):332-6. Epub 2007 Nov 9. PMID:18079064

Tabar MD, Francino O, Altet L, Sánchez A, Ferrer L, Roura X. PCR survey of vectorborne pathogens in dogs living in and around Barcelona, an area endemic for leishmaniasis. Vet Rec. 2009 Jan 24;164(4):112-6. PMID:19168881

Tabar MD, Maggi RG, Altet L, Vilafranca M, Francino O, Roura X. Gammopathy in a Spanish dog infected with Bartonella henselae. J Small Anim Pract. 2011 Apr;52(4):209-12. PMID:21906064

Täger F M, Jahnsen K J, Mediavilla R M, Burgos L R. [Ocular bartonellosis: report of three clinical cases].[Article in Spanish]. Rev Chilena Infectol. 2008 Feb;25(1):58-63. Epub 2008 Feb 8. PMID:18273527

Takazoe I. [Achievement by Hideyo Noguchi].[Article in Japanese]. Nihon Naika Gakkai Zasshi. 2002 Oct 10;91(10):2887-90. PMID:12451642

Takeda N, Ishiwada N, Fukasawa C, Furuya Y, Tsuneoka H, Tsukahara M, Kohno Y. [Pediatric pneumonia, pleural effusion, and pericarditis following cat scratch disease and serological cross-reactions among Bartonella henselae and Rickettsia japonica determined by indirect fluorescence antibodies].[Article in Japanese]. Kansenshogaku Zasshi. 2007 Mar;81(2):206-9. PMID:17447481

Tamir E. Cat scratch disease. Acta Dermatovenerol Croat. 2007;15(1):47. PMID:17582885

Tang YW. Duplex PCR assay simultaneously detecting and differentiating Bartonella quintana, B. henselae, and Coxiella burnetii in surgical heart valve specimens. J Clin Microbiol. 2009 Aug;47(8):2647-50. Epub 2009 Jun 24. PMID:19553582

Tapp RA, Roy AF, Corstvet RE, Wilson VL. Differential detection of Bartonella species and strains in cat scratch disease diagnostics by polymerase chain reaction amplification of 16S ribosomal RNA gene. J Vet Diagn Invest. 2001 May;13(3):219-29. PMID:11482599

Tarasevich IV. [New and emerging rickettsial and bartonella infections]. [Article in Russian]. Vestn Ross Akad Med Nauk. 2001;(11):8-11. PMID:11837209

Tasato D, Tateyama M, Inamine M, Hibiya K, Tamaki Y, Haranaga S, Yara S, Higa F, Maruyama S, Fujita J. [Case report: a case of cat scratch disease in elderly patient needed to differentiate tuberculous lymphadenitis].[Article in Japanese]. Nihon Naika Gakkai Zasshi. 2011 Jul 10;100(7):1969-71. PMID:21863773

Tasher D, Armarnik E, Mizrahi A, Liat BS, Constantini S, Grisaru-Soen G. Cat scratch disease with cervical vertebral osteomyelitis and spinal epidural abscess. Pediatr Infect Dis J. 2009 Sep;28(9):848-50. PMID:19654566

Tate CM, Mead DG, Luttrell MP, Howerth EW, Dugan VG, Munderloh UG, Davidson WR. Experimental infection of white-tailed deer with Anaplasma phagocytophilum, etiologic agent of human granulocytic anaplasmosis. J Clin Microbiol. 2005 Aug;43(8):3595-601. PMID:16081884

Tattevin P, Lellouche F, Bruneel F, Régnier B, De Broucker T. [Bartonella henselae meningoencephalitis].[Article in French]. Rev Neurol (Paris). 2001 Jul;157(6-7):698-700. PMID:11458191

Taye A, Chen H, Duncan K, Zhang Z, Hendrix L, Gonzalez J, Ching W. Production of recombinant protein Pap31 and its application for the diagnosis of Bartonella bacilliformis infection. Ann N Y Acad Sci. 2005 Dec;1063:280-5. PMID:16481528

Taylor RH, Smith RA, Issa M. Possible cat scratch disease causing neuroretinitis and CRVO in a child. Eye (Lond). 2002 Mar;16(2):189-90. PMID:11988821

Tea A, Alexiou-Daniel S, Arvanitidou M, Diza E, Antoniadis A. Occurrence of Bartonella henselae and Bartonella quintana in a healthy Greek population. Am J Trop Med Hyg. 2003 May;68(5):554-6. PMID:12812344

Tea A, Alexiou-Daniel S, Papoutsi A, Papa A, Antoniadis A. Bartonella species isolated from rodents, Greece. Emerg Infect Dis. 2004 May;10(5):963-4. PMID:15216849

Telfer S, Begon M, Bennett M, Bown KJ, Burthe S, Lambin X, Telford G, Birtles R. Contrasting dynamics of Bartonella spp. in cyclic field vole populations: the impact of vector and host dynamics. Parasitology. 2007 Mar;134(Pt 3):413-25. Epub 2006 Nov 13. PMID:17096870

Telfer S, Birtles R, Bennett M, Lambin X, Paterson S, Begon M. Parasite interactions in natural populations: insights from longitudinal data. Parasitology. 2008 Jun;135(7):767-81. Epub 2008 May 12. PMID:18474121

Telfer S, Bown KJ, Sekules R, Begon M, Hayden T, Birtles R. Disruption of a host-parasite system following the introduction of an exotic host species. Parasitology. 2005 Jun;130(Pt 6):661-8. PMID:15977903

Telfer S, Clough HE, Birtles LR, Bennett M, Carslake D, Helyar S, Begon M. Ecological differences and coexistence in a guild of microparasites: Bartonella in wild rodents. Ecology. 2007 Jul;88(7):1841-9. PMID:17645030

Telfer S, Lambin X, Birtles R, Beldomenico P, Burthe S, Paterson S, Begon M. Species interactions in a parasite community drive infection risk in a wildlife population. Science. 2010 Oct 8;330(6001):243-6. PMID:20929776

Telford SR 3rd, Wormser GP. Bartonella spp. transmission by ticks not established. Emerg Infect Dis. 2010 Mar;16(3):379-84. PMID:20202410

ten Hove CH, Gubler FM, Kiezebrink-Lindenhovius HH. Back pain in a child caused by cat scratch disease. Pediatr Infect Dis J. 2009 Mar;28(3):258. PMID:19209087

Teng JL, Yeung MY, Yue G, Au-Yeung RK, Yeung EY, Fung AM, Tse H, Yuen KY, Lau SK, Woo PC. In silico analysis of 16S rRNA gene sequencing based methods for identification of medically important aerobic Gram-negative bacteria. J Med Microbiol. 2011 Sep;60(Pt 9):1281-6. Epub 2011 Apr 15. PMID:21498652

Terrada C, Bodaghi B, Conrath J, Raoult D, Drancourt M. Uveitis: an emerging clinical form of Bartonella infection. Clin Microbiol Infect. 2009 Dec;15 Suppl 2:132-3. Epub 2009 Jun 22. PMID:19548998

Thiam M, Fall PD, Gning SB, Grinda JM, Mainardi JL. [Bartonella Quintana infective endocarditis in an immunocompetent Senegalese man].[Article in French]. Rev Med Interne. 2002 Dec;23(12):1035-7. PMID:12504245

Thudi KR, Kreikemeier JT, Phillips NJ, Salvalaggio PR, Kennedy DJ, Hayashi PH. Cat scratch disease causing hepatic masses after liver transplant. Liver Int. 2007 Feb;27(1):145-8. PMID:17241393

Ticona E, Huaroto L, Garcia Y, Vargas L, Madariaga MG. The pathophysiology of the acute phase of human bartonellosis resembles AIDS. Med Hypotheses. 2010 Jan;74(1):45-9. Epub 2009 Aug 7. PMID:19665314

Tijsse-Klasen E, Fonville M, Gassner F, Nijhof AM, Hovius EK, Jongejan F, Takken W, Reimerink JR, Overgaauw PA, Sprong H. Absence of zoonotic Bartonella species in questing ticks: first detection of Bartonella clarridgeiae and Rickettsia felis in cat fleas in the Netherlands. Parasit Vectors. 2011 Apr 18;4:61. PMID:21501464

Todd S, Xu J, Millar BC, Moore JE, Crowe M, Raoult D, Harrison T, Hill C, Douglas J. Culture-negative Bartonella endocarditis in a patient with renal failure: the value of molecular methods in diagnosis. Br J Biomed Sci. 2004;61(4):190-3. PMID:15649011

Tokodi I, Máj C, Deák J, Gyetvai B, Lakatos B, Simon G. [Unusual manifestations of Bartonella infections].[Article in Hungarian]. Orv Hetil. 2001 Oct 7;142(40):2197-200. PMID:11706512

Toledo A, Olmeda AS, Escudero R, Jado I, Valcárcel F, Casado-Nistal MA, Rodríguez-Vargas M, Gil H, Anda P. Tick-borne zoonotic bacteria in ticks collected from central Spain. Am J Trop Med Hyg. 2009 Jul;81(1):67-74. PMID:19556569

Touyama M, Uezu K, Nakamoto A, Shinzato T, Higa F, Tateyama M, Saito A, Nakamura M, Tsuneoka H, Tsukahara M. [A case of cat scratch disease with encephalopathy].[Article in Japanese]. Kansenshogaku Zasshi. 2002 Feb;76(2):113-7. PMID:11904996

Trafny DJ, Oyama MA, Wormser C, Reynolds CA, Singletary GE, Peddle GD. Cardiac troponin-I concentrations in dogs with bradyarrhythmias before and after artificial pacing. J Vet Cardiol. 2010 Dec;12(3):183-90. Epub 2010 Oct 28. PMID:21030328

Tran TN, Forestier CL, Drancourt M, Raoult D, Aboudharam G. Brief communication: co-detection of Bartonella quintana and Yersinia pestis in an 11th-15th burial site in Bondy, France. Am J Phys Anthropol. 2011 Jul;145(3):489-94. Epub 2011 May 3. PMID:21541920

Tran TN, Signoli M, Fozzati L, Aboudharam G, Raoult D, Drancourt M. High throughput, multiplexed pathogen detection authenticates plague waves in medieval Venice, Italy. PLoS One. 2011 Mar 10;6(3):e16735. PMID:21423736

Triller K, Strus P, Petrovec M, Duh D, Avsic-Zupanc T. Genetic variation of Bartonella henselae detected in lymph nodes from patients with cat scratch disease in Slovenia. Ann N Y Acad Sci. 2003 Jun;990:393-6. PMID:12860661

Trombert-Paolantoni S, Clairet V, Gaulier E, Figarella P. [Evaluation of a in house serology reagent for the diagnosis of cat-scratch disease defined by PCR].[Article in French]. Pathol Biol (Paris). 2007 Nov;55(8-9):441-5. Epub 2007 Oct 1. PMID:17905531

Troncone R, Ventura A, Facchini S, Zennaro F, Bussani R, Lenhardt A, Dal Molin G. Clinical quiz: cat scratch disease. J Pediatr Gastroenterol Nutr. 2003 Feb;36(2):227, 265. PMID:12593397

Trout RT, Steelman CD, Szalanski AL. Phylogenetics and population genetics of the louse fly, Lipoptena mazamae, from Arkansas, USA. Med Vet Entomol. 2010 Sep;24(3):258-65. Epub 2010 Jun 1. PMID:20534010

Truttmann MC, Guye P, Dehio C. BID-F1 and BID-F2 domains of Bartonella henselae effector protein BepF trigger together with BepC the formation of invasome structures. PLoS One. 2011;6(10):e25106. Epub 2011 Oct 17. PMID:22043280

Truttmann MC, Misselwitz B, Huser S, Hardt WD, Critchley DR, Dehio C. Bartonella henselae engages inside-out and outside-in signaling by integrin β1 and talin1 during invasome-mediated bacterial uptake. J Cell Sci. 2011 Nov 1;124(Pt 21):3591-602. Epub 2011 Nov 1. PMID:22045736

Truttmann MC, Rhomberg TA, Dehio C. Combined action of the type IV secretion effector proteins BepC and BepF promotes invasome formation of Bartonella henselae on endothelial and epithelial cells. Cell Microbiol. 2011 Feb;13(2):284-99. Epub 2010 Oct 22. PMID:20964799

Tsai KH, Huang CG, Fang CT, Shu PY, Huang JH, Wu WJ. Prevalence of Rickettsia felis and the first identification of Bartonella henselae Fizz/CAL-1 in cat fleas (Siphonaptera: Pulicidae) from Taiwan. J Med Entomol. 2011 Mar;48(2):445-52. PMID:21485388

Tsai PS, DeAngelis DD, Spencer WH, Seiff SR. Bacillary angiomatosis of the anterior orbit, eyelid, and conjunctiva. Am J Ophthalmol. 2002 Sep;134(3):433-4. PMID:12208256

Tsai YL, Chang CC, Chuang ST, Chomel BB. Bartonella species and their ectoparasites: selective host adaptation or strain selection between the vector and the mammalian host? Comp Immunol Microbiol Infect Dis. 2011 Jul;34(4):299-314. Epub 2011 May 25. PMID:21616536

Tsai YL, Chomel BB, Chang CC, Kass PH, Conrad PA, Chuang ST. Bartonella and Babesia infections in cattle and their ticks in Taiwan. Comp Immunol Microbiol Infect Dis. 2011 Mar;34(2):179-87. Epub 2010 Dec 30. PMID:21194750

Tsai YL, Chuang ST, Chang CC, Kass PH, Chomel BB. Bartonella species in small mammals and their ectoparasites in Taiwan. Am J Trop Med Hyg. 2010 Oct;83(4):917-23. PMID:20889892

Tsai YL, Lin CC, Chomel BB, Chuang ST, Tsai KH, Wu WJ, Huang CG, Yu JC, Sung MH, Kass PH, Chang CC. Bartonella infection in shelter cats and dogs and their ectoparasites. Vector Borne Zoonotic Dis. 2011 Aug;11(8):1023-30. Epub 2010 Dec 13. PMID:21142966

Tsujino K, Tsukahara M, Tsuneoka H, Ichihara K, Furuya T, Kawauchi S, Oga A, Sasaki K. Clinical implication of prolonged fever in children with cat scratch disease. J Infect Chemother. 2004 Aug;10(4):227-33. PMID:15365864

Tsukahara M, Iino H, Ishida C, Murakami K, Tsuneoka H, Uchida M. Bartonella henselae bacteraemia in patients with cat scratch disease. Eur J Pediatr. 2001 May;160(5):316. PMID:11388603

Tsukahara M, Tsuneoka H, Iino H, Murano I, Takahashi H, Uchida M. Bartonella henselae infection as a cause of fever of unknown origin. J Clin Microbiol. 2000 May;38(5):1990-1. PMID:10790137

Tsukahara M, Tsuneoka H, Tateishi H, Fujita K, Uchida M. Bartonella infection associated with systemic juvenile rheumatoid arthritis. Clin Infect Dis. 2001 Jan;32(1):E22-3. Epub 2000 Dec 11. PMID:11112671

Tsukahara M. Cat scratch disease in Japan. J Infect Chemother. 2002 Dec;8(4):321-5. PMID:12525891

Tsuneoka H, Fujii R, Fujisawa K, Iino H, Isida C, Murakami K, Tsukahara M. [Clinical evaluation of commercial serological test for Bartonella infection].[Article in Japanese]. Kansenshogaku Zasshi. 2000 Apr;74(4):387-91. PMID:10835846

Tsuneoka H, Ishida C, Tsukahara M. [Determination of antibody titer to Bartonella henselae by indirect fluorescence antibody assay using B. henselae from domestic cats as antigen].[Article in Japanese]. Kansenshogaku Zasshi. 2005 Oct;79(10):826-8. PMID:16296330

Tsuneoka H, Ishida C, Umeda A, Inokuma H, Tsukahara M. [Evaluation of isolation media for the detection of Bartonella henselae--isolation of Bartonella henselae from domestic cats].[Article in Japanese]. Kansenshogaku Zasshi. 2004 Jul;78(7):574-9. PMID:15359889

Tsuneoka H, Ouchi K, Nagaoka H, Ishida C, Iino H, Murakami K, Tsujino K, Umeda A, Tsukahara M. [Serological cross-reaction among Bartonella henselae, Chlamydia pneumoniae and Coxiella burnetii by indirect fluorescence antibody method].[Article in Japanese]. Kansenshogaku Zasshi. 2001 May;75(5):406-10. PMID:11424490

Tsuneoka H, Tsukahara M. Analysis of data in 30 patients with cat scratch disease without lymphadenopathy. J Infect Chemother. 2006 Aug;12(4):224-6. PMID:16944264

Tsuneoka H, Umeda A, Tsukahara M, Sasaki K. Evaluation of indirect fluorescence antibody assay for detection of Bartonella clarridgeiae and Seroprevalence of B. clarridgeiae among patients with suspected cat scratch disease. J Clin Microbiol. 2004 Jul;42(7):3346-9. PMID:15243113

Tsuneoka H, Yanagihara M, Nojima J, Ichihara K. Antimicrobial susceptibility by Etest of Bartonella henselae isolated from cats and human in Japan. J Infect Chemother. 2010 Dec;16(6):446-8. Epub 2010 Jun 22. PMID:20567991

Tsuneoka H, Yanagihara M, Otani S, Katayama Y, Fujinami H, Nagafuji H, Asari S, Nojima J, Ichihara K. A first Japanese case of Bartonella henselae-induced endocarditis diagnosed by prolonged culture of a specimen from the excised valve. Diagn Microbiol Infect Dis. 2010 Oct;68(2):174-6. PMID:20846591

Tucci E, Della Rocca C, Santilli F. Localized bacillary angiomatosis in the oral cavity: observations about a neoplasm with atypical behavior. Description of a case and review of the literature.[Article in English, Italian]. Minerva Stomatol. 2006 Jan-Feb;55(1-2):67-75. PMID:16495874

Tuerk M, Cheng LS, Konia T, Armstrong AW. Umbilicated erythematous papules in an immunocompromised patient. Lancet Infect Dis. 2011 Jun;11(6):488. PMID:21616459

Turgut M, Alabaz D, Karakaş M, Kavak M, Aksaray N, Alhan E, Cevlik F, Tuncer I. Bacillary angiomatosis in an immunocompetent child with a grafted traumatic wound. J Dermatol. 2004 Oct;31(10):844-7. PMID:15672717

Turner JW, Pien BC, Ardoin SA, Anderson AM, Shieh WJ, Zaki SR, Bhatnagar J, Guarner J, Howell DN, Woods CW. A man with chest pain and glomerulonephritis. Lancet. 2005 Jun 11-17;365(9476):2062. PMID:15950721

Turon Estrada A, Osuna Pulido MT, Colomer Pairés J, Vilanova Busquets JC. [Transverse myelitis associated with cat-scratch disease]. [Article in Spanish]. Med Clin (Barc). 2003 Mar 29;120(11):437. PMID:12681227

Tuttle AD, Birkenheuer AJ, Juopperi T, Levy MG, Breitschwerdt EB. Concurrent bartonellosis and babesiosis in a dog with persistent thrombocytopenia. J Am Vet Med Assoc. 2003 Nov 1;223(9):1306-10, 1280-1. PMID:14621218

Umekoji A, Fukai K, Yanagihara S, Ono E, Sowa J, Ishii M. Rapid detection of Bartonella henselae heat shock protein DNA by nested polymerase chain reaction from swollen lymph nodes of a patient with cat-scratch disease. J Dermatol. 2009 Oct;36(10):548-50. PMID:19785710

Ussery DW, Tindbaek N, Hallin PF. Genome update: promoter profiles. Microbiology. 2004 Sep;150(Pt 9):2791-3. PMID:15347738

Valdesoiro Navarrete L, Pineda Solas V, Martín Martín C, Sanfeliu Sala I, Cabezas Maspoch RM, Sánchez Oespina M. [Splenic abscess and cat-scratch disease].[Article in Spanish]. An Esp Pediatr. 2001 Oct;55(4):365-8. PMID:11578546

Valentine KH, Harms CA, Cadenas MB, Birkenheuer AJ, Marr HS, Braun-McNeill J, Maggi RG, Breitschwerdt EB. Bartonella DNA in loggerhead sea turtles. Emerg Infect Dis. 2007 Jun;13(6):949-50. PMID:17582905

Valerio CR, Murray P, Arlian LG, Slater JE. Bacterial 16S ribosomal DNA in house dust mite cultures. J Allergy Clin Immunol. 2005 Dec;116(6):1296-300. PMID:16337462

Valverde-Gubianas M, Ramos-López JF, López-Torres JA, Toribio-García M, Milla-Peñalver C, Gálvez Torres-Puchol J, Medialdea-Marcos S. [Neuroretinitis. Clinical cases].[Article in Spanish]. Arch Soc Esp Oftalmol. 2009 Aug;84(8):389-94. PMID:19728239

Van Audenhove A, Verhoef G, Peetermans WE, Boogaerts M, Vandenberghe P. Autoimmune haemolytic anaemia triggered by Bartonella henselae infection: a case report. Br J Haematol. 2001 Dec;115(4):924-5. PMID:11843827

van der Veer-Meerkerk M, van Zaanen HC. Visceral involvement in an immunocompetent male: a rare presentation of cat scratch disease. Neth J Med. 2008 Apr;66(4):160-2. PMID:18424863

van Passel MW, Kuramae EE, Luyf AC, Bart A, Boekhout T. The reach of the genome signature in prokaryotes. BMC Evol Biol. 2006 Oct 13;6:84. PMID:17040564

van Tooren RM, van Leusen R, Bosch FH. Culture negative endocarditis combined with glomerulonephritis caused by Bartonella species in two immunocompetent adults. Neth J Med. 2001 Nov;59(5):218-24. PMID:11705641

VanderHeyden TR, Yong SL, Breitschwerdt EB, Maggi RG, Mihalik AR, Parada JP, Fimmel CJ. Granulomatous hepatitis due to Bartonella henselae infection in an immunocompetent patient. BMC Infect Dis. 2012 Jan 23;12:17. PMID:22269175

Varagnol M, Parola P, Jouan R, Beaucournu JC, Rolain JM, Raoult D. First detection of Rickettsia felis and Bartonella clarridgeiae in fleas from Laos. Clin Microbiol Infect. 2009 Dec;15 Suppl 2:334-5. Epub 2009 May 2. PMID:19438611

Varanat M, Broadhurst J, Linder KE, Maggi RG, Breitschwerdt EB. Identification of Bartonella henselae in 2 Cats With Pyogranulomatous Myocarditis and Diaphragmatic Myositis. Vet Pathol. 2011 Apr 13. [Epub ahead of print]. PMID:21490304

Varanat M, Maggi RG, Linder KE, Breitschwerdt EB. Molecular prevalence of Bartonella, Babesia, and hemotropic Mycoplasma sp. in dogs with splenic disease. J Vet Intern Med. 2011 Nov-Dec;25(6):1284-91. Epub 2011 Oct 12. PMID:22092618

Varanat M, Maggi RG, Linder KE, Horton S, Breitschwerdt EB. Cross-contamination in the molecular detection of Bartonella from paraffin-embedded tissues. Vet Pathol. 2009 Sep;46(5):940-4. Epub 2009 May 9. PMID:19429988

Varanat M, Travis A, Lee W, Maggi RG, Bissett SA, Linder KE, Breitschwerdt EB. Recurrent osteomyelitis in a cat due to infection with Bartonella vinsonii subsp. berkhoffii genotype II. J Vet Intern Med. 2009 Nov-Dec;23(6):1273-7. Epub 2009 Aug 26. PMID:19709358

Vasil'eva IS. [Bartonellosis and a possible role of Ixodes ticks (family Ixodidae, order Parasitiformes) in the transmission of pathogenic Bartonella bacteria].[Article in Russian]. Med Parazitol (Mosk). 2005 Apr-Jun;(2):44-8. PMID:15984622

Vásquez T P, Chanqueo C L, García C P, Poggi M H, Ferrés G M, Bustos M M, Piottante B A. [Bacillary angiomatosis caused by Bartonella quintana in an human immunodeficiency virus positive patient].[Article in Spanish]. Rev Chilena Infectol. 2007 Apr;24(2):155-9. Epub 2007 Apr 12. PMID:17453076

Vassallo C, Ardigò M, Brazzelli V, Zecca M, Locatelli F, Alessandrino PE, Lazzarino M, Corona S, Lanzerini P, Benazzo M, Fabbi M, Borroni G. Bartonella-related pseudomembranous angiomatous papillomatosis of the oral cavity associated with allogeneic bone marrow transplantation and oral graft-versus-host disease. Br J Dermatol. 2007 Jul;157(1):174-8. Epub 2007 Jun 6. PMID:17553040

Vassilopoulou A, Betto P, Germi L, Bonoldi E, Fornasa CV. Penile chancre: an unusual presentation of cat-scratch disease. J Eur Acad Dermatol Venereol. 2009 Feb;23(2):212-3. Epub 2008 May 19. PMID:18498339

Vayssier-Taussat M, Le Rhun D, Bonnet S, Cotté V. Insights in Bartonella host specificity. Ann N Y Acad Sci. 2009 May;1166:127-32. PMID:19538272

Vayssier-Taussat M, Le Rhun D, Deng HK, Biville F, Cescau S, Danchin A, Marignac G, Lenaour E, Boulouis HJ, Mavris M, Arnaud L, Yang H, Wang J, Quebatte M, Engel P, Saenz H, Dehio C. The Trw type IV secretion system of Bartonella mediates host-specific adhesion to erythrocytes. PLoS Pathog. 2010 Jun 10;6(6):e1000946. PMID:20548954

Vedam V, Kannenberg EL, Haynes JG, Sherrier DJ, Datta A, Carlson RW. A Rhizobium leguminosarum AcpXL mutant produces lipopolysaccharide lacking 27-hydroxyoctacosanoic acid. J Bacteriol. 2003 Mar;185(6):1841-50. PMID:12618448

Velho PE, Cintra ML, Uthida-Tanaka AM, de Moraes AM, Mariotto A. What do we (not) know about the human bartonelloses? Braz J Infect Dis. 2003 Feb;7(1):1-6. PMID:12807686

Velho PE, de Moraes AM, Uthida-Tanaka AM, Cintra ML, Gigliogi R. Ultrastructural changes in a standard strain of Bartonella henselae after passages through BALB/cAn mice. Ultrastruct Pathol. 2002 May-Jun;26(3):161-9. PMID:12184374

Velho PE, Ericson ME. Cryptogenic hepatitis and bartonellosis. Dig Dis Sci. 2012 Apr;57(4):1107-8. Epub 2012 Feb 4. PMID:22307338

Velho PE, Pimentel V, Del Negro GM, Okay TS, Diniz PP, Breitschwerdt EB. Severe anemia, panserositis, and cryptogenic hepatitis in an HIV patient infected with Bartonella henselae. Ultrastruct Pathol. 2007 Nov-Dec;31(6):373-7. PMID:18098054

Velho PE. Blood transfusion as an alternative bartonellosis transmission in a pediatric liver transplant. Transpl Infect Dis. 2009 Oct;11(5):474. PMID:19804481

Vento A, Pätilä T, Vaara M, Larinkari U, Sipponen J. Bartonella quintana and Bartonella pediococcus Infection after Aortic Valve Replacement. Heart Surg Forum. 2008;11(2):E94-5. PMID:18430664

Verdon R, Geffray L, Collet T, Huet H, Parienti JJ, Debruyne M, Vergnaud M, Bazin C. Vertebral osteomyelitis due to Bartonella henselae in adults: a report of 2 cases. Clin Infect Dis. 2002 Dec 15;35(12):e141-4. Epub 2002 Nov 20. PMID:12471592

Verma A, Davis GE, Ihler GM. Formation of stress fibres in human endothelial cells infected with Bartonella bacilliformis is associated with altered morphology, impaired migration and defects in cell morphogenesis. Cell Microbiol. 2001 Mar;3(3):169-80. PMID:11260140

Verma A, Davis GE, Ihler GM. Infection of human endothelial cells with Bartonella bacilliformis is dependent on Rho and results in activation of Rho. Infect Immun. 2000 Oct;68(10):5960-9. PMID:10992508

Verma A, Ihler GM. Activation of Rac, Cdc42 and other downstream signaling molecules by Bartonella bacilliformis during entry into human endothelial cells. Cell Microbiol. 2002 Sep;4(9):557-69. PMID:12390349

Vermeulen MJ, Diederen BM, Verbakel H, Peeters MF. Low sensitivity of Bartonella henselae PCR in serum samples of patients with cat-scratch disease lymphadenitis. J Med Microbiol. 2008 Aug;57(Pt 8):1049-50. PMID:18628513

Vermeulen MJ, Herremans M, Verbakel H, Bergmans AM, Roord JJ, van Dijken PJ, Peeters MF. Serological testing for Bartonella henselae infections in The Netherlands: clinical evaluation of immunofluorescence assay and ELISA. Clin Microbiol Infect. 2007 Jun;13(6):627-34. Epub 2007 Mar 22. PMID:17378931

Vermeulen MJ, Peeters MF, Verbakel H, de Moor RA, Roord JJ, van Dijken PJ. No etiological role for Bartonella henselae infection in Henoch Schönlein purpura. Pediatr Infect Dis J. 2009 Dec;28(12):1142-3. PMID:19935277

Vermeulen MJ, Rutten GJ, Verhagen I, Peeters MF, van Dijken PJ. Transient paresis associated with cat-scratch disease: case report and literature review of vertebral osteomyelitis caused by Bartonella henselae. Pediatr Infect Dis J. 2006 Dec;25(12):1177-81. PMID:17133166

Vermeulen MJ, Verbakel H, Notermans DW, Reimerink JH, Peeters MF. Evaluation of sensitivity, specificity and cross-reactivity in Bartonella henselae serology. J Med Microbiol. 2010 Jun;59(Pt 6):743-5. Epub 2010 Mar 11. PMID:20223899

Vermi W, Facchetti F, Riboldi E, Heine H, Scutera S, Stornello S, Ravarino D, Cappello P, Giovarelli M, Badolato R, Zucca M, Gentili F, Chilosi M, Doglioni C, Ponzi AN, Sozzani S, Musso T. Role of dendritic cell-derived CXCL13 in the pathogenesis of Bartonella henselae B-rich granuloma. Blood. 2006 Jan 15;107(2):454-62. Epub 2005 Sep 27. PMID:16189275

Verougstraete C. White spots syndromes. Bull Soc Belge Ophtalmol. 2001;(279):67-78. PMID:11344717

Veselinović D. [Bartonella henselae as a cause of optical nerve neuritis]. [Article in Serbian]. Vojnosanit Pregl. 2006 Nov;63(11):971-4. PMID:17144434

Viezens J, Arvand M. Simultaneous presence of two different copies of the 16S rRNA gene in Bartonella henselae. Microbiology. 2008 Sep;154(Pt 9):2881-6. PMID:18757822

Vigil A, Ortega R, Jain A, Nakajima-Sasaki R, Tan X, Chomel BB, Kasten RW, Koehler JE, Felgner PL. Identification of the feline humoral immune response to Bartonella henselae infection by protein microarray. PLoS One. 2010 Jul 6;5(7):e11447. PMID:20625509

Vikram HR, Bacani AK, DeValeria PA, Cunningham SA, Cockerill FR 3rd. Bivalvular Bartonella henselae prosthetic valve endocarditis. J Clin Microbiol. 2007 Dec;45(12):4081-4. Epub 2007 Oct 17. PMID:17942646

Vilcins IM, Kosoy M, Old JM, Deane EM. Bartonella-like DNA detected in Ixodes tasmani ticks (Acari: Ixodida) infesting Koalas (Phascolarctos cinereus) in Victoria, Australia. Vector Borne Zoonotic Dis. 2009 Oct;9(5):499-503. PMID:19271994

Vincent JM, Demers DM, Bass JW. Infectious exanthems and unusual infections. Adolesc Med. 2000 Jun;11(2):327-58. PMID:10916128

Vitale G, Incandela S, Incandela C, Micalizzi A, Mansueto P. Isolation and characterization of Bartonella quintana from the parotid gland of an immunocompetent man. J Clin Microbiol. 2009 Mar;47(3):862-4. Epub 2009 Jan 7. PMID:19129406

Vivekananda J, Kiel JL. Anti-Francisella tularensis DNA aptamers detect tularemia antigen from different subspecies by Aptamer-Linked Immobilized Sorbent Assay. Lab Invest. 2006 Jun;86(6):610-8. PMID:16550191

Vögelin E, Büchler U. An epitrochlear tumour. J R Soc Med. 2001 Aug;94(8):403-5. PMID:11461986

von Felbert V, Meybehm M, Megahed M. [Cat scratch disease].[Article in German]. Hautarzt. 2008 Jun;59(6):457-8. PMID:18470500

von Kobyletzki G, Nordmeier R, Stücker M, Sandmann M, Respondek M, Baier J, Altmeyer P. [Acute generalized cat scratch disease in myelodysplastic syndrome].[Article in German]. Hautarzt. 2001 Oct;52(10 Pt 2):980-4. PMID:11715399

Vorou RM, Papavassiliou VG, Tsiodras S. Emerging zoonoses and vector-borne infections affecting humans in Europe. Epidemiol Infect. 2007 Nov;135(8):1231-47. Epub 2007 Apr 20. PMID:17445320

Vukelić D, Benić B, Bozinović D, Vuković B, Dakovic Rode O, Culig Z, Vuković J, Batinica S, Visnjić S, Puljiz I. An unusual outcome in a child with hepatosplenic cat-scratch disease. Wien Klin Wochenschr. 2006 Oct;118(19-20):615-8. PMID:17136337

Wade NK, Levi L, Jones MR, Bhisitkul R, Fine L, Cunningham ET Jr. Optic disk edema associated with peripapillary serous retinal detachment: an early sign of systemic Bartonella henselae infection. Am J Ophthalmol. 2000 Sep;130(3):327-34. PMID:11020412

Wagner CL, Riess T, Linke D, Eberhardt C, Schäfer A, Reutter S, Maggi RG, Kempf VA. Use of Bartonella adhesin A (BadA) immunoblotting in the serodiagnosis of Bartonella henselae infections. Int J Med Microbiol. 2008 Oct;298(7-8):579-90. Epub 2008 May 22. PMID:18501673

Wallace MR, Persing DH, McCutchan JA, Magara J, Nelson JA, Heaton RK, Tasker SA, Grant I; HNRC Group. HIV Neurobehavioral Research Center. Bartonella henselae serostatus is not correlated with neurocognitive decline in HIV infection. Scand J Infect Dis. 2001;33(8):593-5. PMID:11525353

Walls T, Moshal K, Trounce J, Hartley J, Harris K, Davies G. Broad-range polymerase chain reaction for the diagnosis of Bartonella henselae endocarditis. J Paediatr Child Health. 2006 Jul-Aug;42(7-8):469-71. PMID:16898887

Wang CW, Chang WC, Chao TK, Liu CC, Huang GS. Computed tomography and magnetic resonance imaging of cat-scratch disease: a report of two cases. Clin Imaging. 2009 Jul-Aug;33(4):318-21. PMID:19559357

Wang KY, Vong SC, Lee WJ, Lin HJ. Images in emergency medicine. Right axillary mass. Cat scratch disease. Ann Emerg Med. 2010 Dec;56(6):600, 622. PMID:21111249

Wang YY, Chen Q, Yu Q, Zhang LJ. Prokaryotic expression and immunogenicity of 56-Kilodalton protein of Orientia tsutsugamushi strain Karp. Microbiol Immunol. 2012 Mar 30. [Epub ahead of print]. PMID:22462646

Watanabe H, Mitobe J. [Possible bacterial etiologies for diseases of unknown origin].[Article in Japanese]. Nihon Rinsho. 2003 Mar;61 Suppl 3:285-9. PMID:12717985

Webster JD, Miller MA, DuSold D, Ramos-Vara J. Effects of prolonged formalin fixation on the immunohistochemical detection of infectious agents in formalin-fixed, paraffin-embedded tissues. Vet Pathol. 2010 May;47(3):529-35. Epub 2010 Mar 23. PMID:20332424

Weese JS, Peregrine AS, Armstrong J. Occupational health and safety in small animal veterinary practice: Part I--nonparasitic zoonotic diseases. Can Vet J. 2002 Aug;43(8):631-6. PMID:12170843

Wei YJ, Lou WH, Liu T. [Clinical diagnosis and therapy analysis of cervical lymphadenitis in cat-scratch disease].[Article in Chinese]. Zhonghua Er Bi Yan Hou Tou Jing Wai Ke Za Zhi. 2006 Aug;41(8):626-7. PMID:17039811

Weinspach S, Tenenbaum T, Schönberger S, Schaper J, Engers R, Rueggeberg J, Mackenzie CR, Wolf A, Mayatepek E, Schroten H. Cat scratch disease—heterogeneous in clinical presentation: five unusual cases of an infection caused by Bartonella henselae. Klin Padiatr. 2010 Mar;222(2):73-8. Epub 2009 Sep 29. PMID:19790029

Welc-Faleciak R, Bajer A, Behnke JM, Siński E. The ecology of Bartonella spp. infections in two rodent communities in the Mazury Lake District region of Poland. Parasitology. 2010 Jun;137(7):1069-77. Epub 2010 Apr 14. PMID:20388232

Welc-Faleciak R, Paziewska A, Bajer A, Behnke JM, Siński E. Bartonella spp. infection in rodents from different habitats in the Mazury Lake District, Northeast Poland. Vector Borne Zoonotic Dis. 2008 Aug;8(4):467-74. PMID:18399782

Welc-Faleciak R, Rodo A, Siński E, Bajer A. Babesia canis and other tick-borne infections in dogs in Central Poland. Vet Parasitol. 2009 Dec 23;166(3-4):191-8. Epub 2009 Sep 26. PMID:19837515

Welc-Faleciak R. [Current state of the knowledge of Bartonella infections].[Article in Polish]. Przegl Epidemiol. 2009;63(1):11-7. PMID:19522219

Wellinghausen N, Essig A. [Cat-scratch disease as cause of Lymphadenitis colli].[Article in German]. Laryngorhinootologie. 2005 Dec;84(12):929-36; quiz 937-41. PMID:16358204

Werner GH. [The worldwide challenges of "new" or reemerging communicable diseases at the dawn of the 21st century].[Article in French]. Ann Pharm Fr. 2001 May;59(3):147-75. PMID:11427818

Werner JA, Feng S, Chomel BB, Hodzic E, Kasten RW, Barthold SW. P26-based serodiagnosis for Bartonella spp. infection in cats. Comp Med. 2008 Aug;58(4):375-80. PMID:18724780

Werner JA, Feng S, Kasten RW, Hodzic E, Chomel BB, Barthold SW. Cloning, characterization, and expression of Bartonella henselae p26. Clin Vaccine Immunol. 2006 Aug;13(8):830-6. PMID:16893981

Werner JA, Kasten RW, Feng S, Sykes JE, Hodzic E, Salemi MR, Barthold SW, Chomel BB. Experimental infection of domestic cats with passaged genotype I Bartonella henselae. Vet Microbiol. 2007 Jun 21;122(3-4):290-7. Epub 2007 Jan 31. PMID:17321078

Werner M, Fournier PE, Andersson R, Hogevik H, Raoult D. Bartonella and Coxiella antibodies in 334 prospectively studied episodes of infective endocarditis in Sweden. Scand J Infect Dis. 2003;35(10):724-7. PMID:14606611

Wesslen L, Ehrenborg C, Holmberg M, McGill S, Hjelm E, Lindquist O, Henriksen E, Rolf C, Larsson E, Friman G. Subacute bartonella infection in Swedish orienteers succumbing to sudden unexpected cardiac death or having malignant arrhythmias. Scand J Infect Dis. 2001;33(6):429-38. PMID:11450862

Westling K, Farra A, Jorup C, Nordenberg A, Settergren B, Hjelm E. Bartonella henselae antibodies after cat bite. Emerg Infect Dis. 2008 Dec;14(12):1943-4. PMID:19046527

Weston KD, Tran T, Kimmel KN, Maria BL. Possible role of high-dose corticosteroids in the treatment of cat-scratch disease encephalopathy. J Child Neurol. 2001 Oct;16(10):762-3. PMID:11669351

Whittemore JC, Hawley JR, Radecki SV, Steinberg JD, Lappin MR. Bartonella species antibodies and hyperglobulinemia in privately owned cats. J Vet Intern Med. 2012 May;26(3):639-44. Epub 2012 Apr 10. PMID:22490060

Wikswo ME, Hu R, Metzger ME, Eremeeva ME. Detection of Rickettsia rickettsii and Bartonella henselae in Rhipicephalus sanguineus ticks from California. J Med Entomol. 2007 Jan;44(1):158-62. PMID:17294935

Wilk I, Martirosian G. [Nanobacteria--microbiological characteristics]. [Article in Polish]. Postepy Hig Med Dosw (Online). 2004 Mar 3;58:60-4. PMID:15069381

Williams A, Sheldon CD, Riordan T. Cat scratch disease. BMJ. 2002 May 18;324(7347):1199-200. PMID:12016189

Wilmer JA, de Vries RA, Meijer JW, Richter C. [Fibrosing mediastinitis: a rare cause of fever].[Article in Dutch]. Ned Tijdschr Geneeskd. 2004 Mar 13;148(11):530-3. PMID:15054952

Wilson M. Persistent abdominal pain. Clin Pediatr (Phila). 2005 Jul-Aug;44(6):553. PMID:16015406

Wimmersberger Y, Baglivo E. Bartonella henselae infection presenting as a unilateral acute maculopathy. Klin Monbl Augenheilkd. 2007 Apr;224(4):311-3. PMID:17458800

Windsor JJ. Cat-scratch disease: epidemiology, aetiology and treatment. Br J Biomed Sci. 2001;58(2):101-10. PMID:11440202

Windsor RC, Johnson LR, Sykes JE, Drazenovich TL, Leutenegger CM, De Cock HE. Molecular detection of microbes in nasal tissue of dogs with idiopathic lymphoplasmacytic rhinitis. J Vet Intern Med. 2006 Mar-Apr;20(2):250-6. PMID:16594580

Winkelstein JA, Marino MC, Ochs H, Fuleihan R, Scholl PR, Geha R, Stiehm ER, Conley ME. The X-linked hyper-IgM syndrome: clinical and immunologic features of 79 patients. Medicine (Baltimore). 2003 Nov;82(6):373-84. PMID:14663287

Winoto IL, Goethert H, Ibrahim IN, Yuniherlina I, Stoops C, Susanti I, Kania W, Maguire JD, Bangs MJ, Telford SR 3rd, Wongsrichanalai C. Bartonella species in rodents and shrews in the greater Jakarta area. Southeast Asian J Trop Med Public Health. 2005 Nov;36(6):1523-9. PMID:16610656

Winterberg DH. [Diagnostic imaging (257). A boy with a swollen inguinal gland].[Article in Dutch]. Ned Tijdschr Geneeskd. 2006 Jan 14;150(2):89. PMID:16440563

Wiwanitkit V. Optic neuropathy and cat scratch disease. Arq Bras Oftalmol. 2011 Mar-Apr;74(2):147. PMID:21779676

Woestyn S, Moreau M, Munting E, Bigaignon G, Delmée M. Osteomyelitis caused by Bartonella henselae genotype I in an immunocompetent adult woman. J Clin Microbiol. 2003 Jul;41(7):3430-2. PMID:12843112

Woestyn S, Olivé N, Bigaignon G, Avesani V, Delmée M. Study of genotypes and virB4 secretion gene of Bartonella henselae strains from patients with clinically defined cat scratch disease. J Clin Microbiol. 2004 Apr;42(4):1420-7. PMID:15070983

Wollmann P, Zeth K, Lupas AN, Linke D. Purification of the YadA membrane anchor for secondary structure analysis and crystallization. Int J Biol Macromol. 2006 Aug 15;39(1-3):3-9. Epub 2006 Jan 6. PMID:16405993

Wong AK, Alfert M, Castrillon DH, Shen Q, Holash J, Yancopoulos GD, Chin L. Excessive tumor-elaborated VEGF and its neutralization define a lethal paraneoplastic syndrome. Proc Natl Acad Sci U S A. 2001 Jun 19;98(13):7481-6. Epub 2001 Jun 12. PMID:11404464

Woo SB, Treister N. Ciclosporin-induced fibrovascular polyps vs. bacillary angiomatosis. Br J Dermatol. 2008 Mar;158(3):652-3. Epub 2008 Jan 17. PMID:18205872

Woolley MW, Gordon DL, Wetherall BL. Analysis of the first Australian strains of Bartonella quintana reveals unique genotypes. J Clin Microbiol. 2007 Jun;45(6):2040-3. Epub 2007 Apr 11. PMID:17428928

Wormser GP. Discovery of new infectious diseases - bartonella species. N Engl J Med. 2007 Jun 7;356(23):2346-7. PMID:17554115

Xing F, Gao Z, Tang H, Wu Y, Li L, Luo X, Fan H. [The clinical analysis of cat scratch diseases with enlarged masses].[Article in Chinese]. Lin Chung Er Bi Yan Hou Tou Jing Wai Ke Za Zhi. 2008 Sep;22(18):831-3. PMID:19166029

Xu C, Liu Q, Diao B, Kan B, Song X, Li D. Optimization of pulse-field gel electrophoresis for Bartonella subtyping. J Microbiol Methods. 2009 Jan;76(1):6-11. Epub 2008 Sep 5. PMID:18835302

Yabsley MJ, McKibben J, Macpherson CN, Cattan PF, Cherry NA, Hegarty BC, Breitschwerdt EB, O'Connor T, Chandrashekar R, Paterson T, Perea ML, Ball G, Friesen S, Goedde J, Henderson B, Sylvester W. Prevalence of Ehrlichia canis, Anaplasma platys, Babesia canis vogeli, Hepatozoon canis, Bartonella vinsonii berkhoffii, and Rickettsia spp. in dogs from Grenada. Vet Parasitol. 2008 Feb 14;151(2-4):279-85. Epub 2007 Nov 17. PMID:18160223

Yager JA, Best SJ, Maggi RG, Varanat M, Znajda N, Breitschwerdt EB. Bacillary angiomatosis in an immunosuppressed dog. Vet Dermatol. 2010 Aug;21(4):420-8. Epub 2010 Mar 31. PMID:20374571

Yamada Y, Ohkusu K, Yanagihara M, Tsuneoka H, Ezaki T, Tsuboi J, Okabayashi H, Suwabe A. Prosthetic valve endocarditis caused by Bartonella quintana in a patient during immunosuppressive therapies for collagen vascular diseases. Diagn Microbiol Infect Dis. 2011 Jul;70(3):395-8. Epub 2011 May 10. PMID:21558050

Yamamoto K, Chomel BB, Kasten RW, Hew CM, Weber DK, Lee WI, Droz S, Koehler JE. Experimental infection of domestic cats with Bartonella koehlerae and comparison of protein and DNA profiles with those of other Bartonella species infecting felines. J Clin Microbiol. 2002 Feb;40(2):466-74. PMID:11825958

Yamamoto K, Chomel BB, Kasten RW, Hew CM, Weber DK, Lee WI, Koehler JE, Pedersen NC. Infection and re-infection of domestic cats with various Bartonella species or types: B. henselae type I is protective against heterologous challenge with B. henselae type II. Vet Microbiol. 2003 Mar 20;92(1-2):73-86. PMID:12488072

Yamamoto K, Chomel BB, Kasten RW, Hew CM, Weber DK, Lee WI. Experimental infection of specific pathogen free (SPF) cats with two different strains of bartonella henselae type I: a comparative study. Vet Res. 2002 Nov-Dec;33(6):669-84. PMID:12498568

Yamanouchi H, Izumikawa K, Hisamatsu T, Yoshinaga M, Sasaki E, Izumikawa K, Hayakawa T, Hara K, Maruyama S, Ohtani H, Shimokawa I. [A case of Bartonella henselae infection from a dog]. [Article in Japanese]. Kansenshogaku Zasshi. 2004 Mar;78(3):270-3. PMID:15103910

Yanagihara M, Tsuneoka H, Hoshide S, Ishido E, Umeda A, Tsukahara M, Nojima J, Ichihara K, Hino K, Hirai I, Yamamoto Y. Molecular typing of Bartonella henselae DNA extracted from human clinical specimens and cat isolates in Japan. FEMS Immunol Med Microbiol. 2010 Oct;60(1):44-8. PMID:20602637

Yanagihara M, Tsuneoka H, Sugasaki M, Nojima J, Ichihara K. Multispacer typing of Bartonella henselae isolates from humans and cats, Japan. Emerg Infect Dis. 2010 Dec;16(12):1983-5. PMID:21122238

Yang XR, Liu QY, Cui BY, Wang LX, Peng ZH, Ren DS. [Using direct enzyme linked immunosorbent assay for the detection of IgG antibody on Bartonella henselae among healthy people in Changping, Beijing]. [Article in Chinese]. Zhonghua Liu Xing Bing Xue Za Zhi. 2007 Jul;28(7):688-91. PMID:18069561

Ye X, Li GW, Yao ML, Luo W, Su LQ. [Study on the prevalence and genotypes of Bartonella species in rodent hosts from Fujian coastal regions].[Article in Chinese]. Zhonghua Liu Xing Bing Xue Za Zhi. 2009 Oct;30(10):989-92. PMID:20193373

Yeh SH, Zangwill KM, Hall B, McPhaul L, Keller M. Parapharyngeal abscess due to cat-scratch disease. Clin Infect Dis. 2000 Mar;30(3):599-601. PMID:10722453

Yerebakan C, Westphal B, Aepinus C. Infective endocarditis due to Bartonella quintana: a challenging diagnostic entity. Acta Cardiol. 2008 Aug;63(4):519-21. PMID:18795592

Yilmaz C, Ergin C, Kaleli I. [Investigation of Bartonella henselae seroprevalence and related risk factors in blood donors admitted to Pamukkale University Blood Center].[Article in Turkish]. Mikrobiyol Bul. 2009 Jul;43(3):391-401. PMID:19795614

Ying B, Kosoy MY, Maupin GO, Tsuchiya KR, Gage KL. Genetic and ecologic characteristics of Bartonella communities in rodents in southern China. Am J Trop Med Hyg. 2002 May;66(5):622-7. PMID:12201602

Yinh J, Pilichowska M, Kalish R. A 27-year-old Cambodian woman with fever, lymphadenopathy, and arthritis. Arthritis Care Res (Hoboken). 2010 Aug;62(8):1194-9. PMID:20506551

Yoda M, Hata M, Sezai A, Unosawa S, Furukawa N, Minami K. First report of Bartonella quintana endocarditis in Japan. Circ J. 2008 Jun;72(6):1022-4. PMID:18503234

Yoon HJ, Lee WC, Choi YS, Cho S, Song YG, Choi JY, Kim CO, Kim EJ, Kim JM. Cervical lymphadenitis in a patient coinfected with Toxoplasma gondii and Bartonella henselae. Vector Borne Zoonotic Dis. 2010 May;10(4):415-9. PMID:19874186

Yoshida H, Kusaba N, Sata M. [Clinical analysis of cat scratch disease]. [Article in Japanese]. Kansenshogaku Zasshi. 2010 May;84(3):292-5. PMID:20560420

Yoshida H, Kusaba N, Sumino M, Sata M. [Evaluation of serological response to Bartonella henselae by enzyme immunoassay in cat scratch disease].[Article in Japanese]. Kansenshogaku Zasshi. 2000 Jul;74(7):563-6. PMID:10965658

Yoshida H, Kusaba N. [Cat scratch disease].[Article in Japanese]. Nihon Rinsho. 2003 Feb;61 Suppl 2:464-8. PMID:12722263

Youssef D, Shams WE, El Abbassi A, Moorman JP, Al-Abbadi MA. Combining cytomorphology and serology for the diagnosis of cat scratch disease. Diagn Cytopathol. 2011 Mar;39(3):210-3. PMID:21319324

Yuan C, Zhu C, Bai Y, Yang X, Hua X. Staining of Bartonella henselae with carboxyfluorescein diacetate succinimidyl ester for tracking infection in erythrocytes and epithelial cells. J Microbiol Methods. 2012 May;89(2):102-6. Epub 2012 Feb 21. PMID:22374182

Yuan C, Zhu C, Wu Y, Pan X, Hua X. Bacteriological and molecular identification of Bartonella species in cats from different regions of China. PLoS Negl Trop Dis. 2011 Sep;5(9):e1301. Epub 2011 Sep 6. PMID:21909443

Zaccala G, Rizzo G, Boldorini R, Garavelli PL, Campanini M. [Hepatosplenic cat-scratch disease in the immunocompetent adult].[Article in Italian]. Recenti Prog Med. 2001 Sep;92(9):540. PMID:11552311

Zähringer U, Lindner B, Knirel YA, van den Akker WM, Hiestand R, Heine H, Dehio C. Structure and biological activity of the short-chain lipopolysaccharide from Bartonella henselae ATCC 49882T. J Biol Chem. 2004 May 14;279(20):21046-54. Epub 2004 Feb 7. PMID:14766898

Zarkovic A, McMurray C, Deva N, Ghosh S, Whitley D, Guest S. Seropositivity rates for Bartonella henselae, Toxocara canis and Toxoplasma gondii in New Zealand blood donors. Clin Experiment Ophthalmol. 2007 Mar;35(2):131-4. PMID:17362453

Zarraga M, Rosen L, Herschthal D. Bacillary angiomatosis in an immunocompetent child: a case report and review of the literature. Am J Dermatopathol. 2011 Jul;33(5):513-5. PMID:21285862

Zarzycka B, Pieczara A, Skowron-Kobos J, Krzemiński Z. [Prevalence IgG antibodies against Bartonella henselae in children with lymphadenopathy].[Article in Polish]. Przegl Epidemiol. 2008;62(4):759-65. PMID:19209738

Zeaiter Z, Fournier PE, Greub G, Raoult D. Diagnosis of Bartonella endocarditis by a real-time nested PCR assay using serum. J Clin Microbiol. 2003 Mar;41(3):919-25. PMID:12624010

Zeaiter Z, Fournier PE, Ogata H, Raoult D. Phylogenetic classification of Bartonella species by comparing groEL sequences. Int J Syst Evol Microbiol. 2002 Jan;52(Pt 1):165-71. PMID:11837299

Zeaiter Z, Fournier PE, Raoult D. Genomic variation of Bartonella henselae strains detected in lymph nodes of patients with cat scratch disease. J Clin Microbiol. 2002 Mar;40(3):1023-30. PMID:11880432

Zeaiter Z, Liang Z, Raoult D. Genetic classification and differentiation of Bartonella species based on comparison of partial ftsZ gene sequences. J Clin Microbiol. 2002 Oct;40(10):3641-7. PMID:12354859

Zekraoui Y, Megzari A, El Alloussi T, Berraho A. [Unilateral neuroretinitis revealing cat-scratch disease].[Article in French]. Rev Med Interne. 2011 Apr;32(4):e46-8. Epub 2010 Jun 19. PMID:20646795

Zenone T. Systemic Bartonella henselae Infection in Immunocompetent Adult Presenting as Fever of Unknown Origin. Case Report Med. 2011;2011:183937. Epub 2011 May 5. PMID:21629850

Zhang JB, Wen BH, Chen ML, Li LL, Qiu L, Niu DS. [Development of a quantitative real-time polymerase chain reaction for detecting Bartonella henselae].[Article in Chinese]. Zhonghua Liu Xing Bing Xue Za Zhi. 2007 Mar;28(3):277-81. PMID:17649663

Zhang L, Cui F, Wang L, Zhang L, Zhang J, Wang S, Yang S. Investigation of anaplasmosis in Yiyuan County, Shandong Province, China. Asian Pac J Trop Med. 2011 Jul;4(7):568-72. PMID:21803311

Zhang L, Shan A, Mathew B, Yin J, Fu X, Zhang J, Lu J, Xu J, Dumler JS. Rickettsial Seroepidemiology among farm workers, Tianjin, People's Republic of China. Emerg Infect Dis. 2008 Jun;14(6):938-40. PMID:18507907

Zhang P, Chomel BB, Schau MK, Goo JS, Droz S, Kelminson KL, George SS, Lerche NW, Koehler JE. A family of variably expressed outer-membrane proteins (Vomp) mediates adhesion and autoaggregation in Bartonella quintana. Proc Natl Acad Sci U S A. 2004 Sep 14;101(37):13630-5. Epub 2004 Sep 3. PMID:15347808

Zhang Y, Zhang ZL, Yin JY, Lü J, Yu HL, Liang CW, Wang SW, Zhao JB, Zhang LJ. [Sero-epidemiological investigation on Rickettsia typhi, Bartonella henselae and Orientia tsutsugamushi in farmers from rural areas of Tianjin, 2007 - 2009].[Article in Chinese]. Zhonghua Liu Xing Bing Xue Za Zhi. 2011 Mar;32(3):256-259. PMID:21457660

Zhao SQ, Cai YF, Zhu ZY. Comparative proteomic analysis of B. henselae Houston and B. henselae Marseille by two-dimensional gel electrophoresis. Biomed Environ Sci. 2005 Oct;18(5):341-4. PMID:16370318

Zhu J, Hsu YM, Chang CF, Chang CD, Simpson KW, Tu H, Chang YF. Cloning and characterization of an outer membrane protein (Lip18) from Helicobacter bizzozeronii. DNA Seq. 2003 Apr;14(2):87-94. PMID:12825349

Ziemssen F, Bartz-Schmidt KU, Gelisken F. Secondary unilateral glaucoma and neuroretinitis: atypical manifestation of cat-scratch disease. Jpn J Ophthalmol. 2006 Mar-Apr;50(2):177-9. PMID:16604397

Zimmermann R, Kempf VA, Schiltz E, Oberle K, Sander A. Hemin binding, functional expression, and complementation analysis of Pap 31 from Bartonella henselae. J Bacteriol. 2003 Mar;185(5):1739-44. PMID:12591895

Zimran E, Shilo S, Florescu T, Dotan S, Balag S, Mevorach D, Shibolet O, Amer R. Paradoxical response in ocular bartonellosis. J Ophthalmic Inflamm Infect. 2012 Mar;2(1):53-6. Epub 2011 Nov 5. PMID:22057809

Znazen A, Rolain JM, Hammami N, Kammoun S, Hammami A, Raoult D. High prevalence of Bartonella quintana endocarditis in Sfax, Tunisia. Am J Trop Med Hyg. 2005 May;72(5):503-7. PMID:15891120

Zobba R, Chessa G, Mastrandrea S, Pinna Parpaglia ML, Patta C, Masala G. Serological and molecular detection of Bartonella spp. in humans, cats and dogs from northern Sardinia, Italy. Clin Microbiol Infect. 2009 Dec;15 Suppl 2:134-5. Epub 2009 May 18. PMID:19456814

Zupan S, Poljak M, Avsic-Zupanc T. Prevalence of Bartonella infections in Slovenian intravenous drug users. Ann N Y Acad Sci. 2003 Jun;990:414-8. PMID:12860666

An Extensive Collection of Academic References Focused on Emerging Babesia and Malaria Treatment Options

Introduction — Babesia

I have been studying Babesia and malaria treatments almost full-time for many years. While we have agents for treating malaria, we still have many issues that limit application of effective care throughout the world.

In contrast, research on Babesia is not very advanced and treatment options are overly simplistic. Some researchers and clinicians feel one can simply plug in a malaria treatment with the same dose and duration, and get the same effect in killing Babesia. I am certain this is an error. If Babesia was "just like" malaria, we would call it a sub-type of malaria.

Further, the number of true experts on Babesia, and who have read most of the publications in English print, is possibly under a dozen individuals.

And yet with new issues with Babesia resistance and delivery of malaria care and new unique protozoa like FL1953, we see materials speaking with authority not based on broad scientific curiosity, but a type of simplistic medicine consistent with an emerging infection.

Finally, Babesia has huge impacts in human biochemistry, hormones, weight, energy, sensations, tissue and organs. You cannot do one test and determine if Babesia is present in either an animal or a human. I wish such a comfortable myth was true, but it is just old and ineffective medicine.

The references that follow are a small sample of materials related to treatment.

This book is written for individuals who have a master's degree, a Ph.D. or M.D. in the medical sciences. If you are not trained at least at the master's level in mammalian related science, and doing full-time research on these topics, this text is not useful to you.

Abanyie FA, Arguin PM, Gutman J. State of malaria diagnostic testing at clinical laboratories in the United States, 2010: a nationwide survey. Malar J. 2011 Nov 10;10:340. PMID:22074250

Abba K, Deeks JJ, Olliaro P, Naing CM, Jackson SM, Takwoingi Y, Donegan S, Garner P. Rapid diagnostic tests for diagnosing uncomplicated P. falciparum malaria in endemic countries. Cochrane Database Syst Rev. 2011 Jul 6;(7):CD008122. PMID:21735422

Abbas HM, Brenes RA, Ajemian MS, Scholand SJ. Successful conservative treatment of spontaneous splenic rupture secondary to Babesiosis: a case report and literature review. Conn Med. 2011 Mar;75(3):143-6. PMID:21500704

Abdalla HS, Hussein HS, Kreier JP. Babesia rodhaini: passive protection of mice with immune serum. Tropenmed Parasitol. 1978 Sep;29(3):295-306. PMID:726044

Abdulla S, Sagara I. Dispersible formulation of artemether/lumefantrine: specifically developed for infants and young children. Malar J. 2009 Oct 12;8 Suppl 1:S7. PMID:19818174

Abebe G, Kiros M, Golasa L, Zeynudin A. Schistosoma mansoni infection among patients visiting a health centre near Gilgel Gibe Dam, Jimma, south western Ethiopia. East Afr J Public Health. 2009 Dec;6(3):300-2. PMID:20803923

Abebe G, Kiros M, Golasa L, Zeynudin A. Schistosoma mansoni infection among patients visiting a health centre near Gilgel Gibe Dam, Jimma, south Western Ethiopia. East Afr J Public Health. 2010 Mar;7(1):78-80. PMID:21413578

Ablordeppey SY, Hufford CD, Borne RF, Dwuma-Badu D. 1H-NMR and 13C-NMR Assignments of Cryptolepine, A 3:4-Benz-delta-carboline Derivative Isolated from Cryptolepis sanguinolenta. Planta Med. 1990 Aug;56(4):416-7. PMID:17221441

Aboulaila M, Nakamura K, Govind Y, Yokoyama N, Igarashi I. Evaluation of the in vitro growth-inhibitory effect of epoxomicin on Babesia parasites. Vet Parasitol. 2010 Jan 20;167(1):19-27. Epub 2009 Oct 3. PMID:19896277

Aboulaila M, Yokoyama N, Igarashi I. Inhibitory effects of (-)-epigallocatechin-3-gallate from green tea on the growth of Babesia parasites. Parasitology. 2010 Apr;137(5):785-91. Epub 2009 Dec 22. PMID: 20025823

AbouLaila M, Sivakumar T, Yokoyama N, Igarashi I. Inhibitory effect of terpene nerolidol on the growth of Babesia parasites. Parasitol Int. 2010 Jun;59(2):278-82. Epub 2010 Feb 21. PMID:20178862

Abrams Y. Complications of coinfection with Babesia and Lyme disease after splenectomy. J Am Board Fam Med. 2008 Jan-Feb;21(1):75-7. PMID:18178707

Abubucker S, Martin J, Taylor CM, Mitreva M. HelmCoP: an online resource for helminth functional genomics and drug and vaccine targets prioritization. PLoS One. 2011;6(7):e21832. Epub 2011 Jul 8. PMID:21760913

Adams LG, Todorovic RA. The chemotherapeutic efficacy of imidocarb dihydrochloride on concurrent bovine anaplasmosis and babesiosis. I. The effects of a single treatment. Trop Anim Health Prod. 1974 May;6(2):71-8. PMID:4416121

Adams LG, Todorovic RA. The chemotherapeutic efficacy of imidocarb dihydrochloride on concurrent bovine anaplasmosis and babesiosis. II. The effects of multiple treatments. Trop Anim Health Prod. 1974 May;6(2):79-84. PMID:4416122

Adan GL. Development of malaria control in the Philippines. J Philipp Med Assoc. 1954 Jan;30(1):29-35. PMID:13143503

Adaszek Ł, Górna M, Krzysiak M, Adaszek M, Garbal M, Winiarczyk S. Identification of the piroplasms isolated from horses with clinical piroplasmosis in Poland. Wiad Parazytol. 2011;57(1):21-6. PMID:21634230

Adaszek Ł, Martinez AC, Winiarczyk S. The factors affecting the distribution of babesiosis in dogs in Poland. Vet Parasitol. 2011 Sep 27;181(2-4):160-5. Epub 2011 Apr 12. PMID:21524856

Adaszek Ł, Winiarczyk S, Górna M. [From piroplasmosis to babesiosis--problems with classification of Babesia protozoa isolated from dogs]. [Article in Polish]. Wiad Parazytol. 2010;56(2):111-5. PMID:20707294

Adaszek Ł, Winiarczyk S, Skrzypczak M. The clinical course of babesiosis in 76 dogs infected with protozoan parasites Babesia canis canis. Pol J Vet Sci. 2009;12(1):81-7. PMID:19459444

Adaszek Ł, Winiarczyk S. [Dogs babesiosis--still actually problem].[Article in Polish]. Wiad Parazytol. 2008;54(2):109-15. PMID:18702315

Adebayo JO, Krettli AU. Potential antimalarials from Nigerian plants: a review. J Ethnopharmacol. 2011 Jan 27;133(2):289-302. Epub 2010 Nov 18. PMID:21093570

Adedotun AA, Morenikeji OA, Odaibo AB. Knowledge, attitudes and practices about malaria in an urban community in south-western Nigeria. J Vector Borne Dis. 2010 Sep;47(3):155-9. PMID:20834085

Aderinboye O, Syed SS. Congenital babesiosis in a four-week-old female infant. Pediatr Infect Dis J. 2010 Feb;29(2):188. PMID:20118748

Aditya NP, Patankar S, Madhusudhan B. Assessment of in vivo antimalarial activity of rifampicin, isoniazide, and ethambutol combination therapy. Parasitol Res. 2010 May;106(6):1481-4. Epub 2010 Feb 18. PMID:20165870

A-Elbasit IE, Khalil IF, Elbashir MI, Masuadi EM, Bygbjerg IC, Alifrangis M, Giha HA. High frequency of Plasmodium falciparum CICNI/SGEAA and CVIET haplotypes without association with resistance to sulfadoxine/pyrimethamine and chloroquine combination in the Daraweesh area, in Sudan. Eur J Clin Microbiol Infect Dis. 2008 Aug;27(8):725-32. Epub 2008 Mar 29. PMID:18373107

Aeschlimann A, Suter H. [Apropos of "Babesia" rodhaini].[Article in French]. Acta Trop. 1965;22(4):303-20. PMID:4379113

Afsharpad M, Zakeri S, Pirahmadi S, Djadid ND. Molecular assessment of dhfr/dhps mutations among Plasmodium vivax clinical isolates after introduction of sulfadoxine/pyrimethamine in combination with artesunate in Iran. Infect Genet Evol. 2012 Jan;12(1):38-44. Epub 2011 Oct 14. PMID:22020253

Afsharpad M, Zakeri S, Pirahmadi S, Djadid ND. Molecular monitoring of Plasmodium falciparum resistance to antimalarial drugs after adoption of sulfadoxine-pyrimethamine plus artesunate as the first line treatment in Iran. Acta Trop. 2012 Jan;121(1):13-8. Epub 2011 Oct 2. PMID:22001304

Agbenu E, d'Almeida H, Kolou M, Aho M, Agbetiafa K, Padaro E, Dagnra Y, Redah D, David M. [Evaluation of the Widal-Felix serodiagnostic test in Togo].[Article in French]. Med Trop (Mars). 2010 Feb;70(1):43-8. PMID:20337114

Aghahowa SE, Obianwu HO, Isah AO, Arhewoh IM. Chloroquine-induced Pruritus. Indian J Pharm Sci. 2010 May;72(3):283-9. PMID:21188034

Agnandji ST, Kurth F, Fernandes JF, Soulanoudjingar SA, Abossolo BP, Mombo-Ngoma G, Basra A, Gonzalez R, Kizito G, Mayengue PI, Auer-Hackenberg L, Issifou S, Lell B, Adegnika AA, Ramharter M. The use of paediatric artemisinin combinations in sub-Saharan Africa: a snapshot questionnaire survey of health care personnel. Malar J. 2011 Dec 14;10(1):365. [Epub ahead of print]. PMID:22168234

Agnandji ST, Lell B, Soulanoudjingar SS, Fernandes JF, Abossolo BP, Conzelmann C, Methogo BG, Doucka Y, Flamen A, Mordmüller B, Issifou S, Kremsner PG, Sacarlal J, Aide P, Lanaspa M, Aponte JJ, Nhamuave A, Quelhas D, Bassat Q, Mandjate S, Macete E, Alonso P, Abdulla S, Salim N, Juma O, Shomari M, Shubis K, Machera F, Hamad AS, Minja R, Mtoro A, Sykes A, Ahmed S, Urassa AM, Ali AM, Mwangoka G, Tanner M, Tinto H, D'Alessandro U, Sorgho H, Valea I, Tahita MC, Kaboré W, Ouédraogo S, Sandrine Y, Guiguemdé RT, Ouédraogo JB, Hamel MJ, Kariuki S, Odero C, Oneko M, Otieno K, Awino N, Omoto J, Williamson J, Muturi-Kioi V, Laserson KF, Slutsker L, Otieno W, Otieno L, Nekoye O, Gondi S, Otieno A, Ogutu B, Wasuna R, Owira V, Jones D, Onyango AA, Njuguna P, Chilengi R, Akoo P, Kerubo C, Gitaka J, Maingi C, Lang T, Olotu A, Tsofa B, Bejon P, Peshu N, Marsh K, Owusu-Agyei S, Asante KP, Osei-Kwakye K, Boahen O, Ayamba S, Kayan K, Owusu-Ofori R, Dosoo D, Asante I, Adjei G, Adjei G, Chandramohan D, Greenwood B, Lusingu J, Gesase S, Malabeja A, Abdul O, Kilavo H, Mahende C, Liheluka E, Lemnge M, Theander T, Drakeley C, Ansong D, Agbenyega T, Adjei S, Boateng HO, Rettig T, Bawa J, Sylverken J, Sambian D, Agyekum A, Owusu L, Martinson F, Hoffman I, Mvalo T, Kamthunzi P, Nkomo R, Msika A, Jumbe A, Chome N, Nyakuipa D, Chintedza J, Ballou WR, Bruls M, Cohen J, Guerra Y, Jongert E, Lapierre D, Leach A, Lievens M, Ofori-Anyinam O, Vekemans J, Carter T, Leboulleux D, Loucq C, Radford A, Savarese B, Schellenberg D, Sillman M, Vansadia P; RTS,S Clinical Trials Partnership. First results of phase 3 trial of RTS,S/AS01 malaria vaccine in African children. N Engl J Med. 2011 Nov 17;365(20):1863-75. Epub 2011 Oct 18. PMID:22007715

Ahmed J, Yin H, Schnittger L, Jongejan F. Ticks and tick-borne diseases in Asia with special emphasis on China. Parasitol Res. 2002 May;88(13 Suppl 1):S51-5. PMID:12051612

Ahmed OA, Odunukwe NN, Akinwale OP, Raheem TY, Efienemokwu CE, Ogedengbe O, Salako LA. Knowledge and practices of traditional birth attendants in prenatal services in Lagos State, Nigeria. Afr J Med Med Sci. 2005 Mar;34(1):55-8. PMID:15971555

Ahmed SM, Zerihun A. Possession and usage of insecticidal bed nets among the people of Uganda: is BRAC Uganda Health Programme pursuing a pro-poor path? PLoS One. 2010 Sep 10;5(9). pii: e12660. PMID:20844749

Ahorlu CK, Dunyo SK, Afari EA, Koram KA, Nkrumah FK. Malaria-related beliefs and behaviour in southern Ghana: implications for treatment, prevention and control. Trop Med Int Health. 1997 May;2(5):488-99. PMID:9217705

Aikawa M, Beaudoin RL. Plasmodium fallax: high-resolution autoradiography of exoerythrocytic stages treated with Primaquine in vitro. Exp Parasitol. 1970 Jun;27(3):454-63. PMID:5419455

Aikins MK, Pickering H, Greenwood BM. Attitudes to malaria, traditional practices and bednets (mosquito nets) as vector control measures: a comparative study in five west African countries. J Trop Med Hyg. 1994 Apr;97(2):81-6. PMID:8170007

Ajala TO, Igwilo CI, Oreagba IA, Odeku OA. The antiplasmodial effect of the extracts and formulated capsules of Phyllanthus amarus on Plasmodium yoelii infection in mice. Asian Pac J Trop Med. 2011 Apr;4(4):283-7. Epub 2011 May 29. PMID:21771471

Ajayi IO, Falade CO, Kale OO. An assessment of accuracy of mothers' presumptive diagnosis of fever at home in southwest Nigeria: evidence for switch to parasite-based diagnostic test. East Afr J Public Health. 2009 Dec;6(3):229-34. PMID:20803910

Ajayi IO, Falade CO, Olley BO, Yusuf B, Gbotosho S, Iyiola T, Olaniyan O, Happi C, Munguti K, Pagnoni F. A qualitative study of the feasibility and community perception on the effectiveness of artemether-lumefantrine use in the context of home management of malaria in south-west Nigeria. BMC Health Serv Res. 2008 Jun 1;8:119. PMID:18513447

Akachi Y, Atun R. Effect of investment in malaria control on child mortality in sub-Saharan Africa in 2002-2008. PLoS One. 2011;6(6):e21309. Epub 2011 Jun 30. PMID:21738633

Akiba M, Saeki H, Ishii T, Yamamoto S, Ueda K. Immunological changes in Babesia rodhaini infected BALB/c mice after treated with anti-babesial drug; diminazene diaceturate. J Vet Med Sci. 1991 Jun;53(3):371-7. PMID:1832024

Akinosoglou KA, Pasvo G. The management of malaria in adults. Clin Med. 2011 Oct;11(5):497-501. PMID:22034716

Akogun O. Robotic health assistant (Feverkit) for the rational management of fevers among nomads in Nigeria. Nurs Leadersh (Tor Ont). 2011 Jun;24(2):58-67. PMID:21730769

Al Rohani M, Aljawshaei H, Aduolimi E. Acute renal failure in Yemeni patients. Saudi J Kidney Dis Transpl. 2011 Jul;22(4):829-33. PMID:21743244

Alabay M, Duzgun A, Cerci H, Wright IG, Waltisbuhl DJ, Goodger BV. Ovine babesiosis: induction of a protective immune response with crude extracts of either Babesia bovis or B ovis. Res Vet Sci. 1987 Nov;43(3):401-2. PMID:3444987

Al-Adhroey AH, Nor ZM, Al-Mekhlafi HM, Mahmud R. Ethnobotanical study on some Malaysian anti-malarial plants: a community based survey. J Ethnopharmacol. 2010 Oct 28;132(1):362-4. Epub 2010 Aug 17. PMID:20723596

Alaro JR, Lynch MM, Burns JM Jr. Protective immune responses elicited by immunization with a chimeric blood-stage malaria vaccine persist but are not boosted by Plasmodium yoelii challenge infection. Vaccine. 2010 Oct 4;28(42):6876-84. Epub 2010 Aug 13. PMID:20709001

Aldighieri J, Blancard A, Boizis N, Dupoux R, Sautet G, Sautet J. [Influence of the environmental temperature on the development of Plasmodium berghei infections in white mice treated with nivaquine]. [Article in French]. Bull Soc Pathol Exot Filiales. 1965 May-Jun;58(3):423-8. PMID:5898834

Alekseev AN, Rudakov NV, Dubinina EV. [Possible types of tick-borne diseases and the predictive role of history data in their diagnosis (parasitological aspects of the problem)].[Article in Russian]. Med Parazitol (Mosk). 2004 Oct-Dec;(4):31-6. PMID:15689134

Alekseev AN. [The possibility of the detection of one more tick-borne infection--babesiosis--on the territory of Russia].[Article in Russian]. Zh Mikrobiol Epidemiol Immunobiol. 2003 May-Jun;(3):39-43. PMID:12886630

Alesutan I, Bobbala D, Qadri SM, Estremera A, Föller M, Lang F. Beneficial effect of aurothiomalate on murine malaria. Malar J. 2010 May 7;9:118. PMID:20459650

Alhassan A, Govind Y, Tam NT, Thekisoe OM, Yokoyama N, Inoue N, Igarashi I. Comparative evaluation of the sensitivity of LAMP, PCR and in vitro culture methods for the diagnosis of equine piroplasmosis. Parasitol Res. 2007 Apr;100(5):1165-8. Epub 2007 Jan 11. PMID:17216488

Ali WN, Ahmad R, Nor ZM, Ismail Z, Lim LH. Population dynamics of adult mosquitoes (Diptera: Culicidae) in malaria endemic villages of Kuala Lipis, Pahang, Malaysia. Southeast Asian J Trop Med Public Health. 2011 Mar;42(2):259-67. PMID:21710845

Aliu YO, Odegaard S. Pharmacokinetics of diminazene in sheep. J Pharmacokinet Biopharm. 1985 Apr;13(2):173-84. PMID:4057056

Alker AP, Kazadi WM, Kutelemeni AK, Bloland PB, Tshefu AK, Meshnick SR. dhfr and dhps genotype and sulfadoxine-pyrimethamine treatment failure in children with falciparum malaria in the Democratic Republic of Congo. Trop Med Int Health. 2008 Nov;13(11):1384-91. PMID:19055622

Alkhalil A, Hill DA, Desai SA. Babesia and plasmodia increase host erythrocyte permeability through distinct mechanisms. Cell Microbiol. 2007 Apr;9(4):851-60. Epub 2006 Nov 3. PMID:17087736

Alkizim F, Matheka D, Muriithi A. Childhood Diarrhoea: Failing Conventional Measures, what Next? Pan Afr Med J. 2011;8:47. Epub 2011 Apr 24. PMID:22121455

Allison AC, Eugui EM. Approaches to vaccines against protozoan parasites of cattle. Adv Exp Med Biol. 1981;137:225-37. PMID:6800224

Allison RW, Yeagley TJ, Levis K, Reichard MV. Babesia canis rossi infection in a Texas dog. Vet Clin Pathol. 2011 Sep;40(3):345-50. Epub 2011 Jul 26. PMID:21790699

Allred DR, Al-Khedery B. Antigenic variation as an exploitable weakness of babesial parasites. Vet Parasitol. 2006 May 31;138(1-2):50-60. Epub 2006 Mar 3. PMID:16517078

Almerìa S, Delgado-Neira Y, Adelantado C, Huguet M, Vinent J, Nicolàs A. Mediterranean theileriosis and other tick transmitted piroplasmoses in cattle in Minorca (Balearic Islands, Spain): the effect of tick control on prevalence levels analyzed by reverse line blot (RLB) macroarrays. J Parasitol. 2009 Jun;95(3):598-603. PMID:19086744

Alonso M, Blandino T, Mendoza E, Savon L, Camacho M. Development of a Babesia bovis live attenuated vaccine. Arch Med Res. 1994 Summer;25(2):273-7. PMID:7919825

Alonso PL, Brown G, Arevalo-Herrera M, Binka F, Chitnis C, Collins F, Doumbo OK, Greenwood B, Hall BF, Levine MM, Mendis K, Newman RD, Plowe CV, Rodríguez MH, Sinden R, Slutsker L, Tanner M. A research agenda to underpin malaria eradication. PLoS Med. 2011 Jan 25;8(1):e1000406. PMID:21311579

Alter HJ, Stramer SL, Dodd RY. Emerging infectious diseases that threaten the blood supply. Semin Hematol. 2007 Jan;44(1):32-41. PMID:17198845

Altstatt LB. A clinical view of the biology of Plasmodia. Ann Intern Med. 1969 Jan;70(1):130-4. PMID:4884380

Alvarez JA, Ramos JA, Rojas EE, Mosqueda JJ, Vega CA, Olvera AM, Figueroa JV, Cantó GJ. Field challenge of cattle vaccinated with a combined Babesia bovis and Babesia bigemina frozen immunogen. Ann N Y Acad Sci. 2004 Oct;1026:277-83. PMID:15604506

Alward W, Javaid M, Garner J. Babesiosis in a Connecticut resident. Conn Med. 1990 Aug;54(8):425-7. PMID:2225809

Amer A, Mehlhorn H. Repellency effect of forty-one essential oils against Aedes, Anopheles, and Culex mosquitoes. Parasitol Res. 2006 Sep;99(4):478-90. Epub 2006 Apr 27. PMID:16642384

Amuasi JH, Diap G, Blay-Nguah S, Boakye I, Karikari PE, Dismas B, Karenzo J, Nsabiyumva L, Louie KS, Kiechel JR. Access to artesunate-amodiaquine, quinine and other anti-malarials: policy and markets in Burundi. Malar J. 2011 Feb 10;10:34. PMID:21310057

Amzat J. Assessing the progress of malaria control in Nigeria. World Health Popul. 2011;12(3):42-51. PMID:21677528

An X, Mohandas N. Red cell membrane and malaria. Transfus Clin Biol. 2010 Sep;17(3):197-9. Epub 2010 Jul 31. PMID:20674435

Anantharaman A, Rizvi MS, Sahal D. Synergy with rifampin and kanamycin enhances potency, kill kinetics, and selectivity of de novo-designed antimicrobial peptides. Antimicrob Agents Chemother. 2010 May;54(5):1693-9. Epub 2010 Feb 22. PMID:20176897

Anders JC, Chung H, Theoharides AD. Methemoglobin formation resulting from administration of candidate 8-aminoquinoline antiparasitic drugs in the dog. Fundam Appl Toxicol. 1988 Feb;10(2):270-5. PMID:3356313

Anderson AE, Cassaday PB, Healy GR. Babesiosis in man. Sixth documented case. Am J Clin Pathol. 1974 Nov;62(5):612-8. PMID:4412160

Andriantsoanirina V, Ménard D, Tuseo L, Durand R. History and current status of Plasmodium falciparum antimalarial drug resistance in Madagascar. Scand J Infect Dis. 2010;42(1):22-32. PMID:19883158

Angrisano F, Delves MJ, Sturm A, Mollard V, McFadden GI, Sinden RE, Baum J. A GFP-Actin reporter line to explore microfilament dynamics across the malaria parasite lifecycle. Mol Biochem Parasitol. 2011 Nov 25. [Epub ahead of print]. PMID:22138565

Ankrah NA. Treatment of falciparum malaria with a tea-bag formulation of cryptolepis sanguinolenta root. Ghana Med J. 2010 Mar;44(1):2. PMID:21326983

Annerberg A, Lwin KM, Lindegardh N, Khrutsawadchai S, Ashley E, Day NP, Singhasivanon P, Tarning J, White NJ, Nosten F. A small amount of fat does not affect piperaquine exposure in patients with malaria. Antimicrob Agents Chemother. 2011 Sep;55(9):3971-6. Epub 2011 Jun 27. PMID:21709087

Ansah C, Gooderham NJ. The popular herbal antimalarial, extract of Cryptolepis sanguinolenta, is potently cytotoxic. Toxicol Sci. 2002 Dec;70(2):245-51. PMID:12441369

Ansah C, Khan A, Gooderham NJ. In vitro genotoxicity of the West African anti-malarial herbal Cryptolepis sanguinolenta and its major alkaloid cryptolepine. Toxicology. 2005 Mar 1;208(1):141-7. PMID:15664441

Ansari MA, Razdan RK. Relative efficacy of various oils in repelling mosquitoes. Indian J Malariol. 1995 Sep;32(3):104-11. PMID:8936292

Antinori S, Cigardi B, Galimberti L, Orlando G, Schifanella L, Milazzo L, Viola A, Giuliani G, Ridolfo A, Corbellino M. Diagnosis and therapy for hospitalized imported malaria in adults in Italy. J Travel Med. 2011 Nov-Dec;18(6):379-85. Epub 2011 Oct 17. PMID:22017713

Antonio Alvarez J, Lopez U, Rojas C, Borgonio VM, Sanchez V, Castañeda R, Vargas P, Figueroa JV. Immunization of Bos taurus steers with Babesia bovis recombinant antigens MSA-1, MSA-2c and 12D3. Transbound Emerg Dis. 2010 Apr;57(1-2):87-90. PMID:20537116

Anyaehie UB. Medicinal properties of fractionated acetone/water neem [Azadirachta indica] leaf extract from Nigeria: a review. Niger J Physiol Sci. 2009 Dec;24(2):157-9. PMID:20234757

Anyama NG, Tibenderana JK, Kutyabami P, Kamba PF, Kitutu FE, Adome RO. Participatory healthcare-provider orientation to improve artemether-lumefantrine-based drug treatment of uncomplicated malaria: a cluster quasi-experimental study. BMJ Qual Saf. 2011 Jul 11. [Epub ahead of print]. PMID:21749990

Arai S, Tsuji M, Kaiho I, Murayama H, Zamoto A, Wei Q, Okabe N, Kamiyama T, Ishihara C. Retrospective seroepidemiological survey for human babesiosis in an area in Japan where a tick-borne disease is endemic. J Vet Med Sci. 2003 Mar;65(3):335-40. PMID:12679563

Arai S, Tsuji M, Kim SJ, Nakade T, Kanno Y, Ishihara C. Babesia canis infection in canine-red blood cell-substituted SCID mice. Int J Parasitol. 1998 Sep;28(9):1429-35. PMID:9770629

Arango E, Carmona-Fonseca J, Blair S. [In vitro susceptibility of Colombian Plasmodium falciparum isolates to different antimalarial drugs].[Article in Spanish]. Biomedica. 2008 Jun;28(2):213-23. PMID:18719723

Archinti M, Britto M, Eden G, Furlan F, Murphy R, Degryse B. The urokinase receptor in the central nervous system. CNS Neurol Disord Drug Targets. 2011 Mar;10(2):271-94. PMID:20874700

Ardington PC. Bovine fluid therapy. J S Afr Vet Assoc. 1977 Oct;48(3):215-8. PMID:599536

Aregawi MW, Ali AS, Al-mafazy AW, Molteni F, Katikiti S, Warsame M, Njau RJ, Komatsu R, Korenromp E, Hosseini M, Low-Beer D, Bjorkman A, D'Alessandro U, Coosemans M, Otten M. Reductions in malaria and anaemia case and death burden at hospitals following scale-up of malaria control in Zanzibar, 1999-2008. Malar J. 2011 Feb 18;10:46. PMID:21332989

Arévalo-Pinzón G, Curtidor H, Muñoz M, Patarroyo MA, Bermudez A, Patarroyo ME. A single amino acid change in the Plasmodium falciparum RH5 (PfRH5) human RBC binding sequence modifies its structure and determines species-specific binding activity. Vaccine. 2011 Nov 17. [Epub ahead of print]. PMID:22100885

Armstrong PM, Brunet LR, Spielman A, Telford SR 3rd. Risk of Lyme disease: perceptions of residents of a Lone Star tick-infested community. Bull World Health Organ. 2001;79(10):916-25. PMID:11693973

Arnez M, Luznik-Bufon T, Avsic-Zupanc T, Ruzic-Sabljic E, Petrovec M, Lotric-Furlan S, Strle F. Causes of febrile illnesses after a tick bite in Slovenian children. Pediatr Infect Dis J. 2003 Dec;22(12):1078-83. PMID:14688569

Arnold L, Tyagi RK, Meija P, Swetman C, Gleeson J, Pérignon JL, Druilhe P. Further improvements of the P. falciparum humanized mouse model. PLoS One. 2011 Mar 31;6(3):e18045. PMID:21483851.

Arnold L, Tyagi RK, Mejia P, Van Rooijen N, Pérignon JL, Druilhe P. Analysis of innate defences against Plasmodium falciparum in immunodeficient mice. Malar J. 2010 Jul 9;9:197. PMID:20618960

Arogundade ED, Adebayo SB, Anyanti J, Nwokolo E, Ladipo O, Ankomah A, Meremikwu MM. Relationship between care-givers' misconceptions and non-use of ITNs by under-five Nigerian children. Malar J. 2011 Jun 22;10:170. PMID:21696622

Arora U, Sonal GS, Dhillon GP, Thakor HG. Emergence of drug resistance in India. J Indian Med Assoc. 2008 Oct;106(10):678-81, 683. PMID:19552104

Arulogun OS, Gregory AU. Management practices of childhood malaria among caregivers in Ojo Military Cantonment, Lagos, Nigeria: implication for child survival. Afr J Med Med Sci. 2009 Mar;38(1):45-54. PMID:19722428

Arunkumar JS, Naik AS, Prasad KC, Santhosh SG. Role of nasal endoscopy in chronic osteomyelitis of maxilla and zygoma: a case report. Case Report Med. 2011;2011:802964. Epub 2011 Nov 1. PMID:22110519

Asad S, Sweeney J, Mermel LA. Transfusion-transmitted babesiosis in Rhode Island. Transfusion. 2009 Dec;49(12):2564-73. Epub 2009 Sep 16. PMID:19761547

Asante KP, Abdulla S, Agnandji S, Lyimo J, Vekemans J, Soulanoudjingar S, Owusu R, Shomari M, Leach A, Jongert E, Salim N, Fernandes JF, Dosoo D, Chikawe M, Issifou S, Osei-Kwakye K, Lievens M, Paricek M, Möller T, Apanga S, Mwangoka G, Dubois MC, Madi T, Kwara E, Minja R, Hounkpatin AB, Boahen O, Kayan K, Adjei G, Chandramohan D, Carter T, Vansadia P, Sillman M, Savarese B, Loucq C, Lapierre D, Greenwood B, Cohen J, Kremsner P, Owusu-Agyei S, Tanner M, Lell B. Safety and efficacy of the RTS,S/AS01E candidate malaria vaccine given with expanded-programme-on-immunisation vaccines: 19 month follow-up of a randomised, open-label, phase 2 trial. Lancet Infect Dis. 2011 Oct;11(10):741-9. Epub 2011 Jul 22. PMID:21782519

Ashley EA, Pinoges L, Turyakira E, Dorsey G, Checchi F, Bukirwa H, van den Broek I, Zongo I, Urruta PP, van Herp M, Balkan S, Taylor WR, Olliaro P, Guthmann JP. Different methodological approaches to the assessment of in vivo efficacy of three artemisinin-based combination antimalarial treatments for the treatment of uncomplicated falciparum malaria in African children. Malar J. 2008 Aug 9;7:154. PMID:18691429

Ashton RA, Kyabayinze DJ, Opio T, Auma A, Edwards T, Matwale G, Onapa A, Brooker S, Kolaczinski JH. The impact of mass drug administration and long-lasting insecticidal net distribution on Wuchereria bancrofti infection in humans and mosquitoes: an observational study in northern Uganda. Parasit Vectors. 2011 Jul 15;4:134. PMID:21756371

Asih PB, Dewi RM, Tuti S, Sadikin M, Sumarto W, Sinaga B, van der Ven AJ, Sauerwein RW, Syafruddin D. Efficacy of artemisinin-based combination therapy for treatment of persons with uncomplicated Plasmodium falciparum malaria in West Sumba District, East Nusa Tenggara Province, Indonesia, and genotypic profiles of the parasite. Am J Trop Med Hyg. 2009 Jun;80(6):914-8. PMID:19478248

Asiimwe C, Gelvin D, Lee E, Ben Amor Y, Quinto E, Katureebe C, Sundaram L, Bell D, Berg M. Use of an innovative, affordable, and open-source short message service-based tool to monitor malaria in remote areas of Uganda. Am J Trop Med Hyg. 2011 Jul;85(1):26-33. PMID:21734120

Ataíde R, Mwapasa V, Molyneux ME, Meshnick SR, Rogerson SJ. Antibodies that induce phagocytosis of malaria infected erythrocytes: effect of HIV infection and correlation with clinical outcomes. PLoS One. 2011;6(7):e22491. Epub 2011 Jul 19. PMID:21811621

Atangana J, Bigoga JD, Patchoké S, Ndjemaï MN, Tabue RN, Nem TE, Fondjo E. Anopheline fauna and malaria transmission in four ecologically distinct zones in Cameroon. Acta Trop. 2010 Jul-Aug;115(1-2):131-6. Epub 2010 Mar 3. PMID:20206111

Athri P, Wenzler T, Tidwell R, Bakunova SM, Wilson WD. Pharmacophore model for pentamidine analogs active against Plasmodium falciparum. Eur J Med Chem. 2010 Dec;45(12):6147-51. Epub 2010 Sep 18. PMID:20884090

Avdeeva O, Lazarus JV, Aziz MA, Atun R. The Global Fund's resource allocation decisions for HIV programmes: addressing those in need. J Int AIDS Soc. 2011 Oct 26;14:51. PMID:22029667

Avery RK. Update in management of ganciclovir-resistant cytomegalovirus infection. Curr Opin Infect Dis. 2008 Aug;21(4):433-7. PMID:18594298

Avril M, Cartwright MM, Hathaway MJ, Smith JD. Induction of strain-transcendent antibodies to placental-type isolates with VAR2CSA DBL3 or DBL5 recombinant proteins. Malar J. 2011 Feb 11;10(1):36. PMID:21314945

Avril M, Hathaway MJ, Srivastava A, Dechavanne S, Hommel M, Beeson JG, Smith JD, Gamain B. Antibodies to a full-length VAR2CSA immunogen are broadly strain-transcendent but do not cross-inhibit different placental-type parasite isolates. PLoS One. 2011 Feb 7;6(2):e16622. PMID:21326877

Awasthi S. Taking aim at novel vaccines market. Hum Vaccin. 2009 Oct;5(10):654-7. Epub 2009 Oct 1. PMID:19855156

Ayede IA, Falade AG, Sowunmi A, Jansen FH. An open randomized clinical trial in comparing two artesunate-based combination treatments on Plasmodium falciparum malaria in Nigerian children: artesunate/sulphamethoxypyrazine/pyrimethamine (fixed dose over 24 hours) versus artesunate/amodiaquine (fixed dose over 48 hours). Malar J. 2010 Dec 31;9:378. PMID:21194422

Ayoob AL, Hackner SG, Prittie J. Clinical management of canine babesiosis. J Vet Emerg Crit Care (San Antonio). 2010 Feb;20(1):77-89. PMID:20230437

Ayoob AL, Prittie J, Hackner SG. Feline babesiosis. J Vet Emerg Crit Care (San Antonio). 2010 Feb;20(1):90-7. PMID:20230438

Azouzi S, Morandat S, El Kirat K. The potent antimalarial peptide cyclosporin A induces the aggregation and permeabilization of sphingomyelin-rich membranes. Langmuir. 2011 Aug 2;27(15):9465-72. Epub 2011 Jun 30. PMID:21692492

Baber I, Tamby JP, Manoukis NC, Sangaré D, Doumbia S, Traoré SF, Maiga MS, Dembélé D. A python module to normalize microarray data by the quantile adjustment method. Infect Genet Evol. 2011 Jun;11(4):765-8. Epub 2010 Oct 21. PMID:20970526

Babu RV, Sharma G. A 57-year-old man with abdominal pain, jaundice, and a history of blood transfusion. Chest. 2007 Jul;132(1):347-50. PMID:17625097

Bachmeier B, Fichtner I, Killian PH, Kronski E, Pfeffer U, Efferth T. Development of resistance towards artesunate in MDA-MB-231 human breast cancer cells. PLoS One. 2011;6(5):e20550. Epub 2011 May 26. PMID:21637790

Bacon DJ, McCollum AM, Griffing SM, Salas C, Soberon V, Santolalla M, Haley R, Tsukayama P, Lucas C, Escalante AA, Udhayakumar V. Dynamics of malaria drug resistance patterns in the Amazon basin region following changes in Peruvian national treatment policy for uncomplicated malaria. Antimicrob Agents Chemother. 2009 May;53(5):2042-51. Epub 2009 Mar 2. PMID:19258269

Baguley D, Lim E, Bevan A, Pallet A, Faust SN. Prescribing for children - taste and palatability affect adherence to antibiotics: a review. Arch Dis Child. 2011 Nov 16. [Epub ahead of print]. PMID:22088684

Baiden F, Owusu-Agyei S, Bawah J, Bruce J, Tivura M, Delmini R, Gyaase S, Amenga-Etego S, Chandramohan D, Webster J. An evaluation of the clinical assessments of under-five febrile children presenting to primary health facilities in rural ghana. PLoS One. 2011;6(12):e28944. Epub 2011 Dec 13. PMID:22174932

Bailly C, Laine W, Baldeyrou B, De Pauw-Gillet MC, Colson P, Houssier C, Cimanga K, Van Miert S, Vlietinck AJ, Pieters L. DNA intercalation, topoisomerase II inhibition and cytotoxic activity of the plant alkaloid neocryptolepine. Anticancer Drug Des. 2000 Jun;15(3):191-201. PMID:11049087

Baker JG, Hill SJ, Summers RJ. Evolution of β-blockers: from anti-anginal drugs to ligand-directed signalling. Trends Pharmacol Sci. 2011 Apr;32(4):227-34. Epub 2011 Mar 21. PMID:21429598

Baliraine FN, Rosenthal PJ. Prolonged selection of pfmdr1 polymorphisms after treatment of falciparum malaria with artemether-lumefantrine in Uganda. J Infect Dis. 2011 Oct 1;204(7):1120-4. PMID:21881128

Banek K, Kilian A, Allan R. Evaluation of Interceptor long-lasting insecticidal nets in eight communities in Liberia. Malar J. 2010 Mar 24;9:84. PMID:20334677

Banerjee DP, Singh B, Gautam OP, Sarup S. Cell-mediated immune response in equine babesiosis. Trop Anim Health Prod. 1977 Aug;9(3):153-8. PMID:910301

Baptista FG, Pamplona A, Pena AC, Mota MM, Pied S, Vigário AM. Accumulation of Plasmodium berghei-infected red blood cells in the brain is crucial for the development of cerebral malaria in mice. Infect Immun. 2010 Sep;78(9):4033-9. Epub 2010 Jul 6. PMID:20605973

Baptista MS, Wainwright M. Photodynamic antimicrobial chemotherapy (PACT) for the treatment of malaria, leishmaniasis and trypanosomiasis. Braz J Med Biol Res. 2011 Jan;44(1):1-10. Epub 2010 Dec 10. PMID:21152709

Barboza-Filho CG, Cabrera FC, Dos Santos RJ, De Saja Saez JA, Job AE. The influence of natural rubber/Au nanoparticle membranes on the physiology of Leishmania brasiliensis. Exp Parasitol. 2011 Nov 10. [Epub ahead of print]. PMID:22101110

Barends M, Jaidee A, Khaohirun N, Singhasivanon P, Nosten F. In vitro activity of ferroquine (SSR 97193) against Plasmodium falciparum isolates from the Thai-Burmese border. Malar J. 2007 Jun 27;6:81. PMID:17597537

Barker RH Jr, Metelev V, Rapaport E, Zamecnik P. Inhibition of Plasmodium falciparum malaria using antisense oligodeoxynucleotides. Proc Natl Acad Sci U S A. 1996 Jan 9;93(1):514-8. PMID:8552672

Barnard CJ, Collins SA, Daisley JN, Behnke JM. Odour learning and immunity costs in mice. Behav Processes. 2006 Mar;72(1):74-83. Epub 2006 Jan 26. PMID:16442748

Barr J. A short history of dapsone, or an alternative model of drug development. J Hist Med Allied Sci. 2011 Oct;66(4):425-67. Epub 2010 Oct 21. PMID:20966036

Barratt JL, Harkness J, Marriott D, Ellis JT, Stark D. Importance of nonenteric protozoan infections in immunocompromised people. Clin Microbiol Rev. 2010 Oct;23(4):795-836. PMID:20930074

Barré N, Happold J, Delathière JM, Desoutter D, Salery M, de Vos A, Marchal C, Perrot R, Grailles M, Mortelecque A. A campaign to eradicate bovine babesiosis from New Caledonia. Ticks Tick Borne Dis. 2011 Mar;2(1):55-61. Epub 2011 Jan 26. PMID:21771538

Barrera SM, Pérez MA, Knudson A, Nicholls RS, Guerra AP. [Genotypic survey of Plasmodium falciparum based on the msp1, msp2 and glurp genes by multiplex PCR].[Article in Spanish]. Biomedica. 2010 Oct-Dec;30(4):530-8. PMID:21713358

Barriga OO. A review on vaccination against protozoa and arthropods of veterinary importance. Vet Parasitol. 1994 Oct;55(1-2):29-55. PMID:7886919

Barros FC, Bhutta ZA, Batra M, Hansen TN, Victora CG, Rubens CE; GAPPS Review Group. Global report on preterm birth and stillbirth (3 of 7): evidence for effectiveness of interventions. BMC Pregnancy Childbirth. 2010 Feb 23;10 Suppl 1:S3. PMID:20233384

Barry DN. Metabolism of Babesia parasites in vitro. Change in adenylate energy charge and infectivity of Babesia rodhaini-infected erythrocytes. Aust J Exp Biol Med Sci. 1984 Feb;62 (Pt 1):63-71. PMID:6743142

Bartlett MS, Queener SF, Durkin MM, Shaw MA, Smith JW. Inoculated mouse model of Pneumocystis carinii infection. Diagn Microbiol Infect Dis. 1992 Feb;15(2):129-34. PMID:1572137

Bartlett SL, Abou-Madi N, Messick JB, Birkenheuer A, Kollias GV. Diagnosis and treatment of Babesia odocoilei in captive reindeer (Rangifer tarandus tarandus) and recognition of three novel host species. J Zoo Wildl Med. 2009 Mar;40(1):152-9. PMID:19368255

Bassat Q, Gonzalez R, Machevo S, Nahum A, Lyimo J, Maiga H, Martensson A, Bashraheil M, Ouma P, Ubben D, Walter V, Nwaiwu O, Kipkeu C, Lefevre G, Ogutu B, Menendez C. Similar efficacy and safety of artemether-lumefantrine (Coartem(R)) in African infants and children with uncomplicated falciparum malaria across different body weight ranges. Malar J. 2011 Dec 16;10(1):369. [Epub ahead of print]. PMID:22176931

Basu SK. A health profile of tribal India. Health Millions. 1994 Apr;2(2):12-4. PMID:12287763

Batista TM, Marques JT. RNAi pathways in parasitic protists and worms. J Proteomics. 2011 Aug 24;74(9):1504-14. Epub 2011 Mar 6. PMID:21385631

Batwala V, Magnussen P, Hansen KS, Nuwaha F. Cost-effectiveness of malaria microscopy and rapid diagnostic tests versus presumptive diagnosis: implications for malaria control in Uganda. Malar J. 2011 Dec 19;10(1):372. [Epub ahead of print]. PMID:22182735

Batwala V, Magnussen P, Nuwaha F. Antibiotic use among patients with febrile illness in a low malaria endemicity setting in Uganda. Malar J. 2011 Dec 20;10(1):377. [Epub ahead of print]. PMID:22183039

Batwala V, Magnussen P, Nuwaha F. Comparative feasibility of implementing rapid diagnostic test and microscopy for parasitological diagnosis of malaria in Uganda. Malar J. 2011 Dec 19;10(1):373. [Epub ahead of print]. PMID:22182758

Baumann D, Pusterla N, Péter O, Grimm F, Fournier PE, Schär G, Bossart W, Lutz H, Weber R. [Fever after a tick bite: clinical manifestations and diagnosis of acute tick bite-associated infections in northeastern Switzerland]. [Article in German]. Dtsch Med Wochenschr. 2003 May 9;128(19):1042-7. PMID:12736854

Baumeister S, Wiesner J, Reichenberg A, Hintz M, Bietz S, Harb OS, Roos DS, Kordes M, Friesen J, Matuschewski K, Lingelbach K, Jomaa H, Seeber F. Fosmidomycin uptake into Plasmodium and Babesia-infected erythrocytes is facilitated by parasite-induced new permeability pathways. PLoS One. 2011 May 4;6(5):e19334. PMID:21573242

Bautista CR, Alvarez JA, Mosqueda JJ, Falcon A, Ramos JA, Rojas C, Figueroa JV, Ku M. Enhancement of the Mexican bovine babesiosis vaccine efficacy by using Lactobacillus casei. Ann N Y Acad Sci. 2008 Dec;1149:126-30. PMID:19120190

Bautista CR, Sandoval A, Aguilar BR. Effect of high- and low-molecular-weight components of Lactobacillus casei on resistance against Babesia microti in NIH mice. Ann N Y Acad Sci. 2008 Dec;1149:152-4. PMID:19120196

Bautista-Garfias CR, Gómez MB, Aguilar BR, Ixta O, Martínez F, Mosqueda J. The treatment of mice with Lactobacillus casei induces protection against Babesia microti infection. Parasitol Res. 2005 Dec;97(6):472-7. Epub 2005 Sep 17. PMID:16170567

Bayes M, Rabasseda X, Prous JR. Gateways to clinical trials. Methods Find Exp Clin Pharmacol. 2003 Nov;25(9):747-71. PMID:14685303

Bayés M, Rabasseda X, Prous JR. Gateways to clinical trials. Methods Find Exp Clin Pharmacol. 2005 Jun;27(5):331-72. PMID:16082422

Bayés M, Rabasseda X. Gateways to clinical trials. Methods Find Exp Clin Pharmacol. 2008 Jan-Feb;30(1):67-99. PMID:18389098

Becker JL. Vector-borne illnesses and the safety of the blood supply. Curr Hematol Rep. 2003 Nov;2(6):511-7. PMID:14561396

Becker JV, Mtwisha L, Crampton BG, Stoychev S, van Brummelen AC, Reeksting S, Louw AI, Birkholtz LM, Mancama DT. Plasmodium falciparum spermidine synthase inhibition results in unique perturbation-specific effects observed on transcript, protein and metabolite levels. BMC Genomics. 2010 Apr 12;11:235. PMID:20385001

Becker JV, van der Merwe MM, van Brummelen AC, Pillay P, Crampton BG, Mmutlane EM, Parkinson C, van Heerden FR, Crouch NR, Smith PJ, Mancama DT, Maharaj VJ. In vitro anti-plasmodial activity of Dicoma anomala subsp. Gerrardii (Asteraceae): identification of its main active constituent, structure-activity relationship studies and gene expression profiling. Malar J. 2011 Oct 11;10:295. PMID:21985233

Beez D, Sanchez CP, Stein WD, Lanzer M. Genetic predisposition favors the acquisition of stable artemisinin resistance in malaria parasites. Antimicrob Agents Chemother. 2011 Jan;55(1):50-5. Epub 2010 Nov 1. PMID:21041511

Beiersmann C, Bountogo M, Tiendrébeogo J, De Allegri M, Louis VR, Coulibaly B, Yé M, Mueller O. Falciparum malaria in young children of rural Burkina Faso: comparison of survey data in 1999 with 2009. Malar J. 2011 Oct 11;10:296. PMID:21989335

Bell DJ, Nyirongo SK, Mukaka M, Zijlstra EE, Plowe CV, Molyneux ME, Ward SA, Winstanley PA. Sulfadoxine-pyrimethamine-based combinations for malaria: a randomised blinded trial to compare efficacy, safety and selection of resistance in Malawi. PLoS One. 2008 Feb 13;3(2):e1578. PMID:18270569

Bell SL, Chiang AN, Brodsky JL. Expression of a malarial Hsp70 improves defects in chaperone-dependent activities in ssa1 mutant yeast. PLoS One. 2011;6(5):e20047. Epub 2011 May 19. PMID:21625512

Belloli C, Crescenzo G, Lai O, Carofiglio V, Marang O, Ormas P. Pharmacokinetics of imidocarb dipropionate in horses after intramuscular administration. Equine Vet J. 2002 Sep;34(6):625-9. PMID:12358005

Bellot F, Coslédan F, Vendier L, Brocard J, Meunier B, Robert A. Trioxaferroquines as new hybrid antimalarial drugs. J Med Chem. 2010 May 27;53(10):4103-9. PMID:20443628

Belongia EA, Reed KD, Mitchell PD, Mueller-Rizner N, Vandermause M, Finkel MF, Kazmierczak JJ. Tickborne infections as a cause of nonspecific febrile illness in Wisconsin. Clin Infect Dis. 2001 May 15;32(10):1434-9. Epub 2001 Apr 17. PMID:11317244

Ben Mamoun C, Prigge ST, Vial H. Targeting the Lipid Metabolic Pathways for the Treatment of Malaria. Drug Dev Res. 2010 Feb;71(1):44-55. PMID:20559451

Ben Musa N, Dawoud HA. The protective activity of serum and fractionated serum from rats against Babesia divergens. J Egypt Soc Parasitol. 2004 Aug;34(2):407-22. PMID:15287167

Ben Musa N, Phillips RS. The adaptation of three isolates of Babesia divergens to continuous culture in rat erythrocytes. Parasitology. 1991 Oct;103 Pt 2:165-70. PMID:1745544

Benach JL, Habicht GS, Holbrook TW, Cook JA. Glucan as an adjuvant for a murine Babesia microti immunization trial. Infect Immun. 1982 Mar;35(3):947-51. PMID:7068224

Benavides MV, Sacco AM. Differential Bos taurus cattle response to Babesia bovis infection. Vet Parasitol. 2007 Nov 30;150(1-2):54-64. Epub 2007 Oct 24. PMID:17919816

Beniwal RP, Nichani AK, Rakha NK, Sharma RD, Sarup S. An immunisation trial with in vitro produced Babesia bigemina exoantigens. Trop Anim Health Prod. 1997 Nov;29(4 Suppl):124S-126S. PMID:9512758

Berdelle N, Nikolova T, Quiros S, Efferth T, Kaina B. Artesunate Induces Oxidative DNA Damage, Sustained DNA Double-Strand Breaks, and the ATM/ATR Damage Response in Cancer Cells. Mol Cancer Ther. 2011 Dec;10(12):2224-33. Epub 2011 Oct 13. PMID:21998290

Berg M, Van der Veken P, Goeminne A, Haemers A, Augustyns K. Inhibitors of the purine salvage pathway: a valuable approach for antiprotozoal chemotherapy? Curr Med Chem. 2010;17(23):2456-81. PMID:20491648

Berglund J. [Ticks--a medical topic of current interest which sticks]. [Article in Swedish]. Lakartidningen. 1998 Jun 3;95(23):2695-700. PMID:9656623

Bergmann-Leitner ES, Legler PM, Savranskaya T, Ockenhouse CF, Angov E. Cellular and humoral immune effector mechanisms required for sterile protection against sporozoite challenge induced with the novel malaria vaccine candidate CelTOS. Vaccine. 2011 Aug 11;29(35):5940-9. Epub 2011 Jun 29. PMID:21722682

Bergmann-Leitner ES, Mease RM, De La Vega P, Savranskaya T, Polhemus M, Ockenhouse C, Angov E. Immunization with pre-erythrocytic antigen CelTOS from Plasmodium falciparum elicits cross-species protection against heterologous challenge with Plasmodium berghei. PLoS One. 2010 Aug 19;5(8):e12294. PMID:20808868

Berkman SA. Infectious complications of blood transfusion. Blood Rev. 1988 Sep;2(3):206-10. PMID:3052666

Berkman SA. The spectrum of transfusion reactions. Hosp Pract (Off Ed). 1984 Jun;19(6):205-8, 210-2, 217-9. PMID:6427247

Bern C. Antitrypanosomal therapy for chronic Chagas' disease. N Engl J Med. 2011 Jun 30;364(26):2527-34. PMID:21714649

Bero J, Frédérich M, Quetin-Leclercq J. Antimalarial compounds isolated from plants used in traditional medicine. J Pharm Pharmacol. 2009 Nov;61(11):1401-33. PMID:19903367

Bertin G, Briand V, Bonaventure D, Carrieu A, Massougbodji A, Cot M, Deloron P. Molecular markers of resistance to sulphadoxine-pyrimethamine during intermittent preventive treatment of pregnant women in Benin. Malar J. 2011 Jul 19;10:196. PMID:21767415

Bertinaria M, Guglielmo S, Rolando B, Giorgis M, Aragno C, Fruttero R, Gasco A, Parapini S, Taramelli D, Martins YC, Carvalho LJ. Amodiaquine analogues containing NO-donor substructures: synthesis and their preliminary evaluation as potential tools in the treatment of cerebral malaria. Eur J Med Chem. 2011 May;46(5):1757-67. Epub 2011 Feb 22. PMID:21396743

Bertol CD, Oliveira PR, Kuminek G, Rauber GS, Stulzer HK, Silva MA. Increased bioavailability of primaquine using poly(ethylene oxide) matrix extended-release tablets administered to beagle dogs. Ann Trop Med Parasitol. 2011 Oct;105(7):475-84. PMID:22185941

Beshir KB, Hallett RL, Eziefula AC, Bailey R, Watson J, Wright SG, Chiodini PL, Polley SD, Sutherland CJ. Measuring the efficacy of anti-malarial drugs in vivo: quantitative PCR measurement of parasite clearance. Malar J. 2010 Nov 5;9:312. PMID:21054863

Bethell D, Se Y, Lon C, Socheat D, Saunders D, Teja-Isavadharm P, Khemawoot P, Darapiseth S, Lin J, Sriwichai S, Kuntawungin W, Surasri S, Lee SJ, Sarim S, Tyner S, Smith B, Fukuda MM. Dose-dependent risk of neutropenia after 7-day courses of artesunate monotherapy in Cambodian patients with acute Plasmodium falciparum malaria. Clin Infect Dis. 2010 Dec 15;51(12):e105-14. Epub 2010 Nov 11. PMID:21070142

Bethell D, Se Y, Lon C, Tyner S, Saunders D, Sriwichai S, Darapiseth S, Teja-Isavadharm P, Khemawoot P, Schaecher K, Ruttvisutinunt W, Lin J, Kuntawungin W, Gosi P, Timmermans A, Smith B, Socheat D, Fukuda MM. Artesunate dose escalation for the treatment of uncomplicated malaria in a region of reported artemisinin resistance: a randomized clinical trial. PLoS One. 2011;6(5):e19283. Epub 2011 May 13. PMID:21603629

Bethony JM, Cole RN, Guo X, Kamhawi S, Lightowlers MW, Loukas A, Petri W, Reed S, Valenzuela JG, Hotez PJ. Vaccines to combat the neglected tropical diseases. Immunol Rev. 2011 Jan;239(1):237-70. PMID:21198676

Beveridge E. Babesicidal effect of basically substituted carbanilides. II. Imidocarb in rats and mice: toxicity and activity against Babesia rodhaini. Res Vet Sci. 1969 Nov;10(6):534-9. PMID:5368455

Beveridge E. The rate of development of drug resistance in Babesia rodhaini. Trans R Soc Trop Med Hyg. 1969;63(4):427. PMID:4980625

Bharatham N, Chang MW, Yoon HS. Targeting FK506 binding proteins to fight malarial and bacterial infections: current advances and future perspectives. Curr Med Chem. 2011;18(12):1874-89. PMID:21466465

Bhardwaj A, Scaria V, Raghava GP, Lynn AM, Chandra N, Banerjee S, Raghunandanan MV, Pandey V, Taneja B, Yadav J, Dash D, Bhattacharya J, Misra A, Kumar A, Ramachandran S, Thomas Z; Open Source Drug Discovery Consortium, Brahmachari SK. Open source drug discovery--a new paradigm of collaborative research in tuberculosis drug development. Tuberculosis (Edinb). 2011 Sep;91(5):479-86. Epub 2011 Jul 22. PMID:21782516

Bhat UK, Mahoney DF, Wright IG. The invasion and growth of Babesia bovis in tick tissue culture. Experientia. 1979 Jun 15;35(6):752-3. PMID:467577

Bianchi MW, Barré N, Messad S. Factors related to cattle infestation level and resistance to acaricides in Boophilus microplus tick populations in New Caledonia. Vet Parasitol. 2003 Feb 28;112(1-2):75-89. PMID:12581586

Bienvenu AL, Gonzalez-Rey E, Picot S. Apoptosis induced by parasitic diseases. Parasit Vectors. 2010 Nov 17;3:106. PMID:21083888

Bierer DE, Dubenko LG, Zhang P, Lu Q, Imbach PA, Garofalo AW, Phuan PW, Fort DM, Litvak J, Gerber RE, Sloan B, Luo J, Cooper R, Reaven GM. Antihyperglycemic activities of cryptolepine analogues: an ethnobotanical lead structure isolated from Cryptolepis sanguinolenta. J Med Chem. 1998 Jul 16;41(15):2754-64. PMID:9667966

Bierer DE, Fort DM, Mendez CD, Luo J, Imbach PA, Dubenko LG, Jolad SD, Gerber RE, Litvak J, Lu Q, Zhang P, Reed MJ, Waldeck N, Bruening RC, Noamesi BK, Hector RF, Carlson TJ, King SR. Ethnobotanical-directed discovery of the antihyperglycemic properties of cryptolepine: its isolation from Cryptolepis sanguinolenta, synthesis, and in vitro and in vivo activities. J Med Chem. 1998 Mar 12;41(6):894-901. PMID:9526563

Bigey P, Gnidehou S, Doritchamou J, Quiviger M, Viwami F, Couturier A, Salanti A, Nielsen MA, Scherman D, Deloron P, Tuikue Ndam N. The NTS-DBL2X region of VAR2CSA induces cross-reactive antibodies that inhibit adhesion of several Plasmodium falciparum isolates to chondroitin sulfate A. J Infect Dis. 2011 Oct 1;204(7):1125-33. PMID:21881129

Bin Dajem SM, Al-Qahtani A. Analysis of gene mutations involved in chloroquine resistance in Plasmodium falciparum parasites isolated from patients in the southwest of Saudi Arabia. Ann Saudi Med. 2010 May-Jun;30(3):187-92. PMID:20427933

Birkenheuer AJ, Levy MG, Breitschwerdt EB. Efficacy of combined atovaquone and azithromycin for therapy of chronic Babesia gibsoni (Asian genotype) infections in dogs. J Vet Intern Med. 2004 Jul-Aug;18(4):494-8. PMID:15320586

Birkenheuer AJ, Whittington J, Neel J, Large E, Barger A, Levy MG, Breitschwerdt

EB. Molecular characterization of a Babesia species identified in a North American raccoon. J Wildl Dis. 2006 Apr;42(2):375-80. PMID:16870860

Birkett MA, Hassanali A, Hoglund S, Pettersson J, Pickett JA. Repellent activity of catmint, Nepeta cataria, and iridoid nepetalactone isomers against Afro-tropical mosquitoes, ixodid ticks and red poultry mites. Phytochemistry. 2011 Jan;72(1):109-14. Epub 2010 Nov 4. PMID:21056438

Bishop JP, Adams LG, Thompson KC, Corrier DE. The isolation, separation and preservation of Babesia bigemina. Trop Anim Health Prod. 1973 Aug;5(3):141-5. PMID:4802625

Bishop JP, Adams LG. Babesia bigemina: immune response of cattle inoculated with irradiated parasites. Exp Parasitol. 1974 Feb;35(1):35-43. PMID:4815017

Biswas S, Dicks MD, Long CA, Remarque EJ, Siani L, Colloca S, Cottingham MG, Holder AA, Gilbert SC, Hill AV, Draper SJ. Transgene optimization, immunogenicity and in vitro efficacy of viral vectored vaccines expressing two alleles of Plasmodium falciparum AMA1. PLoS One. 2011;6(6):e20977. Epub 2011 Jun 16. PMID:21698193

Black H. Mosquito gut bacterium may curb malaria. Environ Health Perspect. 2011 Aug;119(8):A337. PMID:21807592

Blagborough AM, Yoshida S, Sattabongkot J, Tsuboi T, Sinden RE. Intranasal and intramuscular immunization with Baculovirus Dual Expression System-based Pvs25 vaccine substantially blocks Plasmodium vivax transmission. Vaccine. 2010 Aug 23;28(37):6014-20. Epub 2010 Jul 14. PMID:20637303

Blue D, Graves V, McCarthy L, Cruz J, Gregurek S, Smith D. Fatal transfusion-transmitted Babesia microti in the Midwest. Transfusion. 2009 Jan;49(1):8. Epub 2008 Aug 6. PMID:18694463

Bobbala D, Alesutan I, Föller M, Huber SM, Lang F. Effect of anandamide in Plasmodium Berghei-infected mice. Cell Physiol Biochem. 2010;26(3):355-62. Epub 2010 Aug 24. PMID:20798520

Bobbala D, Alesutan I, Föller M, Tschan S, Huber SM, Lang F. Protective effect of amiodarone in malaria. Acta Trop. 2010 Oct;116(1):39-44. Epub 2010 May 27. PMID:20510873

Bobenchik AM, Augagneur Y, Hao B, Hoch JC, Ben Mamoun C. Phosphoethanolamine methyltransferases in phosphocholine biosynthesis: functions and potential for antiparasite therapy. FEMS Microbiol Rev. 2011 Jul;35(4):609-19. Epub 2011 Mar 10. PMID:21303393

Bock R, Jackson L, de Vos A, Jorgensen W. Babesiosis of cattle. Parasitology. 2004;129 Suppl:S247-69. PMID:15938514

Bock RE, Blight GW, Kingston TG, de Vos AJ. A survey of cattle producers in the Boophilus microplus endemic area of Queensland to determine attitudes to the control of and vaccination against tick fever. Aust Vet J. 1995 Mar;72(3):88-92. PMID:7611988

Bock RE, de Vos AJ, Kingston TG, Shiels IA, Dalgliesh RJ. Investigations of breakdowns in protection provided by living Babesia bovis vaccine. Vet Parasitol. 1992 Jun;43(1-2):45-56. PMID:1496802

Bock RE, de Vos AJ. Immunity following use of Australian tick fever vaccine: a review of the evidence. Aust Vet J. 2001 Dec;79(12):832-9. PMID:11837905

Böhm M, Leisewitz AL, Thompson PN, Schoeman JP. Capillary and venous Babesia canis rossi parasitaemias and their association with outcome of infection and circulatory compromise. Vet Parasitol. 2006 Oct 10;141(1-2):18-29. Epub 2006 Jun 27. PMID:16806713

Boivin MJ, Giordani B. Neuropsychological assessment of African children: evidence for a universal brain/behavior omnibus within a coconstructivist paradigm. Prog Brain Res. 2009;178:113-35. PMID:19874965

Bomfim MR, Ko A, Koury MC. Evaluation of the recombinant LipL32 in enzyme-linked immunosorbent assay for the serodiagnosis of bovine leptospirosis. Vet Microbiol. 2005 Aug 10;109(1-2):89-94. PMID:15950404

Bompart F, Kiechel JR, Sebbag R, Pecoul B. Innovative public-private partnerships to maximize the delivery of anti-malarial medicines: lessons learned from the ASAQ Winthrop experience. Malar J. 2011 May 23;10:143. PMID:21605364

Bonjean K, De Pauw-Gillet MC, Defresne MP, Colson P, Houssier C, Dassonneville L, Bailly C, Greimers R, Wright C, Quetin-Leclercq J, Tits M, Angenot L. The DNA intercalating alkaloid cryptolepine interferes with topoisomerase II and inhibits primarily DNA synthesis in B16 melanoma cells. Biochemistry. 1998 Apr 14;37(15):5136-46. PMID:9548744

Bonnet M, Broek I, van Herp M, Urrutia PP, van Overmeir C, Kyomuhendo J, Ndosimao CN, Ashley E, Guthmann JP. Varying efficacy of artesunate+amodiaquine and artesunate+sulphadoxine-pyrimethamine for the treatment of uncomplicated falciparum malaria in the Democratic Republic of Congo: a report of two in-vivo studies. Malar J. 2009 Aug 10;8:192. PMID:19664280

Bonnet M, Roper C, Félix M, Coulibaly L, Kankolongo GM, Guthmann JP. Efficacy of antimalarial treatment in Guinea: in vivo study of two artemisinin combination therapies in Dabola and molecular markers of resistance to sulphadoxine-pyrimethamine in N'Zérékoré. Malar J. 2007 May 3;6:54. PMID:17477865

Bono MF, Mangold AJ, Baravalle ME, Valentini BS, Thompson CS, Wilkowsky SE, Echaide IE, Farber MD, Torioni de Echaide SM. Efficiency of a recombinant MSA-2c-based ELISA to establish the persistence of antibodies in cattle vaccinated with Babesia bovis. Vet Parasitol. 2008 Nov 7;157(3-4):203-10. Epub 2008 Aug 5. PMID:18783887

Bonoan JT, Johnson DH, Cunha BA. Life-threatening babesiosis in an asplenic patient treated with exchange transfusion, azithromycin, and atovaquone. Heart Lung. 1998 Nov-Dec;27(6):424-8. PMID:9835673

Bönsch C, Kempf C, Mueller I, Manning L, Laman M, Davis TM, Ros C. Chloroquine and its derivatives exacerbate B19V-associated anemia by promoting viral replication. PLoS Negl Trop Dis. 2010 Apr 27;4(4):e669. PMID:20436917

Booker ML, Bastos CM, Kramer ML, Barker RH Jr, Skerlj R, Sidhu AB, Deng X, Celatka C, Cortese JF, Guerrero Bravo JE, Crespo Llado KN, Serrano AE, Angulo-Barturen I, Jiménez-Díaz MB, Viera S, Garuti H, Wittlin S, Papastogiannidis P, Lin JW, Janse CJ, Khan SM, Duraisingh M, Coleman B, Goldsmith EJ, Phillips MA, Munoz B, Wirth DF, Klinger JD, Wiegand R, Sybertz E. Novel inhibitors of Plasmodium falciparum dihydroorotate dehydrogenase with anti-malarial activity in the mouse model. J Biol Chem. 2010 Oct 22;285(43):33054-64. Epub 2010 Aug 11. PMID:20702404

Bora U, Sahu A, Saikia AP, Ryakala VK, Goswami P. Medicinal plants used by the people of Northeast India for curing malaria. Phytother Res. 2007 Aug;21(8):800-4. PMID:17533627

Borges S, Cravo P, Creasey A, Fawcett R, Modrzynska K, Rodrigues L, Martinelli A, Hunt P. Genomewide scan reveals amplification of mdr1 as a common denominator of resistance to mefloquine, lumefantrine, and artemisinin in Plasmodium chabaudi malaria parasites. Antimicrob Agents Chemother. 2011 Oct;55(10):4858-65. Epub 2011 Jun 27. PMID:21709099

Bork S, Okamura M, Boonchit S, Hirata H, Yokoyama N, Igarashi I. Identification of Babesia bovis L-lactate dehydrogenase as a potential chemotherapeutical target against bovine babesiosis. Mol Biochem Parasitol. 2004 Aug;136(2):165-72. PMID:15478796

Bork S, Yokoyama N, Ikehara Y, Kumar S, Sugimoto C, Igarashi I. Growth-inhibitory effect of heparin on Babesia parasites. Antimicrob Agents Chemother. 2004 Jan;48(1):236-41. PMID:14693545

Bork S, Yokoyama N, Matsuo T, Claveria FG, Fujisaki K, Igarashi I. Growth inhibitory effect of triclosan on equine and bovine Babesia parasites. Am J Trop Med Hyg. 2003 Mar;68(3):334-40. PMID:12685641

Bork S, Yokoyama N, Matsuo T, Claveria FG, Fujisaki K, Igarashi I. Clotrimazole, ketoconazole, and clodinafop-propargyl as potent growth inhibitors of equine Babesia parasites during in vitro culture. J Parasitol. 2003 Jun;89(3):604-6. PMID:12880264

Borrmann S, Matuschewski K. Protective immunity against malaria by 'natural immunization': a question of dose, parasite diversity, or both? Curr Opin Immunol. 2011 Aug;23(4):500-8. Epub 2011 Jun 28. PMID:21719266

Borrmann S, Matuschewski K. Targeting Plasmodium liver stages: better late than never. Trends Mol Med. 2011 Sep;17(9):527-36. Epub 2011 Jul 6. PMID:21737347

Borrmann S, Sasi P, Mwai L, Bashraheil M, Abdallah A, Muriithi S, Frühauf H, Schaub B, Pfeil J, Peshu J, Hanpithakpong W, Rippert A, Juma E, Tsofa B, Mosobo M, Lowe B, Osier F, Fegan G, Lindegårdh N, Nzila A, Peshu N, Mackinnon M, Marsh K. Declining Responsiveness of Plasmodium falciparum Infections to Artemisinin-Based Combination Treatments on the Kenyan Coast. PLoS One. 2011;6(11):e26005. Epub 2011 Nov 10. PMID:22102856

Botros BA, Moch RW, Barsoum IS. Some observations on experimentally induced infection of dogs with Babesia gibsoni. Am J Vet Res. 1975 Mar;36(3):293-6. PMID:1115427

Bouillet LÉ, Dias MO, Dorigo NA, Moura AD, Russell B, Nosten F, Renia L, Braga EM, Gazzinelli RT, Rodrigues MM, Soares IS, Bruna-Romero O. Long-term humoral and cellular immune responses elicited by a heterologous Plasmodium vivax apical membrane antigen 1 protein prime/adenovirus boost immunization protocol. Infect Immun. 2011 Sep;79(9):3642-52. Epub 2011 Jul 5. PMID:21730090

Boulton IC, Nwaka S, Bathurst I, Lanzer M, Taramelli D, Vial H, Doerig C, Chibale K, Ward SA. CRIMALDDI: a co-ordinated, rational, and integrated effort to set logical on priorities in anti-malarial drug discovery initiatives. Malar J. 2010 Jul 13;9:202. PMID:20626844

Bourdoiseau G. Canine babesiosis in France. Vet Parasitol. 2006 May 31;138(1-2):118-25. Epub 2006 Feb 28. PMID:16507334

Bousema T, Drakeley C. Epidemiology and infectivity of Plasmodium falciparum and Plasmodium vivax gametocytes in relation to malaria control and elimination. Clin Microbiol Rev. 2011 Apr;24(2):377-410. PMID:21482730

Bousema T, Okell L, Shekalaghe S, Griffin JT, Omar S, Sawa P, Sutherland C, Sauerwein R, Ghani AC, Drakeley C. Revisiting the circulation time of Plasmodium falciparum gametocytes: molecular detection methods to estimate the duration of gametocyte carriage and the effect of gametocytocidal drugs. Malar J. 2010 May 24;9:136. PMID:20497536

Boustani MR, Lepore TJ, Gelfand JA, Lazarus DS. Acute respiratory failure in patients treated for babesiosis. Am J Respir Crit Care Med. 1994 Jun;149(6):1689-91. PMID:8004331

Bouwman H, van den Berg H, Kylin H. DDT and malaria prevention: addressing the paradox. Environ Health Perspect. 2011 Jun;119(6):744-7. Epub 2011 Jan 18. PMID:21245017

Bouyer G, Cueff A, Egée S, Kmiecik J, Maksimova Y, Glogowska E, Gallagher PG, Thomas SL. Erythrocyte peripheral type benzodiazepine receptor/voltage-dependent anion channels are upregulated by Plasmodium falciparum. Blood. 2011 Aug 25;118(8):2305-12. Epub 2011 Jul 27. PMID:21795748

Bown KJ, Lambin X, Telford GR, Ogden NH, Telfer S, Woldehiwet Z, Birtles RJ. Relative importance of Ixodes ricinus and Ixodes trianguliceps as vectors for Anaplasma phagocytophilum and Babesia microti in field vole (Microtus agrestis) populations. Appl Environ Microbiol. 2008 Dec;74(23):7118-25. Epub 2008 Sep 26. PMID:18820068

Boyom FF, Ngouana V, Kemgne EA, Zollo PH, Menut C, Bessiere JM, Gut J, Rosenthal PJ. Antiplasmodial volatile extracts from Cleistopholis patens Engler & Diels and Uvariastrum pierreanum Engl. (Engl. & Diels) (Annonaceae) growing in Cameroon. Parasitol Res. 2011 May;108(5):1211-7. Epub 2010 Nov 25. PMID:21107862

Boyom FF, Ngouana V, Zollo PH, Menut C, Bessiere JM, Gut J, Rosenthal PJ. Composition and anti-plasmodial activities of essential oils from some Cameroonian medicinal plants. Phytochemistry. 2003 Dec;64(7):1269-75. PMID:14599525

Boysen KE, Matuschewski K. Arrested oocyst maturation in Plasmodium parasites lacking type II NADH:ubiquinone dehydrogenase. J Biol Chem. 2011 Sep 16;286(37):32661-71. Epub 2011 Jul 19. PMID:21771793

Bradbury-Golas K, Washart C. A 56-year-old woman with fever, generalized body aches, and anemia after a tick bite. J Emerg Nurs. 2005 Apr;31(2):137-8. PMID:15856537

Braga W, Venasco J, Willard L, Moro MH. Ultrastructure of Babesia WA1 (Apicomplexa: Piroplasma) during infection of erythrocytes in a hamster model. J Parasitol. 2006 Oct;92(5):1104-7. PMID:17152960

Brasseur P, Badiane M, Cisse M, Agnamey P, Vaillant MT, Olliaro PL. Changing patterns of malaria during 1996-2010 in an area of moderate transmission in southern Senegal. Malar J. 2011 Jul 25;10:203. PMID:21787420

Brasseur P, Gorenflot A. Human babesial infections in Europe. Rocz Akad Med Bialymst. 1996;41(1):117-22. PMID:8673796

Brasseur P, Lecoublet S, Kapel N, Favennec L, Ballet JJ. Quinine in the treatment of Babesia divergens infections in humans. Eur J Clin Microbiol Infect Dis. 1996 Oct;15(10):840-1. PMID:8950568

Brasseur P. [Tolerance of amodiaquine].[Article in French]. Med Trop (Mars). 2007 Jun;67(3):288-90. PMID:17784684

Breitschwerdt EB, Maggi RG. A confusing case of canine vector-borne disease: clinical signs and progression in a dog co-infected with Ehrlichia canis and Bartonella vinsonii ssp. berkhoffii. Parasit Vectors. 2009 Mar 26;2 Suppl 1:S3. PMID:19426442

Brigden ML. Detection, education and management of the asplenic or hyposplenic patient. Am Fam Physician. 2001 Feb 1;63(3):499-506, 508. PMID:11272299

Brizuela CM, Ortellado CA, Sanabria E, Torres O, Ortigosa D. The safety and efficacy of Australian tick-borne disease vaccine strains in cattle in Paraguay. Vet Parasitol. 1998 Mar 31;76(1-2):27-41. PMID:9653988

Brocklesby DW, Harness E, Sellwood SA. The effect of age on the natural immunity of cattle to Babesia divergens. Res Vet Sci. 1971 Jan;12(1):15-7. PMID:4252543

Brocks DR, Mehvar R. Stereoselectivity in the pharmacodynamics and pharmacokinetics of the chiral antimalarial drugs. Clin Pharmacokinet. 2003;42(15):1359-82. PMID:14674788

Brodwall K. [Fewer malaria deaths in Zanzibar].[Article in Norwegian]. Tidsskr Nor Laegeforen. 2011 May 6;131(8):796. PMID:21710705

Brooker S, Okello G, Njagi K, Dubeck MM, Halliday KE, Inyega H, Jukes MC. Improving educational achievement and anaemia of school children: design of a cluster randomised trial of school-based malaria prevention and enhanced literacy instruction in Kenya. Trials. 2010 Oct 7;11:93. PMID:20929566

Brown A, Higgins MK. Carbohydrate binding molecules in malaria pathology. Curr Opin Struct Biol. 2010 Oct;20(5):560-6. Epub 2010 Jul 23. PMID:20655195

Brown A, Nitayaphan S. The Armed Forces Research Institute of Medical Sciences: five decades of collaborative medical research. Southeast Asian J Trop Med Public Health. 2011 May;42(3):477-90. PMID:21706925

Brown KN. Immunity to protozoal infections. Proc R Soc Med. 1969 Mar 3;62(3):301-2. PMID:4181289

Brown WC, McElwain TF, Hötzel I, Suarez CE, Palmer GH. Helper T-cell epitopes encoded by the Babesia bigemina rap-1 gene family in the constant and variant domains are conserved among parasite strains. Infect Immun. 1998 Apr;66(4):1561-9. PMID:9529082

Brown WC, Norimine J, Goff WL, Suarez CE, McElwain TF. Prospects for recombinant vaccines against Babesia bovis and related parasites. Parasite Immunol. 2006 Jul;28(7):315-27. PMID:16842268

Brown WC, Norimine J, Knowles DP, Goff WL. Immune control of Babesia bovis infection. Vet Parasitol. 2006 May 31;138(1-2):75-87. Epub 2006 Feb 28. PMID:16510249

Brown WC, Zhao S, Logan KS, Grab DJ, Rice-Ficht AC. Identification of candidate vaccine antigens of bovine hemoparasites Theileria parva and Babesia bovis by use of helper T cell clones. Vet Parasitol. 1995 Mar;57(1-3):189-203. PMID:7597783

Brown WC. Molecular approaches to elucidating innate and acquired immune responses to Babesia bovis, a protozoan parasite that causes persistent infection. Vet Parasitol. 2001 Nov 22;101(3-4):233-48. PMID:11707299

Bruce-Chwatt LJ. Transfusion associated parasitic infections. Prog Clin Biol Res. 1985;182:101-25. PMID:3929259

Bruce-Hickman D. Oxygen therapy for cerebral malaria. Travel Med Infect Dis. 2011 Sep;9(5):223-30. Epub 2011 Jul 31. PMID:21807563

Bruder JT, Angov E, Limbach KJ, Richie TL. Molecular vaccines for malaria. Hum Vaccin. 2010 Jan;6(1):54-77. Epub 2010 Jan 29. PMID:20061792

Bruder JT, Stefaniak ME, Patterson NB, Chen P, Konovalova S, Limbach K, Campo JJ, Ettyreddy D, Li S, Dubovsky F, Richie TL, King CR, Long CA, Doolan DL. Adenovectors induce functional antibodies capable of potent inhibition of blood stage malaria parasite growth. Vaccine. 2010 Apr 19;28(18):3201-10. Epub 2010 Feb 25. PMID:20188680

Brueckner RP, Coster T, Wesche DL, Shmuklarsky M, Schuster BG. Prophylaxis of Plasmodium falciparum infection in a human challenge model with WR 238605, a new 8-aminoquinoline antimalarial. Antimicrob Agents Chemother. 1998 May;42(5):1293-4. PMID:9593172

Brueckner RP, Fleckenstein L. Simultaneous modeling of the pharmacokinetics and methemoglobin pharmacodynamics of an 8-aminoquinoline candidate antimalarial (WR 238605). Pharm Res. 1991 Dec;8(12):1505-10. PMID:1808614

Brueckner RP, Lasseter KC, Lin ET, Schuster BG. First-time-in-humans safety and pharmacokinetics of WR 238605, a new antimalarial. Am J Trop Med Hyg. 1998 May;58(5):645-9. PMID:9598455

Brüning A. Equine piroplasmosis an update on diagnosis, treatment and prevention. Br Vet J. 1996 Mar;152(2):139-51. PMID:8680838

Brumlik MJ, Pandeswara S, Ludwig SM, Murthy K, Curiel TJ. Parasite mitogen-activated protein kinases as drug discovery targets to treat human protozoan pathogens. J Signal Transduct. 2011;2011:971968. Epub 2011 Feb 27. PMID:21637385

Bryceson AD, Fleming AF, Edington GM. Splenomegaly in Northern Nigeria. Acta Trop. 1976;33(3):185-214. PMID:11654

Bu Jassoum S, Fong IW, Hannach B, Kain KC. Transfusion-transmitted babesiosis in Ontario: first reported case in Canada. [Article in English, French]. Can Commun Dis Rep. 2000 Jan 15;26(2):9-13. PMID:10680253

Buckee CO, Gupta S. Modelling malaria population structure and its implications for control. Adv Exp Med Biol. 2010;673:112-26. PMID:20632533

Buckingham SC. Tick-borne infections in children: epidemiology, clinical manifestations, and optimal management strategies. Paediatr Drugs. 2005;7(3):163-76. PMID:15977962

Buelvas F, Alvis N, Buelvas I, Miranda J, Mattar S. [A high prevalence of antibodies against Bartonella and Babesia microti has been found in villages and urban populations in Cordoba, Colombia].[Article in Spanish]. Rev Salud Publica (Bogota). 2008 Jan-Feb;10(1):168-77. PMID:18368229

Buening GM, Kuttler KL, Rodriguez SD. Evaluation of a cloned Babesia bovis organism as a live immunogen. Vet Parasitol. 1986 Dec;22(3-4):235-42. PMID:3564326

Bugyei KA, Boye GL, Addy ME. Clinical efficacy of a tea-bag formulation of cryptolepis sanguinolenta root in the treatment of acute uncomplicated falciparum malaria. Ghana Med J. 2010 Mar;44(1):3-9. PMID:21326984

Bukhari T, Takken W, Githeko AK, Koenraadt CJ. Efficacy of aquatain, a monomolecular film, for the control of malaria vectors in rice paddies. PLoS One. 2011;6(6):e21713. Epub 2011 Jun 29. PMID:21738774

Bukhari T, Takken W, Koenraadt CJ. Development of Metarhizium anisopliae and Beauveria bassiana formulations for control of malaria mosquito larvae. Parasit Vectors. 2011 Feb 22;4:23. PMID:21342492

Bulterys PL, Chao A, Dalai SC, Zink MC, Dushimimana A, Katzenstein D, Saah AJ, Bulterys M. Placental malaria and mother-to-child transmission of human immunodeficiency virus-1 in rural Rwanda. Am J Trop Med Hyg. 2011 Aug;85(2):202-6. PMID:21813835

Bulusu V, Thakur SS, Venkatachala R, Balaram H. Mechanism of growth inhibition of intraerythrocytic stages of Plasmodium falciparum by 5-aminoimidazole-4-carboxamide ribonucleoside (AICAR). Mol Biochem Parasitol. 2011 May;177(1):1-11. Epub 2011 Jan 18. PMID:21251933

Buma AH, van Thiel P. Experiences with malaria chemoprophylaxis in Dutch troops. Med Trop (Mars). 2001;61(1):77-8. PMID:11584661

Bunin KV. [A brief essay on the development of chemotherapy of malaria and recurrent typhus in Russia].[Article in Russian]. Zh Mikrobiol Epidemiol Immunobiol. 1957 Feb;28(2):122-7. PMID:13423825

Burchard G. [Therapeutic management of malaria].[Article in German]. Internist (Berl). 2011 Nov 11. [Epub ahead of print]. PMID:22071912

Burgess RW, Young MD. The development of pyrimethamine resistance by Plasmodium falciparum. Bull World Health Organ. 1959;20(1):37-46. PMID:13638788

Burki T. From quinine to artesunate in Africa. Lancet Infect Dis. 2011 Jun;11(6):428-9. PMID:21770055

Burrows JN, Chibale K, Wells TN. The state of the art in anti-malarial drug discovery and development. Curr Top Med Chem. 2011;11(10):1226-54. PMID:21401508

Butler CM, Nijhof AM, van der Kolk JH, de Haseth OB, Taoufik A, Jongejan F, Houwers DJ. Repeated high dose imidocarb dipropionate treatment did not eliminate Babesia caballi from naturally infected horses as determined by PCR-reverse line blot hybridization. Vet Parasitol. 2008 Feb 14;151(2-4):320-2. Epub 2007 Nov 17. PMID:18160222

Butler CM, van Gils JA, van der Kolk JH. [A literature review of equine piroplasmosis after an episode of acute babesiosis in a Dutch Standardbred foal after a stay in Normandy].[Article in Dutch]. Tijdschr Diergeneeskd. 2005 Dec 1;130(23):726-31. PMID:16363205

Butler D. Mosquitoes score in chemical war. Nature. 2011 Jul 5;475(7354):19. PMID:21734682

Butler NS, Schmidt NW, Vaughan AM, Aly AS, Kappe SH, Harty JT. Superior antimalarial immunity after vaccination with late liver stage-arresting genetically attenuated parasites. Cell Host Microbe. 2011 Jun 16;9(6):451-62. PMID:21669394

Butler SE, Augostini P, Secor WE. Mycoplasma hominis infection of Trichomonas vaginalis is not associated with metronidazole-resistant trichomoniasis in clinical isolates from the United States. Parasitol Res. 2010 Sep;107(4):1023-7. Epub 2010 Jul 21. PMID:20652315

Butler T, Warren KS, Mahmoud AA. Algorithms in the diagnosis and management of exotic diseases. XIII. Malaria. J Infect Dis. 1976 Jun;133(6):721-6. PMID:932498

Button C. Fluid therapy in canine babesiosis. J S Afr Vet Assoc. 1976 Dec;47(4):284-7. PMID:1035270

Byrnes C, Terry Lee Y, Donahue RE, Miller JL. Identification of a cross-reacting, monoclonal anti-human CD233 antibody for identification and sorting of rhesus macaque erythrocytes. Cytometry A. 2011 Dec 13. [Epub ahead of print]. PMID:22170815

Byrnes V, Chopra S, Koziel MJ. Resolution of chronic hepatitis C following parasitosis. World J Gastroenterol. 2007 Aug 21;13(31):4268-9. PMID:17696260

Cable RG, Leiby DA. Risk and prevention of transfusion-transmitted babesiosis and other tick-borne diseases. Curr Opin Hematol. 2003 Nov;10(6):405-11. PMID:14564169

Cacciò S, Cammà C, Onuma M, Severini C. The beta-tubulin gene of Babesia and Theileria parasites is an informative marker for species discrimination. Int J Parasitol. 2000 Oct;30(11):1181-5. PMID:11027785

Cahill KM, Benach JL, Reich LM, Bilmes E, Zins JH, Siegel FP, Hochweis S. Red cell exchange: treatment of babesiosis in a splenectomized patient. Transfusion. 1981 Mar-Apr;21(2):193-8. PMID:7194528

Cahill KM. Babesiosis: unappreciated even in endemic areas. J Community Health. 1995 Aug;20(4):315-20. PMID:7593737

Cairns M, Gosling R, Carneiro I, Gesase S, Mosha JF, Hashim R, Kaur H, Lemnge M, Mosha FW, Greenwood B, Chandramohan D. Duration of protection against clinical malaria provided by three regimens of intermittent preventive treatment in Tanzanian infants. PLoS One. 2010 Mar 1;5(3):e9467. PMID:20209126

Callender DM, Hsue G. Artesunate: investigational drug for the treatment of severe falciparum malaria in Hawai'i. Hawaii Med J. 2011 Apr;70(4):77-9. PMID:21785506

Callow LL, Dalgliesh RJ, de Vos AJ. Development of effective living vaccines against bovine babesiosis--the longest field trial? Int J Parasitol. 1997 Jul;27(7):747-67. PMID:9279577

Callow LL, McGregor W. Vaccination against Babesia argentina infection in cattle during chemoprophylaxis with a quinuronium compound. Aust Vet J. 1969 Sep;45(9):408-10. PMID:5389523

Callow LL, Stewart NP. Immunosuppression by Babesia bovis against its tick vector, Boophilus microplus. Nature. 1978 Apr 27;272(5656):818-9. PMID:643072

Callow LL. Some aspects of the epidemiology and control of bovine babesiosis in Australia. J S Afr Vet Assoc. 1979 Dec;50(4):353-6. PMID:399977

Callow LL. Vaccination against bovine babesiosis. Adv Exp Med Biol. 1977;93:121-49. PMID:596295

Cambournac FJ. [The development of the eradication of malaria. A practical public health lesson].[Article in French]. An Esc Nacl Saude Publica Med Trop (Lisb). 1969 Jan-Dec;3(1):33-46. PMID:5404998

Campagna AM, Patnaik MM. Advances in global biotechnology and local resources to treat malaria. Minn Med. 2009 Feb;92(2):44-5. PMID:19331290

Campbell DD, Moran B. Sustaining the vision for Millennium Development Goal 6, to halt and reverse the spread of HIV/AIDS and other infections. J Obstet Gynecol Neonatal Nurs. 2010 Sep-Oct;39(5):600-5. Epub 2010 Jul 29. PMID:20673317

Campo JJ, Dobaño C, Sacarlal J, Guinovart C, Mayor A, Angov E, Dutta S, Chitnis C, Macete E, Aponte JJ, Alonso PL. Impact of the RTS,S malaria vaccine candidate on naturally acquired antibody responses to multiple asexual blood stage antigens. PLoS One. 2011;6(10):e25779. Epub 2011 Oct 12. PMID:22022448

Canfield CJ, Rozman RS. Clinical testing of new antimalarial compounds. Bull World Health Organ. 1974;50(3-4):203-12.PMID: 4613503

Cangelosi JJ, Sarvat B, Sarria JC, Herwaldt BL, Indrikovs AJ. Transmission of Babesia microti by blood transfusion in Texas. Vox Sang. 2008 Nov;95(4):331-4. PMID:19138264

Cantey PT, Roy S, Lee B, Cronquist A, Smith K, Liang J, Beach MJ. Study of nonoutbreak giardiasis: novel findings and implications for research. Am J Med. 2011 Dec;124(12):1175.e1-8. Epub 2011 Oct 18. PMID:22014792

Canto GJ, Figueroa JV, Ramos JA, Rojas EE, Garcia-Tapia D, Alvarez JA, Allred DR, Carson CA. Evaluation of cattle inoculated with Babesia bovis clones adhesive in vitro to bovine brain endothelial cells. Ann N Y Acad Sci. 2006 Oct;1081:397-404. PMID:17135543

Cantu A, Ortega JA, Garcia-Vazquez Z, Mosqueda J, Henke SE, George J. EPIDEMIOLOGY OF Babesia bovis AND Babesia bigemina IN FREE-RANGING WHITE-TAILED DEER IN NORTHEASTERN MEXICO. J Parasitol. 2008 Sep 16:1. [Epub ahead of print]. PMID:18795810

Cantu-C A, Ortega-S JA, García-Vázquez Z, Mosqueda J, Henke SE, George JE. Epizootiology of Babesia bovis and Babesia bigemina in free-ranging white-tailed deer in northeastern Mexico. J Parasitol. 2009 Jun;95(3):536-42. PMID:19642800

Capan M, Mombo-Ngoma G, Makristathis A, Ramharter M. Anti-bacterial activity of intermittent preventive treatment of malaria in pregnancy: comparative in vitro study of sulphadoxine-pyrimethamine, mefloquine, and azithromycin. Malar J. 2010 Oct 29;9:303. PMID:21029476

Capela R, Cabal GG, Rosenthal PJ, Gut J, Mota MM, Moreira R, Lopes F, Prudêncio M. Design and evaluation of primaquine-artemisinin hybrids as a multistage antimalarial strategy. Antimicrob Agents Chemother. 2011 Oct;55(10):4698-706. Epub 2011 Aug 1. PMID:21807973

Caprio V, Guyen B, Opoku-Boahen Y, Mann J, Gowan SM, Kelland LM, Read MA, Neidle S. A novel inhibitor of human telomerase derived from 10H-indolo[3,2-b]quinoline. Bioorg Med Chem Lett. 2000 Sep 18;10(18):2063-6. PMID:10999471

Carbrey EA, Avery RJ, Knowles RC, Sash SC. Chemotherapy of equine babesiosis. J Am Vet Med Assoc. 1971 Dec 1;159(11):1538-45. PMID:5005185

Carcy B, Précigout E, Schetters T, Gorenflot A. Genetic basis for GPI-anchor merozoite surface antigen polymorphism of Babesia and resulting antigenic diversity. Vet Parasitol. 2006 May 31;138(1-2):33-49. Epub 2006 Mar 23. PMID:16551492

Cardoso L, Tuna J, Vieira L, Yisaschar-Mekuzas Y, Baneth G. Molecular detection of Anaplasma platys and Ehrlichia canis in dogs from the North of Portugal. Vet J. 2010 Feb;183(2):232-3. Epub 2008 Dec 3. PMID:19056304

Carey JB, Pearson FE, Vrdoljak A, McGrath MG, Crean AM, Walsh PT, Doody T, O'Mahony C, Hill AV, Moore AC. Microneedle array design determines the induction of protective memory CD8+ T cell responses induced by a recombinant live malaria vaccine in mice. PLoS One. 2011;6(7):e22442. Epub 2011 Jul 25. PMID:21799855

Carlsson AM, Ngasala BE, Dahlstrom S, Membi C, Veiga IM, Rombo L, Abdullah S, Premji Z, Gil P, Bjorkman A, Martensson A. Plasmodium falciparum population dynamics during the early phase of anti-malarial drug treatment in Tanzanian children with acute uncomplicated malaria. Malar J. 2011 Dec 20;10(1):380. [Epub ahead of print]. PMID:22185672

Carlsson T, Bergqvist L, Hellgren U. Homeopathic Resistant Malaria. J Travel Med. 1996 Mar 1;3(1):62. PMID:9815426

Carlton JM, Sina BJ, Adams JH. Why is Plasmodium vivax a neglected tropical disease? PLoS Negl Trop Dis. 2011 Jun;5(6):e1160. Epub 2011 Jun 28. PMID:21738804

Carmichael M. Halting the world's most lethal parasite. Sci Am. 2010 Nov;303(5):68-75. PMID:21033287

Carrara VI, Zwang J, Ashley EA, Price RN, Stepniewska K, Barends M, Brockman A, Anderson T, McGready R, Phaiphun L, Proux S, van Vugt M, Hutagalung R, Lwin KM, Phyo AP, Preechapornkul P, Imwong M, Pukrittayakamee S, Singhasivanon P, White NJ, Nosten F. Changes in the treatment responses to artesunate-mefloquine on the northwestern border of Thailand during 13 years of continuous deployment. PLoS One. 2009;4(2):e4551. Epub 2009 Feb 23. PMID:19234601

Carter WJ, Yan Z, Cassai ND, Sidhu GS. Detection of extracellular forms of babesia in the blood by electron microscopy: a diagnostic method for differentiation from Plasmodium falciparum. Ultrastruct Pathol. 2003 Jul-Aug;27(4):211-6. PMID:12907365

Carvalho BO, Matsuda JS, Luz SL, Martinez-Espinosa FE, Leite JA, Franzin F, Orlandi PP, Gregoracci GB, Lacerda MV, Nogueira PA, Costa FT. Gestational malaria associated to Plasmodium vivax and Plasmodium falciparum placental mixed-infection followed by foetal loss: a case report from an unstable transmission area in Brazil. Malar J. 2011 Jun 27;10:178. PMID:21708032

Carvalho L, Luque-Ortega JR, Manzano JI, Castanys S, Rivas L, Gamarro F. Tafenoquine, an antiplasmodial 8-aminoquinoline, targets leishmania respiratory complex III and induces apoptosis. Antimicrob Agents Chemother. 2010 Dec;54(12):5344-51. Epub 2010 Sep 13. PMID:20837758

Cassera MB, Hazleton KZ, Merino EF, Obaldia N 3rd, Ho MC, Murkin AS, Depinto R, Gutierrez JA, Almo SC, Evans GB, Babu YS, Schramm VL. Plasmodium falciparum Parasites Are Killed by a Transition State Analogue of Purine Nucleoside Phosphorylase in a Primate Animal Model. PLoS One. 2011;6(11):e26916. Epub 2011 Nov 11. PMID:22096507

Castellini MA, Buguliskis JS, Casta LJ, Butz CE, Clark AB, Kunkel TA, Taraschi TF. Malaria drug resistance is associated with defective DNA mismatch repair. Mol Biochem Parasitol. 2011 Jun;177(2):143-7. Epub 2011 Feb 21. PMID:21315772

Cech PG, Aebi T, Abdallah MS, Mpina M, Machunda EB, Westerfeld N, Stoffel SA, Zurbriggen R, Pluschke G, Tanner M, Daubenberger C, Genton B, Abdulla S. Virosome-formulated Plasmodium falciparum AMA-1 & CSP derived peptides as malaria vaccine: randomized phase 1b trial in semi-immune adults & children. PLoS One. 2011;6(7):e22273. Epub 2011 Jul 22. PMID:21799810

Centeno-Lima S, do Rosário V, Parreira R, Maia AJ, Freudenthal AM, Nijhof AM, Jongejan F. A fatal case of human babesiosis in Portugal: molecular and phylogenetic analysis. Trop Med Int Health. 2003 Aug;8(8):760-4. PMID:12869099

Centers for Disease Control and Prevention (CDC). Ten great public health achievements--worldwide, 2001-2010. MMWR Morb Mortal Wkly Rep. 2011 Jun 24;60(24):814-8. PMID:21697806

Cessay SJ, Bojang KA, Nwakanma D, Conway DJ, Koita OA, Doumbia SO, Ndiaye D, Coulibaly TF, Diakité M, Traoré SF, Coulibaly M, Ndiaye JL, Sarr O, Gaye O, Konaté L, Sy N, Faye B, Faye O, Sogoba N, Jawara M, Dao A, Poudiougou B, Diawara S, Okebe J, Sangaré L, Abubakar I, Sissako A, Diarra A, Kéita M, Kandeh B, Long CA, Fairhurst RM, Duraisingh M, Perry R, Muskavitch MA, Valim C, Volkman SK, Wirth DF, Krogstad DJ. Sahel, savana, riverine and urban malaria in West Africa: Similar control policies with different outcomes. Acta Trop. 2011 Nov 19. [Epub ahead of print]. PMID:22119584

Chadwick J, Amewu RK, Marti F, Garah FB, Sharma R, Berry NG, Stocks PA, Burrell-Saward H, Wittlin S, Rottmann M, Brun R, Taramelli D, Parapini S, Ward SA, O'Neill PM. Antimalarial mannoxanes: hybrid antimalarial drugs with outstanding oral activity profiles and a potential dual mechanism of action. ChemMedChem. 2011 Aug 1;6(8):1357-61. Epub 2011 Jun 20. PMID:21692184

Chaijaroenkul W, Wisedpanichkij R, Na-Bangchang K. Monitoring of in vitro susceptibilities and molecular markers of resistance of Plasmodium falciparum isolates from Thai-Myanmar border to chloroquine, quinine, mefloquine and artesunate. Acta Trop. 2010 Feb;113(2):190-4. Epub 2009 Oct 30. PMID:19879850

Chalyĭ VF, Mirzoaliev IuIu, Daburov KN. [The specific features of the development of the malaria mosquitoes Anopheles superpictus (Grassi 1899) in Tajikistan].[Article in Russian]. Med Parazitol (Mosk). 2010 Jan-Mar;(1):30-3. PMID:20361634

Chambers JA. Military aviators, special operations forces, and causal malaria prophylaxis. Mil Med. 2003 Dec;168(12):1001-6. PMID:14719625

Chandler CI, Hall-Clifford R, Asaph T, Pascal M, Clarke S, Mbonye AK. Introducing malaria rapid diagnostic tests at registered drug shops in Uganda: limitations of diagnostic testing in the reality of diagnosis. Soc Sci Med. 2011 Mar;72(6):937-44. Epub 2011 Feb 3. PMID:21349623

Chansiri K, Sarataphan N. Molecular phylogenetic study of Theileria sp. (Thung Song) based on the thymidylate synthetase gene. Parasitol Res. 2002 May;88(13 Suppl 1):S33-5. PMID:12051604

Chapman WE, Ward PA. Babesia rodhaini: requirement of complement for penetration of human erythrocytes. Science. 1977 Apr 1;196(4285):67-70. PMID:841340

Chapman WE, Ward PA. The complement profile in babesiosis. J Immunol. 1976 Sep;117(3):935-8. PMID:956661

Chapman WL Jr, Hanson W. Plasmodium berghei infection in neonatallythymectomized hamsters. J Parasitol. 1971 Feb;57(1):24-8. PMID:4101132

Charles BG, Miller AK, Nasveld PE, Reid MG, Harris IE, Edstein MD. Population pharmacokinetics of tafenoquine during malaria prophylaxis in healthy subjects. Antimicrob Agents Chemother. 2007 Aug;51(8):2709-15. Epub 2007 May 21. PMID:17517850

Charman SA, Arbe-Barnes S, Bathurst IC, Brun R, Campbell M, Charman WN, Chiu FC, Chollet J, Craft JC, Creek DJ, Dong Y, Matile H, Maurer M, Morizzi J, Nguyen T, Papastogiannidis P, Scheurer C, Shackleford DM, Sriraghavan K, Stingelin L, Tang Y, Urwyler H, Wang X, White KL, Wittlin S, Zhou L, Vennerstrom JL. Synthetic ozonide drug candidate OZ439 offers new hope for a single-dose cure of uncomplicated malaria. Proc Natl Acad Sci U S A. 2011 Mar 15;108(11):4400-5. Epub 2011 Feb 7. PMID:21300861

Chatel G, Gulletta M, Matteelli A, Marangoni A, Signorini L, Oladeji O, Caligaris S. Short report: Diagnosis of tick-borne relapsing fever by the quantitative buffy coat fluorescence method. Am J Trop Med Hyg. 1999 May;60(5):738-9. PMID:10344644

Chattopadhyay R, Majam VF, Kumar S. Survival of Plasmodium falciparum in human blood during refrigeration. Transfusion. 2011 Mar;51(3):630-5. Epub 2010 Sep 16. PMID:20849405

Chattopadhyay R, Velmurugan S, Chakiath C, Andrews Donkor L, Milhous W, Barnwell JW, Collins WE, Hoffman SL. Establishment of an in vitro assay for assessing the effects of drugs on the liver stages of Plasmodium vivax malaria. PLoS One. 2010 Dec 9;5(12):e14275. PMID:21151554

Chaudhary SC, Sonkar SK, Kumar V, Gupta A. Falciparum malaria presenting as subdural hematoma. J Assoc Physicians India. 2011 May;59:325-6. PMID:21751613

Chaudhuri S, Varshney JP. Clinical management of babesiosis in dogs with homeopathic Crotalus horridus 200C. Homeopathy. 2007 Apr;96(2):90-4. PMID:17437935

Chaykovsky M, Rosowsky A, Papathanasopoulos N, Chen KK, Modest EJ, Kisliuk RL, Gaumont Y. Methotrexate analogs. 3. Synthesis and biological properties of some side-chain altered analogs. J Med Chem. 1974 Nov;17(11):1212-6. PMID:4213249

Chebbi Mahjoub R, Khemiss M, Dhidah M, Dellaï A, Bouraoui A, Khemiss F. Chloroformic and Methanolic Extracts of Olea europaea L. Leaves Present Anti-Inflammatory and Analgesic Activities. ISRN Pharmacol. 2011;2011:564972. Epub 2011 May 26. PMID:22084717

Cheema B, Molyneux EM, Emmanuel JC, M'baya B, Esan M, Kamwendo H, Kalilani-Phiri L, Boele van Hensbroek M. Development and evaluation of a new paediatric blood transfusion protocol for Africa. Transfus Med. 2010 Jun;20(3):140-51. Epub 2010 Feb 23. PMID:20210924

Chema S, Chumo RS, Dolan TT, Gathuma JM, Irvin AD, James AD, Young AS. Clinical trial of halofuginone lactate for the treatment of East Coast fever in Kenya. Vet Rec. 1987 Jun 13;120(24):575-7. PMID:3303642

Chen LH, Keystone JS. New strategies for the prevention of malaria in travelers. Infect Dis Clin North Am. 2005 Mar;19(1):185-210. PMID:15701554

Chen X, Orser BA, MacDonald JF. Design and screening of ASIC inhibitors based on aromatic diamidines for combating neurological disorders. Eur J Pharmacol. 2010 Dec 1;648(1-3):15-23. Epub 2010 Sep 18. PMID:20854810

Chen Y, Li S, Sun F, Han H, Zhang X, Fan Y, Tai G, Zhou Y. In vivo antimalarial activities of glycoalkaloids isolated from Solanaceae plants. Pharm Biol. 2010 Sep;48(9):1018-24. PMID:20731554

Chêne A, Nylén S, Donati D, Bejarano MT, Kironde F, Wahlgren M, Falk KI. Effect of acute Plasmodium falciparum malaria on reactivation and shedding of the eight human herpes viruses. PLoS One. 2011;6(10):e26266. Epub 2011 Oct 24. PMID:22039454

Cheng C, Ho WE, Goh FY, Guan SP, Kong LR, Lai WQ, Leung BP, Wong WS. Anti-malarial drug artesunate attenuates experimental allergic asthma via inhibition of the phosphoinositide 3-kinase/Akt pathway. PLoS One. 2011;6(6):e20932. Epub 2011 Jun 9. PMID:21695271

Cheun HI, Cho SH, Lee HI, Shin EH, Lee JS, Kim TS, Lee WJ. Seasonal prevalence of mosquitoes, including vectors of Brugian filariasis, in southern islands of the Republic of Korea. Korean J Parasitol. 2011 Mar;49(1):59-64. Epub 2011 Mar 18. PMID:21461270

Chevalley S, Coste A, Lopez A, Pipy B, Valentin A. Flow cytometry for the evaluation of anti-plasmodial activity of drugs on Plasmodium falciparum gametocytes. Malar J. 2010 Feb 11;9:49. PMID:20149239

Chiang E, Haller N. Babesiosis: an emerging infectious disease that can affect those who travel to the northeastern United States. Travel Med Infect Dis. 2011 Sep;9(5):238-42. Epub 2011 Sep 8. PMID:21862413

Chico RM, Chandramohan D. Azithromycin plus chloroquine: combination therapy for protection against malaria and sexually transmitted infections in pregnancy. Expert Opin Drug Metab Toxicol. 2011 Sep;7(9):1153-67. Epub 2011 Jul 7. PMID:21736423

Chothani DL, Vaghasiya HU. A review on Balanites aegyptiaca Del (desert date): phytochemical constituents, traditional uses, and pharmacological activity. Pharmacogn Rev. 2011 Jan;5(9):55-62. PMID:22096319

Chotivanich K, Sattabongkot J, Choi YK, Park JS, Sritabal J, Lim CS, Udomsangpetch R, White NJ, Lee WJ. Antimalarial drug susceptibility of Plasmodium vivax in the Republic of Korea. Am J Trop Med Hyg. 2009 Jun;80(6):902-4. PMID:19478246

Chou S, Marousek G, Auerochs S, Stamminger T, Milbradt J, Marschall M. The unique antiviral activity of artesunate is broadly effective against human cytomegaloviruses including therapy-resistant mutants. Antiviral Res. 2011 Nov;92(2):364-8. Epub 2011 Aug 6. PMID:21843554

Christensen NO, Furu P, Kurtzhals J, Odaibo A. Heterologous synergistic interactions in concurrent experimental infection in the mouse with Schistosoma mansoni, Echinostoma revolutum, Plasmodium yoelii, Babesia microti, and Trypanosoma brucei. Parasitol Res. 1988;74(6):544-51. PMID:3143108

Christensson DA, Morén T. Seroresponse (IgG) after vaccination and natural infection of cattle with Babesia divergens. Acta Vet Scand. 1987;28(3-4):393-402. PMID:3454550

Chrubasik C, Jacobson RL. The development of artemisinin resistance in malaria: reasons and solutions. Phytother Res. 2010 Jul;24(7):1104-6. PMID:20578122

Chung HC, Wang JT, Sun HY, Wang JL, Lo YC, Sheng WH, Hsieh SM, Fang CT, Hsueh PR, Chen YC, Chang SC. Clinical experience of 17 cases of imported malaria at a Taiwan university hospital, 1999-2005. J Microbiol Immunol Infect. 2007 Jun;40(3):209-15. PMID:17639160

Churcher TS, Dawes EJ, Sinden RE, Christophides GK, Koella JC, Basáñez MG. Population biology of malaria within the mosquito: density-dependent processes and potential implications for transmission-blocking interventions. Malar J. 2010 Nov 4;9:311. PMID:21050427

Cichocka A, Skotarczak B. [Babesosis--difficulty of diagnosis].[Article in Polish]. Wiad Parazytol. 2001;47(3):527-33. PMID:16894770

Cimanga K, De Bruyne T, Lasure A, Van Poel B, Pieters L, Claeys M, Berghe DV, Kambu K, Tona L, Vlietinck AJ. In vitro biological activities of alkaloids from Cryptolepis sanguinolenta. Planta Med. 1996 Feb;62(1):22-7. PMID:8720383

Cimanga K, De Bruyne T, Pieters L, Vlietinck AJ, Turger CA. In vitro and in vivo antiplasmodial activity of cryptolepine and related alkaloids from Cryptolepis sanguinolenta. J Nat Prod. 1997 Jul;60(7):688-91. PMID:9249972

Clark DL, Chrisey LA, Campbell JR, Davidson EA. Non-sequence-specific antimalarial activity of oligodeoxynucleotides. Mol Biochem Parasitol. 1994 Jan;63(1):129-34. PMID:8183311

Clark IA, Allison AC, Cox FE. Protection of mice against Babesia and Plasmodium with BCG. Nature. 1976 Jan 29;259(5541):309-11. PMID:765838

Clark IA, Budd AC, Hsue G, Haymore BR, Joyce AJ, Thorner R, Krause PJ. Absence of erythrocyte sequestration in a case of babesiosis in a splenectomized human patient. Malar J. 2006 Aug 4;5:69. PMID:16887045

Clark IA, Cox FE, Allison AC. Protection of mice against Babesia spp. and Plasmodium spp. with killed Corynebacterium parvum. Parasitology. 1977 Feb;74(1):9-18. PMID:320544

Clark IA. Resistance to Babesia spp. and Plasmodium sp. in mice pretreated with an extract of Coxiella burnetii. Infect Immun. 1979 May;24(2):319-25. PMID:378850

Clark RL. Effects of artemisinins on reticulocyte count and relationship to possible embryotoxicity in confirmed and unconfirmed malarial patients. Birth Defects Res A Clin Mol Teratol. 2011 Nov 28. [Epub ahead of print]. PMID:22125126

Cliff J, Lewin S, Woelk G, Fernandes B, Mariano A, Sevene E, Daniels K, Matinhure S, Oxman A, Lavis J. Policy development in malaria vector management in Mozambique, South Africa and Zimbabwe. Health Policy Plan. 2010 Sep;25(5):372-83. Epub 2010 Feb 21. PMID:20176574

Clyde DF, McCarthy VC, Rebert CC, Miller RM. Prophylactic activity of a phenanthrene methanol (WR 33063) and a quinoline methanol (WR 30090) in human malaria. Antimicrob Agents Chemother. 1973 Feb;3(2):220-3. PMID:4597716

Clyde DF, Shute GT, McCarthy VC, Sangalang RP. Characterization of a drug resistant strain of Plasmodium falciparum from the Philippines. J Trop Med Hyg. 1971 May;74(5):101-5. PMID:4931686

Clyde DF. The problem of drug-resistant malaria. Am J Trop Med Hyg. 1972 Sep;21(5):736-43. PMID:4561521

Cockburn IA, Chen YC, Overstreet MG, Lees JR, van Rooijen N, Farber DL, Zavala F. Prolonged antigen presentation is required for optimal CD8+ T cell responses against malaria liver stage parasites. PLoS Pathog. 2010 May 6;6(5):e1000877. PMID:20463809

Cocquyt K, Cos P, Herdewijn P, Maes L, Van den Steen PE, Laekeman G. Ajuga remota Benth.: from ethnopharmacology to phytomedical perspective in the treatment of malaria. Phytomedicine. 2011 Nov 15;18(14):1229-37. Epub 2011 Oct 19. PMID:22015320

Codd A, Teuscher F, Kyle DE, Cheng Q, Gatton ML. Artemisinin-induced parasite dormancy: a plausible mechanism for treatment failure. Malar J. 2011 Mar 8;10:56. PMID:21385409

Cohen J, Benns S, Vekemans J, Leach A. [The malaria vaccine candidate RTS,S/AS is in phase III clinical trials].[Article in French]. Ann Pharm Fr. 2010 Nov;68(6):370-9. Epub 2010 Oct 13. PMID:21073995

Cohen S, Butcher GA. Serum antibody in acquired malarial immunity. Trans R Soc Trop Med Hyg. 1971;65(2):125-35. PMID:4934028

Coleman RE, Clavin AM, Milhous WK. Gametocytocidal and sporontocidal activity of antimalarials against Plasmodium berghei ANKA in ICR Mice and Anopheles stephensi mosquitoes. Am J Trop Med Hyg. 1992 Feb;46(2):169-82. PMID:1539752

Coleman RE. Sporontocidal activity of the antimalarial WR-238605 against Plasmodium berghei ANKA in Anopheles stephensi. Am J Trop Med Hyg. 1990 Mar;42(3):196-205. PMID:2180334

Collett MG. Survey of canine babesiosis in South Africa. J S Afr Vet Assoc. 2000 Sep;71(3):180-6. PMID:11205168

Collins WE, Contacos PG, Garnham PC, Warren M, Skinner JC. Plasmodium hylobati: a malaria parasite of the gibbon. J Parasitol. 1972 Feb;58(1):123-8. PMID:4335047

Collins WE, Contacos PG, Skinner JC, Chin W, Guinn E. Fluorescent antibody studies on simian malaria. I. Development of antibodies to Plasmodium knowlesi. Am J Trop Med Hyg. 1967 Jan;16(1):1-6. PMID:4960484

Collins WE, Contacos PG. Immunization of monkeys against Plasmodium cynomolgi by X-irradiated sporozoites. Nat New Biol. 1972 Apr 12;236(67):176-7. PMID:4624244

Collins WE, Jeffrey GM, Skinner JC. Fluorescent Antibody Studies In Human Malaria. II. Development And Persistence Of Antibodies To Plasmodium Falciparum. Am J Trop Med Hyg. 1964 Mar;13:256-60. PMID:14125876

Collins WE, Skinner JC, Contacos PG, Guinn EG. Fluorescent-antibody studies on simian malaria. II. Development of antibodies to Plasmodium cynomolgi. Am J Trop Med Hyg. 1967 May;16(3):267-72. PMID:4960704

Colly LP, Nesbit JW. Fatal acute babesiosis in a juvenile wild dog (Lycaon pictus). J S Afr Vet Assoc. 1992 Mar;63(1):36-8. PMID:1569540

Combrink MP, Troskie PC, Du Plessis F, Latif AA. Serological responses to Babesia bovis vaccination in cattle previously infected with Babesia bigemina. Vet Parasitol. 2010 May 28;170(1-2):30-6. Epub 2010 Feb 18. PMID:20207488

Combrink MP, Troskie PC. Effect of diminazene block treatment on live redwater vaccine reactions. Onderstepoort J Vet Res. 2004 Jun;71(2):113-7. PMID:15373333

Commins MA, Goodger BV, Wright IG. Proteinases in the lysate of bovine erythrocytes infected with Babesia bovis: initial vaccination studies. Int J Parasitol. 1985 Oct;15(5):491-5. PMID:3905658

Congpuong K, Bualombai P, Banmairuroi V, Na-Bangchang K. Compliance with a three-day course of artesunate-mefloquine combination and baseline anti-malarial treatment in an area of Thailand with highly multidrug resistant falciparum malaria. Malar J. 2010 Feb 4;9:43. PMID:20132537

Conly GN. The impact of malaria on economic development. A case study. Am J Trop Med Hyg. 1972 Sep;21(5):668-74. PMID:5074689

Conrad PA, Kjemtrup AM, Carreno RA, Thomford J, Wainwright K, Eberhard M, Quick R, Telford SR 3rd, Herwaldt BL. Description of Babesia duncani n.sp. (Apicomplexa: Babesiidae) from humans and its differentiation from other piroplasms. Int J Parasitol. 2006 Jun;36(7):779-89. Epub 2006 May 4. PMID:16725142

Cooke BM, Mohandas N, Coppel RL. The malaria-infected red blood cell: structural and functional changes. Adv Parasitol. 2001;50:1-86. PMID:11757330

Cooper PE, Watson PM. Discontinuation of redwater treatments. Vet Rec. 1989 Jun 17;124(24):643. PMID:2773215

Cooper RD, Milhous WK, Rieckmann KH. The efficacy of WR238605 against the blood stages of a chloroquine resistant strain of Plasmodium vivax. Trans R Soc Trop Med Hyg. 1994 Nov-Dec;88(6):691-2. PMID:7886774

Corash L. Inactivation of infectious pathogens in labile blood components: meeting the challenge. Transfus Clin Biol. 2001 Jun;8(3):138-45. PMID:11499954

Corash L. Inactivation of viruses, bacteria, protozoa and leukocytes in platelet and red cell concentrates. Vox Sang. 2000;78 Suppl 2:205-10. PMID: 10938954

Corash L. Inactivation of viruses, bacteria, protozoa, and leukocytes in platelet concentrates. Vox Sang. 1998;74 Suppl 2:173-6. PMID:9704443

Corash L. New technologies for the inactivation of infectious pathogens in cellular blood components and the development of platelet substitutes. Baillieres Best Pract Res Clin Haematol. 2000 Dec;13(4):549-63. PMID:11102276

Corbett KD, Berger JM. Structure of the ATP-binding domain of Plasmodium falciparum Hsp90. Proteins. 2010 Oct;78(13):2738-44. PMID:20635416

Corpelet C, Vacher P, Coudore F, Laurichesse H, Conort N, Souweine B. Role of quinine in life-threatening Babesia divergens infection successfully treated with clindamycin. Eur J Clin Microbiol Infect Dis. 2005 Jan;24(1):74-5. PMID:15616840

Corradetti A. Some remarks on the use of avian malaria parasites in research. Ann Parasitol Hum Comp. 1973 Mar-Apr;48(2):217-9. PMID:4785849

Corrier DE, Vizcaino O, Terry M, Betancourt A, Kuttler KL, Carson CA, Trevino G, Ristic M. Mortality, weight loss and anaemia in Bos taurus calves exposed to Boophilus microplus ticks in the tropics of Colombia. Trop Anim Health Prod. 1979 Nov;11(4):215-21. PMID:552671

Corrier DE, Wagner GG, Kuttler KL. Viability and virulence of Babesia rodhaini eight years after cryogenic preservation with dimethyl sulfoxide. Vet Parasitol. 1985 Jun;18(1):71-3. PMID:4049729

Corrier DE, Wagner GG. Comparison of the effect of T-2 toxin with that of dexamethasone or cyclophosphamide on resistance to Babesia microti infection in mice. Am J Vet Res. 1988 Nov;49(11):2000-3. PMID:3247926

Costa-Júnior LM, Rabelo EM, Martins Filho OA, Ribeiro MF. Comparison of different direct diagnostic methods to identify Babesia bovis and Babesia bigemina in animals vaccinated with live attenuated parasites. Vet Parasitol. 2006 Jun 30;139(1-3):231-6. Epub 2006 Mar 31. PMID:16580136

Cottrell BJ, Playfair JH, de Sousa B. Plasmodium yoelii and Plasmodium vinckei: the effects of nonspecific immunostimulation on murine malaria. Exp Parasitol. 1977 Oct;43(1):45-53. PMID:330190

Covell G. A brief review of the history and development of the more important antimalarial drugs. Indian J Malariol. 1947 Jun;1(2):231-41. PMID:18901444

Cox FE. Heterologous immunity between piroplasms and malaria parasites: the simultaneous elimination of Plasmodium vinckei and Babesia microti from the blood of doubly infected mice. Parasitology. 1978 Feb;76(1):55-60. PMID:622306

Cox HW, Saleh SM. Anemia and thrombocytopenia from Corynebacterium parvum-stimulated resistance against malaria, trypanosomiasis, and babesiosis. J Parasitol. 1983 Aug;69(4):654-9. PMID:6355427

Cramer JP, López-Vélez R, Burchard GD, Grobusch MP, de Vries PJ. Treatment of imported severe malaria with artesunate instead of quinine—more evidence needed? Malar J. 2011 Sep 7;10:256. PMID:21899729

Cranwell MP. Efficacy of long-acting oxytetracycline for the prevention of tick-borne fever in calves. Vet Rec. 1990 Apr 7;126(14):334-6. PMID:2339491

Criado-Fornelio A, Martinez-Marcos A, Buling-Saraña A, Barba-Carretero JC. Presence of Mycoplasma haemofelis, Mycoplasma haemominutum and piroplasmids in cats from southern Europe: a molecular study. Vet Microbiol. 2003 Jun 10;93(4):307-17. PMID:12713893

Criado-Fornelio A. A review of nucleic-acid-based diagnostic tests for Babesia and Theileria, with emphasis on bovine piroplasms. Parassitologia. 2007 May;49 Suppl 1:39-44. PMID:17691606

Crockett M, Kain KC. Tafenoquine: a promising new antimalarial agent. Expert Opin Investig Drugs. 2007 May;16(5):705-15. PMID:17461742

Crompton PD, Pierce SK, Miller LH. Advances and challenges in malaria vaccine development. J Clin Invest. 2010 Dec 1;120(12):4168-78. Epub 2010 Dec 1. PMID:21123952

Cui X, Wang Y, Kokudo N, Fang D, Tang W. Traditional Chinese medicine and related active compounds against hepatitis B virus infection. Biosci Trends. 2010 Apr;4(2):39-47. PMID:20448340

Cunha BA, Cohen YZ, McDermott B. Fever of unknown origin (FUO) due to babesiosis in a immunocompetent host. Heart Lung. 2008 Nov-Dec;37(6):481-4. Epub 2008 Sep 30. PMID:18992633

Cunha BA, Nausheen S, Szalda D. Pulmonary complications of babesiosis: case report and literature review. Eur J Clin Microbiol Infect Dis. 2007 Jul;26(7):505-8. PMID:17558489

Cunnington AJ, de Souza JB, Walther M, Riley EM. Malaria impairs resistance to Salmonella through heme- and heme oxygenase-dependent dysfunctional granulocyte mobilization. Nat Med. 2011 Dec 18. [Epub ahead of print]. PMID:22179318

Curley JM, Mody RM, Gasser RA Jr. Malaria caused by Plasmodium vivax complicated by acalculous cholecystitis. Am J Trop Med Hyg. 2011 Jul;85(1):42-9. PMID:21734122

Czajkowsky DM, Salanti A, Ditlev SB, Shao Z, Ghumra A, Rowe JA, Pleass RJ. IgM, Fc mu Rs, and malarial immune evasion. J Immunol. 2010 May 1;184(9):4597-603. PMID:20410497

da Silva RA, Corrêa Fdo N, Botteon Rde C, Botteon Pde T. [Natural infection by hemoparasites in calves submitted to chemoprophylaxis at 30 days of age].[Article in Portuguese]. Rev Bras Parasitol Vet. 2007 Jul-Sep;16(3):163-5. PMID:18078605

D'Acquarica I, Gasparrini F, Kotoni D, Pierini M, Villani C, Cabri W, Di Mattia M, Giorgi F. Stereodynamic investigation of labile stereogenic centres in dihydroartemisinin. Molecules. 2010 Mar 5;15(3):1309-23. PMID:20335983

D'Acremont V, Greub G, Genton B. [Rapid diagnostic tests (RDT): the cure-all for the practitioner?].[Article in French]. Rev Med Suisse. 2011 May 11;7(294):984-6, 988-90. PMID:21692310

Dahlbäck M, Nielsen MA, Salanti A. Can any lessons be learned from the ambiguous glycan binding of PfEMP1 domains? Trends Parasitol. 2010 May;26(5):230-5. Epub 2010 Feb 26. PMID:20189879

Dahlström S, Ferreira PE, Veiga MI, Sedighi N, Wiklund L, Mårtensson A, Färnert A, Sisowath C, Osório L, Darban H, Andersson B, Kaneko A, Conseil G, Björkman A, Gil JP. Plasmodium falciparum multidrug resistance protein 1 and artemisinin-based combination therapy in Africa. J Infect Dis. 2009 Nov 1;200(9):1456-64. PMID:19807279

Dai M, Reznik SE, Spray DC, Weiss LM, Tanowitz HB, Gulinello M, Desruisseaux MS. Persistent cognitive and motor deficits after successful antimalarial treatment in murine cerebral malaria. Microbes Infect. 2010 Dec;12(14-15):1198-207. Epub 2010 Aug 26. PMID:20800692

Dalgliesh RJ, Callow LL, Mellors LT, McGregor W. Development of a highly infective Babesia bigemina vaccine of reduced virulence. Aust Vet J. 1981 Jan;57(1):8-11. PMID:7236153

Dalgliesh RJ, Jorgensen WK, de Vos AJ. Australian frozen vaccines for the control of babesiosis and anaplasmosis in cattle--a review. Trop Anim Health Prod. 1990 Feb;22(1):44-52. PMID:2181745

Dalgliesh RJ, Mellors LT. Survival of the parasitic protozoan, Babesia bigemina, in blood cooled at widely different rates to -196 degrees C. Int J Parasitol. 1974 Apr;4(2):169-72. PMID:4822484

Dalgliesh RJ. Dimethyl sulphoxide in the low-temperature preservation of Babesia bigemina. Res Vet Sci. 1971 Sep;12(5):469-71. PMID:4999644

Dalgliesh RJ. Effects of low temperature preservation and route of inoculation on infectivity of Babesia bigemina in blood diluted with glycerol. Res Vet Sci. 1972 Nov;13(6):540-5. PMID:4630813

Dalgliesh RJ. Field observations on Babesia argentina vaccination in Queensland. Aust Vet J. 1968 Mar;44(3):103-4. PMID:5689432

Danner R, Chaudhari SN, Rosenberger J, Surls J, Richie TL, Brumeanu TD, Casares S. Expression of HLA class II molecules in humanized NOD.Rag1KO.IL2RgcKO mice is critical for development and function of human T and B cells. PLoS One. 2011;6(5):e19826. Epub 2011 May 17. PMID:21611197

Dantas-Torres F, Figueredo LA. Canine babesiosis: a Brazilian perspective. Vet Parasitol. 2006 Nov 5;141(3-4):197-203. Epub 2006 Sep 8. PMID:16962707

Dantas-Torres F. The brown dog tick, Rhipicephalus sanguineus (Latreille, 1806) (Acari: Ixodidae): from taxonomy to control. Vet Parasitol. 2008 Apr 15;152(3-4):173-85. Epub 2008 Jan 3. PMID:18280045

Dantrakool A, Somboon P, Hashimoto T, Saito-Ito A. Identification of a new type of Babesia species in wild rats (Bandicota indica) in Chiang Mai Province, Thailand. J Clin Microbiol. 2004 Feb;42(2):850-4. PMID:14766871

Dao AH. Human babesiosis. Compr Ther. 1996 Nov;22(11):713-8. PMID:8978977

DaRe JT, Kouri DP, Zimmerman PA, Thomas PJ. Differentiating Plasmodium falciparum alleles by transforming Cartesian X,Y data to polar coordinates. BMC Genet. 2010 Jun 29;11:57. PMID:20587031

Das A, Ravindran TS. Factors affecting treatment-seeking for febrile illness in a malaria endemic block in Boudh district, Orissa, India: policy implications for malaria control. Malar J. 2010 Dec 30;9:377. PMID:21192825

Das Gupta RK, Thakor HG, Sonal GS, Dhillon GP. New perspectives of malaria control in India under World Bank Project. J Indian Med Assoc. 2009 Dec;107(12):870, 879-80, 882-3. PMID:20509472

Das MK, Lumb V, Mittra P, Singh SS, Dash AP, Sharma YD. High chloroquine treatment failure rates and predominance of mutant genotypes associated with chloroquine and antifolate resistance among falciparum malaria patients from the island of Car Nicobar, India. J Antimicrob Chemother. 2010 Jun;65(6):1258-61. Epub 2010 Apr 2. PMID:20363804

Dassonneville L, Bonjean K, De Pauw-Gillet MC, Colson P, Houssier C, Quetin-Leclercq J, Angenot L, Bailly C. Stimulation of topoisomerase II-mediated DNA cleavage by three DNA-intercalating plant alkaloids: cryptolepine, matadine, and serpentine. Biochemistry. 1999 Jun 15;38(24):7719-26. PMID:10387011

Dassonneville L, Lansiaux A, Wattelet A, Wattez N, Mahieu C, Van Miert S, Pieters L, Bailly C. Cytotoxicity and cell cycle effects of the plant alkaloids cryptolepine and neocryptolepine: relation to drug-induced apoptosis. Eur J Pharmacol. 2000 Dec 1;409(1):9-18. PMID:11099695

Dattani JJ, Rajput DK, Moid N, Highland HN, George LB, Desai KR. Ameliorative effect of curcumin on hepatotoxicity induced by chloroquine phosphate. Environ Toxicol Pharmacol. 2010 Sep;30(2):103-9. Epub 2010 May 20. PMID:21787638

Dauvillée D, Delhaye S, Gruyer S, Slomianny C, Moretz SE, d'Hulst C, Long CA, Ball SG, Tomavo S. Engineering the chloroplast targeted malarial vaccine antigens in Chlamydomonas starch granules. PLoS One. 2010 Dec 15;5(12):e15424. PMID:21179538

Davidson RN, Wall RA. Prevention and management of infections in patients without a spleen. Clin Microbiol Infect. 2001 Dec;7(12):657-60. PMID:11843905

Davis SP, Amrein M, Gillrie MR, Lee K, Muruve DA, Ho M. Plasmodium falciparum-induced CD36 clustering rapidly strengthens cytoadherence via p130CAS-mediated actin cytoskeletal rearrangement. FASEB J. 2011 Nov 21. [Epub ahead of print]. PMID:22106368

Dawson PA, Cochran DA, Emmerson BT, Gordon RB. Inhibition of Plasmodium falciparum hypoxanthine-guanine phosphoribosyltransferase mRNA by antisense oligodeoxynucleotide sequence. Mol Biochem Parasitol. 1993 Jul;60(1):153-6. PMID:8366890

de Almeida RR, Souto RN, Bastos CN, da Silva MH, Maia JG. Chemical variation in Piper aduncum and biological properties of its dillapiole-rich essential oil. Chem Biodivers. 2009 Sep;6(9):1427-34. PMID:19774604

de Caprariis D, Dantas-Torres F, Capelli G, Mencke N, Stanneck D, Breitschwerdt EB, Otranto D. Evolution of clinical, haematological and biochemical findings in young dogs naturally infected by vector-borne pathogens. Vet Microbiol. 2011 Apr 21;149(1-2):206-12. Epub 2010 Oct 16. PMID:21106311

de Cassan SC, Forbes EK, Douglas AD, Milicic A, Singh B, Gupta P, Chauhan VS, Chitnis CE, Gilbert SC, Hill AV, Draper SJ. The requirement for potent adjuvants to enhance the immunogenicity and protective efficacy of protein vaccines can be overcome by prior immunization with a recombinant adenovirus. J Immunol. 2011 Sep 1;187(5):2602-16. Epub 2011 Aug 3. PMID:21813775

de Jong YP, Rice CM, Ploss A. New horizons for studying human hepatotropic infections. J Clin Invest. 2010 Mar 1;120(3):650-3. Epub 2010 Feb 22. PMID:20179350

de la Fuente J, Rodríguez M, Montero C, Redondo M, García-García JC, Méndez L, Serrano E, Valdés M, Enríquez A, Canales M, Ramos E, Boué O, Machado H, Lleonart R. Vaccination against ticks (Boophilus spp.): the experience with the Bm86-based vaccine Gavac. Genet Anal. 1999 Nov;15(3-5):143-8. PMID:10596754 de la Fuente J, Rodríguez M, Redondo M, Montero C, García-García JC, Méndez L, Serrano E, Valdés M, Enriquez A, Canales M, Ramos E, Boué O, Machado H, Lleonart R, de Armas CA, Rey S, Rodríguez JL, Artiles M, García L. Field studies and cost-effectiveness analysis of vaccination with Gavac against the cattle tick Boophilus microplus. Vaccine. 1998 Feb;16(4):366-73. PMID:9607057

de Sousa A, Rabarijaona LP, Ndiaye JL, Sow D, Ndyiae M, Hassan J, Lambo N, Adovohekpe P, Guidetti F, Recht J, Affo A. Acceptability of coupling Intermittent Preventive Treatment in infants with the Expanded Programme on Immunization in three francophone countries in Africa. Trop Med Int Health. 2011 Nov 29. [Epub ahead of print]. PMID:22128893

de Sousa BC, Cunha C. Development of mathematical models for the analysis of hepatitis delta virus viral dynamics. PLoS One. 2010 Sep 16;5(9). pii: e12512. PMID:20862328

De Souza CM, Silva ED, Ano Bom AP, Bastos RC, Nascimento HJ, Da Silva Junior JG. Evaluation of an ELISA for canine leishmaniasis immunodiagnostic using recombinant proteins. Parasite Immunol. 2012 Jan;34(1):1-7. PMID:21929686

de Souza JB, Okomo U, Alexander ND, Aziz N, Owens BM, Kaur H, Jasseh M, Muangnoicharoen S, Sumariwalla PF, Warhurst DC, Ward SA, Conway DJ, Ulloa L, Tracey KJ, Foxwell BM, Kaye PM, Walther M. Oral activated charcoal prevents experimental cerebral malaria in mice and in a randomized controlled clinical trial in man did not interfere with the pharmacokinetics of parenteral artesunate. PLoS One. 2010 Apr 15;5(4):e9867. PMID:20419161

de Souza NB, Carmo AM, Lagatta DC, Alves MJ, Fontes AP, Coimbra ES, da Silva AD, Abramo C. 4-aminoquinoline analogues and its platinum (II) complexes as antimalarial agents. Biomed Pharmacother. 2011 Jul;65(4):313-6. Epub 2011 May 30. PMID:21704476

De Vos AJ, Bessenger R, Fourie CG. Virulence and heterologous strain immunity of South African and Australian Babesia bovis strains with reduced pathogenicity. Onderstepoort J Vet Res. 1982 Sep;49(3):133-6. PMID:7177589

De Vos AJ, Bock RE. Vaccination against bovine babesiosis. Ann N Y Acad Sci. 2000;916:540-5. PMID:11193669

de Vos AJ. Epidemiology and control of bovine babesiosis in South Africa. J S Afr Vet Assoc. 1979 Dec;50(4):357-62. PMID:576018

de Waal DT, Combrink MP. Live vaccines against bovine babesiosis. Vet Parasitol. 2006 May 31;138(1-2):88-96. Epub 2006 Feb 28. PMID:16504404

Deiana S, Watanabe A, Yamasaki Y, Amada N, Arthur M, Fleming S, Woodcock H, Dorward P, Pigliacampo B, Close S, Platt B, Riedel G. Plasma and brain pharmacokinetic profile of cannabidiol (CBD), cannabidivarine (CBDV), Δ(9)-tetrahydrocannabivarin (THCV) and cannabigerol (CBG) in rats and mice following oral and intraperitoneal administration and CBD action on obsessive-compulsive behaviour. Psychopharmacology (Berl). 2011 Jul 28. [Epub ahead of print]. PMID:21796370

Delbecq S, Precigout E, Schetters T, Gorenflot A. Babesia divergens: cloning of a Ran binding protein 1 homologue. Vet Parasitol. 2003 Jul 29;115(3):205-11. PMID:12935735

Della-Giustina D, Laird TW Jr, Smith T. Transfusion-acquired babesiosis in a nonendemic area. Mil Med. 2005 Apr;170(4):295-6. PMID:15916297

Dennig HK. [Babesia galagolata n.sp., a Babesia of the galago (Galago crassicaudatus) (author's transl)].[Article in German]. Z Parasitenkd. 1973 Jul 16;41(4):281-90. PMID:4742782

Depinay N, Franetich JF, Grüner AC, Mauduit M, Chavatte JM, Luty AJ, van Gemert GJ, Sauerwein RW, Siksik JM, Hannoun L, Mazier D, Snounou G, Rénia L. Inhibitory effect of TNF-α on malaria pre-erythrocytic stage development: influence of host hepatocyte/parasite combinations. PLoS One. 2011 Mar 4;6(3):e17464. PMID:21394207

Deplaine G, Lavazec C, Bischoff E, Natalang O, Perrot S, Guillotte-Blisnick M, Coppée JY, Pradines B, Mercereau-Puijalon O, David PH. Artesunate tolerance in transgenic Plasmodium falciparum parasites overexpressing a tryptophan-rich protein. Antimicrob Agents Chemother. 2011 Jun;55(6):2576-84. Epub 2011 Apr 4. PMID:21464256

Derieg NJ, Sangaumphai A, Bruederle LP. Genetic diversity and endemism in North American Carex section Ceratocystis (Cyperaceae). Am J Bot. 2008 Oct;95(10):1287-96. PMID:21632333

Desai M, Dellicour S. Effects of malaria and its treatment in early pregnancy. Lancet Infect Dis. 2011 Dec 12. [Epub ahead of print]. PMID:22169410

Deschermeier C, Hecht LS, Bach F, Rützel K, Stanway RR, Nagel A, Seeber F, Heussler VT. Mitochondrial lipoic acid scavenging is essential for Plasmodium berghei liver stage development. Cell Microbiol. 2011 Nov 30. [Epub ahead of print]. PMID:22128915

de-Thé G, Geser A. [Prospective epidemiologic studies and the nature of the association between Epstein-Barr virus (EBV) and Burkitt's lymphoma (BL)].[Article in French]. C R Acad Sci Hebd Seances Acad Sci D. 1976 Apr 5;282(14):1387-90. PMID:181158

Devine GJ, Killeen GF. The potential of a new larviciding method for the control of malaria vectors. Malar J. 2010 May 25;9:142. PMID:20500865

Deye GA, Miller RS, Miller L, Salas CJ, Tosh D, Macareo L, Smith BL, Fracisco S, Clemens EG, Murphy J, Sousa JC, Dumler JS, Magill AJ. Prolonged Protection Provided by a Single Dose of Atovaquone-Proguanil for the Chemoprophylaxis of Plasmodium falciparum Malaria in a Human Challenge Model. Clin Infect Dis. 2011 Nov 3. [Epub ahead of print]. PMID:22052893

Dhanawat M, Das N, Nagarwal RC, Shrivastava SK. Antimalarial drug development: past to present scenario. Mini Rev Med Chem. 2009 Oct;9(12):1447-69. PMID:19929818

Dharia NV, Plouffe D, Bopp SE, González-Páez GE, Lucas C, Salas C, Soberon V, Bursulaya B, Kochel TJ, Bacon DJ, Winzeler EA. Genome scanning of Amazonian Plasmodium falciparum shows subtelomeric instability and clindamycin-resistant parasites. Genome Res. 2010 Nov;20(11):1534-44. Epub 2010 Sep 9. PMID:20829224

Dhiman S, Goswami D, Rabha B, Gopalakrishnan R, Baruah I, Singh L. Malaria epidemiology along Indo-Bangladesh border in Tripura State, India. Southeast Asian J Trop Med Public Health. 2010 Nov;41(6):1279-89. PMID:21329299

Diawara HZ, Gbaguidi F, Evrard B, Leclercq JQ, Moudachirou M, Debrus B, Hubert P, Rozet E. Validation, transfer and measurement uncertainty estimation of an HPLC-UV method for the quantification of artemisinin in hydro alcoholic extracts of Artemisia annua L. J Pharm Biomed Anal. 2011 Aug 25;56(1):7-15. Epub 2011 Apr 21. PMID:21570794

Dicko A, Doumbo O. Efficacy of RTS,S malaria vaccine given with EPI vaccines. Lancet Infect Dis. 2011 Oct;11(10):722-3. Epub 2011 Jul 22. PMID:21782518

Dicko A, Toure SO, Traore M, Sagara I, Toure OB, Sissoko MS, Diallo AT, Rogier C, Salomon R, de Sousa A, Doumbo OK. Increase in EPI vaccines coverage after implementation of intermittent preventive treatment of malaria in infant with Sulfadoxine -pyrimethamine in the district of Kolokani, Mali: results from a cluster randomized control trial. BMC Public Health. 2011 Jul 18;11:573. PMID:21767403

Diggs CL, Osler AG. Humoral immunity in rodent malaria. III: Studies on the site of antibody action. J Immunol. 1975 Apr;114(4):1243-7. PMID:1090670

Dimmock CK, Bell K. Haemolytic disease of the newborn in calves. Aust Vet J. 1970 Feb;46(2):44-7. PMID:5463721

Dimmock CK. Blood group antibody production in cattle by a vaccine against Babesia argentina. Res Vet Sci. 1973 Nov;15(3):305-9. PMID:4792010

Dinter D, Gajski G, Garaj-Vrhovac V. An alkaline comet assay study on the antimalarial drug atovaquone in human peripheral blood lymphocytes: a study based on clinically relevant concentrations. J Appl Toxicol. 2011 Jul 7. [Epub ahead of print]. PMID:21735454

Diou J, Tardif MR, Barat C, Tremblay MJ. Dendritic cells derived from hemozoin-loaded monocytes display a partial maturation phenotype that promotes HIV-1 trans-infection of CD4+ T cells and virus replication. J Immunol. 2010 Mar 15;184(6):2899-907. Epub 2010 Feb 10. PMID:20147629

Dippmann AK, Bienzle U, Harms G, Mockenhaupt FP. pfmdr1 mutations in imported African Plasmodium falciparum isolates. Trans R Soc Trop Med Hyg. 2008 Nov;102(11):1148-50. Epub 2008 May 29. PMID:18513774

Distiller GB, Little F, Barnes KI. Nonlinear mixed effects modeling of gametocyte carriage in patients with uncomplicated malaria. Malar J. 2010 Feb 26;9:60. PMID:20187935

Djimdé AA, Fofana B, Sagara I, Sidibe B, Toure S, Dembele D, Dama S, Ouologuem D, Dicko A, Doumbo OK. Efficacy, safety, and selection of molecular markers of drug resistance by two ACTs in Mali. Am J Trop Med Hyg. 2008 Mar;78(3):455-61. PMID:18337343

Dlamini SV, Beshir K, Sutherland CJ. Markers of anti-malarial drug resistance in Plasmodium falciparum isolates from Swaziland: identification of pfmdr1-86F in natural parasite isolates. Malar J. 2010 Mar 3;9:68. PMID:20199676

DoAmaral JR, French FA, Blanz EJ Jr, French DA. Antimalarial activity of guanylhydrazone salts of aromatic ketones. 2. Development of active polyhalo derivatives. J Med Chem. 1971 Sep;14(9):862-6. PMID:5140015

Dobaño C, Quelhas D, Quintó L, Puyol L, Serra-Casas E, Mayor A, Nhampossa T, Macete E, Aide P, Mandomando I, Sanz S, Puniya SK, Singh B, Gupta P, Bhattacharya A, Chauhan VS, Aponte JJ, Chitnis CE, Alonso PL, Menéndez C. Age-Dependent IgG Subclass Responses to Plasmodium falciparum EBA-175 are Differentially Associated with Incidence of Malaria in Mozambican Children. Clin Vaccine Immunol. 2011 Dec 14. [Epub ahead of print]. PMID:22169088

Dobroszycki J, Herwaldt BL, Boctor F, Miller JR, Linden J, Eberhard ML, Yoon JJ, Ali NM, Tanowitz HB, Graham F, Weiss LM, Wittner M. A cluster of transfusion-associated babesiosis cases traced to a single asymptomatic donor. JAMA. 1999 Mar 10;281(10):927-30. PMID:10078490

Dodd JD, Aquino SL, Sharma A. Babesiosis: CT and hematologic findings. J Thorac Imaging. 2007 Aug;22(3):271-3. PMID:17721341

Dodd RY. Current risk for transfusion transmitted infections. Curr Opin Hematol. 2007 Nov;14(6):671-6. PMID:17898573

Dodd RY. Emerging pathogens in transfusion medicine. Clin Lab Med. 2010 Jun;30(2):499-509. Epub 2010 May 6. PMID:20513567

Dodd RY. Transmission of parasites by blood transfusion. Vox Sang. 1998;74 Suppl 2:161-3. PMID:9704440

Dondorp AM, Fairhurst RM, Slutsker L, Macarthur JR, M D JG, Guerin PJ, Wellems TE, Ringwald P, Newman RD, Plowe CV. The threat of artemisinin-resistant malaria. N Engl J Med. 2011 Sep 22;365(12):1073-5. PMID:21992120

Dondorp AM, Fanello CI, Hendriksen IC, Gomes E, Seni A, Chhaganlal KD, Bojang K, Olaosebikan R, Anunobi N, Maitland K, Kivaya E, Agbenyega T, Nguah SB, Evans J, Gesase S, Kahabuka C, Mtove G, Nadjm B, Deen J, Mwanga-Amumpaire J, Nansumba M, Karema C, Umulisa N, Uwimana A, Mokuolu OA, Adedoyin OT, Johnson WB, Tshefu AK, Onyamboko MA, Sakulthaew T, Ngum WP, Silamut K, Stepniewska K, Woodrow CJ, Bethell D, Wills B, Oneko M, Peto TE, von Seidlein L, Day NP, White NJ; AQUAMAT group. Artesunate versus quinine in the treatment of severe falciparum malaria in African children (AQUAMAT): an open-label, randomised trial. Lancet. 2010 Nov 13;376(9753):1647-57. Epub 2010 Nov 7. PMID:21062666

Dondorp AM, Nosten F, Yi P, Das D, Phyo AP, Tarning J, Lwin KM, Ariey F, Hanpithakpong W, Lee SJ, Ringwald P, Silamut K, Imwong M, Chotivanich K, Lim P, Herdman T, An SS, Yeung S, Singhasivanon P, Day NP, Lindegardh N, Socheat D, White NJ. Artemisinin resistance in Plasmodium falciparum malaria. N Engl J Med. 2009 Jul 30;361(5):455-67. PMID:19641202

Dorman SE, Cannon ME, Telford SR 3rd, Frank KM, Churchill WH. Fulminant babesiosis treated with clindamycin, quinine, and whole-blood exchange transfusion. Transfusion. 2000 Mar;40(3):375-80. PMID:10738042

Douradinha B, Doolan DL. Harnessing immune responses against Plasmodium for rational vaccine design. Trends Parasitol. 2011 Jun;27(6):274-83. Epub 2011 Apr 30. PMID:21531627

Dow GS, Gettayacamin M, Hansukjariya P, Imerbsin R, Komcharoen S, Sattabongkot J, Kyle D, Milhous W, Cozens S, Kenworthy D, Miller A, Veazey J, Ohrt C. Radical curative efficacy of tafenoquine combination regimens in Plasmodium cynomolgi-infected Rhesus monkeys (Macaca mulatta). Malar J. 2011 Jul 29;10:212. PMID:21801400

Dowling DP, Ilies M, Olszewski KL, Portugal S, Mota MM, Llinás M, Christianson DW. Crystal structure of arginase from Plasmodium falciparum and implications for L-arginine depletion in malarial infection. Biochemistry. 2010 Jul 6;49(26):5600-8. PMID:20527960

Dowsett KF, Dimmock CK, Hill MW. Haemolytic disease in new born calves. Aust Vet J. 1978 Feb;54(2):65-7. PMID:566099

Doyle E, Fowles SE, Summerfield S, White TJ. Rapid determination of tafenoquine in small volume human plasma samples by high-performance liquid chromatography-tandem mass spectrometry. J Chromatogr B Analyt Technol Biomed Life Sci. 2002 Mar 25;769(1):127-32. PMID:11936685

Drame PM, Poinsignon A, Besnard P, Le Mire J, Dos-Santos MA, Sow CS, Cornelie S, Foumane V, Toto JC, Sembene M, Boulanger D, Simondon F, Fortes F, Carnevale P, Remoue F. Human antibody response to Anopheles gambiae saliva: an immuno-epidemiological biomarker to evaluate the efficacy of insecticide-treated nets in malaria vector control. Am J Trop Med Hyg. 2010 Jul;83(1):115-21. PMID:20595489

Draper SJ, Biswas S, Spencer AJ, Remarque EJ, Capone S, Naddeo M, Dicks MD, Faber BW, de Cassan SC, Folgori A, Nicosia A, Gilbert SC, Hill AV. Enhancing blood-stage malaria subunit vaccine immunogenicity in rhesus macaques by combining adenovirus, poxvirus, and protein-in-adjuvant vaccines. J Immunol. 2010 Dec 15;185(12):7583-95. Epub 2010 Nov 22. PMID:21098232

Dreyer K, Fourie LJ, Kok DJ. The efficacy of used engine oil against ticks on cattle. Onderstepoort J Vet Res. 1998 Dec;65(4):275-9. PMID:10192839

Dua VK, Pandey AC, Dash AP. Adulticidal activity of essential oil of Lantana camara leaves against mosquitoes. Indian J Med Res. 2010 Mar;131:434-9. PMID:20418559

Duda RB, Anarfi JK, Adanu RM, Seffah J, Darko R, Hill AG. The health of the "older women" in Accra, Ghana: results of the Women's Health Study of Accra. J Cross Cult Gerontol. 2011 Sep;26(3):299-314. PMID:21695397

Duh D, Jelovsek M, Avsic-Zupanc T. Evaluation of an indirect fluorescence immunoassay for the detection of serum antibodies against Babesia divergens in humans. Parasitology. 2007 Feb;134(Pt 2):179-85. Epub 2006 Oct 11. PMID:17032478

Duncan CJ, Sheehy SH, Ewer KJ, Douglas AD, Collins KA, Halstead FD, Elias SC, Lillie PJ, Rausch K, Aebig J, Miura K, Edwards NJ, Poulton ID, Hunt-Cooke A, Porter DW, Thompson FM, Rowland R, Draper SJ, Gilbert SC, Fay MP, Long CA, Zhu D, Wu Y, Martin LB, Anderson CF, Lawrie AM, Hill AV, Ellis RD. Impact on malaria parasite multiplication rates in infected volunteers of the protein-in-adjuvant vaccine AMA1-C1/Alhydrogel+CPG 7909. PLoS One. 2011;6(7):e22271. Epub 2011 Jul 22. PMID:21799809

Dunn MA, Quinn TC, Terwedow HA Jr. Pre-erythrocytic rodent malaria, Plasmodium berghei--prevention of development in the ethionine fatty liver. Am J Trop Med Hyg. 1972 May;21(3):288-92. PMID:5025613

Duthaler U, Smith TA, Keiser J. In vivo and in vitro sensitivity of Fasciola hepatica to triclabendazole combined with artesunate, artemether, or OZ78. Antimicrob Agents Chemother. 2010 Nov;54(11):4596-604. Epub 2010 Aug 23. PMID:20733042

Dutta S, Sullivan JS, Grady KK, Haynes JD, Komisar J, Batchelor AH, Soisson L, Diggs CL, Heppner DG, Lanar DE, Collins WE, Barnwell JW. High antibody titer against apical membrane antigen-1 is required to protect against malaria in the Aotus model. PLoS One. 2009 Dec 3;4(12):e8138. PMID:19997632

Dvoraková HM, Dvoráckova M. [Babesiosis, a little known zoonosis]. [Article in Czech]. Epidemiol Mikrobiol Imunol. 2007 Nov;56(4):176-80. PMID:18072299

Dy FJ. Present status of malaria control in Asia. Bull World Health Organ. 1954;11(4-5):725-63. PMID:13209318

Dye C, Bourdin Trunz B, Lönnroth K, Roglic G, Williams BG. Nutrition, diabetes and tuberculosis in the epidemiological transition. PLoS One. 2011;6(6):e21161. Epub 2011 Jun 21. PMID:21712992

East IJ, Zakrzewski H, Gale KR, Leatch G, Dimmock CM, Thomas MB, Waltisbuhl DJ. Vaccination against Babesia bovis: T cells from protected and unprotected animals show different cytokine profiles. Int J Parasitol. 1997 Dec;27(12):1537-45. PMID:9467739

Eberhard ML, Walker EM, Steurer FJ. Survival and infectivity of Babesia in blood maintained at 25 C and 2-4 C. J Parasitol. 1995 Oct;81(5):790-2. PMID:7472878

Echaide IE, de Echaide ST, Guglielmone AA. Live and soluble antigens for cattle protection to Babesia bigemina. Vet Parasitol. 1993 Dec;51(1-2):35-40. PMID:8128585

Eder AF, Dy BA, Barton J, Kennedy JM, Benjamin RJ. The American Red Cross Hemovigilance Program: advancing the safety of blood donation and transfusion. Immunohematology. 2009;25(4):179-85. PMID:20406027

Edstein MD, Kocisko DA, Brewer TG, Walsh DS, Eamsila C, Charles BG. Population pharmacokinetics of the new antimalarial agent tafenoquine in Thai soldiers. Br J Clin Pharmacol. 2001 Dec;52(6):663-70. PMID:11736877

Edstein MD, Kocisko DA, Walsh DS, Eamsila C, Charles BG, Rieckmann KH. Plasma concentrations of tafenoquine, a new long-acting antimalarial agent, in thai soldiers receiving monthly prophylaxis. Clin Infect Dis. 2003 Dec 15;37(12):1654-8. Epub 2003 Nov 20. PMID:14689348

Edstein MD, Nasveld PE, Kocisko DA, Kitchener SJ, Gatton ML, Rieckmann KH. Gender differences in gastrointestinal disturbances and plasma concentrations of tafenoquine in healthy volunteers after tafenoquine administration for post-exposure vivax malaria prophylaxis. Trans R Soc Trop Med Hyg. 2007 Mar;101(3):226-30. Epub 2006 Jun 30. PMID:16814823

Edstein MD, Walsh DS, Eamsila C, Sasiprapha T, Nasveld PE, Kitchener S, Rieckmann KH. Malaria prophylaxis/radical cure: recent experiences of the Australian Defence Force. Med Trop (Mars). 2001;61(1):56-8. PMID:11584657

Efferth T, Giaisi M, Merling A, Krammer PH, Li-Weber M. Artesunate induces ROS-mediated apoptosis in doxorubicin-resistant T leukemia cells. PLoS One. 2007 Aug 1;2(8):e693. PMID:17668070

Egdell HG, Stanfield JP. Paediatric neurology in Africa: a Ugandan report. Br Med J. 1972 Feb 26;1(5799):548-52. PMID:5015052

Eisele TP, Larsen D, Steketee RW. Protective efficacy of interventions for preventing malaria mortality in children in Plasmodium falciparum endemic areas. Int J Epidemiol. 2010 Apr;39 Suppl 1:i88-101. PMID:20348132

Eisele TP, Miller JM, Moonga HB, Hamainza B, Hutchinson P, Keating J. Malaria infection and anemia prevalence in Zambia's Luangwa District: an area of near-universal insecticide-treated mosquito net coverage. Am J Trop Med Hyg. 2011 Jan;84(1):152-7. PMID:21212219

El Bardicy S, El Sayed I, Yousif F, Van der Veken P, Haemers A, Augustyns K, Pieters L. Schistosomicidal and molluscicidal activities of aminoalkylamino substituted neo- and norneocryptolepine derivatives. . Pharm Biol. 2012 Feb;50(2):134-40. PMID:22338119

El Sahly HM, Patel SM, Atmar RL, Lanford TA, Dube T, Thompson D, Sim BK, Long C, Keitel WA. Safety and immunogenicity of a recombinant nonglycosylated erythrocyte binding antigen 175 Region II malaria vaccine in healthy adults living in an area where malaria is not endemic. Clin Vaccine Immunol. 2010 Oct;17(10):1552-9. Epub 2010 Aug 11. PMID:20702657

El-Bahnasawy MM, Morsy TA. Egyptian human babesiosis and general review. J Egypt Soc Parasitol. 2008 Apr;38(1):265-72. PMID:19143136

Ellis RD, Sagara I, Doumbo O, Wu Y. Blood stage vaccines for Plasmodium falciparum: current status and the way forward. Hum Vaccin. 2010 Aug;6(8):627-34. PMID:20519960

Ellis RD, Fay MP, Sagara I, Dicko A, Miura K, Guindo MA, Guindo A, Sissoko MS, Doumbo OK, Diallo D. Anaemia in a phase 2 study of a blood stage falciparum malaria vaccine. Malar J. 2011 Jan 19;10:13. PMID:21247484

Ellis RD, Sagara I, Durbin A, Dicko A, Shaffer D, Miller L, Assadou MH, Kone M, Kamate B, Guindo O, Fay MP, Diallo DA, Doumbo OK, Emanuel EJ, Millum J. Comparing the understanding of subjects receiving a candidate malaria vaccine in the United States and Mali. Am J Trop Med Hyg. 2010 Oct;83(4):868-72. PMID:20889881

Elmes NJ, Nasveld PE, Kitchener SJ, Kocisko DA, Edstein MD. The efficacy and tolerability of three different regimens of tafenoquine versus primaquine for post-exposure prophylaxis of Plasmodium vivax malaria in the Southwest Pacific. Trans R Soc Trop Med Hyg. 2008 Nov;102(11):1095-101. Epub 2008 Jun 9. PMID:18541280

Emmerson FR, Knott SG, Callow LL. Vaccination with Babesia argentina in 5 beef herds in south-eastern Queensland. Aust Vet J. 1976 Oct;52(10):451-4. PMID:1016135

Enato EF, Sounyo AA, Einarson TR. Medication utilization and illness management study in Nigeria. Ann Pharmacother. 2011 Jul;45(7-8):924-30. Epub 2011 Jun 28. PMID:21712507

Englund L, Pringle J. New diseases and increased risk of diseases in companion animals and horses due to transport. Acta Vet Scand Suppl. 2003-2004;100:19-25. PMID:16429803

Enosse S, Magnussen P, Abacassamo F, Gómez-Olivé X, Rønn AM, Thompson R, Alifrangis M. Rapid increase of Plasmodium falciparum dhfr/dhps resistant haplotypes, after the adoption of sulphadoxine-pyrimethamine as first line treatment in 2002, in southern Mozambique. Malar J. 2008 Jul 1;7:115. PMID:18590577

Enwere OO. Herbs in orthodox practice: a view by medical students. Afr J Tradit Complement Altern Med. 2009 Mar 7;6(2):203-6. PMID:20209013

Erah PO, Aghayere PA, Suleman IA, Osahon TP. Treatment of uncomplicated malaria in Africa: evaluation of randomized clinical trials. Nig Q J Hosp Med. 2010 Oct-Dec;20(4):214-22. PMID:21913531

Erbsloh JK. Babesiosis in the newborn foal. J Reprod Fertil Suppl. 1975 Oct;(23):725-6. PMID:1060872

Erol E, Kumar N, Carson CA. Immunogenicity of recombinant Babesia microti hsp70 homologue in mice. Int J Parasitol. 1999 Feb;29(2):263-6. PMID:10221626

Erp EE, Smith RD, Ristic M, Osorno BM. Optimization of the suspension culture method for in vitro cultivation of Babesia bovis. Am J Vet Res. 1980 Dec;41(12):2059-62. PMID:7212439

Esimone CO, Omeje EO, Okoye FB, Obonga WO, Onah BU. Evidence for the spectroscopic determination of artesunate in dosage form. J Vector Borne Dis. 2008 Dec;45(4):281-6. PMID:19248654

Eskow ES, Krause PJ, Spielman A, Freeman K, Aslanzadeh J. Southern extension of the range of human babesiosis in the eastern United States. J Clin Microbiol. 1999 Jun;37(6):2051-2. PMID:10325378

Esteve M, Loras C, García-Planella E. Inflammatory bowel disease in travelers: choosing the right vaccines and check-ups. World J Gastroenterol. 2011 Jun 14;17(22):2708-14. PMID:21734778

Evenson DA, Perry E, Kloster B, Hurley R, Stroncek DF. Therapeutic apheresis for babesiosis. J Clin Apher. 1998;13(1):32-6. PMID:9590496

Ezzelarab M, Yeh P, Wagner R, Cooper DK. Babesia as a complication of immunosuppression following pig-to-baboon heart transplantation. Xenotransplantation. 2007 Mar;14(2):162-5. PMID:17381691

Falagas ME, Klempner MS. Babesiosis in patients with AIDS: a chronic infection presenting as fever of unknown origin. Clin Infect Dis. 1996 May;22(5):809-12. PMID:8722936

Fall B, Diawara S, Sow K, Baret E, Diatta B, Fall KB, Mbaye PS, Fall F, Diémé Y, Rogier C, Wade B, Bercion R, Pradines B. Ex vivo susceptibility of Plasmodium falciparum isolates from Dakar, Senegal, to seven standard anti-malarial drugs. Malar J. 2011 Oct 20;10:310. PMID:22014157

Famanta A, Diakite M, Diawara SI, Diakité SA, Doumbia S, Traoré K, Konaté DS, Doumbia M, Keita AS, Thiéro D, Traoré SF, Doumbia S, Tounkara A. [Prevalence of maternal and placental malaria and of neonatal low birth weight in a semi-urban area of Bamako (Mali)]. [Article in French]. Sante. 2011 Jan-Mar;21(1):3-7. PMID:21700554

Fanello CI, Karema C, Ngamije D, Uwimana A, Ndahindwa V, Van Overmeir C, Van Doren W, Curtis J, D'Alessandro U. A randomised trial to assess the efficacy and safety of chlorproguanil/dapsone + artesunate for the treatment of uncomplicated Plasmodium falciparum malaria. Trans R Soc Trop Med Hyg. 2008 May;102(5):412-20. Epub 2008 Mar 6. PMID:18328518

Farenhorst M, Knols BG. A novel method for standardized application of fungal spore coatings for mosquito exposure bioassays. Malar J. 2010 Jan 20;9:27. PMID:20089180

Farrance CE, Rhee A, Jones RM, Musiychuk K, Shamloul M, Sharma S, Mett V, Chichester JA, Streatfield SJ, Roeffen W, van de Vegte-Bolmer M, Sauerwein RW, Tsuboi T, Muratova OV, Wu Y, Yusibov V. A plant-produced Pfs230 vaccine candidate blocks transmission of Plasmodium falciparum. Clin Vaccine Immunol. 2011 Aug;18(8):1351-7. Epub 2011 Jun 29. PMID:21715576

Farzad E, Cator M, Giulivi A, Zhang J. Physician survey on knowledge and reporting practices of transfusion-transmitted infections in Canada. Can J Public Health. 2004 Nov-Dec;95(6):451-5. PMID:15622796

Fasan PO. The control of malaria in a holoendemic region. Niger Med J. 1973 Jul;3(3):124-7. PMID:16366343

Faucher B, Zaegel O, Niang A, Ba Fall K, Mbaye PS. [Permanent deafness following typhoid fever: case report from Dakar, Senegal]. [Article in French]. Med Trop (Mars). 2009 Feb;69(1):73-4. PMID:19499740

Fawole OI, Akinboye DO, Falade CO, Arulogun OS, Adeniyi JD. Case management of childhood fever by traditional healers in southwest Nigeria: identification of training and collaborative needs. Int Q Community Health Educ. 2007-2008;28(4):319-35. PMID:19193526

Fawole OI, Onadeko MO. Knowledge and home management of malaria fever by mothers and care givers of under five children. West Afr J Med. 2001 Apr-Jun;20(2):152-7. PMID:11768016

Faye A, Manga NM, Seck I, Niang K, Leye MM, Diagne-Camara M, Diongue M, Ba M, Ndiaye P, Tal-Dia A. [Access to intermittent preventive treatment (IPt) in a situation of abolition of user's fee: role of economic welfare].[Article in French]. Bull Soc Pathol Exot. 2011 Dec 6. [Epub ahead of print]. PMID:22147304

Faye B, Ndiaye JL, Ndiaye D, Dieng Y, Faye O, Gaye O. Efficacy and tolerability of four antimalarial combinations in the treatment of uncomplicated Plasmodium falciparum malaria in Senegal. Malar J. 2007 Jun 14;6:80. PMID:17570848

Feachem RG. The Global Fund: getting the reforms right. Lancet. 2011 Nov 19;378(9805):1764-5. PMID:22098844

Fedosov DA, Pan W, Caswell B, Gompper G, Karniadakis GE. Predicting human blood viscosity in silico. Proc Natl Acad Sci U S A. 2011 Jul 19;108(29):11772-7. Epub 2011 Jul 5. PMID:21730178

Fehintola FA, Balogun ST, Adeoye SB. Intermittent Preventive Treatment during Pregnancy with Sulphadoxine-Pyrimethamine May Promote Plasmodium falciparum Gametocytogenesis. Med Princ Pract. 2012;21(1):63-7. Epub 2011 Oct 21. PMID:22025224

Fell E. An update on Lyme disease and other tick-borne illnesses. Nurse Pract. 2000 Oct;25(10):38-40, 43-4, 47-8 passim; quiz 56-7. PMID:11068777

Fendel R, Brandts C, Rudat A, Kreidenweiss A, Steur C, Appelmann I, Ruehe B, Schröder P, Berdel WE, Kremsner PG, Mordmüller B. Hemolysis is associated with low reticulocyte production index and predicts blood transfusion in severe malarial anemia. PLoS One. 2010 Apr 6;5(4):e10038. PMID:20386613

Feng TS, Guantai EM, Nell M, van Rensburg CE, Ncokazi K, Egan TJ, Hoppe HC, Chibale K. Effects of highly active novel artemisinin-chloroquinoline hybrid compounds on β-hematin formation, parasite morphology and endocytosis in Plasmodium falciparum. Biochem Pharmacol. 2011 Aug 1;82(3):236-47. Epub 2011 May 8. PMID:21596024

Fernandes Fde F, Freitas Ede P. Analysis of the use of fenthion via epicutaneous in dogs for Rhipicephalus sanguineus control. Rev Soc Bras Med Trop. 2001 Jul-Aug;34(4):339-42. PMID:11562726

Fernández-Villegas A, Pinazo MJ, Marañón C, Thomas MC, Posada E, Carrilero B, Segovia M, Gascon J, López MC. Short-term follow-up of chagasic patients after benznidazole treatment using multiple serological markers. BMC Infect Dis. 2011 Jul 31;11:206. PMID:21801456

Fernando D, Rodrigo C, Rajapakse S. Primaquine in vivax malaria: an update and review on management issues. Malar J. 2011 Dec 12;10(1):351. [Epub ahead of print]. PMID:22152065

Ferreira ID, Martinelli A, Rodrigues LA, do Carmo EL, do Rosário VE, Póvoa MM, Cravo P. Plasmodium falciparum from Pará state (Brazil) shows satisfactory in vitro response to artemisinin derivatives and absence of the S769N mutation in the ERCA-type PfATPase6. PMID:18304266

Fidock DA. Drug discovery: Priming the antimalarial pipeline. Nature. 2010 May 20;465(7296):297-8. PMID:20485420

Figueroa JV, Alvarez JA, Rojas EE, Ramos JA, Mosqueda JJ, Cantó GJ, Vega CA, Buening GM. Use of a duplex PCR/DNA probe assay to monitor Babesia bovis and Babesia bigemina in cattle during a vaccination trial. Rev Latinoam Microbiol. 1998 Jan-Jun;40(1-2):39-44. PMID:10932733

Figueroa JV, Buening GM. In vitro inhibition of multiplication of Babesia bigemina by using monoclonal antibodies. J Clin Microbiol. 1991 May;29(5):997-1003. PMID:2056067

Filbin MR, Mylonakis EE, Callegari L, Legome E. Babesiosis. J Emerg Med. 2001 Jan;20(1):21-4. PMID:11165832

Finerty JF, Krehl EP. Cyclophosphamide pretreatment and protection against malaria. Infect Immun. 1976 Oct;14(4):1103-5. PMID:791863

Fink E, Dann O. [Further development of the Roehl test for testing antimalarial agents on Plasmodium cathemerium in the canary by intravenous administration].[Article in German]. Z Tropenmed Parasitol. 1967 Dec;18(4):466-74. PMID:5613461

Fink E. Assessment of causal prophylactic activity in Plasmodium berghei yoelii and its value for the development of new antimalarial drugs. Bull World Health Organ. 1974;50(3-4):213-22. PMID: 4155355

Fish L, Leibovich B, Krigel Y, McElwain T, Shkap V. Vaccination of cattle against B. bovis infection with live attenuated parasites and non-viable immunogens. Vaccine. 2008 Dec 19;26 Suppl 6:G29-33. PMID:19178890

Fish L, Pipano E, Indrakamhang P. Lyophilised bovine serum as a substitute for frozen serum in the cultivation of Babesia bigemina and B bovis. Res Vet Sci. 1992 Jan;52(1):115-6. PMID:1553430

Flateau C, Le Loup G, Pialoux G. Consequences of HIV infection on malaria and therapeutic implications: a systematic review. Lancet Infect Dis. 2011 Jul;11(7):541-56. PMID:21700241

Flateau C. [Artemether-lumefantrine: another choice for the treatment of malaria in pregnant women].[Article in French]. Med Mal Infect. 2011 May;41(5):276-7. PMID:21728261

Flaxman AD, Fullman N, Otten MW Jr, Menon M, Cibulskis RE, Ng M, Murray CJ, Lim SS. Rapid scaling up of insecticide-treated bed net coverage in Africa and its relationship with development assistance for health: a systematic synthesis of supply, distribution, and household survey data. PLoS Med. 2010 Aug 17;7(8):e1000328. PMID:20808957

Fleck SL, Robinson BL, Peters W. The chemotherapy of rodent malaria. LIV. Combinations of 'Fenozan B07' (Fenozan-50F), a difluorinated 3,3'-spirocyclopentane 1,2,4-trioxane, with other drugs against drug-sensitive and drug-resistant parasites. Ann Trop Med Parasitol. 1997 Jan;91(1):33-9. PMID:9093427

Flegg JA, Guerin PJ, White NJ, Stepniewska K. Standardizing the measurement of parasite clearance in falciparum malaria: the parasite clearance estimator. Malar J. 2011 Nov 10;10:339. PMID:22074219

Fletcher TI, Wigg JL, Rolls PJ, de Vos AJ. Viability assays of intra-erythrocytic organisms using fluorescent dyes. Vet Parasitol. 2009 Jul 7;163(1-2):144-7. Epub 2009 Mar 31. PMID:19380205

Floch H. [Development of the malaria campaign in French Guiana from 1950 to 1954].[Article in French]. Publ Inst Pasteur Guyane Fr Inini. 1954 Nov;15(345):1-8. PMID:14377655

Florent I, Maréchal E, Gascuel O, Bréhélin L. Bioinformatic strategies to provide functional clues to the unknown genes in Plasmodium falciparum genome. Parasite. 2010 Dec;17(4):273-83. PMID:21275233

Flores W, Chang J, Barillas E. Rapid assessment of the performance of malaria control strategies implemented by countries in the Amazon subregion using adequacy criteria: case study. Malar J. 2011 Dec 20;10(1):379. [Epub ahead of print]. PMID:22185638

Florescu D, Sordillo PP, Glyptis A, Zlatanic E, Smith B, Polsky B, Sordillo E. Splenic infarction in human babesiosis: two cases and discussion. Clin Infect Dis. 2008 Jan 1;46(1):e8-11. PMID:18171204

Florin-Christensen M, Schnittger L, Dominguez M, Mesplet M, Rodríguez A, Ferreri L, Asenzo G, Wilkowsky S, Farber M, Echaide I, Suarez C. Search for Babesia bovis vaccine candidates. Parassitologia. 2007 May;49 Suppl 1:9-12. PMID:17691600

Folarin OA, Bustamante C, Gbotosho GO, Sowunmi A, Zalis MG, Oduola AM, Happi CT. In vitro amodiaquine resistance and its association with mutations in pfcrt and pfmdr1 genes of Plasmodium falciparum isolates from Nigeria. Acta Trop. 2011 Dec;120(3):224-30. Epub 2011 Sep 6. PMID:21920347

Fonjungo PN, Kebede Y, Messele T, Ayana G, Tibesso G, Abebe A, Nkengasong JN, Kenyon T. Laboratory equipment maintenance: A critical bottleneck for strengthening health systems in sub-Saharan Africa? J Public Health Policy. 2011 Nov 10. [Epub ahead of print]. PMID:22071568

Foppa IM, Krause PJ, Spielman A, Goethert H, Gern L, Brand B, Telford SR 3rd. Entomologic and serologic evidence of zoonotic transmission of Babesia microti, eastern Switzerland. Emerg Infect Dis. 2002 Jul;8(7):722-6. PMID:12095442

Fort DM, Litvak J, Chen JL, Lu Q, Phuan PW, Cooper R, Bierer DE. Isolation and unambiguous synthesis of cryptolepinone: An oxidation artifact of cryptolepine. J Nat Prod. 1998 Dec;61(12):1528-30. PMID:9868157

Four Artemisinin-Based Combinations (4ABC) Study Group. A Head-to-Head Comparison of Four Artemisinin-Based Combinations for Treating Uncomplicated Malaria in African Children: A Randomized Trial. PLoS Med. 2011 Nov;8(11):e1001119. Epub 2011 Nov 8. PMID:22087077

Fowler JL, Ruff MD, Fernau RC, Furusho Y. Babesia gibsoni: chemotherapy in dogs. Am J Vet Res. 1972 Jun;33(6):1109-14. PMID:5022393

Fox LM, Wingerter S, Ahmed A, Arnold A, Chou J, Rhein L, Levy O. Neonatal babesiosis: case report and review of the literature. Pediatr Infect Dis J. 2006 Feb;25(2):169-73. PMID:16462298

Frank M, Lehners N, Mayengue PI, Gabor J, Dal-Bianco M, Kombila DU, Ngoma GM, Supan C, Lell B, Ntoumi F, Grobusch MP, Dietz K, Kremsner PG. A thirteen-year analysis of Plasmodium falciparum populations reveals high conservation of the mutant pfcrt haplotype despite the withdrawal of chloroquine from national treatment guidelines in Gabon. Malar J. 2011 Oct 17;10:304. PMID:22004584

Freeman MJ, Kirby BM, Panciera DL, Henik RA, Rosin E, Sullivan LJ. Hypotensive shock syndrome associated with acute Babesia canis infection in a dog. J Am Vet Med Assoc. 1994 Jan 1;204(1):94-6. PMID:8125828

Frerichs WM, Allen PC, Holbrook AA. Equine piroplasmosis (Babesia equi): therapeutic trials of imidocarb dihydrochloride in horses and donkeys. Vet Rec. 1973 Jul 21;93(3):73-5. PMID:4748680

Frerichs WM, Holbrook AA. Treatment of equine piroplasmosis (B caballi) with imidocarb dipropionate. Vet Rec. 1974 Aug 31;95(9):188-9. PMID:4450446

Friedhoff KT. [Piroplasmas of horses--impact on the international horse trade].[Article in German]. Berl Munch Tierarztl Wochenschr. 1982 Oct 1;95(19):368-74. PMID:6756387

Friesen J, Borrmann S, Matuschewski K. Induction of antimalaria immunity by pyrimethamine prophylaxis during exposure to sporozoites is curtailed by parasite resistance. Antimicrob Agents Chemother. 2011 Jun;55(6):2760-7. Epub 2011 Mar 28. PMID:21444698

Friesen J, Silvie O, Putrianti ED, Hafalla JC, Matuschewski K, Borrmann S. Natural immunization against malaria: causal prophylaxis with antibiotics. Sci Transl Med. 2010 Jul 14;2(40):40ra49. PMID:20630856

Froberg MK, Dannen D, Bakken JS. Babesiosis and HIV. Lancet. 2004 Feb 28;363(9410):704. PMID:15001329

Froberg MK, Dannen D, Bernier N, Shieh WJ, Guarner J, Zaki S. Case report: spontaneous splenic rupture during acute parasitemia of Babesia microti. Ann Clin Lab Sci. 2008 Autumn;38(4):390-2. PMID:18988934

Frölich S, Entzeroth R, Wallach M. Comparison of protective immune responses to apicomplexan parasites. J Parasitol Res. 2012;2012:852591. Epub 2011 Aug 18. PMID:21876783

Fukumoto S, Tamaki Y, Igarashi I, Suzuki H, Xuan X. Immunogenicity and growth inhibitory efficacy of the prime-boost immunization regime with DNA followed by recombinant vaccinia virus carrying the P29 gene of Babesia gibsoni in dogs. Exp Parasitol. 2009 Dec;123(4):296-301. Epub 2009 Aug 25. PMID:19712674

Fukumoto S, Tamaki Y, Okamura M, Bannai H, Yokoyama N, Suzuki T, Igarashi I, Suzuki H, Xuan X. Prime-boost immunization with DNA followed by a recombinant vaccinia virus expressing P50 induced protective immunity against Babesia gibsoni infection in dogs. Vaccine. 2007 Jan 26;25(7):1334-41. Epub 2006 Oct 10. PMID:17055131

Fukumoto S, Tamaki Y, Shirafuji H, Harakawa S, Suzuki H, Xuan X. Immunization with recombinant surface antigen P50 of Babesia gibsoni expressed in insect cells induced parasite growth inhibition in dogs. Clin Diagn Lab Immunol. 2005 Apr;12(4):557-9. PMID:15817768

Fukumoto S, Xuan X, Igarashi I, Zhang S, Mugisha J, Ogata T, Nagasawa H, Fujisaki K, Suzuki N, Mikami T. Morphological changes of Babesia gibsoni grown in canine red blood cell-substituted severe combined immune deficiency mice. J Parasitol. 2000 Oct;86(5):956-8. PMID:11128518

Fukumoto S, Xuan X, Kadota K, Igarashi I, Sugimoto C, Fujisaki K, Nagasawa H, Mikami T, Suzuki H. High-level expression of truncated surface antigen P50 of Babesia gibsoni in insect cells by baculovirus and evaluation of its immunogenicity and antigenicity. Clin Diagn Lab Immunol. 2003 Jul;10(4):596-601. PMID:12853391

Fukumoto S, Xuan X, Takabatake N, Igarashi I, Sugimoto C, Fujisaki K, Nagasawa H, Mikami T, Suzuki H. Inhibitory effect of antiserum to surface antigen P50 of Babesia gibsoni on growth of parasites in severe combined immunodeficiency mice given canine red blood cells. Infect Immun. 2004 Mar;72(3):1795-8. PMID:14977989

Gachohi JM, Ngumi PN, Kitala PM, Skilton RA. Estimating seroprevalence and variation to four tick-borne infections and determination of associated risk factors in cattle under traditional mixed farming system in Mbeere District, Kenya. Prev Vet Med. 2010 Jul 1;95(3-4):208-23. PMID: 20434227

Gahutu JB, Musemakweri A, Harms G, Mockenhaupt FP. Prevalence of classic erythrocyte polymorphisms among 749 children in southern highland Rwanda. Trans R Soc Trop Med Hyg. 2012 Jan;106(1):63-5. Epub 2011 Oct 20. PMID:22018599

Gajski G, Dinter D, Garaj-Vrhovac V. In vitro effect of the antimalarial drug proguanil hydrochloride on viability and DNA damage in human peripheral blood lymphocytes. Environ Toxicol Pharmacol. 2010 Nov;30(3):257-63. Epub 2010 Jul 16. PMID:21787658

Galay RL, Maeda H, Aung KM, Umemiya-Shirafuji R, Xuan X, Igarashi I, Tsuji N, Tanaka T, Fujisaki K. Anti-babesial activity of a potent peptide fragment derived from longicin of Haemaphysalis longicornis. Trop Anim Health Prod. 2011 Nov 20. [Epub ahead of print]. PMID:22102016

Gallagher LG, Chau S, Owaisi AS, Konczyk M, Bishop HS, Arguin PM, Trenholme GM. An 84-year-old woman with fever and dark urine. Clin Infect Dis. 2009 Jul 15;49(2):278, 310-1. PMID:19538064

Gama BE, Pereira-Carvalho GA, Lutucuta Kosi FJ, Almeida de Oliveira NK, Fortes F, Rosenthal PJ, Daniel-Ribeiro CT, de Fátima Ferreira-da-Cruz M. Plasmodium falciparum isolates from Angola show the StctVMNT haplotype in the pfcrt gene. Malar J. 2010 Jun 18;9:174. PMID:20565881

Gamo FJ, Sanz LM, Vidal J, de Cozar C, Alvarez E, Lavandera JL, Vanderwall DE, Green DV, Kumar V, Hasan S, Brown JR, Peishoff CE, Cardon LR, Garcia-Bustos JF. Thousands of chemical starting points for antimalarial lead identification. Nature. 2010 May 20;465(7296):305-10. PMID:20485427

Gandhi A, Garg K, Wadhwa N. Neonatal Plasmodium vivax malaria: an overlooked entity. J Infect Dev Ctries. 2011 Jul 4;5(6):489-92. PMID:21727650

Gangopadhyay R, Karoshi M, Keith L. Anemia and pregnancy: A link to maternal chronic diseases. Int J Gynaecol Obstet. 2011 Nov;115 Suppl 1:S11-5. PMID:22099433

Garcia LS. Malaria. Clin Lab Med. 2010 Mar;30(1):93-129. PMID:20513543

Garnham PC, Warren M, Killick-Kendrick R. The action of 'terramycin' on the primary exoerythrocytic development of Plasmodium vivax and Plasmodium cynomolgi ceylonensis. J Trop Med Hyg. 1971 Feb;74(2):32-5. PMID:4993964

Garren H. Gene Based Vaccines: Optimising Development and Delivery - A marcus evans Conference. IDrugs. 2010 Nov;13(11):759-61. PMID:21046520

Garrett-Jones C, Gramiccia G. Evidence of the development of resistance to DDT by Anopheles sacharovi in the Levant. Bull World Health Organ. 1954;11(4-5):865-83. PMID:13209325

Gary AT, Webb JA, Hegarty BC, Breitschwerdt EB. The low seroprevalence of tick-transmitted agents of disease in dogs from southern Ontario and Quebec. Can Vet J. 2006 Dec;47(12):1194-200. PMID:17217089

Gautam A, Ahmed T, Batra V, Paliwal J. Pharmacokinetics and pharmacodynamics of endoperoxide antimalarials. Curr Drug Metab. 2009 Mar;10(3):289-306. PMID:19442090

Gbotosho GO, Happi CT, Sijuade AO, Sowunmi A, Oduola AM. A simple cost-effective high performance liquid chromatographic assay of sulphadoxine in whole blood spotted on filter paper for field studies. Malar J. 2009 Oct 24;8:238. PMID:19852850

Gbotosho GO, Okuboyejo T, Happi CT, Sowunmi A. Fall in Hematocrit per 1000 Parasites Cleared From Peripheral Blood: A Simple Method for Estimating Drug-Related Fall in Hematocrit After Treatment of Malaria Infections. Am J Ther. 2011 Oct 17. [Epub ahead of print]. PMID:22020083

Gbotosho GO, Sowunmi A, Happi CT, Okuboyejo TM. Plasmodium falciparum gametocyte carriage, sex ratios and asexual parasite rates in Nigerian children before and after a treatment protocol policy change instituting the use of artemisinin-based combination therapies. Mem Inst Oswaldo Cruz. 2011 Sep;106(6):685-90. PMID:22012222

Gear JH. The occurrence and diagnosis of malaria. S Afr Med J. 1974 May 25;48(25):1078-84. PMID:4602110

Gebresilassie FE, Mariam DH. Factors influencing people's willingness-to-buy insecticide-treated bednets in Arbaminch Zuria District, southern Ethiopia. J Health Popul Nutr. 2011 Jun;29(3):200-6. PMID:21766555

Gemma S, Travagli V, Savini L, Novellino E, Campiani G, Butini S. Malaria chemotherapy: recent advances in drug development. Recent Pat Antiinfect Drug Discov. 2010 Nov 1;5(3):195-225. PMID:20738242

Gerber MA, Shapiro ED, Krause PJ, Cable RG, Badon SJ, Ryan RW. The risk of acquiring Lyme disease or babesiosis from a blood transfusion. J Infect Dis. 1994 Jul;170(1):231-4. PMID:8014507

Gerena Y, Gonzalez-Pons M, Serrano AE. Cytofluorometric detection of rodent malaria parasites using red-excited fluorescent dyes. Cytometry A. 2011 Nov;79(11):965-72. Epub 2011 Aug 25. PMID:22015734

German PI, Aweeka FT. Clinical pharmacology of artemisinin-based combination therapies. Clin Pharmacokinet. 2008;47(2):91-102. PMID:18193915

Gern L, Lienhard R, Péter O. [Diseases and pathogenic agents transmitted by ticks in Switzerland].[Article in French]. Rev Med Suisse. 2010 Oct 13;6(266):1906-9. PMID:21089555

Gero AM, Wood AM. New nucleoside transport pathways induced in the host erythrocyte membrane of malaria and Babesia infected cells. Adv Exp Med Biol. 1991;309A:169-72. PMID:1789200

Gething PW, Smith DL, Patil AP, Tatem AJ, Snow RW, Hay SI. Climate change and the global malaria recession. Nature. 2010 May 20;465(7296):342-5. PMID:20485434

Geurts N, Opdenakker G, Van den Steen PE. Matrix metalloproteinases as therapeutic targets in protozoan parasitic infections. Pharmacol Ther. 2011 Nov 28. [Epub ahead of print]. PMID:22138604

Gharoro EP, Igbafe AA. Pattern of drug use amongst antenatal patients in Benin City, Nigeria. Med Sci Monit. 2000 Jan-Feb;6(1):84-7. PMID:11208289

Gholizadeh S, Basseri HR, Zakeri S, Ladoni H, Djadid ND. Cloning, expression and transmission-blocking activity of anti-PvWARP, malaria vaccine candidate, in Anopheles stephensi mysorensis. Malar J. 2010 Jun 11;9:158. PMID:20537198

Ghosh SK, Chakaravarthy P, Panch SR, Krishnappa P, Tiwari S, Ojha VP, Manjushree R, Dash AP. Comparative efficacy of two poeciliid fish in indoor cement tanks against chikungunya vector Aedes aegypti in villages in Karnataka, India. BMC Public Health. 2011 Jul 28;11:599. PMID:21798018

Ghumra A, Khunrae P, Ataide R, Raza A, Rogerson SJ, Higgins MK, Rowe JA. Immunisation with recombinant PfEMP1 domains elicits functional rosette-inhibiting and phagocytosis-inducing antibodies to Plasmodium falciparum. PLoS One. 2011 Jan 31;6(1):e16414. PMID:21305024

Gibbons S, Fallah F, Wright CW. Cryptolepine hydrochloride: a potent antimycobacterial alkaloid derived from Cryptolepis sanguinolenta. Phytother Res. 2003 Apr;17(4):434-6. PMID:12722159

Giha HA. Artemisinin derivatives for treatment of uncomplicated Plasmodium falciparum malaria in Sudan: too early for too much hope. Parasitol Res. 2010 Feb;106(3):549-52. Epub 2009 Dec 15. PMID:20012990

Gilbert IH, Leroy D, Frearson JA. Finding new hits in neglected disease projects: target or phenotypic based screening? Curr Top Med Chem. 2011;11(10):1284-91. PMID:21401505

Gill AC, Cowman AF, Stewart NP, Kemp DJ, Timms P. Babesia bovis: molecular and biological characteristics of cloned parasite lines. Exp Parasitol. 1987 Apr;63(2):180-8. PMID:3032666

Gillet J, Herman F. [Development of Plasmodium berghei berghei in mice embryos].[Article in French]. C R Seances Soc Biol Fil. 1971;165(9):2029-31. PMID:4263149

Ginsburg H, Deharo E. A call for using natural compounds in the development of new antimalarial treatments - an introduction. Malar J. 2011 Mar 15;10 Suppl 1:S1. [Epub ahead of print]. PMID:21411010

Giri S, Sykes EA, Jennings TL, Chan WC. Rapid screening of genetic biomarkers of infectious agents using quantum dot barcodes. ACS Nano. 2011 Mar 22;5(3):1580-7. Epub 2011 Feb 28. PMID:21355538

Gitau EN, Kokwaro GO, Newton CR, Ward SA. Global proteomic analysis of plasma from mice infected with Plasmodium berghei ANKA using two dimensional gel electrophoresis and matrix assisted laser desorption ionization-time of flight mass spectrometry. Malar J. 2011 Jul 26;10:205. PMID:21791037

Gleason NN, Wolf RE. Entopolypoides macaci (Babesiidae) in Macaca mulatta. J Parasitol. 1974 Oct;60(5):844-7. PMID:4214908

Gleckman RA, Roth RM. Fever following abdominal surgery. Unusual infectious causes. Postgrad Med. 1986 Feb 1;79(2):287-94. PMID:3945600

Goel S, Gowda DC. How specific is Plasmodium falciparum adherence to chondroitin 4-sulfate? Trends Parasitol. 2011 Sep;27(9):375-81. Epub 2011 Apr 18. PMID:21507719

Goel S, Valiyaveettil M, Achur RN, Goyal A, Mattei D, Salanti A, Trenholme KR, Gardiner DL, Gowda DC. Dual stage synthesis and crucial role of cytoadherence-linked asexual gene 9 in the surface expression of malaria parasite var proteins. Proc Natl Acad Sci U S A. 2010 Sep 21;107(38):16643-8. Epub 2010 Sep 7. PMID:20823248

Goethert HK, Telford SR 3rd. Enzootic transmission of Babesia divergens among cottontail rabbits on Nantucket Island, Massachusetts. Am J Trop Med Hyg. 2003 Nov;69(5):455-60. PMID:14695079

Goheen MP, Bartlett MS, Shaw MM, Queener SF, Smith JW. Effects of 8-aminoquinolines on the ultrastructural morphology of Pneumocystis carinii. Int J Exp Pathol. 1993 Aug;74(4):379-87. PMID:8398811

Gohil S, Kats LM, Sturm A, Cooke BM. Recent insights into alteration of red blood cells by Babesia bovis: moovin' forward. Trends Parasitol. 2010 Dec;26(12):591-9. Epub 2010 Jul 2. PMID:20598944

Golightly LM, Hirschhorn LR, Weller PF. Fever and headache in a splenectomized woman. Rev Infect Dis. 1989 Jul-Aug;11(4):629-37. PMID:2772469

Gonçalves PM, Passos LM, Ribeiro MF. Detection of IgM antibodies against Babesia bovis in cattle. Vet Parasitol. 1999 Mar 22;82(1):11-7. PMID:10223346

González EF, Todorovic RA, Thompson KC. Immunization against anaplasmosis and babesiosis: Part I. Evaluation of immunization using minimum infective doses under laboratory conditions. Tropenmed Parasitol. 1976 Dec;27(4):427-37. PMID:1006801

González IJ. [Metacaspases and their role in the life cycle of human protozoan parasites].[Article in Spanish]. Biomedica. 2009 Sep;29(3):485-93. PMID:20436999

González-Bulnes P, Bobenchik AM, Augagneur Y, Cerdan R, Vial HJ, Llebaria A, Ben Mamoun C. PG12, a phospholipid analog with potent antimalarial activity, inhibits Plasmodium falciparum CTP:phosphocholine cytidylyltransferase activity. J Biol Chem. 2011 Aug 19;286(33):28940-7. Epub 2011 Jun 25. PMID:21705805

Goo YK, Terkawi MA, Jia H, Aboge GO, Ooka H, Nelson B, Kim S, Sunaga F, Namikawa K, Igarashi I, Nishikawa Y, Xuan X. Artesunate, a potential drug for treatment of Babesia infection. Parasitol Int. 2010 Sep;59(3):481-6. Epub 2010 Jun 9. PMID:20541037

Goodger BV, Commins MA, Waltisbuhl DJ, Wright IG, Rode-Bramanis K. Babesia bovis: immunity induced by vaccination with a lipid enriched fraction. Int J Parasitol. 1990 Aug;20(5):685-7. PMID:2228430

Goodger BV, Commins MA, Wright IG, Mirre GB, Waltisbuhl DJ, White M. Babesia bovis: vaccination trial with a dominant immunodiffusion antigen in splenectomised calves. Z Parasitenkd. 1986;72(6):715-22. PMID:3099492

Goodger BV, Commins MA, Wright IG, Waltisbuhl DJ, Mirre GB. Successful homologous vaccination against Babesia bovis using a heparin-binding fraction of infected erythrocytes. Int J Parasitol. 1987 Apr;17(4):935-40. PMID:3583543

Goodger BV, Waltisbuhl DJ, Commins MA, Wright IG. Babesia bovis: dextran sulphate as an adjuvant for and precipitant of protective immunogens. Int J Parasitol. 1992 Jul;22(4):465-9. PMID:1644521

Goodger BV, Waltisbuhl DJ, Wright IG, Mahoney DF, Commins MA. Babesia bovis--analysis and vaccination trial with the cryoprecipitable immune complex. Vet Immunol Immunopathol. 1987 Jan;14(1):57-65. PMID:3103316

Goodger BV, Waltisbuhl DJ, Wright IG, White M. Babesia bovis: analysis of and preliminary vaccination studies with a defined infected erythrocyte membrane binding antigen. Int J Parasitol. 1992 Jul;22(4):533-5. PMID:1644530

Goodger BV, Wright IG, Mahoney DF. The use of pathophysiological reactions to assess the efficacy of the immune response to Babesia bovis in cattle. Z Parasitenkd. 1981;66(1):41-8. PMID:6172907

Goodger BV, Wright IG, Waltisbuhl DJ, Mirre GB. Babesia bovis: successful vaccination against homologous challenge in splenectomised calves using a fraction of haemagglutinating antigen. Int J Parasitol. 1985 Apr;15(2):175-9. PMID:3997349

Goodger BV, Wright IG, Waltisbuhl DJ. The lysate from bovine erythrocytes infected with Babesia bovis. Analysis of antigens and a report on their immunogenicity when polymerized with glutaraldehyde. Z Parasitenkd. 1983;69(4):473-82. PMID:6414195

Goodman AL, Draper SJ. Blood-stage malaria vaccines - recent progress and future challenges. Ann Trop Med Parasitol. 2010 Apr;104(3):189-211. PMID:20507694

Goodyer L, Rice L, Martin A. Choice of and adherence to prophylactic antimalarials. J Travel Med. 2011 Jul-Aug;18(4):245-9. PMID:21722235

Gordon S, Cordon RA, Mazdzer EJ, Valigorsky JM, Blagg NA, Barnes SJ. Adult respiratory distress syndrome in babesiosis. Chest. 1984 Oct;86(4):633-4. PMID:6541117

Gorenflot A, Bazin C, Ambroise-Thomas P. [Human babesiosis. Treatment of severe forms].[Article in French]. Presse Med. 1987 Jun 13;16(22):1099. PMID:2955343

Gorenflot A, Brasseur P, Bonmarchand G, Laneele D, Simonin D. [2 cases of severe human babesiosis treated successfully].[Article in French]. Presse Med. 1990 Feb 24;19(7):335. PMID:2138308

Gorenflot A, Moubri K, Precigout E, Carcy B, Schetters TP. Human babesiosis. Ann Trop Med Parasitol. 1998 Jun;92(4):489-501. PMID:9683900

Gorenflot A, Precigout E, Bissuel G, Lecointre O, Brasseur P, Vidor E, L'Hostis M, Schrevel J. Identification of major Babesia divergens polypeptides that induce protection against homologous challenge in gerbils. Infect Immun. 1990 Dec;58(12):4076-82. PMID:2254031

Gorenflot A, Precigout E, Valentin A, Bissuel G, Carcy B, Brasseur P, Moreau Y, Schrevel J. Babesia divergens vaccine. Mem Inst Oswaldo Cruz. 1992;87 Suppl 3:279-81. PMID:1343703

Govindarajan M, Sivakumar R, Rajeswari M, Yogalakshmi K. Chemical composition and larvicidal activity of essential oil from Mentha spicata (Linn.) against three mosquito species. Parasitol Res. 2011 Dec 6. [Epub ahead of print]. PMID:22139403

Grabowski EF, Giardina PJ, Goldberg D, Masur H, Read SE, Hirsch RL, Benach JL. Babesiosis transmitted by a transfusion of frozen-thawed blood. Ann Intern Med. 1982 Apr;96(4):466-7. PMID:7199884

Graham HA, Palczuk NC, Stauber LA. Immunity to exoerythrocytic forms of malaria. II. Passive transfer of immunity to exoerythrocytic forms. Exp Parasitol. 1973 Dec;34(3):372-81. PMID:4773576

Graham HA, Stauber LA, Palczuk NC, Barnes WD. Immunity to exoerythrocytic forms of malaria. I. Course of infection of Plasmodium fallax in turkeys. Exp Parasitol. 1973 Dec;34(3):364-71. PMID:4773575

Graham SM. Nontyphoidal salmonellosis in Africa. Curr Opin Infect Dis. 2010 Oct;23(5):409-14. PMID:20736739

Gray GD, Phillips RS. Suppression of primary and secondary antibody responses and inhibition of antigen priming during Babesia microti infections in mice. Parasite Immunol. 1983 Mar;5(2):123-34. PMID:6844029

Gray GD, Phillips RS. Use of sorbitol in the cryopreservation of babesia. Res Vet Sci. 1981 May;30(3):388-9. PMID:7255935

Gray J, Zintl A, Hildebrandt A, Hunfeld KP, Weiss L. Zoonotic babesiosis: overview of the disease and novel aspects of pathogen identity. Ticks Tick Borne Dis. 2010 Mar;1(1):3-10. Epub 2009 Dec 24. PMID:21771506

Gray JS, Gannon P. Preliminary development of a live drug-controlled vaccine against bovine babesiosis using the Mongolian gerbil, Meriones unguiculatus. Vet Parasitol. 1992 May;42(3-4):179-88. PMID:1496778

Gray JS, Langley RJ, Brophy PO, Gannon P. Vaccination against bovine babesiosis with drug-controlled live parasites. Vet Rec. 1989 Sep 30;125(14):369-72. PMID:2683338

Gray JS, Pudney M. Activity of atovaquone against Babesia microti in the Mongolian gerbil, Meriones unguiculatus. J Parasitol. 1999 Aug;85(4):723-8. PMID:10461956

Graz B, Willcox ML, Diakite C, Falquet J, Dackuo F, Sidibe O, Giani S, Diallo D. Argemone mexicana decoction versus artesunate-amodiaquine for the management of malaria in Mali: policy and public-health implications. Trans R Soc Trop Med Hyg. 2010 Jan;104(1):33-41. Epub 2009 Sep 5. PMID:19733875

Greenwood B. Anti-malarial drugs and the prevention of malaria in the population of malaria endemic areas. Malar J. 2010 Dec 13;9 Suppl 3:S2. PMID:21144082

Greenwood B, Bojang K, Tagbor H, Pagnoni F. Combining community case management and intermittent preventive treatment for malaria. Trends Parasitol. 2011 Nov;27(11):477-80. Epub 2011 Jul 27. PMID:21802363

Greenwood B, Salisbury D, Hill AV. Vaccines and global health. Philos Trans R Soc Lond B Biol Sci. 2011 Oct 12;366(1579):2733-42. PMID:21893534

Greenwood B. Anti-malarial drugs and the prevention of malaria in the population of malaria endemic areas. Malar J. 2010 Dec 13;9 Suppl 3:S2. PMID:21144082

Gregory KG, Peters W. The chemotherapy of rodent malaria. IX. Causal prophylaxis. I. A method for demonstrating drug action on exo-erythrocytic stages. Ann Trop Med Parasitol. 1970 Mar;64(1):15-24. PMID:5485706

Grellier P, Benach J, Labaied M, Charneau S, Gil H, Monsalve G, Alfonso R, Sawyer L, Lin L, Steiert M, Dupuis K. Photochemical inactivation with amotosalen and long-wavelength ultraviolet light of Plasmodium and Babesia in platelet and plasma components. Transfusion. 2008 Aug;48(8):1676-84. Epub 2008 May 22. PMID:18503613

Grellier P, Santus R, Mouray E, Agmon V, Mazière JC, Rigomier D, Dagan A, Gatt S, Schrével J. Photosensitized inactivation of Plasmodium falciparum- and Babesia divergens-infected erythrocytes in whole blood by lipophilic pheophorbide derivatives. Vox Sang. 1997;72(4):211-20. PMID:9228710

Griffing SM, Mixson-Hayden T, Sridaran S, Alam MT, McCollum AM, Cabezas C, Marquiño Quezada W, Barnwell JW, De Oliveira AM, Lucas C, Arrospide N, Escalante AA, Bacon DJ, Udhayakumar V. South American Plasmodium falciparum after the malaria eradication era: clonal population expansion and survival of the fittest hybrids. PLoS One. 2011;6(9):e23486. Epub 2011 Sep 16. PMID:21949680

Grima KM. Therapeutic apheresis in hematological and oncological diseases. J Clin Apher. 2000;15(1-2):28-52. PMID:10767050

Grimberg BT. Methodology and application of flow cytometry for investigation of human malaria parasites. J Immunol Methods. 2011 Mar 31;367(1-2):1-16. Epub 2011 Feb 4. PMID:21296083

Grimble RF, Tappia PS. Modulation of pro-inflammatory cytokine biology by unsaturated fatty acids. Z Ernahrungswiss. 1998;37 Suppl 1:57-65. PMID:9558730

Grosse SD, Odame I, Atrash HK, Amendah DD, Piel FB, Williams TN. Sickle cell disease in Africa a neglected cause of early childhood mortality. Am J Prev Med. 2011 Dec;41(6 Suppl 4):S398-405. PMID:22099364

Grover WH, Bryan AK, Diez-Silva M, Suresh S, Higgins JM, Manalis SR. Measuring single-cell density. Proc Natl Acad Sci U S A. 2011 Jul 5;108(27):10992-6. Epub 2011 Jun 20. PMID:21690360

Gruber M, Wernsdorfer G, Satimai W, Wiedermann U, Congpuong K, Wernsdorfer WH. Pharmacodynamic interaction between mefloquine and retinol in Plasmodium falciparum in vitro. Wien Klin Wochenschr. 2009 Oct;121 Suppl 3:27-31. PMID:19915813

Guan G, Chauvin A, Luo J, Inoue N, Moreau E, Liu Z, Gao J, Thekisoe OM, Ma M, Liu A, Dang Z, Liu J, Ren Q, Jin Y, Sugimoto C, Yin H. The development and evaluation of a loop-mediated isothermal amplification (LAMP) method for detection of Babesia spp. infective to sheep and goats in China. Exp Parasitol. 2008 Sep;120(1):39-44. Epub 2008 Apr 18. PMID:18504039

Guan G, Chauvin A, Yin H, Luo J, Moreau E. Course of infection by Babesia sp. BQ1 (Lintan) and B. divergens in sheep depends on the production of IFNgamma and IL10. Parasite Immunol. 2010 Feb;32(2):143-52. PMID:20070828

Guay D. Update on clindamycin in the management of bacterial, fungal and protozoal infections. Expert Opin Pharmacother. 2007 Oct;8(14):2401-44. PMID:17927492

Gubernot DM, Lucey CT, Lee KC, Conley GB, Holness LG, Wise RP. Babesia infection through blood transfusions: reports received by the US Food and Drug Administration, 1997-2007. Clin Infect Dis. 2009 Jan 1;48(1):25-30. PMID:19035776

Gubernot DM, Nakhasi HL, Mied PA, Asher DM, Epstein JS, Kumar S. Transfusion-transmitted babesiosis in the United States: summary of a workshop. Transfusion. 2009 Dec;49(12):2759-71. Epub 2009 Oct 10. PMID:19821952

Guerrero FD, Miller RJ, Rousseau ME, Sunkara S, Quackenbush J, Lee Y, Nene V. BmiGI: a database of cDNAs expressed in Boophilus microplus, the tropical/southern cattle tick. Insect Biochem Mol Biol. 2005 Jun;35(6):585-95. Epub 2005 Mar 27. PMID:15857764

Guglielmone AA, de Echaide ST, Pérez y Santaella M, Iglesias JA, Vanzini VR, Lugaresi CI, Dellepiane EL. Cross-sectional estimation of Babesia bovis antibody prevalence in an area of Argentina used for extensive cattle breeding as an aid to control babesiosis. Prev Vet Med. 1997 May;30(2):151-4. PMID:9234418

Guglielmone AA, Lugaresi CI, Volpogni MM, Anziani OS, Vanzini VR. Babesial antibody dynamics after cattle immunisation with live vaccines, measured with an indirect immunofluorescence test. Vet Parasitol. 1997 Jun;70(1-3):33-9. PMID:9195707

Guha-Sapir D, van Panhuis WG. Health impact of the 2004 Andaman Nicobar earthquake and tsunami in Indonesia. Prehosp Disaster Med. 2009 Nov-Dec;24(6):493-9. PMID:20301065

Guiguemde WA, Shelat AA, Bouck D, Duffy S, Crowther GJ, Davis PH, Smithson DC, Connelly M, Clark J, Zhu F, Jiménez-Díaz MB, Martinez MS, Wilson EB, Tripathi AK, Gut J, Sharlow ER, Bathurst I, El Mazouni F, Fowble JW, Forquer I, McGinley PL, Castro S, Angulo-Barturen I, Ferrer S, Rosenthal PJ, Derisi JL, Sullivan DJ, Lazo JS, Roos DS, Riscoe MK, Phillips MA, Rathod PK, Van Voorhis WC, Avery VM, Guy RK. Chemical genetics of Plasmodium falciparum. Nature. 2010 May 20;465(7296):311-5. PMID:20485428

Guilbride DL, Gawlinski P, Guilbride PD. Why functional pre-erythrocytic and bloodstage malaria vaccines fail: a meta-analysis of fully protective immunizations and novel immunological model. PLoS One. 2010 May 19;5(5):e10685. PMID:20502667

Guittat L, Alberti P, Rosu F, Van Miert S, Thetiot E, Pieters L, Gabelica V, De Pauw E, Ottaviani A, Riou JF, Mergny JL. Interactions of cryptolepine and neocryptolepine with unusual DNA structures. Biochimie. 2003 May;85(5):535-47. PMID:12763313

Gulia-Nuss M, Mundhalia A, Gakhar SK. Effect of anti-fat body antibodies on reproductive capacity of mosquito Anopheles stephensi and transmission blocking of Plasmodium vivax. Indian J Exp Biol. 2011 Jul;49(7):479-82. PMID:21800498

Gummow B, Swan GE, Du Preez JL. A bioequivalence and pharmacokinetic evaluation of two commercial diminazene aceturate formulations administered intramuscularly to cattle. Onderstepoort J Vet Res. 1994 Dec;61(4):317-26. PMID:7501363

Guo J, Guiguemde AW, Bentura-Marciano A, Clark J, Haynes RK, Chan WC, Wong HN, Hunt N, Guy RK, Golenser J. Synthesis of Artemiside and Its Effects in Combination with Conventional Drugs, Against Severe Murine Malaria. Antimicrob Agents Chemother. 2011 Oct 17. [Epub ahead of print]. PMID:22006004

Gupta P, Hurley RW, Helseth PH, Goodman JL, Hammerschmidt DE. Pancytopenia due to hemophagocytic syndrome as the presenting manifestation of babesiosis. Am J Hematol. 1995 Sep;50(1):60-2. PMID:7668227

Gutman J, Green M, Durand S, Rojas OV, Ganguly B, Quezada WM, Utz GC, Slutsker L, Ruebush TK 2nd, Bacon DJ. Mefloquine pharmacokinetics and mefloquine-artesunate effectiveness in Peruvian patients with uncomplicated Plasmodium falciparum malaria. Malar J. 2009 Apr 9;8:58. PMID:19358697

Gutman JD, Kotton CN, Kratz A. Case records of the Massachusetts General Hospital. Weekly clinicopathological exercises. Case 29-2003. A 60-year-old man with fever, rigors, and sweats. N Engl J Med. 2003 Sep 18;349(12):1168-75. PMID:13679532

Gutteridge WE. Antimalarial drugs currently in development. J R Soc Med. 1989;82 Suppl 17:63-6; discussion 66-8. PMID:2693729

Gwadz RW. Successful immunization against the sexual stages of Plasmodium gallinaceum. Science. 1976 Sep 17;193(4258):1150-1. PMID:959832

Hadden CE, Sharaf MHM, Guido JE, Robins RH, Tackie AN, Phoebe CH Jr, Schiff PL Jr, Martin GE. 11-Isopropylcryptolepine: A novel alkaloid isolated from cryptolepis sanguinolenta characterized using submicro NMR techniques. J Nat Prod. 1999 Feb;62(2):238-40. PMID:10075749

Hadj-Kaddour K, Carcy B, Vallet A, Randazzo S, Delbecq S, Kleuskens J, Schetters T, Gorenflot A, Precigout E. Recombinant protein Bd37 protected gerbils against heterologous challenges with isolates of Babesia divergens polymorphic for the bd37 gene. Parasitology. 2007 Feb;134(Pt 2):187-96. Epub 2006 Oct 13. PMID:17038236

Hafalla JC, Silvie O, Matuschewski K. Cell biology and immunology of malaria. Immunol Rev. 2011 Mar;240(1):297-316. PMID:21349101

Hagimori I, Machida H, Goi R, Mencke N. Efficacy of imidacloprid/ permethrin and fipronil/(S)-methoprene combinations against Haemaphysalis longicornis ticks evaluated under in vitro and in vivo conditions. Parasitol Res. 2005 Oct;97 Suppl 1:S120-6. PMID:16228268

Hale BR, Owusu-Agyei S, Fryauff DJ, Koram KA, Adjuik M, Oduro AR, Prescott WR, Baird JK, Nkrumah F, Ritchie TL, Franke ED, Binka FN, Horton J, Hoffman SL. A randomized, double-blind, placebo-controlled, dose-ranging trial of tafenoquine for weekly prophylaxis against Plasmodium falciparum. Clin Infect Dis. 2003 Mar 1;36(5):541-9. Epub 2003 Feb 14. PMID:12594633

Hamer SA, Tsao JI, Walker ED, Mansfield LS, Foster ES, Hickling GJ. Use of tick surveys and serosurveys to evaluate pet dogs as a sentinel species for emerging Lyme disease. Am J Vet Res. 2009 Jan;70(1):49-56. PMID:19119948

Hampton T. Antimalarial drugs--here and on the horizon. JAMA. 2007 May 23;297(20):2185-6. PMID:17519403

Han JI, Lee SJ, Jang HJ, Na KJ. Asymptomatic Babesia microti-like parasite infection in wild raccoon dogs (Nyctereutes procyonoides) in South Korea. J Wildl Dis. 2010 Apr;46(2):632-5. PMID:20688664

Hanafi-Bojd AA, Vatandoost H, Oshaghi MA, Eshraghian MR, Haghdoost AA, Abedi F, Zamani G, Sedaghat MM, Rashidian A, Madani AH, Raeisi A. Knowledge, attitudes and practices regarding malaria control in an endemic area of southern Iran. Southeast Asian J Trop Med Public Health. 2011 May;42(3):491-501. PMID:21706926

Hanafusa Y, Onuma M, Kamiyama T. Partial protection of severe combined immunodeficient mice against infection with Babesia microti by in vitro-generated CD4+ T cell clones. J Vet Med Sci. 1998 Apr;60(4):401-4. PMID:9592710

Handel TM, Horuk R. Duffy antigen inhibitors: useful therapeutics for malaria? Trends Parasitol. 2010 Jul;26(7):329-33. Epub 2010 Apr 9. PMID:20382562

Hanefeld J. The impact of Global Health Initiatives at national and sub-national level – a policy analysis of their role in implementation processes of antiretroviral treatment (ART) roll-out in Zambia and South Africa. AIDS Care. 2010;22 Suppl 1:93-102. PMID:20680864

Hansen G, Heitmann A, Witt T, Li H, Jiang H, Shen X, Heussler VT, Rennenberg A, Hilgenfeld R. Structural basis for the regulation of cysteine-protease activity by a new class of protease inhibitors in Plasmodium. Structure. 2011 Jul 13;19(7):919-29. PMID:21742259

Hanssen E, Knoechel C, Klonis N, Abu-Bakar N, Deed S, LeGros M, Larabell C, Tilley L. Cryo transmission X-ray imaging of the malaria parasite, P. falciparum. J Struct Biol. 2011 Jan;173(1):161-8. Epub 2010 Sep 6. PMID:20826218

Hansford CF. The use of antimalarial drugs. S Afr Med J. 1974 Jun 22;48(30):1314-6. PMID:4605355

Hanson J, Hasan MM, Royakkers AA, Alam S, Charunwatthana P, Maude RJ, Douthwaite ST, Yunus EB, Mantha ML, Schultz MJ, Faiz MA, White NJ, Day NP, Dondorp AM. Laboratory prediction of the requirement for renal replacement in acute falciparum malaria. Malar J. 2011 Aug 3;10:217. PMID:21813009

Hao GF, Li H, Sun Y, Ge RP, Qiao GQ, Li B, Tian WZ, Shi NX, Yang XY. [Detection of tick and tick-borne pathogen in some ports of Inner Mongolia]. [Article in Chinese]. Zhonghua Liu Xing Bing Xue Za Zhi. 2009 Apr;30(4):365-7. PMID: 19731529

Haque A, Best SE, Amante FH, Mustafah S, Desbarrieres L, de Labastida F, Sparwasser T, Hill GR, Engwerda CR. CD4+ natural regulatory T cells prevent experimental cerebral malaria via CTLA-4 when expanded in vivo. PLoS Pathog. 2010 Dec 9;6(12):e1001221. PMID:21170302

Haque A, Best SE, Ammerdorffer A, Desbarrieres L, de Oca MM, Amante FH, de Labastida Rivera F, Hertzog P, Boyle GM, Hill GR, Engwerda CR. Type I interferons suppress CD4+ T-cell-dependent parasite control during blood-stage Plasmodium infection. Eur J Immunol. 2011 Sep;41(9):2688-98. Epub 2011 Aug 8. PMID:21674481

Haque A, Best SE, Unosson K, Amante FH, de Labastida F, Anstey NM, Karupiah G, Smyth MJ, Heath WR, Engwerda CR. Granzyme B expression by CD8+ T cells is required for the development of experimental cerebral malaria. J Immunol. 2011 Jun 1;186(11):6148-56. Epub 2011 Apr 27. PMID:21525386

Harandi AM, Medaglini D, Shattock RJ; Working Group convened by EUROPRISE. Vaccine adjuvants: a priority for vaccine research. Vaccine. 2010 Mar 11;28(12):2363-6. Epub 2010 Jan 9. PMID:20064476

Harijanto PN. Malaria treatment by using artemisinin in Indonesia. Acta Med Indones. 2010 Jan;42(1):51-6. PMID:20305333

Harrington WE, Mutabingwa TK, Kabyemela E, Fried M, Duffy PE. Intermittent treatment to prevent pregnancy malaria does not confer benefit in an area of widespread drug resistance. Clin Infect Dis. 2011 Aug 1;53(3):224-30. PMID:21765070

Harris P, Price S, Senthuran S, Cochupanachimootil J, Norton R. Automated erythrocytapheresis for severe falciparum malaria. Intern Med J. 2011 Jan;41(1a):60-3. PMID:21265962

Harrison KA, Ibeziako PA. Maternal anaemia and fetal birthweight. J Obstet Gynaecol Br Commonw. 1973 Sep;80(9):798-804. PMID:4743068

Harvey WT, Martz D. Motor neuron disease recovery associated with IV ceftriaxone and anti-Babesia therapy. Acta Neurol Scand. 2007 Feb;115(2):129-31. PMID:17212618

Harwin RM. Gametocytes, sporozoites and liver schizonts. S Afr Med J. 1974 Jun 1;48(26):1123-4. PMID:4135674

Häselbarth K, Kurz M, Hunfeld KP, Krieger G. [Babesiosis in an immunocompromised German patient].[Article in German]. Med Klin (Munich). 2008 Feb 15;103(2):104-7. PMID:18270666

Häselbarth K, Tenter AM, Brade V, Krieger G, Hunfeld KP. First case of human babesiosis in Germany - Clinical presentation and molecular characterisation of the pathogen. Int J Med Microbiol. 2007 Jun;297(3):197-204. Epub 2007 Mar 12. PMID:17350888

Hashemi-Fesharki R. Ovine and caprine babesiosis in Iran: treatment with imidocarb. Vet Rec. 1991 Oct 26;129(17):383-4. PMID:1746117

Hassan V, Arash R, Mehdi J, Ahmad R, Ali HB, Wali YA, Ali D, Abdulrasool M, Abbas P. Demonstration of malaria situation analysis, stratification and planning in Minab District, southern Iran. Asian Pac J Trop Med. 2011 Jan;4(1):67-71. Epub 2011 Jan 15. PMID:21771420

Hatcher JC, Greenberg PD, Antique J, Jimenez-Lucho VE. Severe babesiosis in Long Island: review of 34 cases and their complications. Clin Infect Dis. 2001 Apr 15;32(8):1117-25. Epub 2001 Mar 26. PMID:11283800

Hawkes M, Opoka RO, Namasopo S, Miller C, Conroy AL, Serghides L, Kim H, Thampi N, Liles WC, John CC, Kain KC. Nitric oxide for the adjunctive treatment of severe malaria: hypothesis and rationale. Med Hypotheses. 2011 Sep;77(3):437-44. Epub 2011 Jul 13. PMID:21745716

Hawkes M, Opoka RO, Namasopo S, Miller C, Thorpe KE, Lavery JV, Conroy AL, Liles WC, John CC, Kain KC. Inhaled nitric oxide for the adjunctive therapy of severe malaria: protocol for a randomized controlled trial. Trials. 2011 Jul 13;12:176. PMID:21752262

Hawking F. Entopolypoides macaci, a Babesia-like parasite in Cercopithecus monkeys. Parasitology. 1972 Aug;65(1):89-109. PMID:4626455

Haynes RK, Chan WC, Wong HN, Li KY, Wu WK, Fan KM, Sung HH, Williams ID, Prosperi D, Melato S, Coghi P, Monti D. Facile oxidation of leucomethylene blue and dihydroflavins by artemisinins: relationship with flavoenzyme function and antimalarial mechanism of action. ChemMedChem. 2010 Aug 2;5(8):1282-99. PMID:20629071

Heal KG, Taylor-Robinson AW. Tomatine adjuvantation of protective immunity to a major pre-erythrocytic vaccine candidate of malaria is mediated via CD8+ T cell release of IFN-gamma. J Biomed Biotechnol. 2010;2010:834326. Epub 2010 Mar 11. PMID:20300588

Healy GR. Babesia infections in man. Hosp Pract. 1979 Jun;14(6):107-11, 115-6. PMID:376427

Heidari S, Mofenson LM, Hobbs CV, Cotton MF, Marlink R, Katabira E. Unresolved Antiretroviral Treatment Management Issues in HIV-Infected Children. J Acquir Immune Defic Syndr. 2011 Dec 1. [Epub ahead of print]. PMID:22138766

Heidari S, Mofenson LM, Hobbs CV, Cotton MF, Marlink R, Katabira E. Unresolved Antiretroviral Treatment Management Issues in HIV-Infected Children. J Acquir Immune Defic Syndr. 2011 Nov 30. [Epub ahead of print]. PMID:22134147

Held J, Zanger P, Issifou S, Kremsner PG, Mordmüller B. In vitro activity of tigecycline in Plasmodium falciparum culture-adapted strains and clinical isolates from Gabon. Int J Antimicrob Agents. 2010 Jun;35(6):587-9. Epub 2010 Mar 15. PMID:20227854

Hemmer RM, Wozniak EJ, Lowenstine LJ, Plopper CG, Wong V, Conrad PA. Endothelial cell changes are associated with pulmonary edema and respiratory distress in mice infected with the WA1 human Babesia parasite. J Parasitol. 1999 Jun;85(3):479-89. PMID:10386441

Hemshekhar M, Sebastin Santhosh M, Kemparaju K, Girish KS. Emerging Roles of Anacardic Acid and Its Derivatives: A Pharmacological Overview. Basic Clin Pharmacol Toxicol. 2011 Nov 21. [Epub ahead of print]. PMID:22103711

Henschler R, Seifried E, Mufti N. Development of the S-303 Pathogen Inactivation Technology for Red Blood Cell Concentrates. Transfus Med Hemother. 2011;38(1):33-42. Epub 2011 Jan 31. PMID:21779204

Hensen B, Paintain LS, Shretta R, Bruce J, Jones C, Webster J. Taking stock: provider prescribing practices in the presence and absence of ACT stock. Malar J. 2011 Aug 3;10:218. PMID:21812948

Hentrich B, Böse R, Doherr M. Cryopreservation of Babesia caballi cultures. Int J Parasitol. 1994 Apr;24(2):253-4. PMID:8026902

Hentrich B, Böse R. Cryopreservation of Babesia divergens from jirds as a live vaccine for cattle. Int J Parasitol. 1993 Sep;23(6):771-6. PMID:8300287

Herbas MS, Ueta YY, Ichikawa C, Chiba M, Ishibashi K, Shichiri M, Fukumoto S, Yokoyama N, Takeya M, Xuan X, Arai H, Suzuki H. Alpha-tocopherol transfer protein disruption confers resistance to malarial infection in mice. Malar J. 2010 Apr 19;9:101. PMID:20403155

Herman JH, Ayache S, Olkowska D. Autoimmunity in transfusion babesiosis: a spectrum of clinical presentations. J Clin Apher. 2010;25(6):358-61. Epub 2010 Sep 7. PMID:20824620

Herman R, Shiroishi T, Buckler CE. Viral interference with exoerythrocytic forms of malaria (Plasmodium gallinaceum) in ovo. J Infect Dis. 1973 Aug;128(2):148-55. PMID:4353044

Herman R, Shiroishi T. Plasmodium gallinaceum: selective immunosuppression by cyclophosphamide in preerythrocytic malaria. Exp Parasitol. 1973 Oct;34(2):295-305. PMID:4583057

Hermanowska-Szpakowicz T, Skotarczak B, Kondrusik M, Rymaszewska A, Sawczuk M, Maciejewska A, Adamska M, Pancewicz S, Zajkowska J. Detecting DNAs of Anaplasma phagocytophilum and Babesia in the blood of patients suspected of Lyme disease. Ann Agric Environ Med. 2004;11(2):351-4. PMID:15627349

Herod E, Clark IA, Allison AC. Protection of mice against haemoprotozoan Babesia microti with Brucella abortus strain 19. Clin Exp Immunol. 1978 Mar;31(3):518-23. PMID:95914

Herwaldt BL, Cacciò S, Gherlinzoni F, Aspöck H, Slemenda SB, Piccaluga P, Martinelli G, Edelhofer R, Hollenstein U, Poletti G, Pampiglione S, Löschenberger , Tura S, Pieniazek NJ. Molecular characterization of a non-Babesia divergens organism causing zoonotic babesiosis in Europe. Emerg Infect Dis. 2003 Aug;9(8):942-8. PMID:12967491

Herwaldt BL, Kjemtrup AM, Conrad PA, Barnes RC, Wilson M, McCarthy MG, Sayers MH, Eberhard ML. Transfusion-transmitted babesiosis in Washington State: first reported case caused by a WA1-type parasite. J Infect Dis. 1997 May;175(5):1259-62. PMID:9129100

Herwaldt BL, Linden JV, Bosserman E, Young C, Olkowska D, Wilson M. Transfusion-associated babesiosis in the United States: a description of cases. Ann Intern Med. 2011 Oct 18;155(8):509-19. Epub 2011 Sep 5. PMID:21893613

Herwaldt BL, McGovern PC, Gerwel MP, Easton RM, MacGregor RR. Endemic babesiosis in another eastern state: New Jersey. Emerg Infect Dis. 2003 Feb;9(2):184-8. PMID:12603988

Herwaldt BL, Neitzel DF, Gorlin JB, Jensen KA, Perry EH, Peglow WR, Slemenda SB,

Won KY, Nace EK, Pieniazek NJ, Wilson M. Transmission of Babesia microti in Minnesota through four blood donations from the same donor over a 6-month period. Transfusion. 2002 Sep;42(9):1154-8. PMID:12430672

Herwaldt BL, Springs FE, Roberts PP, Eberhard ML, Case K, Persing DH, Agger WA. Babesiosis in Wisconsin: a potentially fatal disease. Am J Trop Med Hyg. 1995 Aug;53(2):146-51. PMID:7677215

Heyman P, Cochez C, Hofhuis A, van der Giessen J, Sprong H, Porter SR, Losson B, Saegerman C, Donoso-Mantke O, Niedrig M, Papa A. A clear and present danger: tick-borne diseases in Europe. Expert Rev Anti Infect Ther. 2010 Jan;8(1):33-50. PMID:20014900

Hien TT, Truong NT, Minh NH, Dat HD, Dung NT, Hue NT, Dung TK, Tuan PQ, Campbell JI, Farrar JJ, Day JN. A randomized controlled pilot study of artesunate versus triclabendazole for human fascioliasis in central Vietnam. Am J Trop Med Hyg. 2008 Mar;78(3):388-92. PMID:18337331

Higuchi M, Okumura J, Aoyama A, Suryawati S, Porter J. Application of standard treatment guidelines in rural community health centres, Timor-Leste. Health Policy Plan. 2011 Jul 11. [Epub ahead of print]. PMID:21746735

Hildebrandt A, Hunfeld KP, Baier M, Krumbholz A, Sachse S, Lorenzen T, Kiehntopf M, Fricke HJ, Straube E. First confirmed autochthonous case of human Babesia microti infection in Europe. Eur J Clin Microbiol Infect Dis. 2007 Aug;26(8):595-601. PMID:17587072

Hill AV. Vaccines against malaria. Philos Trans R Soc Lond B Biol Sci. 2011 Oct 12;366(1579):2806-14. PMID:21893544

Hill K, Amouzou A. Trends in Child Mortality, 1960 to 2000. In: Jamison DT, Feachem RG, Makgoba MW, Bos ER, Baingana FK, Hofman KJ, Rogo KO, editors. Disease and Mortality in Sub-Saharan Africa. 2nd edition. Washington(DC): World Bank; 2006. Chapter 3. PMID:21290657

Hilton E, DeVoti J, Benach JL, Halluska ML, White DJ, Paxton H, Dumler JS. Seroprevalence and seroconversion for tick-borne diseases in a high-risk population in the northeast United States. Am J Med. 1999 Apr;106(4):404-9. PMID:10225242

Hinaidy HK. [Bovine babesiasis in Austria. IV. Studies with killed vaccines].[Article in German]. Berl Munch Tierarztl Wochenschr. 1981 Apr 1;94(7):121-5. PMID:7247917

Hines SA, Palmer GH, Jasmer DP, Goff WL, McElwain TF. Immunization of cattle with recombinant Babesia bovis merozoite surface antigen-1. Infect Immun. 1995 Jan;63(1):349-52. PMID:7806376

Hjelm K, Mufunda E. Zimbabwean diabetics' beliefs about health and illness: an interview study. BMC Int Health Hum Rights. 2010 May 12;10:7. PMID:20462425

Hobbs C, Duffy P. Drugs for malaria: something old, something new, something borrowed. F1000 Biol Rep. 2011;3:24. Epub 2011 Nov 1. PMID:22076126

Hodel EM, Marfurt J, Müller D, Rippert A, Borrmann S, Müller I, Reeder JC, Siba P, Genton B, Beck HP. Lack of multiple copies of pfmdr1 gene in Papua New Guinea. Trans R Soc Trop Med Hyg. 2008 Nov;102(11):1151-3. Epub 2008 Jul 2. PMID:18599099

Hohenschild S. [Babesiosis--a dangerous infection for splenectomized children and adults].[Article in German]. Klin Padiatr. 1999 May-Jun;211(3):137-40. PMID:10412122

Hollenberg D, Zakus D, Cook T, Xu XW. Re-positioning the role of traditional, complementary and alternative medicine as essential health knowledge in global health: do they still have a role to play? World Health Popul. 2008;10(4):62-75. PMID:19550163

Holman PJ, Backlund BB, Wilcox AL, Stone R, Stricklin AL, Bardin KE. Detection of a large unnamed Babesia piroplasm originally identified in dogs in North Carolina in a dog with no history of travel to that state. J Am Vet Med Assoc. 2009 Oct 1;235(7):851-4. PMID:19793016

Holman PJ, Frerichs WM, Chieves L, Wagner GG. Culture confirmation of the carrier status of Babesia caballi-infected horses. J Clin Microbiol. 1993 Mar;31(3):698-701. PMID:8458966

Holman PJ, Petrini K, Rhyan J, Wagner GG. In vitro isolation and cultivation of a Babesia from an American woodland caribou (Rangifer tarandus caribou). J Wildl Dis. 1994 Apr;30(2):195-200. PMID:7913142

Holman PJ, Snowden KF. Canine hepatozoonosis and babesiosis, and feline cytauxzoonosis. Vet Clin North Am Small Anim Pract. 2009 Nov;39(6):1035-53, v. PMID:19932361

Holman PJ, Spencer AM, Droleskey RE, Goethert HK, Telford SR 3rd. In vitro cultivation of a zoonotic Babesia sp. isolated from eastern cottontail rabbits (Sylvilagus floridanus) on Nantucket Island, Massachusetts. J Clin Microbiol. 2005 Aug;43(8):3995-4001. PMID:16081941

Holman PJ, Spencer AM, Telford SR 3rd, Goethert HK, Allen AJ, Knowles DP, Goff WL. Comparative infectivity of Babesia divergens and a zoonotic Babesia divergens-like parasite in cattle. Am J Trop Med Hyg. 2005 Nov;73(5):865-70. PMID:16282295

Holman PJ, Waldrup KA, Droleskey RE, Corrier DE, Wagner GG. In vitro growth of Babesia bovis in white-tailed deer (Odocoileus virginianus) erythrocytes. J Parasitol. 1993 Apr;79(2):233-7. PMID:8459334

Holman PJ, Waldrup KA, Wagner GG. In vitro cultivation of a Babesia isolated from a white-tailed deer (Odocoileus virginianus). J Parasitol. 1988 Feb;74(1):111-5. PMID:3357095

Holtel A, Troye-Blomberg M, Penas-Jimenez I. EU-funded malaria research under the 6th and 7th Framework Programmes for research and technological development. Malar J. 2011 Jan 14;10:11. PMID:21235784

Homer MJ, Aguilar-Delfin I, Telford SR 3rd, Krause PJ, Persing DH. Babesiosis. Clin Microbiol Rev. 2000 Jul;13(3):451-69. PMID:10885987

Homer MJ, Lodes MJ, Reynolds LD, Zhang Y, Douglass JF, McNeill PD, Houghton RL, Persing DH. Identification and characterization of putative secreted antigens from Babesia microti. J Clin Microbiol. 2003 Feb;41(2):723-9. PMID:12574273

Hopkins A. Beyond providing drugs, the mectizan ® donation creating paradigm shifts in health care and health systems strengthening. Curr Pharm Biotechnol. 2011 Oct 31. [Epub ahead of print]. PMID:22039801

Horii T, Shirai H, Jie L, Ishii KJ, Palacpac NQ, Tougan T, Hato M, Ohta N, Bobogare A, Arakaki N, Matsumoto Y, Namazue J, Ishikawa T, Ueda S, Takahashi M. Evidences of protection against blood-stage infection of Plasmodium falciparum by the novel protein vaccine SE36. Parasitol Int. 2010 Sep;59(3):380-6. Epub 2010 May 20. PMID:20493274

Hornok S, Edelhofer R, Szotáczky I, Hajtós I. Babesia divergens becoming extinct in cattle of Northeast Hungary: new data on the past and present situation. Acta Vet Hung. 2006 Dec;54(4):493-501. PMID:17278721

Horowitz ML, Coletta F, Fein AM. Delayed onset adult respiratory distress syndrome in babesiosis. Chest. 1994 Oct;106(4):1299-301. PMID:7924525

Hotez P. Enlarging the "Audacious Goal": Elimination of the World's high prevalence neglected tropical diseases. Vaccine. 2011 Dec 19. [Epub ahead of print]. PMID:22188933

Houghton RL, Homer MJ, Reynolds LD, Sleath PR, Lodes MJ, Berardi V, Leiby DA, Persing DH. Identification of Babesia microti-specific immunodominant epitopes and development of a peptide EIA for detection of antibodies in serum. Transfusion. 2002 Nov;42(11):1488-96. PMID:12421223

Howard AF, N'Guessan R, Koenraadt CJ, Asidi A, Farenhorst M, Akogbéto M, Knols BG, Takken W. First report of the infection of insecticide-resistant malaria vector mosquitoes with an entomopathogenic fungus under field conditions. Malar J. 2011 Feb 2;10:24. PMID:21288359

Howard N, Durrani N, Sanda S, Beshir K, Hallett R, Rowland M. Clinical trial of extended-dose chloroquine for treatment of resistant falciparum malaria among Afghan refugees in Pakistan. Malar J. 2011 Jun 23;10:171. PMID:21699697

Hsu LY, Jin J, Ang BS, Kurup A, Tambyah PA. Hand hygiene and infection control survey pre- and peri-H1N1-2009 pandemic: knowledge and perceptions of final year medical students in Singapore. Singapore Med J. 2011 Jul;52(7):486-90. PMID:21808958

Huang HL, Chiu TY, Huang KC, Cheng SY, Yao CA, Lee LT. Travel-related mosquito-transmitted disease questionnaire survey among health professionals in Taiwan. J Travel Med. 2011 Jan-Feb;18(1):34-8. Epub 2010 Dec 9. PMID:21199140

Huang X, Xuan X, Yokoyama N, Katayama Y, Anzai T, Igarashi I. Evaluation of enzyme-linked immunosorbent assays with recombinant antigens for the serodiagnosis of equine Babesia infections. Vet Parasitol. 2006 Aug 31;140(1-2):158-61. Epub 2006 Apr 18. PMID:16621293

Huffman SA, Veen J, Hennink MM, McFarland DA. Exploitation, vulnerability to tuberculosis and access to treatment among Uzbek labor migrants in Kazakhstan. Soc Sci Med. 2011 Aug 24. [Epub ahead of print]. PMID:22094009

Hughes CC, Hunter JM. Disease and "development" in Africa. Soc Sci Med. 1970 Apr;3(4):443-93. PMID:5483543

Hughes LM, Lanteri CA, O'Neil MT, Johnson JD, Gribble GW, Trumpower BL. Design of anti-parasitic and anti-fungal hydroxy-naphthoquinones that are less susceptible to drug resistance. Mol Biochem Parasitol. 2011 May;177(1):12-9. Epub 2011 Jan 18. PMID:21251932

Hughes WT, Oz HS. Successful prevention and treatment of babesiosis with atovaquone. J Infect Dis. 1995 Oct;172(4):1042-6. PMID:7561178

Hugoson G, Vennström R, Henriksson K. The occurrence of bovine leukosis following the introduction of babesiosis vaccination. Bibl Haematol. 1968;30:157-61. PMID:5695478

Hugoson G. Studies on lymphocytosis in regions with high and low incidences of bovine leukosis and babesiosis. Bibl Haematol. 1970;(36):537-43. PMID:5538363.

Huijben S, Nelson WA, Wargo AR, Sim DG, Drew DR, Read AF. Chemotherapy, within-host ecology and the fitness of drug-resistant malaria parasites. Evolution. 2010 Oct;64(10):2952-68. Epub 2010 Aug 19. PMID:20584075

Humeniuk R, Kaczmarek L, Peczyńska-Czoch W, Marcinkowska E. Cytotoxicity and cell cycle effects of novel indolo[2,3-b]quinoline derivatives. Oncol Res. 2003;13(5):269-77. PMID:12688678

Hunfeld KP, Allwinn R, Peters S, Kraiczy P, Brade V. Serologic evidence for tick-borne pathogens other than Borrelia burgdorferi (TOBB) in Lyme borreliosis patients from midwestern Germany. Wien Klin Wochenschr. 1998 Dec 23;110(24):901-8. PMID:10048174

Hunfeld KP, Brade V. Zoonotic Babesia: possibly emerging pathogens to be considered for tick-infested humans in Central Europe. Int J Med Microbiol. 2004 Apr;293 Suppl 37:93-103. PMID:15146990

Hunfeld KP, Hildebrandt A, Gray JS. Babesiosis: recent insights into an ancient disease. Int J Parasitol. 2008 Sep;38(11):1219-37. Epub 2008 Mar 20. PMID:18440005

Hunfeld KP, Lambert A, Kampen H, Albert S, Epe C, Brade V, Tenter AM. Seroprevalence of Babesia infections in humans exposed to ticks in Midwestern Germany. J Clin Microbiol. 2002 Jul;40(7):2431-6. PMID:12089258

Hunt P, Afonso A, Creasey A, Culleton R, Sidhu AB, Logan J, Valderramos SG, McNae I, Cheesman S, do Rosario V, Carter R, Fidock DA, Cravo P. Gene encoding a deubiquitinating enzyme is mutated in artesunate- and chloroquine-resistant rodent malaria parasites. Mol Microbiol. 2007 Jul;65(1):27-40. PMID:17581118

Hunt PW. Molecular diagnosis of infections and resistance in veterinary and human parasites. Vet Parasitol. 2011 Aug 4;180(1-2):12-46. Epub 2011 May 27. PMID:21700392

Hutchings CL, Li A, Fernandez KM, Fletcher T, Jackson LA, Molloy JB, Jorgensen WK, Lim CT, Cooke BM. New insights into the altered adhesive and mechanical properties of red blood cells parasitized by Babesia bovis. Mol Microbiol. 2007 Aug;65(4):1092-105. Epub 2007 Jul 19. PMID:17640278

Huthmacher C, Hoppe A, Bulik S, Holzhütter HG. Antimalarial drug targets in Plasmodium falciparum predicted by stage-specific metabolic network analysis. BMC Syst Biol. 2010 Aug 31;4:120. PMID:20807400

Huwer M, Schwarzmaier A, Hamel HD, Will R. [The occurrence of Babesia divergens in the Freiburg i. Br. district and piroplasmosis prevention trials in cattle].[Article in German]. Berl Munch Tierarztl Wochenschr. 1994 Jun;107(6):198-202. PMID:8067991

Hwang J, Alemayehu BH, Hoos D, Melaku Z, Tekleyohannes SG, Teshi T, Birhanu SG, Demeke L, Gobena K, Kassa M, Jima D, Reithinger R, Nettey H, Green M, Malone JL, Kachur SP, Filler S. In vivo efficacy of artemether-lumefantrine against uncomplicated Plasmodium falciparum malaria in Central Ethiopia. Malar J. 2011 Jul 28;10:209. PMID:21798054

Hwang SJ, Yamasaki M, Nakamura K, Sasaki N, Murakami M, Wickramasekara Rajapakshage BK, Ohta H, Maede Y, Takiguchi M. Development and characterization of a strain of Babesia gibsoni resistant to diminazene aceturate in vitro. J Vet Med Sci. 2010 Jun;72(6):765-71. Epub 2010 Feb 16. PMID:20160418

Ibanga IA, Nwokocha CR. Malaria: morbidity, mortality and its associated complications. West Indian Med J. 2011 Jan;60(1):1-2. PMID:21809702

Ibidapo CA. Perception of causes of malaria and treatment-seeking behaviour of nursing mothers in a rural community. Aust J Rural Health. 2005 Aug;13(4):214-8. PMID:16048462

Idowu ET, Mafe MA, Otubanjo OA, Adeneye AK. Herbal remedy in the treatment of malaria: cross sectional survey of residents of Lagos State, Nigeria. Afr J Med Med Sci. 2006 Jun;35(2):149-53. PMID:17209310

Idowu OR, Peggins JO, Brewer TG, Kelley C. Metabolism of a candidate 8-aminoquinoline antimalarial agent, WR 238605, by rat liver microsomes. Drug Metab Dispos. 1995 Jan;23(1):1-17. PMID:7720510

Igarashi I, Njonge FK, Kaneko Y, Nakamura Y. Babesia bigemina: in vitro and in vivo effects of curdlan sulfate on growth of parasites. Exp Parasitol. 1998 Nov;90(3):290-3. PMID:9806875

Igarashi I, Suzuki R, Waki S, Tagawa Y, Seng S, Tum S, Omata Y, Saito A, Nagasawa H, Iwakura Y, Suzuki N, Mikami T, Toyoda Y. Roles of CD4(+) T cells and gamma interferon in protective immunity against Babesia microti infection in mice. Infect Immun. 1999 Aug;67(8):4143-8. PMID:10417185

Ijarotimi SO, Agbedahunsi JM, Onyeji CO, Adewunmi CO. Chemotherapeutic interaction between Khaya grandifoliola (WELW) CDC stem bark extract and two anti-malarial drugs in mice. Afr J Tradit Complement Altern Med. 2010;7(4):370-6. Epub 2010 Jul 3. PMID:21731168

Ilchmann G. [New findings on the immunology of protozoan blood parasitoses in domestic animals].[Article in German]. Beitr Trop Landwirtsch Veterinarmed. 1978;16(3):305-12. PMID:373747

Imam M, Devi YS, Verma AK, Chauhan VS. Comparative Immunogenicities of full-length Plasmodium falciparum merozoite surface protein 3 and a 24-kilodalton N-terminal fragment. Clin Vaccine Immunol. 2011 Aug;18(8):1221-8. Epub 2011 Jun 1. PMID:21632889

Imbahale SS, Fillinger U, Githeko A, Mukabana WR, Takken W. An exploratory survey of malaria prevalence and people's knowledge, attitudes and practices of mosquito larval source management for malaria control in western Kenya. Acta Trop. 2010 Sep;115(3):248-56. Epub 2010 Apr 24. PMID:20399739

Imwong M, Dondorp AM, Nosten F, Yi P, Mungthin M, Hanchana S, Das D, Phyo AP, Lwin KM, Pukrittayakamee S, Lee SJ, Saisung S, Koecharoen K, Nguon C, Day NP, Socheat D, White NJ. Exploring the contribution of candidate genes to artemisinin resistance in Plasmodium falciparum. Antimicrob Agents Chemother. 2010 Jul;54(7):2886-92. Epub 2010 Apr 26. PMID:20421395

Infectious Diseases Chapter, Indian Academy of Pediatrics, Kundu R, Ganguly N, Ghosh TK. Collaborators: Shah RC, Kundu R, Nandy A, Ugra D, Narain NP, Shah NK, Ganguly N, Choudhury P, Shivananda, Ghosh TK, Govindaraj M. Management of malaria in children: update 2008. Indian Pediatr. 2008 Sep;45(9):731-5. PMID:18820376

Innocent E, Joseph CC, Gikonyo NK, Nkunya MH, Hassanali A. Constituents of the essential oil of Suregada zanzibariensis leaves are repellent to the mosquito, Anopheles gambiae s.s. J Insect Sci. 2010;10:57. PMID:20569134

Inoue M, Culleton RL. The intradermal route for inoculation of sporozoites of rodent malaria parasites for immunological studies. Parasite Immunol. 2011 Feb;33(2):137-42. PMID:21226727

Institute of Medicine (US) Forum on Microbial Threats. Antibiotic Resistance: Implications for Global Health and Novel Intervention Strategies: Workshop Summary. Washington (DC): National Academies Press (US); 2010. PMID:21595116

Ioset JR, Chang S. Drugs for Neglected Diseases initiative model of drug development for neglected diseases: current status and future challenges. Future Med Chem. 2011 Sep;3(11):1361-71. PMID:21879842

Irvin AD. Control of tick-borne diseases. Int J Parasitol. 1987 Feb;17(2):649-57. PMID:3294675

Irwin PJ. Canine babesiosis. Vet Clin North Am Small Anim Pract. 2010 Nov;40(6):1141-56. PMID:20933141

Irwin PJ. Canine babesiosis: from molecular taxonomy to control. Parasit Vectors. 2009 Mar 26;2 Suppl 1:S4. PMID:19426443

Isacchi B, Bergonzi MC, Grazioso M, Righeschi C, Pietretti A, Severini C, Bilia AR. Artemisinin and artemisinin plus curcumin liposomal formulations: Enhanced antimalarial efficacy against Plasmodium berghei-infected mice. Eur J Pharm Biopharm. 2011 Nov 28. [Epub ahead of print]. PMID:22142592

Isah AY, Amanabo MA, Ekele BA. Prevalence of malaria parasitemia amongst asymptomatic pregnant women attending a Nigerian teaching hospital. Ann Afr Med. 2011 Apr-Jun;10(2):171-4. PMID:21691026

Iseki H, Takabatake N, Ota N, Ishigame T, Yokoyama N, Igarashi I. Babesia: the protective effects of killed Propionibacterium acnes on the infections of two rodent Babesia parasites in mice. Exp Parasitol. 2008 Apr;118(4):543-8. Epub 2007 Nov 19. PMID:18164706

Ishengoma DS, Francis F, Mmbando BP, Lusingu JP, Magistrado P, Alifrangis M, Theander TG, Bygbjerg IC, Lemnge MM. Accuracy of malaria rapid diagnostic tests in community studies and their impact on treatment of malaria in an area with declining malaria burden in north-eastern Tanzania. Malar J. 2011 Jun 26;10:176. PMID:21703016

Israili ZH, Lyoussi B. Ethnopharmacology of the plants of genus Ajuga. Pak J Pharm Sci. 2009 Oct;22(4):425-62. PMID:19783524

Ito S, Shimura K. A double screening trial for the development of drugs against Theileria sergenti in cattle using Babesia rodhaini and Plasmodium berghei in mice. Nihon Juigaku Zasshi. 1985 Feb;47(1):101-9. PMID:3884864

Ittarat I, Webster HK, Yuthavong Y. High-performance liquid chromatographic determination of dihydroorotate dehydrogenase of Plasmodium falciparum and effects of antimalarials on enzyme activity. J Chromatogr. 1992 Nov 6;582(1-2):57-64. PMID:1491058

Iwatsuki M, Takada S, Mori M, Ishiyama A, Namatame M, Nishihara-Tsukashima A, Nonaka K, Masuma R, Otoguro K, Shiomi K, Omura S. In vitro and in vivo antimalarial activity of puberulic acid and its new analogs, viticolins A-C, produced by Penicillium sp. FKI-4410. J Antibiot (Tokyo). 2011 Feb;64(2):183-8. Epub 2010 Nov 10. PMID:21063422

Iwelunmor J, Idris O, Adelakun A, Airhihenbuwa CO. Child malaria treatment decisions by mothers of children less than five years of age attending an outpatient clinic in south-west Nigeria: an application of the PEN-3 cultural model. Malar J. 2010 Dec 8;9:354. PMID:21143854

Jack RM, Ward PA. Babesia rodhaini interactions with complement: relationship to parasitic entry into red cells. J Immunol. 1980 Apr;124(4):1566-73. PMID:6767771

Jack RM, Ward PA. The role in vivo of C3 and the C3b receptor in babesial infection in the rat. J Immunol. 1980 Apr;124(4):1574-8. PMID:6965951

Jackson LA, Waldron SJ, Weier HM, Nicoll CL, Cooke BM. Babesia bovis: culture of laboratory-adapted parasite lines and clinical isolates in a chemically defined medium. Exp Parasitol. 2001 Nov;99(3):168-74. PMID:11846527

Jacobs RL, Koontz LC. Plasmodium berghei: development of resistance to clindamycin and minocycline in mice. Exp Parasitol. 1976 Aug;40(1):116-23. PMID:780118

Jacobs RT, Plattner JJ, Keenan M. Boron-based drugs as antiprotozoals. Curr Opin Infect Dis. 2011 Dec;24(6):586-92. PMID:22001943

Jacoby GA, Hunt JV, Kosinski KS, Demirjian ZN, Huggins C, Etkind P, Marcus LC, Spielman A. Treatment of transfusion-transmitted babesiosis by exchange transfusion. N Engl J Med. 1980 Nov 6;303(19):1098-100. PMID:7191475

Jahangir A, Kolbert C, Edwards W, Mitchell P, Dumler JS, Persing DH. Fatal pancarditis associated with human granulocytic Ehrlichiosis in a 44-year-old man. Clin Infect Dis. 1998 Dec;27(6):1424-7. PMID:9868655

Jahiel RI, Nussenzweig RS, Vanderberg J, Vilcek J. Anti-malarial effect of interferon inducers at different stages of development of Plasmodium berghei in the mouse. Nature. 1968 Nov 16;220(5168):710-1. PMID:5688147

Jahiel RI, Vilcek J, Nussenzweig R, Vanderberg J. Interferon inducers protect mice against plasmodium berghei malaria. Science. 1968 Aug 23;161(3843):802-4. PMID:5663811

Jain R, Jordanova R, Müller IB, Wrenger C, Groves MR. Purification, crystallization and preliminary X-ray analysis of the aspartate aminotransferase of Plasmodium falciparum. Acta Crystallogr Sect F Struct Biol Cryst Commun. 2010 Apr 1;66(Pt 4):409-12. Epub 2010 Mar 31. PMID:20383010

Jambou R, Le Bras J, Randrianarivelojosia M. Pitfalls in new artemisinin-containing antimalarial drug development. Trends Parasitol. 2011 Feb;27(2):82-90. Epub 2010 Oct 26. PMID:21030307

James B. Control of malaria cycle. Lancet. 1968 Apr 6;1(7545):758. PMID:4170998

James MA, Kuttler KL, Levy MG, Ristic M. Antibody kinetics in response to vaccination against Babesia bovis. Am J Vet Res. 1981 Nov;42(11):1999-2001. PMID:7337297

James MA. Antibody levels during bovine hemoparasitic diseases: trypanosomiasis, anaplasmosis, and babesiosis. Acta Cient Venez. 1983;34(3-4):185-90. PMID:6399967

James MA. Application of exoantigens of Babesia and Plasmodium in vaccine development. Trans R Soc Trop Med Hyg. 1989;83 Suppl:67-72. PMID:2696163

Jamsen KM, Duffull SB, Tarning J, Lindegardh N, White NJ, Simpson JA. Optimal designs for population pharmacokinetic studies of oral artesunate in patients with uncomplicated falciparum malaria. Malar J. 2011 Jul 1;10:181. PMID:21722356

Jansen FH. Effectiveness of ACTs in cases of resistance to partner drugs. Lancet Infect Dis. 2011 Jul;11(7):498-9. PMID:21700240

Jansen FH. Intermittent preventive therapy for malaria: arguments in favour of artesunate and sulphamethoxypyrazine - pyrimethamine combination. Malar J. 2011 Mar 29;10:70. PMID:21443809

Jayaseelan C, Rahuman AA, Rajakumar G, Vishnu Kirthi A, Santhoshkumar T, Marimuthu S, Bagavan A, Kamaraj C, Zahir AA, Elango G. Synthesis of pediculocidal and larvicidal silver nanoparticles by leaf extract from heartleaf moonseed plant, Tinospora cordifolia Miers. Parasitol Res. 2011 Jul;109(1):185-94. Epub 2011 Jan 7. PMID:21212979

Jefferies R, Ryan UM, Jardine J, Robertson ID, Irwin PJ. Babesia gibsoni: detection during experimental infections and after combined atovaquone and azithromycin therapy. Exp Parasitol. 2007 Oct;117(2):115-23. Epub 2007 Apr 3. PMID:17543304

Jeffery GM, McWilson W, Collins WE, Lobel H. Application of the indirect fluorescent antibody method in a study of malaria endemicity in Mato Grosso, Brazil. Am J Trop Med Hyg. 1975 May;24(3):402-11. PMID:1098491

Jeffrey HC. Morphological changes in lasmodium vivax in patients under treatment with chloroquine. Trans R Soc Trop Med Hyg. 1968;62(1):47-50. PMID:4170613

Jeneby MM, Ngeiywa M, Yole DS, Mwenda JM, Suleman MA, Carlson HE. Enzootic simian piroplasm (Entopolypoides macaci) in wild-caught Kenyan non-human primates. J Med Primatol. 2008 Dec;37(6):329-36. Epub 2008 May 27. PMID:18507704

Jenkins MC. Advances and prospects for subunit vaccines against protozoa of veterinary importance. Vet Parasitol. 2001 Nov 22;101(3-4):291-310. PMID:11707303

Jeong YI, Kim SH, Ju JW, Cho SH, Lee WJ, Park JW, Park YM, Lee SE. Clonorchis sinensis-derived total protein attenuates airway inflammation in murine asthma model by inducing regulatory T cells and modulating dendritic cell functions. Biochem Biophys Res Commun. 2011 Apr 22;407(4):793-800. Epub 2011 Apr 1. PMID:21440530

Jiang B, Qin L, Du Y, Peng N, Chen L, Chen Z, Chen X. Transgenic Plasmodium that expresses HIV-1 Gag elicits immunity and protects mice against vaccinia virus-gag and malarial parasites. Vaccine. 2010 Nov 23;28(50):7915-22. Epub 2010 Oct 8. PMID:20933565

Jirage D, Keenan SM, Waters NC. Exploring novel targets for antimalarial drug discovery: plasmodial protein kinases. Infect Disord Drug Targets. 2010 Jun;10(3):134-46. PMID:20334624

Jittapalapong S, Jansawan W, Barriga OO, Stich RW. Reduced incidence of Babesia bigemina infection in cattle immunized against the cattle tick, Boophilus microplus. Ann N Y Acad Sci. 2004 Oct;1026:312-8. PMID:15604511

Johnson ST, Cable RG, Tonnetti L, Spencer B, Rios J, Leiby DA. Seroprevalence of Babesia microti in blood donors from Babesia-endemic areas of the northeastern United States: 2000 through 2007. Transfusion. 2009 Dec;49(12):2574-82. Epub 2009 Oct 10. PMID:19821951

Jongejan F, Fourie JJ, Chester ST, Manavella C, Mallouk Y, Pollmeier MG, Baggott D. The prevention of transmission of Babesia canis canis by Dermacentor reticulatus ticks to dogs using a novel combination of fipronil, amitraz and (S)-methoprene. Vet Parasitol. 2011 Jul 15;179(4):343-50. PMID:21777737

Jonckers TH, van Miert S, Cimanga K, Bailly C, Colson P, De Pauw-Gillet MC, van den Heuvel H, Claeys M, Lemière F, Esmans EL, Rozenski J, Quirijnen L, Maes L, Dommisse R, Lemière GL, Vlietinck A, Pieters L. Synthesis, cytotoxicity, and antiplasmodial and antitrypanosomal activity of new neocryptolepine derivatives. J Med Chem. 2002 Aug 1;45(16):3497-508. PMID:12139461

Jorgensen WK, De Vos AJ, Dalgliesh RJ. Comparison of immunogenicity and virulence between Babesia bigemina parasites from continuous culture and from a splenectomised calf. Aust Vet J. 1989 Nov;66(11):371-2. PMID:2619652

Jorgensen WK, de Vos AJ, Dalgliesh RJ. Infectivity of cryopreserved Babesia bovis, Babesia bigemina and Anaplasma centrale for cattle after thawing, dilution and incubation at 30 degrees C. Vet Parasitol. 1989 Jun;31(3-4):243-51. PMID:2763444

Joseph JT, Roy SS, Shams N, Visintainer P, Nadelman RB, Hosur S, Nelson J, Wormser GP. Babesiosis in Lower Hudson Valley, New York, USA. Emerg Infect Dis. 2011 May;17(5):843-7. PMID:21529393

Joubert KE, Kettner F, Lobetti RG, Miller DM. The effects of diminazene aceturate on systemic blood pressure in clinically healthy adult dogs. J S Afr Vet Assoc. 2003 Sep;74(3):69-71. PMID:15029949

Jovel IT, Mejia RE, Banegas E, Piedade R, Alger J, Fontecha G, Ferrreira PE, Veiga MI, Enamorado IG, Bjorkman A, Ursing J. Drug resistance associated genetic polymorphisms in Plasmodium falciparum and Plasmodium vivax collected in Honduras, Central America. Malar J. 2011 Dec 19;10(1):376. [Epub ahead of print]. PMID:22183028

Jude PJ, Dharshini S, Vinobaba M, Surendran SN, Ramasamy R. Anopheles culicifacies breeding in brackish waters in Sri Lanka and implications for malaria control. Malar J. 2010 Apr 21;9:106. PMID:20409313

Kabanywanyi AM, Mwita A, Sumari D, Mandike R, Mugittu K, Abdulla S. Efficacy and safety of artemisinin-based antimalarial in the treatment of uncomplicated malaria in children in southern Tanzania. Malar J. 2007 Nov 11;6:146. PMID:17996121

Kachan VI, Tkachova AI, Gvozdeva E, Urbanovich I, Yakusik A, Amico P, Avila-Figueroa C. Resource flows and levels of spending for the response to HIV and AIDS in Belarus. BMC Res Notes. 2011 Jul 21;4:248. PMID:21777473

Kachani M, Oliver RA, Brown CG, Ouhelli H, Spooner RL. Common and stage-specific antigens of Theileria annulata. Vet Immunol Immunopathol. 1992 Nov;34(3-4):221-34. PMID:1280878

Kager PA. [The treatment of falciparum malaria].[Article in Dutch]. Ned Tijdschr Geneeskd. 2007 Oct 6;151(40):2192-4. PMID:17969567

Kahama-Maro J, D'Acremont V, Mtasiwa D, Genton B, Lengeler C. Low quality of routine microscopy for malaria at different levels of the health system in Dar es Salaam. Malar J. 2011 Nov 2;10:332. PMID:22047131

Kain KC, Jassoum SB, Fong IW, Hannach B. Transfusion-transmitted babesiosis in Ontario: first reported case in Canada. CMAJ. 2001 Jun 12;164(12):1721-3. PMID:11450217

Kain KC, Shanks GD, Keystone JS. Malaria chemoprophylaxis in the age of drug resistance. I. Currently recommended drug regimens. Clin Infect Dis. 2001 Jul 15;33(2):226-34. Epub 2001 Jun 14. PMID:11418883

Kakai RM, Nasimiyu J, Odero W. Low reliability of home-based diagnosis of malaria in a rural community in western Kenya. J Infect Dev Ctries. 2011 Feb 1;5(1):54-8. PMID:21330741

Kalilani L, Mofolo I, Chaponda M, Rogerson SJ, Alker AP, Kwiek JJ, Meshnick SR. A randomized controlled pilot trial of azithromycin or artesunate added to sulfadoxine-pyrimethamine as treatment for malaria in pregnant women. PLoS One. 2007 Nov 14;2(11):e1166. PMID:18000538

Kaliyaperumal K, Mengistie E, Dagnew Z, Deboch B. Examining household possession and willingness to pay for the retreatment of ITNs with insecticides among local residences in a malaria endemic area. East Afr J Public Health. 2010 Dec;7(4):305-10. PMID:22066326

Kamani J, Sannusi A, Dogo AG, Tanko JT, Egwu KO, Tafarki AE, Ogo IN, Kemza S, Onovoh E, Shamaki D, Lombin LH, Catto V, Birkenheuer AJ. Babesia canis and Babesia rossi co-infection in an untraveled Nigerian dog. Vet Parasitol. 2010 Oct 29;173(3-4):334-5. Epub 2010 Jul 13. PMID:20705395

Kamaraj C, Bagavan A, Elango G, Zahir AA, Rajakumar G, Marimuthu S, Santhoshkumar T, Rahuman AA. Larvicidal activity of medicinal plant extracts against Anopheles subpictus & Culex tritaeniorhynchus. Indian J Med Res. 2011 Jul;134(1):101-6. PMID:21808141

Kamatou GP, Makunga NP, Ramogola WP, Viljoen AM. South African Salvia species: a review of biological activities and phytochemistry. J Ethnopharmacol. 2008 Oct 28;119(3):664-72. Epub 2008 Jul 2. PMID:18640254

Kambris Z, Blagborough AM, Pinto SB, Blagrove MS, Godfray HC, Sinden RE, Sinkins SP. Wolbachia stimulates immune gene expression and inhibits plasmodium development in Anopheles gambiae. PLoS Pathog. 2010 Oct 7;6(10):e1001143. PMID:20949079

Kamugisha E, Bujila I, Lahdo M, Pello-Esso S, Minde M, Kongola G, Naiwumbwe H, Kiwuwa S, Kaddumukasa M, Kironde F, Swedberg G. Large differences in prevalence of Pfcrt and Pfmdr1 mutations between Mwanza, Tanzania and Iganga, Uganda-A reflection of differences in policies regarding withdrawal of chloroquine? Acta Trop. 2012 Feb;121(2):148-51. Epub 2011 Nov 16. PMID:22118982

Kanagaratnam R, Misiura K, Rebowski G, Ramasamy R. Malaria merozoite surface protein antisense oligodeoxynucleotides lack antisense activity but function as polyanions to inhibit red cell invasion. Int J Biochem Cell Biol. 1998 Sep;30(9):979-85. PMID:9785462

Kania SA, Allred DR, Barbet AF. Babesia bigemina: host factors affecting the invasion of erythrocytes. Exp Parasitol. 1995 Feb;80(1):76-84. PMID:7821413

Kappe SH, Mikolajczak SA. Immunology. Another shot at a malaria vaccine. Science. 2011 Oct 28;334(6055):460-1. PMID:22034421

Kappe SH, Vaughan AM, Boddey JA, Cowman AF. That was then but this is now: malaria research in the time of an eradication agenda. Science. 2010 May 14;328(5980):862-6. PMID:20466924

Kar PK, Bhatt RM, Anvikar A, Dua VK. Malaria - change in therapeutic policy. Indian J Med Res. 2009 Feb;129(2):203-4. PMID:19293450

Kareru PG, Kenji GM, Gachanja AN, Keriko JM, Mungai G. Traditional medicines among the Embu and Mbeere peoples of Kenya. Afr J Tradit Complement Altern Med. 2006 Aug 28;4(1):75-86. PMID:20162075

Karl S, Gurarie D, Zimmerman PA, King CH, St Pierre TG, Davis TM. A sub-microscopic gametocyte reservoir can sustain malaria transmission. PLoS One. 2011;6(6):e20805. Epub 2011 Jun 14. PMID:21695129

Karle JM, Olmeda R, Freeman SG, Schroeder AC. Quantification of the individual enantiomer plasma concentrations of the candidate antimalarial agent N4-[2,6-dimethoxy-4-methyl-5-[(3-trifluoromethyl)phenoxy]-8-quinolinyl] -1,4-pentanediamine (WR 238,605). J Chromatogr B Biomed Appl. 1995 Aug 18;670(2):251-7. PMID:8548015

Karle JM, Olmeda R. Rapid and sensitive quantitative analysis of the new antimalarial N4-[2,6-dimethoxy-4-methyl-5-[(3-trifluoromethyl) phenoxy]-8-quinolinyl]-1,4-pentanediamine in plasma by liquid chromatography and electrochemical detection. J Chromatogr. 1988 Feb 26;424(2):347-56. PMID:3372627

Karunakaran KP, Yu H, Foster LJ, Brunham RC. Development of a Chlamydia trachomatis T cell Vaccine. Hum Vaccin. 2010 Aug;6(8):676-80. Epub 2010 Aug 1. PMID:20523121

Karunamoorthi K. Vector control: a cornerstone in the malaria elimination campaign. Clin Microbiol Infect. 2011 Nov;17(11):1608-16. PMID:21996100

Kasahara K, Nomura S, Subeki, Matsuura H, Yamasaki M, Yamato O, Maede Y, Katakura K, Suzuki M, Trimurningsih, Chairul, Yoshihara T. Anti-babesial compounds from Curcuma zedoaria. Planta Med. 2005 May;71(5):482-4. PMID:15977324

Katz TM, Miller JH, Hebert AA. Insect repellents: historical perspectives and new developments. J Am Acad Dermatol. 2008 May;58(5):865-71. Epub 2008 Feb 13. PMID:18272250

Kaufmann SH, Meinke AL, von Gabain A. [Novel vaccination concepts on the basis of modern insights into immunology].[Article in German]. Bundesgesundheitsblatt Gesundheitsforschung Gesundheitsschutz. 2009 Nov;52(11):1069-82. PMID:19838650

Kaul A, Bani S, Zutshi U, Suri KA, Satti NK, Suri OP. Immunopotentiating properties of Cryptolepis buchanani root extract. Phytother Res. 2003 Dec;17(10):1140-4. PMID:14669245

Kauss T, Fawaz F, Guyot M, Lagueny AM, Dos Santos I, Bonini F, Olliaro P, Caminiti A, Millet P. Fixed artesunate-amodiaquine combined pre-formulation study for the treatment of malaria. Int J Pharm. 2010 Jun 1. [Epub ahead of print]. PMID:20685236

Kauss T, Fawaz F, Guyot M, Lagueny AM, Dos Santos I, Bonini F, Olliaro P, Caminiti A, Millet P. Fixed artesunate-amodiaquine combined pre-formulation study for the treatment of malaria. Int J Pharm. 2010 Aug 16;395(1-2):198-204. PMID:20635516

Kayano AC, Lopes SC, Bueno FG, Cabral EC, Souza-Neiras WC, Yamauchi LM, Foglio MA, Eberlin MN, Mello JC, Costa FT. In vitro and in vivo assessment of the anti-malarial activity of Caesalpinia pluviosa. Malar J. 2011 May 2;10:112. PMID:21535894

Kayentao K, Maiga H, Newman RD, McMorrow ML, Hoppe A, Yattara O, Traore H, Kone Y, Guirou EA, Saye R, Traore B, Djimde A, Doumbo OK. Artemisinin-based combinations versus amodiaquine plus sulphadoxine-pyrimethamine for the treatment of uncomplicated malaria in Faladje, Mali. Malar J. 2009 Jan 7;8:5. PMID:19128455

Kayode J. Conservation of indigenous medicinal botanicals in Ekiti State, Nigeria. J Zhejiang Univ Sci B. 2006 Sep;7(9):713-8. PMID:16909472

Keller TH, Shi PY, Wang QY. Anti-infectives: can cellular screening deliver? Curr Opin Chem Biol. 2011 Aug;15(4):529-33. Epub 2011 Jun 30. PMID:21723774

Keiser J, Veneziano V, Rinaldi L, Mezzino L, Duthaler U, Cringoli G. Anthelmintic activity of artesunate against Fasciola hepatica in naturally infected sheep. Res Vet Sci. 2010 Feb;88(1):107-10. Epub 2009 Jun 5. PMID:19501379

Kelter G, Steinbach D, Konkimalla VB, Tahara T, Taketani S, Fiebig HH, Efferth T. Role of transferrin receptor and the ABC transporters ABCB6 and ABCB7 for resistance and differentiation of tumor cells towards artesunate. PLoS One. 2007 Aug 29;2(8):e798. PMID:17726528

Kengeya-Kayondo JF, Seeley JA, Kajura-Bajenja E, Kabunga E, Mubiru E, Sembajja F, Mulder DW. Recognition, treatment seeking behaviour and perception of cause of malaria among rural women in Uganda. Acta Trop. 1994 Dec;58(3-4):267-73. PMID:7709865

Kern SE, Tiono AB, Makanga M, Gbadoé AD, Premji Z, Gaye O, Sagara I, Ubben D, Cousin M, Oladiran F, Sander O, Ogutu B. Community screening and treatment of asymptomatic carriers of Plasmodium falciparum with artemether-lumefantrine to reduce malaria disease burden: a modelling and simulation analysis. Malar J. 2011 Jul 29;10:210. PMID:21801345

Kerouedan D. [The Global Fund to fight HIV/AIDS, TB and Malaria 5-y: evaluation policy issues].[Article in French]. Bull Soc Pathol Exot. 2010 May;103(2):119-22. Epub 2010 Apr 7. PMID:20376595

Kerouedan D. [The Global Fund to fight HIV/AIDS, TB and malaria policy issues].[Article in French]. Med Trop (Mars). 2010 Feb;70(1):19-27. PMID:20337110

Kerschbaumer G, Wernsdorfer G, Wiedermann U, Congpuong K, Sirichaisinthop J, Wernsdorfer WH. Synergism between mefloquine and artemisinin and its enhancement by retinol in Plasmodium falciparum in vitro. Wien Klin Wochenschr. 2010 Oct;122 Suppl 3:57-60. PMID:20924698

Kessler AD, Maxey JA, Allan N. Infectious disease case: mixed malaria infection with Plasmodium falciparum and Plasmodium vivax in a deployed service member in Afghanistan. Mil Med. 2011 Oct;176(10):1093-5. PMID:22128640

Khai PN, Van NT, Lua TT, Huu VT, Dang DT, Huong PT, Salazar N, Sukthana Y, Singhasivanon P. The situation of malaria along the Vietnam-Lao PDR border and some related factors. Southeast Asian J Trop Med Public Health. 2000;31 Suppl 1:99-105. PMID:11414469

Khalacheva M. [Immunological studies of Babesia ovis strains isolated from various regions of Bulgaria].[Article in Bulgarian]. Vet Med Nauki. 1974;11(8):103-8. PMID:4446350

Khaminsou N, Kritpetcharat O, Daduang J, Charerntanyarak L, Kritpetcharat P. Genetic analysis of the merozoite surface protein-1 block 2 allelic types in Plasmodium falciparum clinical isolates from Lao PDR. Malar J. 2011 Dec 17;10(1):371. [Epub ahead of print]. PMID:22177111

Khan HM, Shujatullah F, Ashfaq M, Raza A. Changing trends in prevalence of different Plasmodium species with dominance of Plasmodium falciparum malaria infection in Aligarh (India). Asian Pac J Trop Med. 2011 Jan;4(1):64-6. Epub 2011 Jan 15. PMID:21771419

Khan MA, Walley JD, Munir MA, Khan MA, Khokar NG, Tahir Z, Nazir A, Shams N. District level external quality assurance (EQA) of malaria microscopy in Pakistan: pilot implementation and feasibility. Malar J. 2011 Feb 17;10(1):45. PMID:21324210

Kheang ST, Duong S, Olkkonen A. Increasing access to early malaria diagnosis and prompted treatment in remote cambodian villages. Am J Public Health. 2011 Dec;101(12):e6-8. Epub 2011 Oct 20. PMID:22021279

Khodzhaeva NM. [Age-related cytokine regulation in children with malaria].[Article in Russian]. Med Parazitol (Mosk). 2011 Apr-Jun;(2):25-8. PMID:21797062

Kift EV, Kredo T, Barnes KI. Parenteral artesunate access programme aims at reducing malaria fatality rates in South Africa. S Afr Med J. 2011 Apr;101(4):240-1. PMID:21786724

Kigadye ES, Nkwengulila G, Magesa SM, Abdulla S. Diversity, spatial and temporal abundance of Anopheles gambiae complex in the Rufiji River basin, south-eastern Tanzania. Tanzan J Health Res. 2010 Jan;12(1):68-72. PMID:20737831

Kikankie CK, Brooke BD, Knols BG, Koekemoer LL, Farenhorst M, Hunt RH, Thomas MB, Coetzee M. The infectivity of the entomopathogenic fungus Beauveria bassiana to insecticide-resistant and susceptible Anopheles arabiensis mosquitoes at two different temperatures. Malar J. 2010 Mar 8;9:71. PMID:20210990

Kilama WL. Health research ethics in malaria vector trials in Africa. Malar J. 2010 Dec 13;9 Suppl 3:S3. PMID:21144083

Kilian A, Boulay M, Koenker H, Lynch M. How many mosquito nets are needed to achieve universal coverage? Recommendations for the quantification and allocation of long-lasting insecticidal nets for mass campaigns. Malar J. 2010 Nov 18;9:330. PMID:21087460

Killeen GF, Chitnis N, Moore SJ, Okumu FO. Target product profile choices for intra-domiciliary malaria vector control pesticide products: repel or kill? Malar J. 2011 Jul 28;10:207. PMID:21798023

Kim CM, Blanco LB, Alhassan A, Iseki H, Yokoyama N, Xuan X, Igarashi I. Development of a rapid immunochromatographic test for simultaneous serodiagnosis of bovine babesioses caused by Babesia bovis and Babesia bigemina. Am J Trop Med Hyg. 2008 Jan;78(1):117-21. PMID:18187794

Kim D, Kwon S, Rhee JW, Kim KD, Kim YE, Park CS, Choi MJ, Suh JG, Kim DS, Lee Y, Kwon HJ. Production of antibodies with peptide-CpG-DNA-liposome complex without carriers. BMC Immunol. 2011 May 18;12:29. PMID:21592346

Kim JY, Cho SH, Joo HN, Tsuji M, Cho SR, Park IJ, Chung GT, Ju JW, Cheun HI, Lee HW, Lee YH, Kim TS. First case of human babesiosis in Korea: detection and characterization of a novel type of Babesia sp. (KO1) similar to ovine babesia. J Clin Microbiol. 2007 Jun;45(6):2084-7. Epub 2007 Mar 28. PMID:17392446

Kim S, Nguon C, Guillard B, Duong S, Chy S, Sum S, Nhem S, Bouchier C, Tichit M, Christophel E, Taylor WR, Baird JK, Menard D. Performance of the CareStart™ G6PD Deficiency Screening Test, a Point-of-Care Diagnostic for Primaquine Therapy Screening. PLoS One. 2011;6(12):e28357. Epub 2011 Dec 2. PMID:22164279

Kim TS, Kim HH, Moon SU, Lee SS, Shin EH, Oh CM, Kang YJ, Kim DK, Sohn Y, Kim H, Lee HW. The role of Pvs28 in sporozoite development in Anopheles sinensis and its longevity in BALB/c mice. Exp Parasitol. 2011 Feb;127(2):346-50. Epub 2010 Aug 27. PMID:20801117

Kim YK, Kim C, Park I, Kim HY, Choi JY, Kim JM. Therapeutic efficacy of chloroquine in Plasmodium vivax and the pvmdr1 polymorphisms in the Republic of Korea under mass chemoprophylaxis. Am J Trop Med Hyg. 2011 Apr;84(4):532-4. PMID:21460004

Kimbi HK, Fagbenro-Beyioku AF, Oyibo WA. Antimalarial herbs against chloroquine-resistant P. yoelii nigeriensis in mice. Indian J Malariol. 1998 Mar;35(1):35-8. PMID:10212890

Kinde-Gazard D, Vignon Makong J, Kossou HD, Sossa CJ. [Evaluation of the use of insecticide-treated nets and intermittent preventive treatment in three health zones in Benin].[Article in French]. Bull Soc Pathol Exot. 2011 Dec 16. [Epub ahead of print]. PMID:22180050

King AC. Regression of mouse sarcoma M(52)B treated with bovine fascia lata extract from animals previously inoculated with Babesia bovis and B. bigemina. S Afr Med J. 1980 Aug 2;58(5):191-3. PMID:7404219

Kinnamon KE, Rothe WE. Biological screening in the U.S. Army antimalarial drug development program. Am J Trop Med Hyg. 1975 Mar;24(2):174-8. PMID:804264

Kinung'hi SM, Mashauri F, Mwanga JR, Nnko SE, Kaatano GM, Malima R, Kishamawe C, Magesa S, Mboera LE. Knowledge, attitudes and practices about malaria among communities: comparing epidemic and non-epidemic prone communities of Muleba district, North-western Tanzania. BMC Public Health. 2010 Jul 5;10:395. PMID:20602778

Kirira PG, Rukunga GM, Wanyonyi AW, Muregi FM, Gathirwa JW, Muthaura CN, Omar SA, Tolo F, Mungai GM, Ndiege IO. Anti-plasmodial activity and toxicity of extracts of plants used in traditional malaria therapy in Meru and Kilifi Districts of Kenya. J Ethnopharmacol. 2006 Jul 19;106(3):403-7. Epub 2006 Mar 13. PMID:16530996

Kiss G. [Contagious diseases in the Austro-Hungarian Army during the First World War].[Article in Hungarian]. Orvostort Kozl. 2010;56(1-4):197-203. PMID:21661262

Kissou SA, Cessouma R, Barro M, Traoré H, Nacro B. [Acute renal failure and Plasmodium falciparum malaria: A case report]. [Article in French]. Arch Pediatr. 2011 Nov 17. [Epub ahead of print]. PMID:22100415

Kitchener S, Nasveld P, Edstein MD. Tafenoquine for the treatment of recurrent Plasmodium vivax malaria. Am J Trop Med Hyg. 2007 Mar;76(3):494-6. PMID:17360873

Kiurtov N. [Deep freezing of Babesia ovis in liquid nitrogen].[Article in Bulgarian]. Vet Med Nauki. 1977;14(6):11-5. PMID:595370

Kiurtov N. [Production of a Babesia ovis extract and its testing for antigenic properties].[Article in Bulgarian]. Vet Med Nauki. 1979;16(4):84-90. PMID:532096

Kiurtov N. [Soluble Babesia ovis antigen].[Article in Bulgarian]. Vet Med Nauki. 1979;16(3):15-22. PMID:93342

Kiurtov N. [Trial of a live vaccine against babesiasis in sheep].[Article in Bulgarian]. Vet Med Nauki. 1977;14(4):25-30. PMID:929961

Kivaria FM, Ruheta MR, Mkonyi PA, Malamsha PC. Epidemiological aspects and economic impact of bovine theileriosis (East Coast fever) and its control: a preliminary assessment with special reference to Kibaha district, Tanzania. Vet J. 2007 Mar;173(2):384-90. Epub 2005 Oct 5. PMID:16169755

Kjemtrup AM, Conrad PA. A review of the small canine piroplasms from California: Babesia conradae in the literature. Vet Parasitol. 2006 May 31;138(1-2):112-7. Epub 2006 Mar 7. PMID:16522352

Kjemtrup AM, Lee B, Fritz CL, Evans C, Chervenak M, Conrad PA. Investigation of transfusion transmission of a WA1-type babesial parasite to a premature infant in California. Transfusion. 2002 Nov;42(11):1482-7. PMID:12421222

Kjemtrup AM, Wainwright K, Miller M, Penzhorn BL, Carreno RA. Babesia conradae, sp. Nov., a small canine Babesia identified in California. Vet Parasitol. 2006 May 31;138(1-2):103-11. Epub 2006 Mar 9. PMID:16524663

Klinkenberg E, Onwona-Agyeman KA, McCall PJ, Wilson MD, Bates I, Verhoeff FH, Barnish G, Donnelly MJ. Cohort trial reveals community impact of insecticide-treated nets on malariometric indices in urban Ghana. Trans R Soc Trop Med Hyg. 2010 Jul;104(7):496-503. Epub 2010 Apr 24. PMID:20417945

Klonis N, Crespo-Ortiz MP, Bottova I, Abu-Bakar N, Kenny S, Rosenthal PJ, Tilley L. Artemisinin activity against Plasmodium falciparum requires hemoglobin uptake and digestion. Proc Natl Acad Sci U S A. 2011 Jul 12;108(28):11405-10. Epub 2011 Jun 27. PMID:21709259

Knight DJ. Babesia rodhaini and Plasmodium berghei. A highly active series of chlorophenoxyalkoxy-substituted diamino-dihydrotriazines against experimental infections in mice. Ann Trop Med Parasitol. 1981 Feb;75(1):1-6. PMID:7023398

Knowles JH. Editorial: American medicine and world health 1976. Ann Intern Med. 1976 Apr;84(4):483-5. PMID:1259295

Kobak S, Deveci H. Retinopathy due to antimalarial drugs in patients with connective tissue diseases: are they so innocent? A single center retrospective study. Int J Rheum Dis. 2010 Aug;13(3):e11-5. PMID:20704603

Kobylinski KC, Sylla M, Chapman PL, Sarr MD, Foy BD. Ivermectin mass drug administration to humans disrupts malaria parasite transmission in Senegalese villages. Am J Trop Med Hyg. 2011 Jul;85(1):3-5. PMID:21734116

Kocan KM. Targeting ticks for control of selected hemoparasitic diseases of cattle. Vet Parasitol. 1995 Mar;57(1-3):121-51. PMID:7597779

Koch HT, Kambeva L, Ocama JG, Munatswa FC, Franssen FF, Uilenberg G, Dolan TT, Norval RA. Immunization of cattle against Theileria parva bovis and their exposure to natural challenge. Vet Parasitol. 1990 Nov;37(3-4):185-96. PMID:2125158

Kocisko DA, Walsh DS, Eamsila C, Edstein MD. Measurement of tafenoquine (WR 238605) in human plasma and venous and capillary blood by high-pressure liquid chromatography. Ther Drug Monit. 2000 Apr;22(2):184-9. PMID:10774631

Kok LD, Wong CK, Leung KN, Tsang SF, Fung KP, Choy YM. Activation of the anti-tumor effector cells by Radix bupleuri. Immunopharmacology. 1995 Jun;30(1):79-87. PMID:7591716

Kolabskiĭ NA, Gaĭdukov AKh, Vorob'ev VV, Sivak DA, Voevoda NI. [Combined chemoprophylaxis of babesiasis in cattle].[Article in Russian]. Veterinariia. 1973 Feb;3:71-3. PMID:4770054

Kolaczinski JH, Robinson E, Finn TP. The cost of antibiotic mass drug administration for trachoma control in a remote area of South Sudan. PLoS Negl Trop Dis. 2011 Oct;5(10):e1362. Epub 2011 Oct 11. PMID:22022632

Kolaczinski K, Durrani N, Rahim S, Rowland M. Sulfadoxine-pyrimethamine plus artesunate compared with chloroquine for the treatment of vivax malaria in areas co-endemic for Plasmodium falciparum and P. vivax: a randomised non-inferiority trial in eastern Afghanistan. Trans R Soc Trop Med Hyg. 2007 Nov;101(11):1081-7. Epub 2007 Aug 17. PMID:17707447

Kolören Z, Avşar C, Şekeroğlu ZA. [Diagnosis of protozoa by loop-mediated isothermal amplification: (LAMP)].[Article in Turkish]. Turkiye Parazitol Derg. 2010;34(4):207-11. PMID:21391196

Komatsu R, McLeod R, Sarkar S, Siripong N, Gupta I, Tangcharoensathien V, Brown T, Jeugmans J, Avila-Figueroa C, Atun R. Asia can afford universal access for AIDS prevention and treatment. AIDS. 2010 Sep;24 Suppl 3:S72-9. PMID:20926931

Kortagere S, Welsh WJ, Morrisey JM, Daly T, Ejigiri I, Sinnis P, Vaidya AB, Bergman LW. Structure-based design of novel small-molecule inhibitors of Plasmodium falciparum. J Chem Inf Model. 2010 May 24;50(5):840-9. PMID:20426475

Kosower NS, Kosower EM. Molecular basis for selective advantage of glucose-6-phosphate-dehydrogenase-deficient individuals exposed to malaria. Lancet. 1970 Dec 26;2(7687):1343-4. PMID:4098912

Kostense S, Mommaas B, Hendriks J, Verhoeven M, Ter Haak M, Tirion F, Wiesken E, Pau MG, Radosevic K, Goudsmit J. A peptide-based Plasmodium falciparum circumsporozoite assay to test for serum antibody responses to pre-erythrocyte malaria vaccines. Clin Vaccine Immunol. 2011 May;18(5):776-82. Epub 2011 Mar 16. PMID:21411600

Köster LS, Van Schoor M, Goddard A, Thompson PN, Matjila PT, Kjelgaard-Hansen M. C-reactive protein in canine babesiosis caused by Babesia rossi and its association with outcome. J S Afr Vet Assoc. 2009 Jun;80(2):87-91. PMID:19831269

Kozlov S, Waters NC, Chavchich M. Leveraging cell cycle analysis in anticancer drug discovery to identify novel plasmodial drug targets. Infect Disord Drug Targets. 2010 Jun;10(3):165-90. PMID:20334621

Krause PJ, Gewurz BE, Hill D, Marty FM, Vannier E, Foppa IM, Furman RR, Neuhaus E, Skowron G, Gupta S, McCalla C, Pesanti EL, Young M, Heiman D, Hsue G, Gelfand JA, Wormser GP, Dickason J, Bia FJ, Hartman B, Telford SR 3rd, Christianson D, Dardick K, Coleman M, Girotto JE, Spielman A. Persistent and relapsing babesiosis in immunocompromised patients. Clin Infect Dis. 2008 Feb 1;46(3):370-6. PMID:18181735

Krause PJ, Gewurz BE, Hill D, Marty FM, Vannier E, Foppa IM, Furman RR, Neuhaus E, Skowron G, Gupta S, McCalla C, Pesanti EL, Young M, Heiman D, Hsue G, Gelfand JA, Wormser GP, Dickason J, Bia FJ, Hartman B, Telford SR 3rd, Christianson D, Dardick K, da Silva RA, Corrêa Fdo N, Botteon Rde C, Botteon Pde T. [Natural infection by hemoparasites in calves submitted to chemoprophylaxis at 30 days of age].[Article in Portuguese]. Rev Bras Parasitol Vet. 2007 Jul-Sep;16(3):163-5. PMID:18078605

Krause PJ, Lepore T, Sikand VK, Gadbaw J Jr, Burke G, Telford SR 3rd, Brassard P, Pearl D, Azlanzadeh J, Christianson D, McGrath D, Spielman A. Atovaquone and azithromycin for the treatment of babesiosis. N Engl J Med. 2000 Nov 16;343(20):1454-8. PMID:11078770

Krause PJ, Spielman A, Telford SR 3rd, Sikand VK, McKay K, Christianson D, Pollack RJ, Brassard P, Magera J, Ryan R, Persing DH. Persistent parasitemia after acute babesiosis. N Engl J Med. 1998 Jul 16;339(3):160-5. PMID:9664092

Krause PJ. Babesiosis diagnosis and treatment. Vector Borne Zoonotic Dis. 2003 Spring;3(1):45-51. PMID:12804380

Krause PJ. Babesiosis. Med Clin North Am. 2002 Mar;86(2):361-73. PMID:11982307

Kreidenweiss A, Kremsner PG, Mordmüller B. Comprehensive study of proteasome inhibitors against Plasmodium falciparum laboratory strains and field isolates from Gabon. Malar J. 2008 Sep 24;7:187. PMID:18816382

Kremsner P. [New preventive antimalaria drug. 3 tables, 2 months of protection. Interview by Petra Eiden].[Article in German]. MMW Fortschr Med. 2000 Sep 21;142(38):13. PMID:11050883

Kremsner PG, Taylor T, Issifou S, Kombila M, Chimalizeni Y, Kawaza K, Bouyou Akotet MK, Duscha M, Mordmüller B, Kösters K, Humberg A, Miller RS, Weina P, Duparc S, Möhrle J, Kun JF, Planche T, Teja-Isavadharm P, Simpson JA, Köhler C, Krishna S. A simplified intravenous artesunate regimen for severe malaria. J Infect Dis. 2012 Jan;205(2):312-9. Epub 2011 Dec 15. PMID:22180622

Kreuels B, Kreuzberg C, Kobbe R, Ayim-Akonor M, Apiah-Thompson P, Thompson B, Ehmen C, Adjei S, Langefeld I, Adjei O, May J. Differing effects of HbS and HbC traits on uncomplicated falciparum malaria, anemia, and child growth. Blood. 2010 Jun 3;115(22):4551-8. Epub 2010 Mar 15. PMID:20231425

Krieg AM. Mechanisms and applications of immune stimulatory CpG oligodeoxynucleotides. Biochim Biophys Acta. 1999 Dec 10;1489(1):107-16. PMID:10807001

Krishnan S, Krishnan AD, Mustafa AS, Talwar GP, Ramalingaswami V. Effect of vitamin A and undernutrition on the susceptibility of rodents to a malarial parasite Plasmodium berghei. J Nutr. 1976 Jun;106(6):784-91. PMID:818347

Kritsiriwuthinan K, Chaotheing S, Shaw PJ, Wongsombat C, Chavalitshewinkoon-Petmitr P, Kamchonwongpaisan S. Global gene expression profiling of Plasmodium falciparum in response to the anti-malarial drug pyronaridine. Malar J. 2011 Aug 18;10:242. PMID:21849091

Krudsood S, Looareesuwan S, Tangpukdee N, Wilairatana P, Phumratanaprapin W, Leowattana W, Chalermrut K, Ramanathan S, Navaratnam V, Olliaro P, Vaillant M, Kiechel JR, Taylor WR. New fixed-dose artesunate-mefloquine formulation against multidrug-resistant Plasmodium falciparum in adults: a comparative phase IIb safety and pharmacokinetic study with standard-dose nonfixed artesunate plus mefloquine. Antimicrob Agents Chemother. 2010 Sep;54(9):3730-7. Epub 2010 Jun 14. PMID:20547795

Kudom AA, Mensah BA. The potential role of the educational system in addressing the effect of inadequate knowledge of mosquitoes on use of insecticide-treated nets in Ghana. Malar J. 2010 Sep 15;9:256. PMID:20843345

Kückelhaus SA, Leite JR, Muniz-Junqueira MI, Sampaio RN, Bloch C Jr, Tosta CE. Antiplasmodial and antileishmanial activities of phylloseptin-1, an antimicrobial peptide from the skin secretion of Phyllomedusa azurea (Amphibia). Exp Parasitol. 2009 Sep;123(1):11-6. Epub 2009 May 19. PMID:19460376

Kuemmerle A, Dodoo AN, Olsson S, Van Erps J, Burri C, Lalvani PS. Assessment of global reporting of adverse drug reactions for anti-malarials, including artemisinin-based combination therapy, to the WHO Programme for International Drug Monitoring. Malar J. 2011 Mar 9;10:57. PMID:21388536

Küttel C, Nascimento E, Demierre N, Silva T, Braschler T, Renaud P, Oliva AG. Label-free detection of Babesia bovis infected red blood cells using impedance spectroscopy on a microfabricated flow cytometer. Acta Trop. 2007 Apr;102(1):63-8. Epub 2007 Mar 12. PMID:17451631

Kueviakoe IM, Segbena AY, Jouault H, Vovor A, Imbert M. Hematological reference values for healthy adults in togo. ISRN Hematol. 2011;2011:736062. Epub 2010 Nov 7. PMID:22084703

Kuhner A. The impact of public health programs on economic development. Report of a study of malaria in Thailand. Int J Health Serv. 1971 Aug;1(3):285-92. PMID:5136231

Kumar S, Gupta AK, Pal Y, Dwivedi SK. In-vivo therapeutic efficacy trial with artemisinin derivative, buparvaquone and imidocarb dipropionate against Babesia equi infection in donkeys. J Vet Med Sci. 2003 Nov;65(11):1171-7. PMID:14665744

Kumar S, Kumar R, Sugimoto C. A perspective on Theileria equi infections in donkeys. Jpn J Vet Res. 2009 Feb;56(4):171-80. PMID:19358444

Kumar S, Malhotra DV, Dhar S, Nichani AK. Vaccination of donkeys against Babesia equi using killed merozoite immunogen. Vet Parasitol. 2002 May 30;106(1):19-33. PMID:11992708

Kumar S, Malhotra DV, Nichani AK. Identification of immunoreactive polypeptides of Babesia equi parasite during immunization. Vet Parasitol. 2002 Aug 22;107(4):295-301. PMID:12163241

Kumari A, Gakhar SK, Hooda V. Antibodies raised against hemolymph of Anopheles culicifacies reduce the fecundity and malaria parasite development. J Vector Borne Dis. 2009 Dec;46(4):255-60. PMID:19959850

Kung'u MW, Goodger BV, Bushell GR, Wright IG, Waltisbuhl DJ. Vaccination of cattle with dextran sulphate-binding Babesia bigemina antigens. Int J Parasitol. 1992 Aug;22(5):621-5. PMID:1399246

Kuppusamy C, Murugan K. Effects of Andrographis paniculata Nees on growth, development and reproduction of malarial vector Anopheles stephensi Liston (Diptera: Culicidae). Trop Biomed. 2010 Dec;27(3):509-16. PMID:21399593

Kurth F, Bélard S, Adegnika AA, Gaye O, Kremsner PG, Ramharter M. Do paediatric drug formulations of artemisinin combination therapies improve the treatment of children with malaria? A systematic review and meta-analysis. Lancet Infect Dis. 2010 Feb;10(2):125-32. PMID:20113981

Kurth F, Pongratz P, Bélard S, Mordmüller B, Kremsner PG, Ramharter M. In vitro activity of pyronaridine against Plasmodium falciparum and comparative evaluation of anti-malarial drug susceptibility assays. Malar J. 2009 Apr 23;8:79. PMID:19389221

Kusi KA, Faber BW, Thomas AW, Remarque EJ. Humoral immune response to mixed PfAMA1 alleles; multivalent PfAMA1 vaccines induce broad specificity. PLoS One. 2009 Dec 1;4(12):e8110. PMID:19956619

Kuttler KL, Johnson LW. Immunization of cattle with a Babesia bigemina antigen in Freund's complete adjuvant. Am J Vet Res. 1980 Apr;41(4):536-8. PMID:7406273

Kuttler KL, Levy MG, James MA, Ristic M. Efficacy of a nonviable culture-derived Babesia bovis vaccine. Am J Vet Res. 1982 Feb;43(2):281-4. PMID:7046534

Kuttler KL, Levy MG, Ristic M. Cell culture-derived Babesia bovis vaccine: sequential challenge exposure of protective immunity during a 6-month postvaccination period. Am J Vet Res. 1983 Aug;44(8):1456-9. PMID:6354014

Kuttler KL, Zaugg JL, Gipson CA. Imidocarb and parvaquone in the treatment of piroplasmosis (Babesia equi) in equids. Am J Vet Res. 1987 Nov;48(11):1613-6. PMID:3434908

Kuttler KL, Zaugg JL, Yunker CE. The pathogenicity and immunologic relationship of a virulent and a tissue-culture-adapted Babesia bovis. Vet Parasitol. 1988 Mar;27(3-4):239-44. PMID:3285573

Kuttler KL. The effect of Imidocarb treatment on Babesia in the bovine and the tick (Boophilus microplus). Res Vet Sci. 1975 Mar;18(2):198-200. PMID:1129539

Kuwayama DP, Briones RJ. Spontaneous splenic rupture caused by Babesia microti infection. Clin Infect Dis. 2008 May 1;46(9):e92-5. PMID:18419430

Kwansa-Bentum B, Ayi I, Suzuki T, Otchere J, Kumagai T, Anyan WK, Asahi H, Akao N, Wilson MD, Boakye DA, Ohta N. Administrative practices of health professionals and use of artesunate-amodiaquine by community members for treating uncomplicated malaria in southern Ghana: implications for artemisinin-based combination therapy deployment. Trop Med Int Health. 2011 Jul 10. [Epub ahead of print]. PMID:21740487

Kwansa-Bentum B, Ayi I, Suzuki T, Otchere J, Kumagai T, Anyan WK, Osei JH, Asahi H, Ofori MF, Akao N, Wilson MD, Boakye DA, Ohta N. Plasmodium falciparum isolates from southern Ghana exhibit polymorphisms in the SERCA-type PfATPase6 though sensitive to artesunate in vitro. Malar J. 2011 Jul 11;10:187. PMID:21745377

Kweka EJ, Mosha F, Lowassa A, Mahande AM, Kitau J, Matowo J, Mahande MJ, Massenga CP, Tenu F, Feston E, Lyatuu EE, Mboya MA, Mndeme R, Chuwa G, Temu EA. Ethnobotanical study of some of mosquito repellent plants in north-eastern Tanzania. Malar J. 2008 Aug 7;7:152. PMID:18687119

Kweka EJ, Mosha FW, Lowassa A, Mahande AM, Mahande MJ, Massenga CP, Tenu F, Lyatuu EE, Mboya MA, Temu EA. Longitudinal evaluation of Ocimum and other plants effects on the feeding behavioral response of mosquitoes (Diptera: Culicidae) in the field in Tanzania. Parasit Vectors. 2008 Oct 22;1(1):42. PMID:18945343

Kweka EJ, Nyindo M, Mosha F, Silva AG. Insecticidal activity of the essential oil from fruits and seeds of Schinus terebinthifolia Raddi against African malaria vectors. Parasit Vectors. 2011 Jul 5;4:129. PMID:21729280

Kwon Y, Kim SH, Ronderos DS, Lee Y, Akitake B, Woodward OM, Guggino WB, Smith DP, Montell C. Drosophila TRPA1 channel is required to avoid the naturally occurring insect repellent citronellal. Curr Biol. 2010 Sep 28;20(18):1672-8. PMID:20797863

Kyabayinze DJ, Asiimwe C, Nakanjako D, Nabakooza J, Counihan H, Tibenderana JK. Use of RDTs to improve malaria diagnosis and fever case management at primary health care facilities in Uganda. Malar J. 2010 Jul 12;9:200. PMID:20624312

Labarthe NV, Remião JO, Sacco AM, Maia LC. Cross-reaction of tick salivary antigens in the Boophilus microplus-cattle system. Vet Parasitol. 1985 Mar;17(3):259-63. PMID:3992881

Labbé AC, Loutfy MR, Kain KC. Recent Advances in the Prophylaxis and Treatment of Malaria. Curr Infect Dis Rep. 2001 Feb;3(1):68-76. PMID:11177733

Lacerda-Queiroz N, Rodrigues DH, Vilela MC, Rachid MA, Soriani FM, Sousa LP, Campos RD, Quesniaux VF, Teixeira MM, Teixeira AL. Platelet-activating factor receptor is essential for the development of experimental cerebral malaria. Am J Pathol. 2012 Jan;180(1):246-55. Epub 2011 Nov 8. PMID:22079430

LaCrue AN, Scheel M, Kennedy K, Kumar N, Kyle DE. Effects of artesunate on parasite recrudescence and dormancy in the rodent malaria model Plasmodium vinckei. PLoS One. 2011;6(10):e26689. Epub 2011 Oct 24. PMID:22039533

Laing AB. Studies on the chemotherapy of malaria. II. Pyrimethamine resistance in The Gambia. Trans R Soc Trop Med Hyg. 1970;64(4):569-80. PMID:4922133

Lança AS, de Sousa KP, Atouguia J, Prazeres DM, Monteiro GA, Silva MS. Trypanosoma brucei: immunisation with plasmid DNA encoding invariant surface glycoprotein gene is able to induce partial protection in experimental African trypanosomiasis. Exp Parasitol. 2011 Jan;127(1):18-24. Epub 2010 Jun 18. PMID:20599996

Lantos PM, Krause PJ. Babesiosis: similar to malaria but different. Pediatr Ann. 2002 Mar;31(3):192-7. PMID:11905293

LaRocque RC, Jentes ES. Health recommendations for international travel: a review of the evidence base of travel medicine. Curr Opin Infect Dis. 2011 Oct;24(5):403-9. PMID:21788892

Larocque RC, Rao SR, Lee J, Ansdell V, Yates JA, Schwartz BS, Knouse M, Cahill J, Hagmann S, Vinetz J, Connor BA, Goad JA, Oladele A, Alvarez S, Stauffer W, Walker P, Kozarsky P, Franco-Paredes C, Dismukes R, Rosen J, Hynes NA, Jacquerioz F, McLellan S, Hale D, Sofarelli T, Schoenfeld D, Marano N, Brunette G, Jentes ES, Yanni E, Sotir MJ, Ryan ET; the Global TravEpiNet Consortium. Global TravEpiNet: A National Consortium of Clinics Providing Care to International Travelers--Analysis of Demographic Characteristics, Travel Destinations, and Pretravel Healthcare of High-Risk US International Travelers, 2009-2011. Clin Infect Dis. 2011 Dec 5. [Epub ahead of print]. PMID:22144534

Larsen DA, Keating J, Miller J, Bennett A, Changufu C, Katebe C, Eisele TP. Barriers to insecticide-treated mosquito net possession 2 years after a mass free distribution campaign in Luangwa District, Zambia. PLoS One. 2010 Nov 10;5(11):e13129. PMID:21085711

Last RD, Hill JM, Matjila PT, Rème CA. A field trial evaluation of the prophylactic efficacy of amitraz-impregnated collars against canine babesiosis (Babesia canis rossi) in South Africa. J S Afr Vet Assoc. 2007 Jun;78(2):63-5. PMID:17941596

Lau AO. An overview of the Babesia, Plasmodium and Theileria genomes: a comparative perspective. Mol Biochem Parasitol. 2009 Mar;164(1):1-8. Epub 2008 Dec 6. PMID:19110007

Lau PK, Woods ML, Ratanjee SK, John GT. Artesunate is ineffective in controlling valganciclovir-resistant cytomegalovirus infection. Clin Infect Dis. 2011 Jan 15;52(2):279. PMID:21288859

Laufer MK, Takala-Harrison S, Dzinjalamala FK, Stine OC, Taylor TE, Plowe CV. Return of chloroquine-susceptible falciparum malaria in Malawi was a reexpansion of diverse susceptible parasites. J Infect Dis. 2010 Sep 1;202(5):801-8. PMID:20662717

Laupattarakasem P, Houghton PJ, Hoult JR, Itharat A. An evaluation of the activity related to inflammation of four plants used in Thailand to treat arthritis. J Ethnopharmacol. 2003 Apr;85(2-3):207-15. PMID:12639742

Laupattarakasem P, Wangsrimongkol T, Surarit R, Hahnvajanawong C. In vitro and in vivo anti-inflammatory potential of Cryptolepis buchanani. J Ethnopharmacol. 2006 Dec 6;108(3):349-54. Epub 2006 Jun 6. PMID:16831527

Lavrado J, Moreira R, Paulo A. Indoloquinolines as scaffolds for drug discovery. Curr Med Chem. 2010;17(22):2348-70. PMID:20491639

Lawrence JA, de Vos AJ. Methods currently used for the control of anaplasmosis and babesiosis: their validity and proposals for future control strategies. Parassitologia. 1990 Apr;32(1):63-71. PMID:2284136

Lawrence JA, Malika J, Whiteland AP, Kafuwa P. Efficacy of an Australian Babesia bovis vaccine strain in Malawi. Vet Rec. 1993 Mar 20;132(12):295-6. PMID:8470344

Lawrence JA, Musisi FL, Mfitilodze MW, Tjornehoj K, Whiteland AP, Kafuwa PT, Chamambala KE. Integrated tick and tick-borne disease control trials in crossbred dairy cattle in Malawi. Trop Anim Health Prod. 1996 Nov;28(4):280-8. PMID:8983132

Lawrence JA, Whiteland AP, Malika J, Kafuwa P, Jongejan F. Use of serological response to evaluate heartwater immunization of cattle. Rev Elev Med Vet Pays Trop. 1993;46(1-2):211-5. PMID:8134634

Lawrence JA. Conventional vaccines for tick-borne haemoparasitic diseases of sheep and goats. Parassitologia. 1997 Jun;39(2):119-21. PMID:9530695

Lazarus JV, Curth N, Bridge J, Atun R. Know your epidemic, know your response: targeting HIV in Asia. AIDS. 2010 Sep;24 Suppl 3:S95-9. PMID:20926934

Le Port A, Watier L, Cottrell G, Ouédraogo S, Dechavanne C, Pierrat C, Rachas A, Bouscaillou J, Bouraima A, Massougbodji A, Fayomi B, Thiébaut A, Chandre F, Migot-Nabias F, Martin-Prevel Y, Garcia A, Cot M. Infections in Infants during the First 12 Months of Life: Role of Placental Malaria and Environmental Factors. PLoS One. 2011;6(11):e27516. Epub 2011 Nov 11. PMID:22096588

Le Roch KG, Chung DW, Ponts N. Genomics and Integrated Systems Biology in Plasmodium falciparum: A Path to Malaria Control and Eradication. Parasite Immunol. 2011 Oct 13. [Epub ahead of print]. PMID:21995286

Leary KJ, Riel MA, Roy MJ, Cantilena LR, Bi D, Brater DC, van de Pol C, Pruett K, Kerr C, Veazey JM Jr, Beboso R, Ohrt C. A randomized, double-blind, safety and tolerability study to assess the ophthalmic and renal effects of tafenoquine 200 mg weekly versus placebo for 6 months in healthy volunteers. Am J Trop Med Hyg. 2009 Aug;81(2):356-62. PMID:19635898

Lee BP. Apnea, bradycardia and thrombocytopenia in a premature infant. Pediatr Infect Dis J. 2001 Aug;20(8):816, 820-2. PMID:11734753

Lee GC, Jeon ES, Le DT, Kim TS, Yoo JH, Kim HY, Chong CK. Development and Evaluation of a Rapid Diagnostic Test for Plasmodium falciparum, P. vivax, and Mixed-Species Malaria Antigens. Am J Trop Med Hyg. 2011 Dec;85(6):989-993. PMID:22144432

Lee S, Carson K, Rice-Ficht A, Good T. Hsp20, a novel alpha-crystallin, prevents Abeta fibril formation and toxicity. Protein Sci. 2005 Mar;14(3):593-601. PMID:15722443

Lee S, Carson K, Rice-Ficht A, Good T. Small heat shock proteins differentially affect Abeta aggregation and toxicity. Biochem Biophys Res Commun. 2006 Aug 25;347(2):527-33. Epub 2006 Jun 30. PMID:16828710

Leiby DA, Chung AP, Cable RG, Trouern-Trend J, McCullough J, Homer MJ, Reynolds LD, Houghton RL, Lodes MJ, Persing DH. Relationship between tick bites and the seroprevalence of Babesia microti and Anaplasma phagocytophila (previously Ehrlichia sp.) in blood donors. Transfusion. 2002 Dec;42(12):1585-91. PMID:12473139

Leiby DA, Chung AP, Gill JE, Houghton RL, Persing DH, Badon S, Cable RG. Demonstrable parasitemia among Connecticut blood donors with antibodies to Babesia microti. Transfusion. 2005 Nov;45(11):1804-10. PMID:16271108

Leiby DA, Gill JE. Transfusion-transmitted tick-borne infections: a cornucopia of threats. Transfus Med Rev. 2004 Oct;18(4):293-306. PMID:15497129

Leiby DA. Babesiosis and blood transfusion: flying under the radar. Vox Sang. 2006 Apr;90(3):157-65. PMID:16507014

Leiby DA. Threats to blood safety posed by emerging protozoan pathogens. Vox Sang. 2004 Jul;87 Suppl 2:120-2. PMID:15209895

Leiby DA. Transfusion-associated babesiosis: shouldn't we be ticked off? Ann Intern Med. 2011 Oct 18;155(8):556-7. Epub 2011 Sep 5. PMID:21893616

Leiby DA. Transfusion-transmitted Babesia spp.: bull's-eye on Babesia microti. Clin Microbiol Rev. 2011 Jan;24(1):14-28. PMID:21233506

Leimanis ML, Jaidee A, Sriprawat K, Kaewpongsri S, Suwanarusk R, Barends M, Phyo AP, Russell B, Renia L, Nosten F. Plasmodium vivax susceptibility to ferroquine. Antimicrob Agents Chemother. 2010 May;54(5):2228-30. Epub 2010 Mar 22. PMID:20308387

Leisewitz AL, Guthrie AJ, Berry WL. Evaluation of the effect of whole-blood transfusion on the oxygen status and acid-base balance of Babesia canis infected dogs using the oxygen status algorithm. J S Afr Vet Assoc. 1996 Mar;67(1):20-6. PMID:8786612

Leisewitz AL, Jacobson LS, de Morais HS, Reyers F. The mixed acid-base disturbances of severe canine babesiosis. J Vet Intern Med. 2001 Sep-Oct;15(5):445-52. PMID:11596731

Leitao R, Rodriguez A. Inhibition of Plasmodium sporozoites infection by targeting the host cell. Exp Parasitol. 2010 Oct;126(2):273-7. Epub 2010 May 21. PMID:20493847

Leitner WW, Bergmann-Leitner ES, Angov E. Comparison of Plasmodium berghei challenge models for the evaluation of pre-erythrocytic malaria vaccines and their effect on perceived vaccine efficacy. Malar J. 2010 May 27;9:145. PMID:20507620

Lekana-Douki JB, Dinzouna Boutamba SD, Zatra R, Zang Edou SE, Ekomy H, Bisvigou U, Toure-Ndouo FS. Increased prevalence of the Plasmodium falciparum Pfmdr1 86N genotype among field isolates from Franceville, Gabon after replacement of chloroquine by artemether-lumefantrine and artesunate-mefloquine. Infect Genet Evol. 2011 Mar;11(2):512-7. Epub 2011 Jan 17. PMID:21251998

Leke RG, Taylor DW. The use of intermittent preventive treatment with sulfadoxine-pyrimethamine for preventing malaria in pregnant women. Clin Infect Dis. 2011 Aug 1;53(3):231-3. PMID:21765071

Lek-Uthai U, Suwanarusk R, Ruengweerayut R, Skinner-Adams TS, Nosten F, Gardiner DL, Boonma P, Piera KA, Andrews KT, Machunter B, McCarthy JS, Anstey NM, Price RN, Russell B. Stronger activity of human immunodeficiency virus type 1 protease inhibitors against clinical isolates of Plasmodium vivax than against those of P. falciparum. Antimicrob Agents Chemother. 2008 Jul;52(7):2435-41. Epub 2008 Apr 28. PMID:18443130

Lell B, Agnandji S, von Glasenapp I, Haertle S, Oyakhiromen S, Issifou S, Vekemans J, Leach A, Lievens M, Dubois MC, Demoitie MA, Carter T, Villafana T, Ballou WR, Cohen J, Kremsner PG. A randomized trial assessing the safety and immunogenicity of AS01 and AS02 adjuvanted RTS,S malaria vaccine candidates in children in Gabon. PLoS One. 2009 Oct 27;4(10):e7611. PMID:19859560

Lell B, Faucher JF, Missinou MA, Borrmann S, Dangelmaier O, Horton J, Kremsner PG. Malaria chemoprophylaxis with tafenoquine: a randomised study. Lancet. 2000 Jun 10;355(9220):2041-5. PMID:10885356

Lemma H, Lofgren C, San Sebastian M. Adherence to a six-dose regimen of artemether-lumefantrine among uncomplicated Plasmodium falciparum patients in the Tigray Region, Ethiopia. Malar J. 2011 Dec 5;10(1):349. [Epub ahead of print]. PMID:22141751

Leoni P, Luchini S. Designing the financial tools to promote universal access to AIDS care. J Health Econ. 2011 Jan;30(1):181-8. Epub 2010 Nov 12. PMID:21126788

Lepes T. Research related to malaria. A review of achievements and further needs. Am J Trop Med Hyg. 1972 Sep;21(5):640-7. PMID:4627544

Leroux-Roels G. Unmet needs in modern vaccinology: adjuvants to improve the immune response. Vaccine. 2010 Aug 31;28 Suppl 3:C25-36. PMID:20713254

Leroy E, Baize S, Gonzalez JP. [Ebola and Marburg hemorrhagic fever viruses: update on filoviruses].[Article in French]. Med Trop (Mars). 2011 Apr;71(2):111-21. PMID:21695865

Lewis BD, Penzhorn BL, López Rebollar LM. Immune responses to South African Babesia canis and the development of a preliminary vaccine. J S Afr Vet Assoc. 1995 Jun;66(2):61-5. PMID:8544162

Lewis BD, Penzhorn BL, Volkmann DH. Could treatment of pregnant mares prevent abortions due to equine piroplasmosis? J S Afr Vet Assoc. 1999 Jun;70(2):90-1. PMID:10855828

Lewis RL. Blood transfusion in a case of bovine piroplasmosis. Vet Rec. 1946 Nov 30;58(48):568. PMID:20279641

L'Hostis M. Epidemiology and vaccination strategy: Babesia divergens bovine babesiosis example. Vet Res. 1995;26(3):240-3. PMID:7795691

Li B, Yao Q, Pan XC, Wang N, Zhang R, Li J, Ding G, Liu X, Wu C, Ran D, Zheng J, Zhou H. Artesunate enhances the antibacterial effect of {beta}-lactam antibiotics against Escherichia coli by increasing antibiotic accumulation via inhibition of the multidrug efflux pump system AcrAB-TolC. J Antimicrob Chemother. 2011 Apr;66(4):769-77. Epub 2011 Feb 9. PMID:21393180

Li J, Zhu JD, Appiah A, McCutchan TF, Long GW, Milhous WK, Hollingdale MR. Plasmodium berghei: quantitation of in vitro effects of antimalarial drugs on exoerythrocytic development by a ribosomal RNA probe. Exp Parasitol. 1991 May;72(4):450-8. PMID:2026219

Li J. [Forty-two cases of malaria treated with ginger-partitioned moxibustion in the Republic of Congo].[Article in Chinese]. Zhongguo Zhen Jiu. 2011 Jun;31(6):559-61. PMID:21739708

Li PN, Khitenkova LP. [Imidocarb, a highly effective preparation in animal piroplasmosis (a survey of the foreign literature)].[Article in Russian]. Veterinariia. 1973 Jan;49(1):117-9. PMID:4756636

Li Q, Weina PJ. Severe embryotoxicity of artemisinin derivatives in experimental animals, but possibly safe in pregnant women. Molecules. 2009 Dec 25;15(1):40-57. PMID:20110870

Li X, Ling V, Li PC. Same-single-cell analysis for the study of drug efflux modulation of multidrug resistant cells using a microfluidic chip. Anal Chem. 2008 Jun 1;80(11):4095-102. Epub 2008 Apr 30. PMID:18447319

Liljander A, Chandramohan D, Kweku M, Olsson D, Montgomery SM, Greenwood B, Färnert A. Influences of intermittent preventive treatment and persistent multiclonal Plasmodium falciparum infections on clinical malaria risk. PLoS One. 2010 Oct 27;5(10):e13649. PMID:21048970

Lim P, Alker AP, Khim N, Shah NK, Incardona S, Doung S, Yi P, Bouth DM, Bouchier C, Puijalon OM, Meshnick SR, Wongsrichanalai C, Fandeur T, Le Bras J, Ringwald P, Ariey F. Pfmdr1 copy number and arteminisin derivatives combination therapy failure in falciparum malaria in Cambodia. Malar J. 2009 Jan 12;8:11. PMID:19138391

Lim P, Wongsrichanalai C, Chim P, Khim N, Kim S, Chy S, Sem R, Nhem S, Yi P, Duong S, Bouth DM, Genton B, Beck HP, Gobert JG, Rogers WO, Coppee JY, Fandeur T, Mercereau-Puijalon O, Ringwald P, Le Bras J, Ariey F. Decreased in vitro susceptibility of Plasmodium falciparum isolates to artesunate, mefloquine, chloroquine, and quinine in Cambodia from 2001 to 2007. Antimicrob Agents Chemother. 2010 May;54(5):2135-42. Epub 2010 Mar 1. PMID:20194689

Lima FM, Oliveira P, Mortara RA, Silveira JF, Bahia D. The challenge of Chagas' disease: has the human pathogen, Trypanosoma cruzi, learned how to modulate signaling events to subvert host cells? N Biotechnol. 2010 Dec 31;27(6):837-43. Epub 2010 Feb 19. PMID:20172059

Limbach K, Aguiar J, Gowda K, Patterson N, Abot E, Sedegah M, Sacci J, Richie T. Identification of two new protective pre-erythrocytic malaria vaccine antigen candidates. Malar J. 2011 Mar 16;10:65. PMID:21410955

Lin MY, Huang HP. Use of a doxycycline-enrofloxacin-metronidazole combination with/without diminazene diaceturate to treat naturally occurring canine babesiosis caused by Babesia gibsoni. Acta Vet Scand. 2010 Apr 24;52:27. PMID:20416095

Linden JV, Wong SJ, Chu FK, Schmidt GB, Bianco C. Transfusion-associated transmission of babesiosis in New York State. Transfusion. 2000 Mar;40(3):285-9. PMID:10738027

Lindgren TG, Deutsch K, Schell E, Bvumbwe A, Hart KB, Laviwa J, Rankin SH. Using mobile clinics to deliver HIV testing and other basic health services in rural Malawi. Rural Remote Health. 2011 Apr-Jun;11(2):1682. Epub 2011 Jun 28. PMID:21787108

Lindholm PF, Annen K, Ramsey G. Approaches to minimize infection risk in blood banking and transfusion practice. Infect Disord Drug Targets. 2011 Feb;11(1):45-56. PMID:21303341

Littman MP. Canine borreliosis. Vet Clin North Am Small Anim Pract. 2003 Jul;33(4):827-62. PMID:12910746

Littrell M, Gatakaa H, Evance I, Poyer S, Njogu J, Solomon T, Munroe E, Chapman S, Goodman C, Hanson K, Zinsou C, Akulayi L, Raharinjatovo J, Arogundade E, Buyungo P, Mpasela F, Adjibabi CB, Agbango JA, Ramarosandratana BF, Coker B, Rubahika D, Hamainza B, Shewchuk T, Chavasse D, O'Connell KA. Monitoring fever treatment behaviour and equitable access to effective medicines in the context of initiatives to improve ACT access: baseline results and implications for programming in six African countries. Malar J. 2011 Oct 31;10:327. PMID:22039892

Littrell M, Gatakaa H, Phok S, Allen H, Yeung S, Chuor CM, Dysoley L, Socheat D, Spiers A, White C, Shewchuk T, Chavasse D, O'Connell KA. Case management of malaria fever in Cambodia: results from national anti-malarial outlet and household surveys. Malar J. 2011 Oct 31;10:328. PMID:22039922

Liu AR, Yu ZY, Lu LL, Sui ZY. [The synergistic action of guanghuoxiang volatile oil and sodium artesunate against Plasmodium berghei and reversal of SA-resistant Plasmodium berghei].[Article in Chinese]. Zhongguo Ji Sheng Chong Xue Yu Ji Sheng Chong Bing Za Zhi. 2000;18(2):76-8. PMID:12567719

Liu J, Obando D, Liao V, Lifa T, Codd R. The many faces of the adamantyl group in drug design. Eur J Med Chem. 2011 Jun;46(6):1949-63. Epub 2011 Feb 3. PMID:21354674

Liu R, Dong HF, Jiang MS. Artemisinin: the gifts from traditional Chinese medicine not only for malaria control but also for schistosomiasis control. Parasitol Res. 2011 Oct 27. [Epub ahead of print]. PMID:22033738

Loa CC, Adelson ME, Mordechai E, Raphaelli I, Tilton RC. Serological diagnosis of human babesiosis by IgG enzyme-linked immunosorbent assay. Curr Microbiol. 2004 Dec;49(6):385-9. PMID:15696612

Lobetti RG, Reyers F, Nesbit JW. The comparative role of haemoglobinaemia and hypoxia in the development of canine babesial nephropathy. J S Afr Vet Assoc. 1996 Dec;67(4):188-98. PMID:9284030

Lodes MJ, Dillon DC, Houghton RL, Skeiky YA. Expression cloning. Methods Mol Med. 2004;94:91-106. PMID:14959824

Lodes MJ, Houghton RL, Bruinsma ES, Mohamath R, Reynolds LD, Benson DR, Krause PJ, Reed SG, Persing DH. Serological expression cloning of novel immunoreactive antigens of Babesia microti. Infect Immun. 2000 May;68(5):2783-90. PMID:10768973

Lohmann J, Wollina U. [Fever in travelers returning from the tropics: outpatient management].[Article in German]. MMW Fortschr Med. 2011 Jun 16;153(24-25):39-41. PMID:21717709

Löhr KF. [Contribution to the problem of the natural resistance of calves to Babesia bigemina].[Article in German]. Zentralbl Veterinarmed B. 1969 Mar;16(2):158-63. PMID:5814189

Löhr KF. [Immunization against babesiasis and anaplasmosis in 40 Charollais cattle imported to Kenya and report the incidence of photosensitization].[Article in German]. Zentralbl Veterinarmed B. 1969 Feb;16(1):40-6. PMID:5389131

Looareesuwan S, Phillips RE, Karbwang J, White NJ, Flegg PJ, Warrell DA. Plasmodium falciparum hyperparasitaemia: use of exchange transfusion in seven patients and a review of the literature. Q J Med. 1990 May;75(277):471-81. PMID:2201995

Lopes NP, Kato MJ, Andrade EH, Maia JG, Yoshida M, Planchart AR, Katzin AM. Antimalarial use of volatile oil from leaves of Virola surinamensis (Rol.) Warb. by Waiãpi Amazon Indians. J Ethnopharmacol. 1999 Nov 30;67(3):313-9. PMID:10617066

López ML, Vommaro R, Zalis M, de Souza W, Blair S, Segura C. Induction of cell death on Plasmodium falciparum asexual blood stages by Solanum nudum steroids. Parasitol Int. 2010 Jun;59(2):217-25. Epub 2010 Feb 11. PMID:20153445

López-Estraño C. Comparative analysis of stage specific gene regulation of apicomplexan parasites: Plasmodium falciparum and Toxoplasma gondii. Infect Disord Drug Targets. 2010 Aug;10(4):240-1. PMID:20687894

Lorenz LM, Koella JC. Maternal environment shapes the life history and susceptibility to malaria of Anopheles gambiae mosquitoes. Malar J. 2011 Dec 21;10(1):382. [Epub ahead of print]. PMID:22188602

Loretti AP, Barros SS. Hemorrhagic disease in dogs infected with an unclassified intraendothelial piroplasm in southern Brazil. Vet Parasitol. 2005 Dec 10;134(3-4):193-213. Epub 2005 Sep 8. PMID:16153781

Losos GJ, Crockett E. Toxicity of beril in the dog. Vet Rec. 1969 Aug 16;85(7):196. PMID:5816642

Losson B, Patz R. [Babesia divergens: activity of long-acting oxytetracycline in the gerbil, Meriones unguiculatus].[Article in French]. Ann Rech Vet. 1989;20(4):501-7. PMID:2619208

Loucoubar C, Goncalves B, Tall A, Sokhna C, Trape JF, Diène Sarr F, Faye J, Badiane A, Ly AB, Diop A, Bar-Hen A, Bureau JF, Sakuntabhai A, Paul R. Impact of changing drug treatment and malaria endemicity on the heritability of malaria phenotypes in a longitudinal family-based cohort study. PLoS One. 2011;6(11):e26364. Epub 2011 Nov 3. PMID:22073159

Lousada-Dietrich S, Jogdand PS, Jepsen S, Pinto VV, Ditlev SB, Christiansen M, Larsen SO, Fox CB, Raman VS, Howard RF, Vedvick TS, Ireton G, Carter D, Reed SG, Theisen M. A synthetic TLR4 agonist formulated in an emulsion enhances humoral and Type 1 cellular immune responses against GMZ2--a GLURP-MSP3 fusion protein malaria vaccine candidate. Vaccine. 2011 Apr 12;29(17):3284-92. Epub 2011 Feb 22. PMID:21349366

Lover AA, Sutton BA, Asy AJ, Wilder-Smith A. An exploratory study of treated-bed nets in Timor-Leste: patterns of intended and alternative usage. Malar J. 2011 Jul 21;10:199. PMID:21777415

Lozano JM, Lesmes LP, Carreño LF, Gallego GM, Patarroyo ME. Development of designed site-directed pseudopeptide-peptido-mimetic immunogens as novel minimal subunit-vaccine candidates for malaria. Molecules. 2010 Dec 6;15(12):8856-89. PMID:21135800

Lu F, Gao Q, Chotivanich K, Xia H, Cao J, Udomsangpetch R, Cui L, Sattabongkot J. In vitro anti-malarial drug susceptibility of temperate Plasmodium vivax from central China. Am J Trop Med Hyg. 2011 Aug;85(2):197-201. PMID:21813834

Lu Z, Ding Y, Li XC, Djigbenou DR, Grimberg BT, Ferreira D, Ireland CM, Van Wagoner RM. 3-bromohomofascaplysin A, a fascaplysin analogue from a Fijian Didemnum sp. ascidian. Bioorg Med Chem. 2011 Nov 15;19(22):6604-7. Epub 2011 Jun 1. PMID:21696970

Lubell Y, Riewpaiboon A, Dondorp AM, von Seidlein L, Mokuolu OA, Nansumba M, Gesase S, Kent A, Mtove G, Olaosebikan R, Ngum WP, Fanello CI, Hendriksen I, Day NP, White NJ, Yeung S. Cost-effectiveness of parenteral artesunate for treating children with severe malaria in sub-Saharan Africa. Bull World Health Organ. 2011 Jul 1;89(7):504-12. Epub 2011 Apr 28. PMID:21734764

Lubin AS, Snydman DR, Miller KB. Persistent babesiosis in a stem cell transplant recipient. Leuk Res. 2011 Jun;35(6):e77-8. Epub 2010 Dec 24. PMID:21185598

Lucantoni L, Yerbanga RS, Lupidi G, Pasqualini L, Esposito F, Habluetzel A. Transmission blocking activity of a standardized neem (Azadirachta indica) seed extract on the rodent malaria parasite Plasmodium berghei in its vector Anopheles stephensi. Malar J. 2010 Mar 2;9:66. PMID:20196858

Lucchi NW, Jain V, Wilson NO, Singh N, Udhayakumar V, Stiles JK. Potential serological biomarkers of cerebral malaria. Dis Markers. 2011 Jan 1;31(6):327-35. PMID:22182805

Lucke K. [Microbiological diagnosis of tuberculosis].[Article in German]. Ther Umsch. 2011 Jul;68(7):376-80. PMID:21728155

Lugada E, Millar D, Haskew J, Grabowsky M, Garg N, Vestergaard M, Kahn JG, Muraguri N, Mermin J. Rapid implementation of an integrated large-scale HIV counseling and testing, malaria, and diarrhea prevention campaign in rural Kenya. PLoS One. 2010 Aug 26;5(8):e12435. PMID:20865049

Lumb V, Das MK, Singh N, Dev V, Khan W, Sharma YD. Multiple origins of Plasmodium falciparum dihydropteroate synthetase mutant alleles associated with sulfadoxine resistance in India. Antimicrob Agents Chemother. 2011 Jun;55(6):2813-7. Epub 2011 Mar 21. PMID:21422213

Lumsden JM, Cranmer MA, Krzych U. An early commitment to expression of a particular TCRVbeta chain on CD8(+) T cells responding to attenuated Plasmodium berghei sporozoites is maintained following challenge with infectious sporozoites. Parasite Immunol. 2010 Sep-Oct;32(9-10):644-55. PMID:20691016

Lumsden JM, Pichyangkul S, Srichairatanakul U, Yongvanitchit K, Limsalakpetch A, Nurmukhambetova S, Klein J, Bertholet S, Vedvick TS, Reed SG, Sattabongkot J, Bennett JW, Polhemus ME, Ockenhouse CF, Howard RF, Yadava A. Evaluation of the safety and immunogenicity in rhesus monkeys of a recombinant malaria vaccine for Plasmodium vivax with a synthetic Toll-like receptor 4 agonist formulated in an emulsion. Infect Immun. 2011 Sep;79(9):3492-500. Epub 2011 Jun 20. PMID:21690242

Luo J, Fort DM, Carlson TJ, Noamesi BK, nii-Amon-Kotei D, King SR, Tsai J, Quan J, Hobensack C, Lapresca P, Waldeck N, Mendez CD, Jolad SD, Bierer DE, Reaven GM. Cryptolepis sanguinolenta: an ethnobotanical approach to drug discovery and the isolation of a potentially useful new antihyperglycaemic agent. Diabet Med. 1998 May;15(5):367-74. PMID:9609357

Luo Y, Jia H, Terkawi MA, Goo YK, Kawano S, Ooka H, Li Y, Yu L, Cao S, Yamagishi J, Fujisaki K, Nishikawa Y, Saito-Ito A, Igarashi I, Xuan X. Identification and characterization of a novel secreted antigen 1 of Babesia microti and evaluation of its potential use in enzyme-linked immunosorbent assay and immunochromatographic test. Parasitol Int. 2011 Jun;60(2):119-25. Epub 2010 Nov 8. PMID:21070864

Lux JZ, Weiss D, Linden JV, Kessler D, Herwaldt BL, Wong SJ, Keithly J, Della-Latta P, Scully BE. Transfusion-associated babesiosis after heart transplant. Emerg Infect Dis. 2003 Jan;9(1):116-9. PMID:12533293

Lykins JD, Ristic M, Weisiger RM. Babesia microti: pathogenesis of parasite of human origin in the hamster. Exp Parasitol. 1975 Jun;37(3):388-97. PMID:805058

Ma C, Wang H, Lu X, Li H, Liu B, Xu G. Analysis of Artemisia annua L. volatile oil by comprehensive two-dimensional gas chromatography time-of-flight mass spectrometry. J Chromatogr A. 2007 May 25;1150(1-2):50-3. Epub 2006 Oct 12. PMID:17045598

Ma DD, Rede T, Naqvi NA, Cook PD. Synthetic oligonucleotides as therapeutics: the coming of age. Biotechnol Annu Rev. 2000;5:155-96. PMID:10875000

Ma H, Yao Q, Zhang AM, Lin S, Wang XX, Wu L, Sun JG, Chen ZT. The Effects of Artesunate on the Expression of EGFR and ABCG2 in A549 Human Lung Cancer Cells and a Xenograft Model. Molecules. 2011 Dec 19;16(12):10556-69. PMID:22183882

Ma X, Zheng C, Hu C, Rahman K, Qin L. The genus Desmodium (Fabaceae)-traditional uses in Chinese medicine, phytochemistry and pharmacology. J Ethnopharmacol. 2011 Nov 18;138(2):314-32. Epub 2011 Oct 17. PMID:22004895

Macchi Bde M, Quaresma JA, Herculano AM, Crespo-López ME, DaMatta RA, do Nascimento JL. Pathogenic action of Plasmodium gallinaceum in chickens: brain histology and nitric oxide production by blood monocyte-derived macrophages. Vet Parasitol. 2010 Aug 27;172(1-2):16-22. Epub 2010 May 6. PMID:20537466

Macgregor JD, Avery JG. Malaria transmission and fetal growth. Br Med J. 1974 Aug 17;3(5928):433-6. PMID:4606777

Machado RZ, McElwain TF, Pancracio HP, Freschi CR, Palmer GH. Babesia bigemina: immunization with purified rhoptries induces protection against acute parasitemia. Exp Parasitol. 1999 Oct;93(2):105-8. PMID:10502474

Machtinger L, Telford SR 3rd, Inducil C, Klapper E, Pepkowitz SH, Goldfinger D. Treatment of babesiosis by red blood cell exchange in an HIV-positive, splenectomized patient. J Clin Apher. 1993;8(2):78-81. PMID:8226709

Macraild CA, Anders RF, Foley M, Norton RS. Apical membrane antigen 1 as an anti-malarial drug target. Curr Top Med Chem. 2011;11(16):2039-47. PMID:21619512

Maggi RG, Mozayeni BR, Pultorak EL, Hegarty BC, Bradley JM, Correa M, Breitschwerdt EB. Bartonella spp. bacteremia and rheumatic symptoms in patients from Lyme disease–endemic region. Emerg Infect Dis. 2012 May;18(5):783-791.

Mahajan B, Berzofsky JA, Boykins RA, Majam V, Zheng H, Chattopadhyay R, de la Vega P, Moch JK, Haynes JD, Belyakov IM, Nakhasi HL, Kumar S. Multiple antigen peptide vaccines against Plasmodium falciparum malaria. Infect Immun. 2010 Nov;78(11):4613-24. Epub 2010 Sep 7. PMID:20823210

Maher D, Harries AD, Nachega JB, Jaffar S. Methodology matters: what type of research is suitable for evaluating community treatment supporters for HIV and tuberculosis treatment? Trop Med Int Health. 2011 Dec 16. [Epub ahead of print]. PMID:22171790

Mahoney DF, Goodger BV. Babesia argentina: immunogenicity of plasma from infected animals. Exp Parasitol. 1972 Aug;32(1):71-85. PMID:4626125

Mahoney DF, Kerr JD, Goodger BV, Wright IG. The immune response of cattle to Babesia bovis (syn. B. argentina). Studies on the nature and specificity of protection. Int J Parasitol. 1979 Aug;9(4):297-306. PMID:489236

Mahoney DF, Mirre GB. Babesia argentina: the infection of splenectomized calves with extracts of larval ticks (Boophilus microplus). Res Vet Sci. 1974 Jan;16(1):112-4. PMID:4819982

Mahoney DF, Wright IG, Goodger BV, Mirre GB, Sutherst RW, Utech KB. The transmission of Babesia bovis in herds of European and Zebu x European cattle infested with the tick, Boophilus microplus. Aust Vet J. 1981 Oct;57(10):461-9. PMID:7337597

Mahoney DF, Wright IG, Goodger BV. Bovine babesiosis: the immunization of cattle with fractions of erythrocytes infected with Babesia bovis (syn B. argentina). Vet Immunol Immunopathol. 1981 Apr;2(2):145-56. PMID:7344266

Mahoney DF, Wright IG, Goodger BV. Changes in the haemolytic activity of serum complement during acute Babesia bovis infection in cattle. Z Parasitenkd. 1980;62(1):39-45. PMID:7395306

Mahoney DF, Wright IG, Goodger BV. Immunity in cattle to Babesia bovis after single infections with parasites of various origin. Aust Vet J. 1979 Jan;55(1):10-2. PMID:435202

Mahoney DF, Wright IG, Ketterer PJ. Babesia argentina: the infectivity and immunogenicity of irradiated blood parasites for splenectomized calves. Int J Parasitol. 1973 Mar;3(2):209-17. PMID:4196318

Maiga OM, Kayentao K, Traoré BT, Djimde A, Traoré B, Traoré M, Ongoiba A, Doumtabé D, Doumbo S, Traoré MS, Dara A, Guindo O, Karim DM, Coulibaly S, Bougoudogo F, Ter Kuile FO, Danis M, Doumbo OK. Superiority of 3 over 2 doses of intermittent preventive treatment with sulfadoxine-pyrimethamine for the prevention of malaria during pregnancy in mali: a randomized controlled trial. Clin Infect Dis. 2011 Aug 1;53(3):215-23. PMID:21765069

malERA Consultative Group on Basic Science and Enabling Technologies. Collaborators: Amino R, Bassat Q, Baum J, Billker O, Bogyo M, Bousema T, Christophides G, Deitsch K, Dinglasan R, Djimde A, Duraisingh M, Dzinjalamala F, Happi C, Heussler V, Kramarik J, de Koning-Ward T, Lacerda M, Laufer M, Lim P, Llinas M, McGovern V, Martinez-Barnetche J, Mota MM, Mueller I, Okumu F, Rasgon J, Serazin A, Sharma P, Sinden R, Wirth D, Gilberger T. A research agenda for malaria eradication: basic science and enabling technologies. PLoS Med. 2011 Jan 25;8(1):e1000399. PMID:21311584

malERA Consultative Group on Diagnoses and Diagnostics. Collaborators: Alonso PL, Bassat Q, Bell D, Berman P, Breman JG, de Savigny D, Drakeley C, Evans T, Block MA, Hanson K, Kachur SP, Kress D, Macdonald M, Newman RD, Nyonator FK, Pagnoni F, Perkins M, Schapira A, Schellenberg D, Slutsker L, Sullivan D, Tanner M, Teklehaimanot A, Teuscher T, Mendis K, Barnwell JW, Moonen B, Brown G. A research agenda for malaria eradication: diagnoses and diagnostics. PLoS Med. 2011 Jan 25;8(1):e1000396. PMID:21311583

malERA Consultative Group on Drugs. Collaborators: Alonso PL, Bassat Q, Binka F, Brewer T, Chandra R, Culpepper J, Dinglasan R, Duncan K, Duparc S, Fukuda M, Laxminarayan R, MacArthur JR, Magill A, Marzetta C, Milman J, Mutabingwa T, Nosten F, Nwaka S, Nyunt M, Ohrt C, Plowe CV, Pottage J, Price R, Ringwald P, Serazin A, Shanks D, Sinden R, Tanner M, Vial H, Ward SA, Wellems TE, Wells T, White N, Wirth D, Yeung S, Yuthavong Y, Alonso PL, Djimde A, Magill A, Milman J, Nájera J, Plowe CV, Wells T, Yeung S, Kremsner P, Mueller I, Newman RD, Rabinovich R. A research agenda for malaria eradication: drugs. PLoS Med. 2011 Jan 25;8(1):e1000402. PMID:21311580

malERA Consultative Group on Health Systems and Operational Research. Collaborators: Alonso PL, Bassat Q, Bell D, Berman P, Breman JG, de Savigny D, Drakeley C, Evans T, Block MA, Hanson K, Kachur SP, Kress D, Macdonald M, Newman RD, Nyonator FK, Pagnoni F, Perkins M, Schapira A, Schellenberg D, Slutsker L, Sullivan D, Tanner M, Teklehaimanot A, Teuscher T, Mendis K, Brown G. A research agenda for malaria eradication: health systems and operational research. PLoS Med. 2011 Jan 25;8(1):e1000397. PMID:21311588

malERA Consultative Group on Integration Strategies. Collaborators: Binka F, Brown G, Alonso PL, Brown G, Tanner M, Abdulla S, Alonso PL, Bart-Plange C, Bassat Q, Binka F, Bojang K, Brooks A, Brown G, Djimde A, Drakeley C, González-Block MA, Hemingway J, Koram K, Keziah M, Macete E, Richards F, de Savigny D, Sinden R, Smith TA, Sirima S, Steketee R, Ogutu B, Owusu-Agyei S, Alonso PL, Brown G, Tanner M. A research agenda for malaria eradication: cross-cutting issues for eradication. PLoS Med. 2011 Jan 25;8(1):e1000404. PMID:21283603

malERA Consultative Group on Modeling. Collaborators: Tanner M, Alonso PL, Eubank S, Ghani A, Hay SI, Sinden R, Smith D, Smith TA, Tanner M, White L, Akhavan D, Antão T, Aultman K, Buchsbaum S, Eckhoff P, Ghani A, Glass G, Hastings I, Hay SI, Kanyok T, Koella J, Lauer J, Maire N, Mordveit H, Schapira A, Sinden R, Smith D, Smith TA, Tanner M, Vounatsou P, White L, Akhavan D, Alonso PL, Antao T, Aponte J, Aultman K, Buchsbaum S, Cárdenas V, Collins F, Cunningham G, Day K, Eckhoff P, Eckstrand I, Eubank S, Ghani A, Glass G, Hall BF, Hastings I, Lauer J, Madey G, Marathe M, McKenzie E, Mortveit HS, Ratcliffe A, Saul A, Sinden R, Smith D, Smith TA, Tanner M, White L, Alonso PL, Eubank S, Ghani A, Hay SI, Sinden R, Smith D, Smith TA, Tanner M, White L, Brown G. A research agenda for malaria eradication: modeling. PLoS Med. 2011 Jan 25;8(1):e1000403. PMID:21283605

malERA Consultative Group on Monitoring, Evaluation, and Surveillance. Collaborators: Steketee R, Voltaire F, Hay SI, Alonso PL, Atta HY, Bassat Q, Bakyaita N, Clark JP, Doumbo OK, Drakeley C, Eckert EL, Eisele T, Gausi K, Guinovart C, Hayes N, Kilian A, Lama M, Meek S, Miller J, Nahlen B, Otten M, Ratcliffe A, López MH, Slutsker L, Greenwood B, Tanner M. A research agenda for malaria eradication: monitoring, evaluation, and surveillance. PLoS Med. 2011 Jan 25;8(1):e1000400. PMID:21311581

malERA Consultative Group on Vaccines. Collaborators: Abdulla S, Agre P, Alonso PL, Arevalo-Herrera M, Bassat Q, Binka F, Chitnis C, Corradin G, Cowman A, Culpepper J, del Portillo H, Dinglasan R, Duffy P, Gargallo D, Greenwood B, Guinovart C, Hall BF, Herrera S, Hoffman S, Lanzavecchia A, Leroy O, Levine MM, Loucq C, Mendis K, Milman J, Moorthy V, Pleuschke G, Plowe CV, Reed S, Sauerwein R, Saul A, Schofield L, Sinden R, Stubbs J, Villafana T, Wirth D, Yadav P, Ballou R, Brown G, Birkett A, Brandt W, Brooks A, Carter T, Golden A, Lee C, Nunes J, Puijalon O, Raphael T, Richards H, Warren C, Woods C. A research agenda for malaria eradication: vaccines. PLoS Med. 2011 Jan 25;8(1):e1000398. PMID:21311586 malERA Consultative Group on Vector Control. Collaborators: Aultman K, Burkot TR, Chandre F, Coetzee M, Collins FH, Corbel V, Dartigues V, Gimnig J, Hawley B, Hemingway J, Jacobs-Lorena M, James AA, Karunaratne P, Killeen G, Lengeler C, Lines J, Macdonald M, Mendez-Galván J, Muskavitch M, Nájera J, Neafsey D, Rosenberg R, Simard F, Sinden R, Subbarao S, Walker N, Williams J, Wirtz R, Alonso PL, Besansky NJ, Burkot TR, Collins FH, Hemingway J, James AA, Lengeler C, Lindsay S, Liu Q, Lobo NF, Mnzava A, Tanner M, Zwiebel L. A research agenda for malaria eradication: vector control. PLoS Med. 2011 Jan 25;8(1):e1000401. PMID:21311587

malERA Consultative Group on Diagnoses and Diagnostics. Collaborators: Alonso PL, Bassat Q, Bell D, Berman P, Breman JG, de Savigny D, Drakeley C, Evans T, Block MA, Hanson K, Kachur SP, Kress D, Macdonald M, Newman RD, Nyonator FK, Pagnoni F, Perkins M, Schapira A, Schellenberg D, Slutsker L, Sullivan D, Tanner M, Teklehaimanot A, Teuscher T, Mendis K, Barnwell JW, Moonen B, Brown G. A research agenda for malaria eradication: diagnoses and diagnostics. PLoS Med. 2011 Jan 25;8(1):e1000396. PMID:21311583

malERA Consultative Group on Drugs. Collaborators: Alonso PL, Bassat Q, Binka F, Brewer T, Chandra R, Culpepper J, Dinglasan R, Duncan K, Duparc S, Fukuda M, Laxminarayan R, MacArthur JR, Magill A, Marzetta C, Milman J, Mutabingwa T, Nosten F, Nwaka S, Nyunt M, Ohrt C, Plowe CV, Pottage J, Price R, Ringwald P, Serazin A, Shanks D, Sinden R, Tanner M, Vial H, Ward SA, Wellems TE, Wells T, White N, Wirth D, Yeung S, Yuthavong Y, Alonso PL, Djimde A, Magill A, Milman J, Nájera J, Plowe CV, Wells T, Yeung S, Kremsner P, Mueller I, Newman RD, Rabinovich R. A research agenda for malaria eradication: drugs. PLoS Med. 2011 Jan 25;8(1):e1000402. PMID:21311580 malERA Consultative Group on Health Systems and Operational Research. Collaborators: Alonso PL, Bassat Q, Bell D, Berman P, Breman JG, de Savigny D, Drakeley C, Evans T, Block MA, Hanson K, Kachur SP, Kress D, Macdonald M, Newman RD, Nyonator FK, Pagnoni F, Perkins M, Schapira A, Schellenberg D, Slutsker L, Sullivan D, Tanner M, Teklehaimanot A, Teuscher T, Mendis K, Brown G. A research agenda for malaria eradication: health systems and operational research. PLoS Med. 2011 Jan 25;8(1):e1000397. PMID:21311588

malERA Consultative Group on Integration Strategies. Collaborators: Binka F, Brown G, Alonso PL, Brown G, Tanner M, Abdulla S, Alonso PL, Bart-Plange C, Bassat Q, Binka F, Bojang K, Brooks A, Brown G, Djimde A, Drakeley C, González-Block MA, Hemingway J, Koram K, Keziah M, Macete E, Richards F, de Savigny D, Sinden R, Smith TA, Sirima S, Steketee R, Ogutu B, Owusu-Agyei S, Alonso PL, Brown G, Tanner M. A research agenda for malaria eradication: cross-cutting issues for eradication. PLoS Med. 2011 Jan 25;8(1):e1000404. PMID:21283603

malERA Consultative Group on Modeling. Collaborators: Tanner M, Alonso PL, Eubank S, Ghani A, Hay SI, Sinden R, Smith D, Smith TA, Tanner M, White L, Akhavan D, Antão T, Aultman K, Buchsbaum S, Eckhoff P, Ghani A, Glass G, Hastings I, Hay SI, Kanyok T, Koella J, Lauer J, Maire N, Mordveit H, Schapira A, Sinden R, Smith D, Smith TA, Tanner M, Vounatsou P, White L, Akhavan D, Alonso PL, Antao T, Aponte J, Aultman K, Buchsbaum S, Cárdenas V, Collins F, Cunningham G, Day K, Eckhoff P, Eckstrand I, Eubank S, Ghani A, Glass G, Hall BF, Hastings I, Lauer J, Madey G, Marathe M, McKenzie E, Mortveit HS, Ratcliffe A, Saul A, Sinden R, Smith D, Smith TA, Tanner M, White L, Alonso PL, Eubank S, Ghani A, Hay SI, Sinden R, Smith D, Smith TA, Tanner M, White L, Brown G. A research agenda for malaria eradication: modeling. PLoS Med. 2011 Jan 25;8(1):e1000403. PMID:21283605

malERA Consultative Group on Monitoring, Evaluation, and Surveillance. Collaborators: Steketee R, Voltaire F, Hay SI, Alonso PL, Atta HY, Bassat Q, Bakyaita N, Clark JP, Doumbo OK, Drakeley C, Eckert EL, Eisele T, Gausi K, Guinovart C, Hayes N, Kilian A, Lama M, Meek S, Miller J, Nahlen B, Otten M, Ratcliffe A, López MH, Slutsker L, Greenwood B, Tanner M. A research agenda for malaria eradication: monitoring, evaluation, and surveillance. PLoS Med. 2011 Jan 25;8(1):e1000400. PMID:21311581

malERA Consultative Group on Vaccines. Collaborators: Abdulla S, Agre P, Alonso PL, Arevalo-Herrera M, Bassat Q, Binka F, Chitnis C, Corradin G, Cowman A, Culpepper J, del Portillo H, Dinglasan R, Duffy P, Gargallo D, Greenwood B, Guinovart C, Hall BF, Herrera S, Hoffman S, Lanzavecchia A, Leroy O, Levine MM, Loucq C, Mendis K, Milman J, Moorthy V, Pleuschke G, Plowe CV, Reed S, Sauerwein R, Saul A, Schofield L, Sinden R, Stubbs J, Villafana T, Wirth D, Yadav P, Ballou R, Brown G, Birkett A, Brandt W, Brooks A, Carter T, Golden A, Lee C, Nunes J, Puijalon O, Raphael T, Richards H, Warren C, Woods C. A research agenda for malaria eradication: vaccines. PLoS Med. 2011 Jan 25;8(1):e1000398. PMID:21311586

malERA Consultative Group on Vector Control. Collaborators: Aultman K, Burkot TR, Chandre F, Coetzee M, Collins FH, Corbel V, Dartigues V, Gimnig J, Hawley B, Hemingway J, Jacobs-Lorena M, James AA, Karunaratne P, Killeen G, Lengeler C, Lines J, Macdonald M, Mendez-Galván J, Muskavitch M, Nájera J, Neafsey D, Rosenberg R, Simard F, Sinden R, Subbarao S, Walker N, Williams J, Wirtz R, Alonso PL, Besansky NJ, Burkot TR, Collins FH, Hemingway J, James AA, Lengeler C, Lindsay S, Liu Q, Lobo NF, Mnzava A, Tanner M, Zwiebel L. A research agenda for malaria eradication: vector control. PLoS Med. 2011 Jan 25;8(1):e1000401. PMID:21311587

Malisa AL, Pearce RJ, Mutayoba BM, Abdullah S, Mshinda H, Kachur PS, Bloland P, Roper C. The evolution of pyrimethamine resistant dhfr in Plasmodium falciparum of south-eastern Tanzania: comparing selection under SP alone vs SP+artesunate combination. Malar J. 2011 Oct 26;10:317. PMID:22029848

Makanga M, Bassat Q, Falade CO, Premji ZG, Krudsood S, Hunt P, Walter V, Beck HP, Marrast AC, Cousin M, Rosenthal PJ. Efficacy and safety of artemether-lumefantrine in the treatment of acute, uncomplicated Plasmodium falciparum malaria: a pooled analysis. Am J Trop Med Hyg. 2011 Nov;85(5):793-804. PMID:22049029

Malagon F, Tapia JL. Experimental transmission of Babesia microti infection by the oral route. Parasitol Res. 1994;80(8):645-8. PMID:7886033

Malik EM, Hanafi K, Ali SH, Ahmed ES, Mohamed KA. Treatment-seeking behaviour for malaria in children under five years of age: implication for home management in rural areas with high seasonal transmission in Sudan. Malar J. 2006 Jul 22;5:60. PMID:16859565

Malimbo M, Mugisha E, Kato F, Karamagi C, Talisuna AO. Caregivers' perceived treatment failure in home-based management of fever among Ugandan children aged less than five years. Malar J. 2006 Dec 15;5:124. PMID:17173675

Malloy P, Paice JA, Ferrell BR, Ali Z, Munyoro E, Coyne P, Smith T. Advancing palliative care in Kenya. Cancer Nurs. 2011 Jan-Feb;34(1):E10-3. PMID:20921889

Mamotte N, Wassenaar D, Koen J, Essack Z. Convergent ethical issues in HIV/AIDS, tuberculosis and malaria vaccine trials in Africa: Report from the WHO/UNAIDS African AIDS Vaccine Programme's Ethics, Law and Human Rights Collaborating Centre consultation, 10-11 February 2009, Durban, South Africa. BMC Med Ethics. 2010 Mar 9;11:3. PMID:20211030

Mangham LJ, Cundill B, Achonduh OA, Ambebila JN, Lele AK, Metoh TN, Ndive SN, Ndong IC, Nguela RL, Nji AM, Orang-Ojong B, Wiseman V, Pamen-Ngako J, Mbacham WF. Malaria prevalence and treatment of febrile patients at health facilities and medicine retailers in Cameroon. Trop Med Int Health. 2011 Nov 21. [Epub ahead of print]. PMID:22098135

Mangham LJ, Cundill B, Ezeoke O, Nwala E, Uzochukwu BS, Wiseman V, Onwujekwe O. Treatment of uncomplicated malaria at public health facilities and medicine retailers in south-eastern Nigeria. Malar J. 2011 Jun 8;10:155. PMID:21651787

Mangia CM, Kissoon N, Branchini OA, Andrade MC, Kopelman BI, Carcillo J. Bacterial sepsis in Brazilian children: a trend analysis from 1992 to 2006. PLoS One. 2011;6(6):e14817. Epub 2011 Jun 3. PMID:21674036

Mangold AJ, Aguirre DH, Cafrune MM, de Echaide ST, Guglielmone AA. Evaluation of the infectivity of a vaccinal and a pathogenic Babesia bovis strain from Argentina to Boophilus microplus. Vet Parasitol. 1993 Dec;51(1-2):143-8. PMID:8128578

Mangold AJ, Aguirre DH, Guglielmone AA. Post-thawing viability of vaccines for bovine babesiosis and anaplasmosis cryopreserved with glycerol. Vet Parasitol. 1990 Nov;37(3-4):301-6. PMID:2267730

Mangold AJ, Vanzini VR, Echaide IE, de Echaide ST, Volpogni MM, Guglielmone AA. Viability after thawing and dilution of simultaneously cryopreserved vaccinal Babesia bovis and Babesia bigemina strains cultured in vitro. Vet Parasitol. 1996 Feb;61(3-4):345-8. PMID:8720572

Mantel PY, Schmidt-Weber CB. Transforming growth factor-beta: recent advances on its role in immune tolerance. Methods Mol Biol. 2011;677:303-38. PMID:20941619

Manyando C, Mkandawire R, Puma L, Sinkala M, Mpabalwani E, Njunju E, Gomes M, Ribeiro I, Walter V, Virtanen M, Schlienger R, Cousin M, Chipimo M, Sullivan FM. Safety of artemether-lumefantrine in pregnant women with malaria: results of a prospective cohort study in Zambia. Malar J. 2010 Sep 1;9:249. PMID:20809964

Manzano JI, Carvalho L, García-Hernández R, Poveda JA, Ferragut JA, Castanys S, Gamarro F. Uptake of the antileishmania drug tafenoquine follows a sterol-dependent diffusion process in Leishmania. J Antimicrob Chemother. 2011 Nov;66(11):2562-5. Epub 2011 Aug 16. PMID:21846675

Manzano JI, Carvalho L, Pérez-Victoria JM, Castanys S, Gamarro F. Increased glycolytic ATP synthesis is associated with tafenoquine resistance in Leishmania major. Antimicrob Agents Chemother. 2011 Mar;55(3):1045-52. Epub 2011 Jan 3. PMID:21199921

Marais BJ, Raviglione MC, Donald PR, Harries AD, Kritski AL, Graham SM, El-Sadr WM, Harrington M, Churchyard G, Mwaba P, Sanne I, Kaufmann SH, Whitty CJ, Atun R, Zumla A. Scale-up of services and research priorities for diagnosis, management, and control of tuberculosis: a call to action. Lancet. 2010 Jun 19;375(9732):2179-91. Epub 2010 May 18. PMID:20488521

Marathe A, Tripathi J, Handa V, Date V. Human babesiosis--a case report. Indian J Med Microbiol. 2005 Oct;23(4):267-9. PMID:16327127

Marco I, Velarde R, Castellà J, Ferrer D, Lavín S. Presumptive Babesia ovis infection in a spanish ibex (Capra pyrenaica). Vet Parasitol. 2000 Jan;87(2-3):217-21. PMID:10622613

Marcotty T, Berkvens D, Besa RK, Losson B, Dolan TT, Madder M, Chaka G, Van den Bossche P, Brandt J. Lyophilisation and resuscitation of sporozoites of Theileria parva: preliminary experiments. Vaccine. 2003 Dec 12;22(2):213-6. PMID:14615148

Marcu CB, Caracciolo E, Libertin C, Donohue T. Fulminant babesiosis manifested soon after coronary bypass surgery. Conn Med. 2005 Feb;69(2):67-8. PMID:15779600

Marcus LC, Mabray CJ, Sturgis GH. Babesia microti infection in the hamster: failure of quinine and pyrimethamine in chemotherapeutic trials. Am J Trop Med Hyg. 1984 Jan;33(1):21-3. PMID:6696180

Marcus LC, Valigorsky JM, Fanning WL, Joseph T, Glick B. A case report of transfusion-induced babesiosis. JAMA. 1982 Jul 23;248(4):465-7. PMID:7201036

Margout D, Gattacceca F, Moarbess G, Wein S, Tran van Ba C, Le Pape S, Berger O, Escale R, Vial HJ, Bressolle FM. Pharmacokinetic properties and metabolism of a new potent antimalarial N-alkylamidine compound, M64, and its corresponding bioprecursors. Eur J Pharm Sci. 2011 Jan 18;42(1-2):81-90. Epub 2010 Nov 2. PMID:21050886

Marley SE, Eberhard ML, Steurer FJ, Ellis WL, McGreevy PB, Ruebush TK 2nd. Evaluation of selected antiprotozoal drugs in the Babesia microti-hamster model. Antimicrob Agents Chemother. 1997 Jan;41(1):91-4. PMID:8980761

Marois E. The multifaceted mosquito anti-Plasmodium response. Curr Opin Microbiol. 2011 Aug;14(4):429-35. Epub 2011 Jul 27. PMID:21802348

Marshall CL. Health, nutrition, and the roots of world population growth. Int J Health Serv. 1974 Fall;4(4):677-90. PMID:4463173

Martinot M, Zadeh MM, Hansmann Y, Grawey I, Christmann D, Aguillon S, Jouglin M, Chauvin A, De Briel D. Babesiosis in immunocompetent patients, Europe. Emerg Infect Dis. 2011 Jan;17(1):114-6. PMID:21192869

Masanja IM, de Bethune X, Jacobs J. Implementing ideal health policy in a fragile health system: the example of expanding the use of malaria rapid diagnostic tests in mainland Tanzania. Malar J. 2011 Oct 28;10:322. PMID:22035466

Mata E, Igartua M, Hernández RM, Rosas JE, Patarroyo ME, Pedraz JL. Comparison of the adjuvanticity of two different delivery systems on the induction of humoral and cellular responses to synthetic peptides. Drug Deliv. 2010 Sep-Oct;17(7):490-9. PMID:20500129

Mathanga DP, Walker ED, Wilson ML, Ali D, Taylor TE, Laufer MK. Malaria control in Malawi: Current status and directions for the future. Acta Trop. 2011 Jul 8. [Epub ahead of print]. PMID:21763670

Máthé A, Dobos-Kovács M, Vörös K. Histological and ultrastructural studies of renal lesions in Babesia canis infected dogs treated with imidocarb. Acta Vet Hung. 2007 Dec;55(4):511-23. PMID:18277710

Máthé A, Vörös K, Németh T, Biksi I, Hetyey C, Manczur F, Tekes L. Clinicopathological changes and effect of imidocarb therapy in dogs experimentally infected with Babesia canis. Acta Vet Hung. 2006 Mar;54(1):19-33. PMID:16613023

Máthé A, Vörös K, Papp L, Reiczigel J. Clinical manifestations of canine babesiosis in Hungary (63 cases). Acta Vet Hung. 2006 Sep;54(3):367-85. PMID:17020140

Matijatko V, Mrljak V, Kis I, Kucer N, Forsek J, Zivicnjak T, Romić Z, Simec Z, Ceron JJ. Evidence of an acute phase response in dogs naturally infected with Babesia canis. Vet Parasitol. 2007 Mar 31;144(3-4):242-50. Epub 2006 Nov 20. PMID:17116368

Matjila PT, Penzhorn BL, Leisewitz AL, Bhoora R, Barker R. Molecular characterisation of Babesia gibsoni infection from a pit-bull terrier pup recently imported into South Africa. J S Afr Vet Assoc. 2007 Mar;78(1):2-5. PMID:17665757

Matjila TP, Nijhof AM, Taoufik A, Houwers D, Teske E, Penzhorn BL, de Lange T, Jongejan F. Autochthonous canine babesiosis in The Netherlands. Vet Parasitol. 2005 Jul 15;131(1-2):23-9. PMID:15923085

Matsui T, Inoue R, Kajimoto K, Tamekane A, Okamura A, Katayama Y, Shimoyama M, Chihara K, Saito-Ito A, Tsuji M. [First documentation of transfusion-associated babesiosis in Japan].[Article in Japanese]. Rinsho Ketsueki. 2000 Aug;41(8):628-34. PMID:11020989

Matsuu A, Koshida Y, Kawahara M, Inoue K, Ikadai H, Hikasa Y, Okano S, Higuchi S. Efficacy of atovaquone against Babesia gibsoni in vivo and in vitro. Vet Parasitol. 2004 Sep 20;124(1-2):9-18. PMID:15350657

Matsuu A, Miyamoto K, Ikadai H, Okano S, Higuchi S. Short report: cloning of the Babesia gibsoni cytochrome B gene and isolation of three single nucleotide polymorphisms from parasites present after atovaquone treatment. Am J Trop Med Hyg. 2006 Apr;74(4):593-7. PMID:16606990

Matsuzaki-Moriya C, Tu L, Ishida H, Imai T, Suzue K, Hirai M, Tetsutani K, Hamano S, Shimokawa C, Hisaeda H. A critical role for phagocytosis in resistance to malaria in iron-deficient mice. Eur J Immunol. 2011 May;41(5):1365-75. PMID:21469097

Matthews J, Rattigan E, Yee H. Case 29-2003: a 60-year-old man with fever, rigors, and sweats. N Engl J Med. 2003 Dec 18;349(25):2467; author reply 2467. PMID:14681519

Mattioli RC, Dampha K, Bah M, Verhulst A, Pandey VS. Effect of controlling natural field-tick infestation on the growth of N'Dama and Gobra zebu cattle in the Gambia. Prev Vet Med. 1998 Feb 27;34(2-3):137-46. PMID:9604263

Matuschewski K, Hafalla JC, Borrmann S, Friesen J. Arrested Plasmodium liver stages as experimental anti-malaria vaccines. Hum Vaccin. 2011 Jan-Feb;7 Suppl:16-21. Epub 2011 Jan 1. PMID:21266857

Maude RJ, Hoque G, Hasan MU, Sayeed A, Akter S, Samad R, Alam B, Yunus EB, Rahman R, Rahman W, Chowdhury R, Seal T, Charunwatthana P, Chang CC, White NJ, Faiz MA, Day NP, Dondorp AM, Hossain A. Timing of enteral feeding in cerebral malaria in resource-poor settings: a randomized trial. PLoS One. 2011;6(11):e27273. Epub 2011 Nov 16. PMID:22110624

Maude RJ, Saralamba S, Lewis A, Sherwood D, White NJ, Day NP, Dondorp AM, White LJ. Modelling malaria elimination on the internet. Malar J. 2011 Jul 14;10:191. PMID:21756319

Maude RJ, Woodrow CJ, White LJ. Artemisinin Antimalarials: Preserving the "Magic Bullet". Drug Dev Res. 2010 Feb;71(1):12-19. PMID:21399699

Mazumdar S. Prevalence, risk factors and treatment-seeking behaviour for malaria: the results of a case study from the Terai region of West Bengal, India. Ann Trop Med Parasitol. 2011 Apr;105(3):197-208. PMID:21801498

Mbati PA, Hlatshwayo M, Mtshali MS, Mogaswane KR, De Waal TD, Dipeolu OO. Ticks and tick-borne diseases of livestock belonging to resource-poor farmers in the eastern Free State of South Africa. Exp Appl Acarol. 2002;28(1-4):217-24. PMID:14570134

Mbonye AK, Neema S, Magnussen P. Malaria in pregnancy, risk perceptions and care seeking practices among adolescents in Mukono district Uganda. Int J Adolesc Med Health. 2006 Oct-Dec;18(4):561-73. PMID:17340848

Mbonye AK, Neema S, Magnussen P. Treatment-seeking practices for malaria in pregnancy among rural women in Mukono district, Uganda. J Biosoc Sci. 2006 Mar;38(2):221-37. PMID:16490155

Mbulaiteye SM, Bhatia K, Adebamowo C, Sasco AJ. HIV and cancer in Africa: mutual collaboration between HIV and cancer programs may provide timely research and public health data. Infect Agent Cancer. 2011 Oct 17;6(1):16. PMID:22004990

McCall MB, Roestenberg M, Ploemen I, Teirlinck A, Hopman J, de Mast Q, Dolo A, Doumbo OK, Luty A, van der Ven AJ, Hermsen CC, Sauerwein RW. Memory-like IFN-γ response by NK cells following malaria infection reveals the crucial role of T cells in NK cell activation by P. falciparum. Eur J Immunol. 2010 Dec;40(12):3472-7. PMID:21072880

McCarthy VC, Clyde DF. Influence of sulfalene upon gametocytogenesis of Plasmodium falciparum and subsequent infection patterns in Anopheles stephensi. Exp Parasitol. 1973 Feb;33(1):73-8. PMID:4570982

McElroy B, Wiseman V, Matovu F, Mwengee W. Malaria prevention in north-eastern Tanzania: patterns of expenditure and determinants of demand at the household level. Malar J. 2009 May 7;8:95. PMID:19422704

McElwain TF, Perryman LE, Musoke AJ, McGuire TC. Molecular characterization and immunogenicity of neutralization-sensitive Babesia bigemina merozoite surface proteins. Mol Biochem Parasitol. 1991 Aug;47(2):213-22. PMID:1944418

McGowan S, Oellig CA, Birru WA, Caradoc-Davies TT, Stack CM, Lowther J, Skinner-Adams T, Mucha A, Kafarski P, Grembecka J, Trenholme KR, Buckle AM, Gardiner DL, Dalton JP, Whisstock JC. Structure of the Plasmodium falciparum M17 aminopeptidase and significance for the design of drugs targeting the neutral exopeptidases. Proc Natl Acad Sci U S A. 2010 Feb 9;107(6):2449-54. Epub 2010 Jan 21. PMID:20133789

McGready R, Lee S, Wiladphaingern J, Ashley E, Rijken M, Boel M, Simpson J, Paw M, Pimanpanarak M, Mu O, Singhasivanon P, White N, Nosten F. Adverse effects of falciparum and vivax malaria and the safety of antimalarial treatment in early pregnancy: a population-based study. Lancet Infect Dis. 2011 Dec 12. [Epub ahead of print]. PMID:22169409

McGregor IA. Immunity to plasmodial infections; consideration of factors relevant to malaria in man. Int Rev Trop Med. 1971;4:1-52. PMID:4944095

McHardy N, Simpson RM. Imidocarb dipropionate therapy in Kenyan anaplasmosis and babesiosis. Trop Anim Health Prod. 1974 May;6(2):63-70. PMID:4413774

McHardy N. Effects of stimulating erythropoiesis in mice infected with Babesia rodhaini. Ann Trop Med Parasitol. 1973 Sep;67(3):301-6. PMID:4761938

McHardy N. Immunization of rats against Babesia (Nuttalia) rodhaini. Nature. 1967 May 20;214(5090):805. PMID:4963880

McHardy N. Protective effect of haemolytic serum on mice infected with Babesia rodhaini. Ann Trop Med Parasitol. 1972 Mar;66(1):1-5. PMID:5021569

McLaughlin GL, Montenegro-James S, Vodkin MH, Howe D, Toro M, Leon E, Armijos R, Kakoma I, Greenwood BM, Hassan-King M, et al. Molecular approaches to malaria and babesiosis diagnosis. Mem Inst Oswaldo Cruz. 1992;87 Suppl 3:57-68. PMID:1343727

McQuillan JA, Mitchell AJ, Ho YF, Combes V, Ball HJ, Golenser J, Grau GE, Hunt NH. Coincident parasite and CD8 T cell sequestration is required for development of experimental cerebral malaria. Int J Parasitol. 2011 Feb;41(2):155-63. Epub 2010 Sep 7. PMID:20828575

McQuiston JH, Childs JE, Chamberland ME, Tabor E. Transmission of tick-borne agents of disease by blood transfusion: a review of known and potential risks in the United States. Transfusion. 2000 Mar;40(3):274-84. PMID:10738026

Meer-Scherrer L, Adelson M, Mordechai E, Lottaz B, Tilton R. Babesia microti infection in Europe. Curr Microbiol. 2004 Jun;48(6):435-7. PMID:15170239

Meeusen E, Lloyd S, Soulsby EJ. Antibody levels in adoptively immunized mice after infection with Babesia microti or injection with antigen fractions. Aust J Exp Biol Med Sci. 1985 Jun;63 (Pt 3):261-72. PMID:2415100

Meeusen E, Lloyd S, Soulsby EJ. Babesia microti in mice. Adoptive transfer of immunity with serum and cells. Aust J Exp Biol Med Sci. 1984 Oct;62 (Pt 5):551-66. PMID:6335965

Meeusen E, Lloyd S, Soulsby EJ. Babesia microti in mice. Subpopulations of cells involved in the adoptive transfer of immunity with immune spleen cells. Aust J Exp Biol Med Sci. 1984 Oct;62 (Pt 5):567-75. PMID:6442859

Mehlhorn H, Schein E. Redescription of Babesia equi Laveran, 1901 as Theileria equi Mehlhorn, Schein 1998. Parasitol Res. 1998 Jun;84(6):467-75. PMID:9660136

Mehta U, Allen E, Barnes KI. Establishing pharmacovigilance programs in resource-limited settings: the example of treating malaria. Expert Rev Clin Pharmacol. 2010 Jul;3(4):509-25. PMID:22111680

Meister J. Human babesiosis: a case study. Clin Excell Nurse Pract. 1999 Jul;3(4):214-6. PMID:10711060

Meliani P, Khatibi S, Randazzo S, Gorenflot A, Marchou B. [Human babesiosis].[Article in French]. Med Mal Infect. 2006 Oct;36(10):499-504. Epub 2006 Oct 4. PMID:17027216

Mellors LT, Dalgliesh RJ, Timms P, Rodwell BJ, Callow LL. Preparation and laboratory testing of a frozen vaccine containing Babesia bovis, Babesia bigemina and Anaplasma centrale. Res Vet Sci. 1982 Mar;32(2):194-7. PMID:7079601

Menan H, Faye O, Same-Ekobo A, Oga AS, Faye B, Kiki Barro CP, Kuete T, N'diaye JL, Vicky AM, Tine R, Yavo W, Kane D, Kassi KF, Kone M. Comparative study of the efficacy and tolerability of dihydroartemisinin-piperaquine-trimethoprim versus artemether-lumefantrine in the treatment of uncomplicated Plasmodium falciparum malaria in Cameroon, Ivory Coast and Senegal. Malar J. 2011 Jul 8;10:185. PMID:21740570

Ménard D, Barnadas C, Bouchier C, Henry-Halldin C, Gray LR, Ratsimbasoa A, Thonier V, Carod JF, Domarle O, Colin Y, Bertrand O, Picot J, King CL, Grimberg BT, Mercereau-Puijalon O, Zimmerman PA. Plasmodium vivax clinical malaria is commonly observed in Duffy-negative Malagasy people. Proc Natl Acad Sci U S A. 2010 Mar 30;107(13):5967-71. Epub 2010 Mar 15. PMID:20231434

Ménard D, Ratsimbasoa A, Randrianarivelojosia M, Rabarijaona LP, Raharimalala L, Domarle O, Randrianasolo L, Randriamanantena A, Jahevitra M, Andriantsoanirina V, Rason MA, Raherinjafy R, Rakotomalala E, Tuseo L, Raveloson A. Assessment of the efficacy of antimalarial drugs recommended by the National Malaria Control Programme in Madagascar: up-dated baseline data from randomized and multi-site clinical trials. Malar J. 2008 Apr 4;7:55. PMID:18394169

Mendoza A, Pérez-Silanes S, Quiliano M, Pabón A, Galiano S, González G, Garavito G, Zimic M, Vaisberg A, Aldana I, Monge A, Deharo E. Aryl piperazine and pyrrolidine as antimalarial agents. Synthesis and investigation of structure-activity relationships. Exp Parasitol. 2011 Jun;128(2):97-103. Epub 2011 Feb 24. PMID:21354139

Menemedengue V, Sahnouni K, Basco L, Tahar R. Molecular epidemiology of malaria in Cameroon. XXX. sequence analysis of Plasmodium falciparum ATPase 6, dihydrofolate reductase, and dihydropteroate synthase resistance markers in clinical isolates from children treated with an artesunate-sulfadoxine-pyrimethamine combination. Am J Trop Med Hyg. 2011 Jul;85(1):22-5. PMID:21734119

Menegon M, Talha AA, Severini C, Elbushra SM, Mohamedani AA, Malik EM, Mohamed TA, Wernsdorfer WH, Majori G, Nour BY. Frequency distribution of antimalarial drug resistance alleles among Plasmodium falciparum isolates from Gezira State, central Sudan, and Gedarif State, eastern Sudan. Am J Trop Med Hyg. 2010 Aug;83(2):250-7. PMID:20682863

Menemedengue V, Sahnouni K, Basco L, Tahar R. Molecular epidemiology of malaria in Cameroon. XXX. sequence analysis of Plasmodium falciparum ATPase 6, dihydrofolate reductase, and dihydropteroate synthase resistance markers in clinical isolates from children treated with an artesunate-sulfadoxine-pyrimethamine combination. Am J Trop Med Hyg. 2011 Jul;85(1):22-5. PMID:21734119

Menéndez C, Serra-Casas E, Scahill MD, Sanz S, Nhabomba A, Bardají A, Sigauque B, Cisteró P, Mandomando I, Dobaño C, Alonso PL, Mayor A. HIV and placental infection modulate the appearance of drug-resistant Plasmodium falciparum in pregnant women who receive intermittent preventive treatment. Clin Infect Dis. 2011 Jan 1;52(1):41-8. PMID:21148518

Mens PF, Scheelbeek PF, Al Atabbi H, Enato EF. Peer education: the effects on knowledge of pregnancy related malaria and preventive practices in women of reproductive age in Edo State, Nigeria. BMC Public Health. 2011 Aug 1;11:610. PMID:21801460

Mercer AE, Sarr Sallah M. The pharmacokinetic evaluation of artemisinin drugs for the treatment of malaria in paediatric populations. Expert Opin Drug Metab Toxicol. 2011 Apr;7(4):427-39. Epub 2011 Feb 15. PMID:21320023

Mercereau-Puijalon O, Ménard D. Plasmodium vivax and the Duffy antigen: a paradigm revisited. Transfus Clin Biol. 2010 Sep;17(3):176-83. Epub 2010 Jul 23. PMID:20655790

Mesfin A, Giday M, Animut A, Teklehaymanot T. Ethnobotanical study of antimalarial plants in Shinile District, Somali Region, Ethiopia, and in vivo evaluation of selected ones against Plasmodium berghei. J Ethnopharmacol. 2012 Jan 6;139(1):221-7. Epub 2011 Nov 11. PMID:22101085

Mesfin F, Demissew S, Teklehaymanot T. An ethnobotanical study of medicinal plants in Wonago Woreda, SNNPR, Ethiopia. J Ethnobiol Ethnomed. 2009 Oct 12;5:28. PMID:19821994

Mesia K, Cimanga K, Tona L, Mampunza MM, Ntamabyaliro N, Muanda T, Muyembe T, Totté J, Mets T, Pieters L, Vlietinck A. Assessment of the short-term safety and tolerability of a quantified 80 % ethanol extract from the stem bark of Nauclea pobeguinii (PR 259 CT1) in healthy volunteers: a clinical phase I study. Planta Med. 2011 Jan;77(2):111-6. Epub 2010 Jul 21. PMID:20665369

Mesia K, Cimanga RK, Dhooghe L, Cos P, Apers S, Totté J, Tona GL, Pieters L, Vlietinck AJ, Maes L. Antimalarial activity and toxicity evaluation of a quantified Nauclea pobeguinii extract. J Ethnopharmacol. 2010 Aug 19;131(1):10-6. Epub 2010 May 12. PMID:20470876

Mesia K, Tona L, Mampunza MM, Ntamabyaliro N, Muanda T, Muyembe T, Cimanga K, Totté J, Mets T, Pieters L, Vlietinck AJ. Antimalarial Efficacy of a Quantified Extract of Nauclea pobeguinii Stem Bark in Human Adult Volunteers with Diagnosed Uncomplicated Falciparum Malaria. Part 1: A Clinical Phase IIA Trial. Planta Med. 2011 Nov 17. [Epub ahead of print]. PMID:22095262

Metcalf ES. The role of international transport of equine semen on disease transmission. Anim Reprod Sci. 2001 Dec 3;68(3-4):229-37. PMID:11744267

Meyer C, Guthrie AJ, Stevens KB. Clinical and clinicopathological changes in 6 healthy ponies following intramuscular administration of multiple doses of imidocarb dipropionate. J S Afr Vet Assoc. 2005 Mar;76(1):26-32. PMID:15900897

Mgone CS. Strengthening of the clinical research capacity for malaria: a shared responsibility. Malar J. 2010 Dec 13;9 Suppl 3:S5. PMID:21144085

Michael OS, Gbotosho GO, Folarin OA, Okuboyejo T, Sowunmi A, Oduola AM, Happi CT. Early variations in plasmodium falciparum dynamics in Nigerian children after treatment with two artemisinin-based combinations: implications on delayed parasite clearance. Malar J. 2010 Nov 22;9:335. PMID:21092220

Michaelis M, Kleinschmidt MC, Barth S, Rothweiler F, Geiler J, Breitling R, Mayer B, Deubzer H, Witt O, Kreuter J, Doerr HW, Cinatl J, Cinatl J Jr. Anti-cancer effects of artesunate in a panel of chemoresistant neuroblastoma cell lines. Biochem Pharmacol. 2010 Jan 15;79(2):130-6. Epub 2009 Aug 19. PMID:19698702

Midzi N, Mtapuri-Zinyowera S, Sangweme D, Paul NH, Makware G, Mapingure MP, Brouwer KC, Mudzori J, Hlerema G, Chadukura V, Mutapi F, Kumar N, Mduluza T. Efficacy of integrated school based de-worming and prompt malaria treatment on helminths -Plasmodium falciparum co-infections: A 33 months follow up study. BMC Int Health Hum Rights. 2011 Jun 22;11:9. PMID:21696629

Miguel CA, Manderson L, Lansang MA. Patterns of treatment for malaria in Tayabas, The Philippines: implications for control. Trop Med Int Health. 1998 May;3(5):413-21. PMID:9623948

Miguel CA, Tallo VL, Manderson L, Lansang MA. Local knowledge and treatment of malaria in Agusan del Sur, The Philippines. Soc Sci Med. 1999 Mar;48(5):607-18. PMID:10080362

Mikhail AF, Leslie TJ, Mayan MI, Zekria R, Mohammad N, Hasanzai MA, Safi N, Whitty CJ, Rowland M. Field trial of three different Plasmodium vivax-detecting rapid diagnostic tests with and without evaporative cool box storage in Afghanistan. Malar J. 2011 Jun 22;10:169. PMID:21696587

Milhous W. Development of new drugs for chemoprophylaxis of malaria. Bull Soc Pathol Exot. 2001 Jul;94(2 Pt 2):149-51. PMID:16579068

Milstien J, Cárdenas V, Cheyne J, Brooks A. WHO policy development processes for a new vaccine: case study of malaria vaccines. Malar J. 2010 Jun 24;9:182. PMID:20576114

Mimche PN, Taramelli D, Vivas L. The plant-based immunomodulator curcumin as a potential candidate for the development of an adjunctive therapy for cerebral malaria. Malar J. 2011 Mar 15;10 Suppl 1:S10. [Epub ahead of print]. PMID:21411011

Minodier P, Noël G, Blanc P, Tsaregorodtseva N, Retornaz K, Garnier JM. [Malaria chemoprophylaxis in traveling children].[Article in French]. Arch Pediatr. 2005 Jan;12(1):53-8. PMID:15653056

Min-Oo G, Fortin A, Poulin JF, Gros P. Cysteamine, the molecule used to treat cystinosis, potentiates the antimalarial efficacy of artemisinin. Antimicrob Agents Chemother. 2010 Aug;54(8):3262-70. Epub 2010 May 17. PMID:20479197

Mintz ED, Anderson JF, Cable RG, Hadler JL. Transfusion-transmitted babesiosis: a case report from a new endemic area. Transfusion. 1991 May;31(4):365-8. PMID:2021001

Mishra N, Anvikar AR, Shah NK, Kamal VK, Sharma SK, Srivastava HC, Das MK, Pradhan K, Kumar H, Gupta YK, Gupta P, Dash AP, Valecha N. Prescription practices and availability of artemisinin monotherapy in India: where do we stand? Malar J. 2011 Dec 13;10(1):360. [Epub ahead of print]. PMID:22166073

Mishra SK, Singh P, Rath SK. A study of toxicity and differential gene expression in murine liver following exposure to anti-malarial drugs: amodiaquine and sulphadoxine-pyrimethamine. Malar J. 2011 May 2;10:109. PMID:21529379

Mishra VS, Stephens EB, Dame JB, Perryman LE, McGuire TC, McElwain TF. Immunogenicity and sequence analysis of recombinant p58: a neutralization-sensitive, antigenically conserved Babesia bigemina merozoite surface protein. Mol Biochem Parasitol. 1991 Aug;47(2):207-12. PMID:1944417

Mitchell GF, Handman E, Howard RJ. Protection of mice against plasmodium and babesia infections: attempts to raise host-protective sera. Aust J Exp Biol Med Sci. 1978 Oct;56(5):553-9. PMID:375903

Mitchell GH, Butcher GA, Cohen S. A merozoite vaccine effective against Plasmodium knowlesi malaria. Nature. 1974 Nov 22;252(5481):311-3. PMID:4431452

Mitrović S, Kranjcić-Zec I, Arsić-Arsenijević V, Dzamić A, Radonjić I. [Human babesiosis--recent discoveries].[Article in Serbian]. Med Pregl. 2004 Jul-Aug;57(7-8):349-53. PMID:15626291

Miura K, Perera S, Brockley S, Zhou H, Aebig JA, Moretz SE, Miller LH, Doumbo OK, Sagara I, Dicko A, Ellis RD, Long CA. Non-apical membrane antigen 1 (AMA1) IgGs from Malian children interfere with functional activity of AMA1 IgGs as judged by growth inhibition assay. PLoS One. 2011;6(6):e20947. Epub 2011 Jun 13. PMID:21695140

Miura K, Zhou H, Diouf A, Tullo G, Moretz SE, Aebig JA, Fay MP, Miller LH, Doumbo OK, Sagara I, Dicko A, Long CA, Ellis RD. Immunological responses against Plasmodium falciparum Apical Membrane Antigen 1 vaccines vary depending on the population immunized. Vaccine. 2011 Mar 9;29(12):2255-61. Epub 2011 Jan 31. PMID:21277408

Miyata T, Harakuni T, Sugawa H, Sattabongkot J, Kato A, Tachibana M, Torii M, Tsuboi T, Arakawa T. Adenovirus-vectored Plasmodium vivax ookinete surface protein, Pvs25, as a potential transmission-blocking vaccine. Vaccine. 2011 Mar 24;29(15):2720-6. Epub 2011 Feb 11. PMID:21315699

Miyata T, Harakuni T, Tsuboi T, Sattabongkot J, Ikehara A, Tachibana M, Torii M, Matsuzaki G, Arakawa T. Tricomponent immunopotentiating system as a novel molecular design strategy for malaria vaccine development. Infect Immun. 2011 Oct;79(10):4260-75. Epub 2011 Aug 1. PMID:21807905

Mlambo G, Kumar N, Yoshida S. Functional immunogenicity of baculovirus expressing Pfs25, a human malaria transmission-blocking vaccine candidate antigen. Vaccine. 2010 Oct 8;28(43):7025-9. Epub 2010 Aug 13. PMID:20709008

Mng'ong'o FC, Sambali JJ, Sabas E, Rubanga J, Magoma J, Ntamatungiro AJ, Turner EL, Nyogea D, Ensink JH, Moore SJ. Repellent plants provide affordable natural screening to prevent mosquito house entry in tropical rural settings--results from a pilot efficacy study. PLoS One. 2011;6(10):e25927. Epub 2011 Oct 12. PMID:22022471

Mnyone LL, Kirby MJ, Lwetoijera DW, Mpingwa MW, Knols BG, Takken W, Russell TL. Infection of the malaria mosquito, Anopheles gambiae, with two species of entomopathogenic fungi: effects of concentration, co-formulation, exposure time and persistence. Malar J. 2009 Dec 23;8:309. PMID:20030834

Mnyone LL, Kirby MJ, Mpingwa MW, Lwetoijera DW, Knols BG, Takken W, Koenraadt CJ, Russell TL. Infection of Anopheles gambiae mosquitoes with entomopathogenic fungi: effect of host age and blood-feeding status. Parasitol Res. 2011 Feb;108(2):317-22. Epub 2010 Sep 25. PMID:20872014

Mnyone LL, Koenraadt CJ, Lyimo IN, Mpingwa MW, Takken W, Russell TL. Anopheline and culicine mosquitoes are not repelled by surfaces treated with the entomopathogenic fungi Metarhizium anisopliae and Beauveria bassiana. Parasit Vectors. 2010 Aug 27;3:80. PMID:20799937

Mohammadi D. Public health insecticide development: a status of hiatus. Lancet. 2010 Oct 9;376(9748):1207. PMID:20934581

Mohanty S, Mishra SK, Patnaik R, Dutt AK, Pradhan S, Das B, Patnaik J, Mohanty AK, Lee SJ, Dondorp AM. Brain swelling and mannitol therapy in adult cerebral malaria: a randomized trial. Clin Infect Dis. 2011 Aug;53(4):349-55. PMID:21810747

Mohapatra MK, Ghosh A. Suboptimal erythropoietin production in adult severe falciparum malaria. J Assoc Physicians India. 2011 Jun;59:392-3. PMID:21751602

Mok S, Imwong M, Mackinnon MJ, Sim J, Ramadoss R, Yi P, Mayxay M, Chotivanich K, Liong KY, Russell B, Socheat D, Newton PN, Day NP, White NJ, Preiser PR, Nosten F, Dondorp AM, Bozdech Z. Artemisinin resistance in Plasmodium falciparum is associated with an altered temporal pattern of transcription. BMC Genomics. 2011 Aug 3;12:391. PMID:21810278

Molinar E, James MA, Kakoma I, Holland C, Ristic M. Antigenic and immunogenic studies on cell culture-derived Babesia canis. Vet Parasitol. 1982 Mar;10(1):29-40. PMID:6179286

Molloy JB, Bock RE, Templeton JM, Bruyeres AG, Bowles PM, Blight GW, Jorgensen WK. Identification of antigenic differences that discriminate between cattle vaccinated with Anaplasma centrale and cattle naturally infected with Anaplasma marginale. Int J Parasitol. 2001 Feb;31(2):179-86. PMID:11239938

Mombo-Ngoma G, Supan C, Dal-Bianco MP, Missinou MA, Matsiegui PB, Ospina Salazar CL, Issifou S, Ter-Minassian D, Ramharter M, Kombila M, Kremsner PG, Lell B. Phase I randomized dose-ascending placebo-controlled trials of ferroquine—a candidate anti-malarial drug--in adults with asymptomatic Plasmodium falciparum infection. Malar J. 2011 Mar 1;10:53. PMID:21362162

Moneriz C, Marín-García P, Bautista JM, Diez A, Puyet A. Parasitostatic effect of maslinic acid. II. Survival increase and immune protection in lethal Plasmodium yoelii-infected mice. Malar J. 2011 Apr 25;10:103. PMID:21518429

Moneriz C, Marín-García P, García-Granados A, Bautista JM, Diez A, Puyet A. Parasitostatic effect of maslinic acid. I. Growth arrest of Plasmodium falciparum intraerythrocytic stages. Malar J. 2011 Apr 10;10:82. PMID:21477369

Moneriz C, Mestres J, Bautista JM, Diez A, Puyet A. Multi-targeted activity of maslinic acid as an antimalarial natural compound. FEBS J. 2011 Aug;278(16):2951-61. Epub 2011 Jul 7. PMID:21689375

Monks D, Fisher M, Forbes NA. Ixodes frontalis and avian tick-related syndrome in the United Kingdom. J Small Anim Pract. 2006 Aug;47(8):451-5. PMID:16911113

Montenegro-James S, Ristic M, Toro Benitez M, Leon E, Lopez R. Heterologous strain immunity in bovine babesiosis using a culture-derived soluble Babesia bovis immunogen. Vet Parasitol. 1985 Dec;18(4):321-37.PMID:4090242

Montenegro-James S, Toro Benitez M, Leon E, Lopez R, Ristic M. Bovine babesiosis: induction of protective immunity with culture-derived Babesia bovis and Babesia bigemina immunogens. Parasitol Res. 1987;74(2):142-50. PMID:3325981

Montenegro-James S, Toro M, Leon E, Guillen AT, Lopez R, Lopez W. Immunization of cattle with an inactivated polyvalent vaccine against anaplasmosis and babesiosis. Ann N Y Acad Sci. 1992 Jun 16;653:112-21. PMID:1626861

Montenegro-James S, Toro M, Leon E, Guillen AT. Field evaluation of an exoantigen-containing Babesia vaccine in Venezuela. Mem Inst Oswaldo Cruz. 1992;87 Suppl 3:283-8. PMID:1343704

Montenegro-James S. Immunoprophylactic control of bovine babesiosis: role of exoantigens of Babesia. Trans R Soc Trop Med Hyg. 1989;83 Suppl:85-94. PMID:2696166

Montenegro-James S. Prevalence and control of babesiosis in the Americas. Mem Inst Oswaldo Cruz. 1992;87 Suppl 3:27-36. PMID:1343700

Montero E, Rodriguez M, Gonzalez LM, Lobo CA. Babesia divergens: identification and characterization of BdHSP-20, a small heat shock protein. Exp Parasitol. 2008 Jun;119(2):238-45. Epub 2008 Feb 13. PMID:18346739

Montero E, Rodriguez M, Oksov Y, Lobo CA. Babesia divergens apical membrane antigen 1 and its interaction with the human red blood cell. Infect Immun. 2009 Nov;77(11):4783-93. Epub 2009 Aug 31. PMID:19720759

Moore DJ. Therapeutic implications of Babesia canis infection in dogs. J S Afr Vet Assoc. 1979 Dec;50(4):346-52. PMID:553976

Moore EM, Lockwood DN. Treatment of visceral leishmaniasis. J Glob Infect Dis. 2010 May;2(2):151-8. PMID:20606971

Moore SJ, Hill N, Ruiz C, Cameron MM. Field evaluation of traditionally used plant-based insect repellents and fumigants against the malaria vector Anopheles darlingi in Riberalta, Bolivian Amazon. J Med Entomol. 2007 Jul;44(4):624-30. PMID:17695017

Moore SJ, Lenglet A, Hill N. Field evaluation of three plant-based insect repellents against malaria vectors in Vaca Diez Province, the Bolivian Amazon. J Am Mosq Control Assoc. 2002 Jun;18(2):107-10. PMID:12083351

Moreau Y, Vidor E, Bissuel G, Dubreuil N. Vaccination against canine babesiosis: an overview of field observations. Trans R Soc Trop Med Hyg. 1989;83 Suppl:95-6. PMID:2623757

Mordmüller B. New medicines for malaria. Wien Klin Wochenschr. 2010 Mar;122 Suppl 1:19-22. PMID:20376719

Moreno Giménez JC, Jiménez Puya R, Galán Gutiérrez M, Ortega Salas R, Dueñas Jurado JM. Erythema figuratum in septic babesiosis. J Eur Acad Dermatol Venereol. 2006 Jul;20(6):726-8. PMID:16836504

Morita T, Saeki H, Imai S, Ishii T. Reactivity of anti-erythrocyte antibody induced by Babesia gibsoni infection against aged erythrocytes. Vet Parasitol. 1995 Jul;58(4):291-9. PMID:8533268

Morrell CN, Srivastava K, Swaim A, Lee MT, Chen J, Nagineni C, Hooks JJ, Detrick B. Beta interferon suppresses the development of experimental cerebral malaria. Infect Immun. 2011 Apr;79(4):1750-8. Epub 2011 Jan 18. PMID:21245265

Morzaria SP, Brocklesby DW, Harradine DL, Barnett SF. Babesia major in Britain: infectivity of suspensions derived from ground-up Haemaphysalis punct at a nymphs. Int J Parasitol. 1974 Aug;4(4):437-8. PMID:4448585

Morzaria SP, Brocklesby DW, Harradine DL, Luther PD. Babesia major in Britain: infectivity for cattle of cryopreserved parasites derived from Haemaphysalis punctata nymphs. Res Vet Sci. 1977 Mar;22(2):190-3. PMID:860093

Morzaria SP, Young AS, Hudson EB. Babesia bigemina in Kenya: experimental transmission by Boophilus decoloratus and the production of tick-derived stabilates. Parasitology. 1977 Jun;74(3):291-8. PMID:876684

Moshkovskiĭ ShD, Tareev EM, Dukhanina NN, Stavrovskaia VI, Ozeretskovskaia NN, Rabinovich SA. [Development of the main trends of malariology in the USSR].[Article in Russian]. Med Parazitol (Mosk). 1967 Nov-Dec;36(6):643-63. PMID:4887958

Mosqueda J, Figueroa JV, Alvarez A, Bautista R, Falcon A, Ramos A, Canto G, Vega CA. Advances in the development of molecular tools for the control of bovine babesiosis in Mexico. Parassitologia. 2007 May;49 Suppl 1:19-22. PMID:17691602

Mosqueira B, Duchon S, Chandre F, Hougard JM, Carnevale P, Mas-Coma S. Efficacy of an insecticide paint against insecticide-susceptible and resistant mosquitoes - part 1: laboratory evaluation. Malar J. 2010 Nov 25;9:340. PMID:21108819

Motabar M, Tabibzadeh I, Manouchehri AV. Malaria and its control in Iran. Trop Geogr Med. 1975 Mar;27(1):71-8. PMID:1094644

Mott GA, Wilson R, Fernando A, Robinson A, MacGregor P, Kennedy D, Schaap D, Matthews JB, Matthews KR. Targeting cattle-borne zoonoses and cattle pathogens using a novel trypanosomatid-based delivery system. PLoS Pathog. 2011 Oct;7(10):e1002340. Epub 2011 Oct 27. PMID:22046137

Mounier-Jack S, Rudge JW, Phetsouvanh R, Chanthapadith C, Coker R. Critical interactions between Global Fund-supported programmes and health systems: a case study in Lao People's Democratic Republic. Health Policy Plan. 2010 Nov;25 Suppl 1:i37-42. PMID:20966107

Moxon ER, Siegrist CA. The next decade of vaccines: societal and scientific challenges. Lancet. 2011 Jul 23;378(9788):348-59. Epub 2011 Jun 12. PMID:21664685

Mubi M, Janson A, Warsame M, Mårtensson A, Källander K, Petzold MG, Ngasala B, Maganga G, Gustafsson LL, Massele A, Tomson G, Premji Z, Björkman A. Malaria rapid testing by community health workers is effective and safe for targeting malaria treatment: randomised cross-over trial in Tanzania. PLoS One. 2011;6(7):e19753. Epub 2011 Jul 5. PMID:21750697

Mubyazi G, Bloch P, Kamugisha M, Kitua A, Ijumba J. Intermittent preventive treatment of malaria during pregnancy: a qualitative study of knowledge, attitudes and practices of district health managers, antenatal care staff and pregnant women in Korogwe District, North-Eastern Tanzania. Malar J. 2005 Jul 20;4:31. PMID:16033639

Müller GC, Beier JC, Traore SF, Toure MB, Traore MM, Bah S, Doumbia S, Schlein Y. Field experiments of Anopheles gambiae attraction to local fruits/seedpods and flowering plants in Mali to optimize strategies for malaria vector control in Africa using attractive toxic sugar bait methods. Malar J. 2010 Sep 20;9:262. PMID:20854666

Müller GC, Beier JC, Traore SF, Toure MB, Traore MM, Bah S, Doumbia S, Schlein Y. Successful field trial of attractive toxic sugar bait (ATSB) plant-spraying methods against malaria vectors in the Anopheles gambiae complex in Mali, West Africa. Malar J. 2010 Jul 21;9:210. PMID:20663142

Müller IB, Hyde JE. Antimalarial drugs: modes of action and mechanisms of parasite resistance. Future Microbiol. 2010 Dec;5(12):1857-73. PMID:21155666

Müller O, Sié A, Meissner P, Schirmer RH, Kouyaté B. Artemisinin resistance on the Thai-Cambodian border. Lancet. 2009 Oct 24;374(9699):1419. PMID:19854368

Mugwaneza P, Umutoni NW, Ruton H, Rukundo A, Lyambabaje A, Bizimana Jde D, Tsague L, Wagner CM, Nyankesha E, Muita J, Mutabazi V, Nyemazi JP, Nsanzimana S, Karema C, Binagwaho A. Under-two child mortality according to maternal HIV status in Rwanda: assessing outcomes within the National PMTCT Program. Pan Afr Med J. 2011;9:37. Epub 2011 Aug 3. PMID:22145068

Muhamad P, Chaijaroenkul W, Congpuong K, Na-Bangchang K. SYBR Green I and TaqMan quantitative real-time polymerase chain reaction methods for the determination of amplification of Plasmodium falciparum multidrug resistance-1 gene (pfmdr1). J Parasitol. 2011 Oct;97(5):939-42. Epub 2011 May 9. PMID:21554069

Muhamad P, Phompradit P, Sornjai W, Maensathian T, Chaijaroenkul W, Rueangweerayut R, Na-Bangchang K. Polymorphisms of molecular markers of antimalarial drug resistance and relationship with artesunate-mefloquine combination therapy in patients with uncomplicated Plasmodium falciparum malaria in Thailand. Am J Trop Med Hyg. 2011 Sep;85(3):568-72. PMID:21896824

Mukanga D, Babirye R, Peterson S, Pariyo GW, Ojiambo G, Tibenderana JK, Nsubuga P, Kallander K. Can lay community health workers be trained to use diagnostics to distinguish and treat malaria and pneumonia in children? Lessons from rural Uganda. Trop Med Int Health. 2011 Jul 14. [Epub ahead of print]. PMID:21752163

Mula P, Fernández-Martínez A, de Lucio A, Ramos JM, Reyes F, González V, Benito A, Berzosa P. Detection of high levels of mutations involved in anti-malarial drug resistance in Plasmodium falciparum and Plasmodium vivax at a rural hospital in southern Ethiopia. Malar J. 2011 Aug 2;10:214. PMID:21810256

Munro JB, Silva JC. Ribonucleotide Reductase as a Target to Control Apicomplexan Diseases. Curr Issues Mol Biol. 2011 Jul 26;14(1):9-26. [Epub ahead of print]. PMID:21791713

Muregi FW, Kano S, Kino H, Ishih A. Plasmodium berghei: efficacy of 5-fluoroorotate in combination with commonly used antimalarial drugs in a mouse model. Exp Parasitol. 2009 Apr;121(4):376-80. PMID:19271282

Muregi FW, Kirira PG, Ishih A. Novel rational drug design strategies with potential to revolutionize malaria chemotherapy. Curr Med Chem. 2011;18(1):113-43. PMID:21110811

Muregi FW, Ohta I, Masato U, Kino H, Ishih A. Resistance of a rodent malaria parasite to a thymidylate synthase inhibitor induces an apoptotic parasite death and imposes a huge cost of fitness. PLoS One. 2011;6(6):e21251. Epub 2011 Jun 16. PMID:21698180

Muregi FW. Antimalarial drugs and their useful therapeutic lives: rational drug design lessons from pleiotropic action of quinolines and artemisinins. Curr Drug Discov Technol. 2010 Dec 1;7(4):280-316. PMID:21034413

Murnigsih T, Subeki, Matsuura H, Takahashi K, Yamasaki M, Yamato O, Maede Y, Katakura K, Suzuki M, Kobayashi S, Chairul, Yoshihara T. Evaluation of the inhibitory activities of the extracts of Indonesian traditional medicinal plants against Plasmodium falciparum and Babesia gibsoni. J Vet Med Sci. 2005 Aug;67(8):829-31. PMID:16141673

Musila N, Opiyo N, English M. Treatment of African children with severe malaria - towards evidence-informed clinical practice using GRADE. Malar J. 2011 Jul 21;10:201. PMID:21777441

Musoke AJ, McKeever D, Nene V. Subunit vaccines for the control of tick-borne diseases: implications for the future. Parassitologia. 1997 Jun;39(2):131-7. PMID:9530697

Mustofa, Sholikhah EN, Wahyuono S. In vitro and in vivo antiplasmodial activity and cytotoxicity of extracts of Phyllanthus niruri L. herbs traditionally used to treat malaria in Indonesia. Southeast Asian J Trop Med Public Health. 2007 Jul;38(4):609-15. PMID:17882995

Mutabingwa TK, Muze K, Ord R, Briceño M, Greenwood BM, Drakeley C, Whitty CJ. Randomized trial of artesunate+amodiaquine, sulfadoxine-pyrimethamine+amodiaquine, chlorproguanal-dapsone and SP for malaria in pregnancy in Tanzania. PLoS One. 2009;4(4):e5138. Epub 2009 Apr 8. PMID:19352498

Muthee JK, Gakuya DW, Mbaria JM, Kareru PG, Mulei CM, Njonge FK. Ethnobotanical study of anthelmintic and other medicinal plants traditionally used in Loitoktok district of Kenya. J Ethnopharmacol. 2011 Apr 26;135(1):15-21. Epub 2011 Feb 22. PMID:21349318

Myint HY, Berman J, Walker L, Pybus B, Melendez V, Baird JK, Ohrt C. Review: improving the therapeutic index of 8-aminoquinolines by the use of drug combinations: review of the literature and proposal for future investigations. Am J Trop Med Hyg. 2011 Dec;85(6):1010-4. PMID:22144436

Myint NW, Kaewkungwal J, Singhasivanon P, Chaisiri K, Panjapiyakul P, Siriwan P, Mallik AK, Nyein SL, Mu TT. Are there any changes in burden and management of communicable diseases in areas affected by Cyclone Nargis? Confl Health. 2011 Jun 28;5(1):9. PMID:21708044

Mylonakis E. When to suspect and how to monitor babesiosis. Am Fam Physician. 2001 May 15;63(10):1969-74. PMID:11388711

Na-Bangchang K, Ruengweerayut R, Mahamad P, Ruengweerayut K, Chaijaroenkul W. Declining in efficacy of a three-day combination regimen of mefloquine-artesunate in a multi-drug resistance area along the Thai-Myanmar border. Malar J. 2010 Oct 8;9:273. PMID:20929590

Nadembega P, Boussim JI, Nikiema JB, Poli F, Antognoni F. Medicinal plants in Baskoure, Kourittenga Province, Burkina Faso: an ethnobotanical study. J Ethnopharmacol. 2011 Jan 27;133(2):378-95. Epub 2010 Oct 13. PMID:20950680

Nagao E, Arie T, Dorward DW, Fairhurst RM, Dvorak JA. The avian malaria parasite Plasmodium gallinaceum causes marked structural changes on the surface of its host erythrocyte. J Struct Biol. 2008 Jun;162(3):460-7. Epub 2008 Mar 21. PMID:18442920

Naha K, Dasari S, Prabhu M. Spectrum of complications associated with Plasmodium vivax infection in a tertiary hospital in South-Western India. Asian Pac J Trop Med. 2012 Jan;5(1):79-82. PMID:22182650

Nahum A, Erhart A, Ahounou D, Bonou D, Van Overmeir C, Menten J, Akogbeto M, Coosemans M, Massougbodji A, D'Alessandro U. Extended high efficacy of the combination sulphadoxine-pyrimethamine with artesunate in children with uncomplicated falciparum malaria on the Benin coast, West Africa. Malar J. 2009 Mar 3;8:37. PMID:19257898

Naidoo S, London L, Burdorf A, Naidoo RN, Kromhout H. Occupational activities associated with a reported history of malaria among women working in small-scale agriculture in South Africa. Am J Trop Med Hyg. 2011 Nov;85(5):805-10. PMID:22049030

Naidoo V, Mulders MS, Swan GE. The intravenous pharmacokinetics of diminazene in healthy dogs. J S Afr Vet Assoc. 2009 Dec;80(4):215-9. PMID:20458860

Naidoo V, Zweygarth E, Eloff JN, Swan GE. Identification of anti-babesial activity for four ethnoveterinary plants in vitro. Vet Parasitol. 2005 Jun 10;130(1-2):9-13. Epub 2005 Apr 12. PMID:15893064

Nain V, Sahi S, Verma A. CPP-ZFN: a potential DNA-targeting anti-malarial drug. Malar J. 2010 Sep 16;9:258. PMID:20846404

Naing C, Aung K, Win DK, Wah MJ. Efficacy and safety of chloroquine for treatment in patients with uncomplicated Plasmodium vivax infections in endemic countries. Trans R Soc Trop Med Hyg. 2010 Nov;104(11):695-705. Epub 2010 Sep 20. PMID:20850161

Nájera JA, González-Silva M, Alonso PL. Some lessons for the future from the Global Malaria Eradication Programme (1955-1969). PLoS Med. 2011 Jan 25;8(1):e1000412. PMID:21311585

Nakamura K, Yokoyama N, Igarashi I. Cyclin-dependent kinase inhibitors block erythrocyte invasion and intraerythrocytic development of Babesia bovis in vitro. Parasitology. 2007 Sep;134(Pt 10):1347-53. Epub 2007 Jul 18. PMID:17634158

Nakamura Y, Tsuji M, Arai S, Ishihara C. A method for rapid and complete substitution of the circulating erythrocytes in SCID mice with bovine erythrocytes and use of the substituted mice for bovine hemoprotozoa infections. J Immunol Methods. 1995 Dec 27;188(2):247-54. PMID:8551053

Nakao R, Mizukami C, Kawamura Y, Subeki, Bawm S, Yamasaki M, Maede Y, Matsuura H, Nabeta K, Nonaka N, Oku Y, Katakura K. Evaluation of efficacy of bruceine A, a natural quassinoid compound extracted from a medicinal plant, Brucea javanica, for canine babesiosis. J Vet Med Sci. 2009 Jan;71(1):33-41. PMID:19194074

Namangala B, Inoue N, Sugimoto C. Preliminary studies on the effects of orally-administered Transforming Growth Factor-beta on protozoan diseases in mice. Jpn J Vet Res. 2009 Aug;57(2):101-8. PMID:19827745

Namsa ND, Mandal M, Tangjang S. Anti-malarial herbal remedies of northeast India, Assam: an ethnobotanical survey. J Ethnopharmacol. 2011 Jan 27;133(2):565-72. Epub 2010 Oct 26. PMID:21029768

Nankabirwa V, Tylleskar T, Nankunda J, Engebretsen IM, Sommerfelt H, Tumwine JK; PROMISE EBF Research Consortium et al. Malaria parasitaemia among infants and its association with breastfeeding peer counselling and vitamin A supplementation: a secondary analysis of a cluster randomized trial. PLoS One. 2011;6(7):e21862. Epub 2011 Jul 7. PMID:21760916

Nansera D, Max I, Annet K, Gessner BD. Bacterial meningitis among children under the age of 2 years in a high human immunodeficiency virus prevalence area after Haemophilus influenzae type b vaccine introduction. J Paediatr Child Health. 2011 Nov 14. [Epub ahead of print]. PMID:22077853

Narasimhan S, Montgomery RR, DePonte K, Tschudi C, Marcantonio N, Anderson JF, Sauer JR, Cappello M, Kantor FS, Fikrig E. Disruption of Ixodes scapularis anticoagulation by using RNA interference. Proc Natl Acad Sci U S A. 2004 Feb 3;101(5):1141-6. Epub 2004 Jan 26. PMID:14745044

Nardin E. The past decade in malaria synthetic peptide vaccine clinical trials. Hum Vaccin. 2010 Jan;6(1):27-38. Epub 2010 Jan 23. PMID:20173408

Nari A. Strategies for the control of one-host ticks and relationship with tick-borne diseases in South America. Vet Parasitol. 1995 Mar;57(1-3):153-65. PMID:7597780

Nasveld P, Kitchener S, Edstein M, Rieckmann K. Comparison of tafenoquine (WR238605) and primaquine in the post-exposure (terminal) prophylaxis of vivax malaria in Australian Defence Force personnel. Trans R Soc Trop Med Hyg. 2002 Nov-Dec;96(6):683-4. PMID:12625150

Nasveld P, Kitchener S. Treatment of acute vivax malaria with tafenoquine. Trans R Soc Trop Med Hyg. 2005 Jan;99(1):2-5. PMID:15550254

Nasveld PE, Edstein MD, Reid M, Brennan L, Harris IE, Kitchener SJ, Leggat PA, Pickford P, Kerr C, Ohrt C, Prescott W; Tafenoquine Study Team. Randomized, double-blind study of the safety, tolerability, and efficacy of tafenoquine versus mefloquine for malaria prophylaxis in nonimmune subjects. Antimicrob Agents Chemother. 2010 Feb;54(2):792-8. Epub 2009 Dec 7. PMID:19995933

Nau JY. [Malaria and trypanosomiasis: good news].[Article in French]. Rev Med Suisse. 2011 Sep 28;7(310):1890-1. PMID:22029130

Nawaz F, Nsobya SL, Kiggundu M, Joloba M, Rosenthal PJ. Selection of parasites with diminished drug susceptibility by amodiaquine-containing antimalarial regimens in Uganda. J Infect Dis. 2009 Dec 1;200(11):1650-7. PMID:19905933

Ndao M. Biomarker discovery in serum/plasma using surface enhanced laser desorption ionization time of flight (SELDI-TOF) mass spectrometry. Methods Mol Biol. 2012;818:67-79. PMID:22083816

Ndiaye D, Patel V, Demas A, LeRoux M, Ndir O, Mboup S, Clardy J, Lakshmanan V, Daily JP, Wirth DF. A non-radioactive DAPI-based high-throughput in vitro assay to assess Plasmodium falciparum responsiveness to antimalarials--increased sensitivity of P. falciparum to chloroquine in Senegal. Am J Trop Med Hyg. 2010 Feb;82(2):228-30. PMID:20133997

Ndjinga JK, Minakawa N. The importance of education to increase the use of bed nets in villages outside of Kinshasa, Democratic Republic of the Congo. Malar J. 2010 Oct 12;9:279. PMID:20937157

Neal AT, Jordan SJ, Oliveira AL, Hernandez JN, Branch OH, Rayner JC. Limited variation in vaccine candidate Plasmodium falciparum Merozoite Surface Protein-6 over multiple transmission seasons. Malar J. 2010 May 24;9:138. PMID:20497564

Neal RA, Garnham PC, Cohen S. [Immunization against protozoal diseases].[Article in Spanish]. Bol Oficina Sanit Panam. 1973 Oct;75(4):337-53. PMID:4272727

Neal RA, Garnham PC, Cohen S. Immunization against protozoal diseases. Br Med Bull. 1969 May;25(2):194-201. PMID:4918534

Nehrbass-Stuedli A, Boykin D, Tidwell RR, Brun R. Novel diamidines with activity against Babesia divergens in vitro and Babesia microti in vivo. Antimicrob Agents Chemother. 2011 Jul;55(7):3439-45. Epub 2011 May 2. PMID:21537025

Neill US. From branch to bedside: Youyou Tu is awarded the 2011 Lasker~DeBakey Clinical Medical Research Award for discovering artemisinin as a treatment for malaria. J Clin Invest. 2011 Oct 3;121(10):3768-73. PMID:22059236

Nelson DA, Bradley JK, Arya R, Ianosi-Irimie M, Marques-Baptista A, Merlin MA. Babesiosis as a rare cause of fever in the immunocompromised patient: a case report. Cases J. 2009 Jul 10;2:7420. PMID:19829959

Németh K, Tárkányi G, Varga E, Imre T, Mizsei R, Iványi R, Visy J, Szemán J, Jicsinszky L, Szente L, Simonyi M. Enantiomeric separation of antimalarial drugs by capillary electrophoresis using neutral and negatively charged cyclodextrins. J Pharm Biomed Anal. 2011 Feb 20;54(3):475-81. Epub 2010 Sep 19. PMID:20943339

Newton PN, Fernández FM, Plançon A, Mildenhall DC, Green MD, Ziyong L, Christophel EM, Phanouvong S, Howells S, McIntosh E, Laurin P, Blum N, Hampton CY, Faure K, Nyadong L, Soong CW, Santoso B, Zhiguang W, Newton J, Palmer K. A collaborative epidemiological investigation into the criminal fake artesunate trade in South East Asia. PLoS Med. 2008 Feb;5(2):e32. PMID:18271620

Newton PN, Green MD, Mildenhall DC, Plancon A, Nettey H, Nyadong L, Hostetler DM, Swamidoss I, Harris GA, Powell K, Timmermans AE, Amin AA, Opuni SK, Barbereau S, Faurant C, Soong RC, Faure K, Thevanayagam J, Fernandes P, Kaur H, Angus B, Stepniewska K, Guerin PJ, Fernandez FM. Poor quality vital anti-malarials in Africa - an urgent neglected public health priority. Malar J. 2011 Dec 13;10(1):352. [Epub ahead of print]. PMID:22152094

Ngo V, Civen R. Babesiosis acquired through blood transfusion, California, USA. Emerg Infect Dis. 2009 May;15(5):785-7. PMID:19402969

Nguta JM, Mbaria JM, Gakuya DW, Gathumbi PK, Kiama SG. Traditional antimalarial phytotherapy remedies used by the South Coast community, Kenya. J Ethnopharmacol. 2010 Sep 15;131(2):256-67. Epub 2010 Jun 30. PMID:20600756

Nguta JM, Mbaria JM, Gathumbi PK, Gakuya D, Kabasa JD, Kiama SG. Ethnodiagnostic skills of the digo community for malaria: a lead to traditional bioprospecting. Front Pharmacol. 2011;2:30. Epub 2011 Jun 24. PMID:21738507

Nicholson GT, Walsh CA, Madan RP. Transfusion-associated babesiosis in a 7-month-old infant after bidirectional Glenn procedure. Congenit Heart Dis. 2010 Nov-Dec;5(6):607-13. PMID:21106022

Nicolas X, Granier H, Laborde JP, Talarmin F, Klotz F. [Plasmodium vivax: therapy update].[Article in French]. Presse Med. 2001 Apr 21;30(15):767-71. PMID:11360746

Nishisaka M, Yokoyama N, Xuan X, Inoue N, Nagasawa H, Fujisaki K, Mikami T, Igarashi I. Characterisation of the gene encoding a protective antigen from Babesia microti identified it as eta subunit of chaperonin containing T-complex protein 1. Int J Parasitol. 2001 Dec;31(14):1673-9. PMID:11730795

Njuguna J, Qader S. Challenges Associated with Scaling up Artemisinin Combination Therapy in Sub-Saharan Africa A Review Article. Libyan J Med. 2008 Mar 1;3(1):42-8. PMID:21499481

No authors listed. Antigenic variation in African trypanosomiasis: a memorandum. Bull World Health Organ. 1977;55(6):703-13. PMID:74295

No authors listed. Artemisinin derivatives and malaria: useful, in combination with other antimalarials. Prescrire Int. 2008 Aug;17(96):162-8. PMID:19492494

No authors listed. Artemisinins in malaria treatment in the UK. Drug Ther Bull. 2010 Nov;48(11):129-32. PMID:21057033

No authors listed. DEVELOPMENT of the antimalarial paludrine. Am Prof Pharm. 1946 Apr;12:352-4. PMID:21027189

No authors listed. Developments in malaria immunology. Report of a WHO scientific group. World Health Organ Tech Rep Ser. 1975;(579):1-68. PMID:813400

No authors listed. Exotic animal diseases bulletin: equine piroplasmosis. Aust Vet J. 2008 Nov;86(11):N20-1. PMID:19058427

No authors listed. Intravenous artesunate for severe malaria. Prescrire Int. 2008 Aug;17(96):168-70. PMID:19492495

No authors listed. Malaria and economic development in Papua New Guinea. Med J Aust. 1972 Dec 30;2(27):1473-4. PMID:4655125

No authors listed. Malaria progress report shows that development aid for health is working. Neurosciences (Riyadh). 2010 Apr;15(2):144-5. PMID:20672509

No authors listed. Malaria progress report shows that development aid for health is working. Saudi Med J. 2010 Feb;31(2):225-7. PMID:20198752

No authors listed. Molecule of the month. Tafenoquine succinate. Drug News Perspect. 2003 May;16(4):238. PMID:12942153

No authors listed. OSHA's bloodborne pathogens standard: analysis and recommendations. Health Devices. 1993 Feb;22(2):35-92. PMID:8444629

No authors listed. Research needs on internal parasites of horses. Am J Vet Res. 1984 Aug;45(8):1614-8. PMID:6383147

No authors listed. Resistance to artemisinin derivatives along the Thai-Cambodian border. [Article in English, French]. Wkly Epidemiol Rec. 2007 Oct 12;82(41):360. PMID:17933087

No authors listed. The Global Fund and a new modus operandi. Lancet. 2011 Dec 3;378(9807):1896. PMID:22137831

No authors listed. Timing antimalarial prophylaxis: when to start and how long to go on. Drug Ther Bull. 1974 Aug 16;12(17):65-7. PMID:4457297

No authors listed. Vaccines against malaria and babesiosis. Lancet. 1983 Nov 26;2(8361):1232-3. PMID:6139575

Noedl H, Se Y, Sriwichai S, Schaecher K, Teja-Isavadharm P, Smith B, Rutvisuttinunt W, Bethell D, Surasri S, Fukuda MM, Socheat D, Chan Thap L. Artemisinin resistance in Cambodia: a clinical trial designed to address an emerging problem in Southeast Asia. Clin Infect Dis. 2010 Dec 1;51(11):e82-9. Epub 2010 Oct 28. PMID:21028985

Nogueira FH, Moreira-Campos LM, Santos RL, Pianetti GA. Quality of essential drugs in tropical countries: evaluation of antimalarial drugs in the Brazilian Health System. Rev Soc Bras Med Trop. 2011 Oct;44(5):582-6. PMID:22031073

Nohýnková E, Kubek J, Měst'ánková O, Chalupa P, Hubálek Z. [A case of Babesia microti imported into the Czech Republic from the USA]. [Article in Czech]. Cas Lek Cesk. 2003;142(6):377-81. PMID:12924039

Noland GS, Chowdhury DR, Urban JF Jr, Zavala F, Kumar N. Helminth infection impairs the immunogenicity of a Plasmodium falciparum DNA vaccine, but not irradiated sporozoites, in mice. Vaccine. 2010 Apr 9;28(17):2917-23. Epub 2010 Feb 25. PMID:20188676

Noonpakdee W, Pothikasikorn J, Nimitsantiwong W, Wilairat P. Inhibition of Plasmodium falciparum proliferation in vitro by antisense oligodeoxynucleotides against malarial topoisomerase II. Biochem Biophys Res Commun. 2003 Mar 21;302(4):659-64. PMID:12646219

Nonaka D, Vongseththa K, Kobayashi J, Bounyadeth S, Kano S, Phompida S, Jimba M. Public and private sector treatment of malaria in Lao PDR. Acta Trop. 2009 Dec;112(3):283-7. Epub 2009 Aug 14. PMID:19683502

Norheim AJ. [Medicinal plants against malaria?].[Article in Norwegian]. Tidsskr Nor Laegeforen. 2011 Sep 20;131(18):1736. PMID:22043476

Norimine J, Mosqueda J, Palmer GH, Lewin HA, Brown WC. Conservation of Babesia bovis small heat shock protein (Hsp20) among strains and definition of T helper cell epitopes recognized by cattle with diverse major histocompatibility complex class II haplotypes. Infect Immun. 2004 Feb;72(2):1096-106. PMID:14742557

Nosten F, White NJ. Artemisinin-based combination treatment of falciparum malaria. Am J Trop Med Hyg. 2007 Dec;77(6 Suppl):181-92. PMID:18165491

Nsagha DS, Njunda AL, Kamga HL, Nsagha SM, Nguedia Assob JC, Wiysonge CS, Tabah EN, Njamnshi AK. Knowledge and practices relating to malaria in a semi-urban area of Cameroon: choices and sources of antimalarials, self-treatment and resistance. Pan Afr Med J. 2011;9:8. Epub 2011 May 25. PMID:22145055

Nsagha DS, Nsagha SM, Shey CU, Njunda AL, Kamga HL, Njamnshi AK. Knowledge, attitudes and practices relating to malaria in a semi-urban area of Cameroon: choices and sources of antimalarials, self-treatment and resistance. East Afr J Public Health. 2011 Jun;8(2):98-102. PMID:22066294

Nsanzimana S, Ruton H, Lowrance DW, Cishahayo S, Nyemazi JP, Muhayimpundu R, Karema C, Raghunathan PL, Binagwaho A, Riedel DJ. Cell Phone- and Internet-based Monitoring and Evaluation of the National Antiretroviral Treatment Program during Rapid Scale-up in Rwanda: TRACnet, 2004--2010. J Acquir Immune Defic Syndr. 2011 Nov 7. [Epub ahead of print]. PMID:22067668

Nsimba B, Guiyedi V, Mabika-Mamfoumbi M, Mourou-Mbina JR, Ngoungou E, Bouyou-Akotet M, Loembet R, Durand R, Le Bras J, Kombila M. Sulphadoxine/pyrimethamine versus amodiaquine for treating uncomplicated childhood malaria in Gabon: a randomized trial to guide national policy. PMID:18267042

Nsobya SL, Dokomajilar C, Joloba M, Dorsey G, Rosenthal PJ. Resistance-mediating Plasmodium falciparum pfcrt and pfmdr1 alleles after treatment with artesunate-amodiaquine in Uganda. Antimicrob Agents Chemother. 2007 Aug;51(8):3023-5. Epub 2007 Jun 11. PMID:17562798

Nurul AA, Norazmi MN. Immunogenicity and in vitro protective efficacy of recombinant Mycobacterium bovis bacille Calmette Guerin (rBCG) expressing the 19 kDa merozoite surface protein-1 (MSP-1(19)) antigen of Plasmodium falciparum. Parasitol Res. 2011 Apr;108(4):887-97. Epub 2010 Nov 6. PMID:21057812

Nurul Aiezzah Z, Noor E, Hasidah MS. Suppression of Plasmodium berghei parasitemia by LiCl in an animal infection model. Trop Biomed. 2010 Dec;27(3):624-31. PMID:21399604

Nussenzweig RS, Vanderberg J, Spitalny GL, Rivera CI, Orton C, Most H. Sporozoite-induced immunity in mammalian malaria. A review. Am J Trop Med Hyg. 1972 Sep;21(5):722-8. PMID:4561520

Nwokocha CR, Ajayi IO, Ebeigbe AB. Altered vascular reactivity induced by malaria parasites. West Indian Med J. 2011 Jan;60(1):13-8. PMID:21809705

Nyadong L, Harris GA, Balayssac S, Galhena AS, Malet-Martino M, Martino R, Parry RM, Wang MD, Fernández FM, Gilard V. Combining two-dimensional diffusion-ordered nuclear magnetic resonance spectroscopy, imaging desorption electrospray ionization mass spectrometry, and direct analysis in real-time mass spectrometry for the integral investigation of counterfeit pharmaceuticals. Anal Chem. 2009 Jun 15;81(12):4803-12. PMID:19453162

Nyunt MM, Plowe CV. Pharmacologic advances in the global control and treatment of malaria: combination therapy and resistance. Clin Pharmacol Ther. 2007 Nov;82(5):601-5. Epub 2007 Sep 26. PMID:17898709

Nzila A, Chilengi R. Modulators of the efficacy and toxicity of drugs in malaria treatment. Trends Pharmacol Sci. 2010 Jun;31(6):277-83. Epub 2010 Apr 9. PMID:20381886

Nzila A, Rottmann M, Chitnumsub P, Kiara SM, Kamchonwongpaisan S, Maneeruttanarungroj C, Taweechai S, Yeung BK, Goh A, Lakshminarayana SB, Zou B, Wong J, Ma NL, Weaver M, Keller TH, Dartois V, Wittlin S, Brun R, Yuthavong Y, Diagana TT. Preclinical evaluation of the antifolate QN254, 5-chloro-N'6'-(2,5-dimethoxy-benzyl)-quinazoline-2,4,6-triamine, as an antimalarial drug candidate. Antimicrob Agents Chemother. 2010 Jun;54(6):2603-10. Epub 2010 Mar 29. PMID:20350951

Obaldia N 3rd, Rossan RN, Cooper RD, Kyle DE, Nuzum EO, Rieckmann KH, Shanks GD. WR 238605, chloroquine, and their combinations as blood schizonticides against a chloroquine-resistant strain of Plasmodium vivax in Aotus monkeys. Am J Trop Med Hyg. 1997 May;56(5):508-10. PMID:9180599

Obodozie OO, Ebeshi BU, Mustapha KB, Kirim RA, Ekpenyong M, Inyang US. The effects of an investigational antimalarial agent, NIPRD-AM1 on the single dose pharmacokinetics of metronidazole in healthy human volunteers. Eur J Drug Metab Pharmacokinet. 2011 Jan;35(3-4):103-8. Epub 2010 Oct 12. PMID:21302036

O'Brien C, Henrich PP, Passi N, Fidock DA. Recent clinical and molecular insights into emerging artemisinin resistance in Plasmodium falciparum. Curr Opin Infect Dis. 2011 Dec;24(6):570-7. PMID:22001944

O'Connell KA, Gatakaa H, Poyer S, Njogu J, Evance I, Munroe E, Solomon T, Goodman C, Hanson K, Zinsou C, Akulayi L, Raharinjatovo J, Arogundade E, Buyungo P, Mpasela F, Adjibabi CB, Agbango JA, Ramarosandratana BF, Coker B, Rubahika D, Hamainza B, Chapman S, Shewchuk T, Chavasse D. Got ACTs? Availability, price, market share and provider knowledge of anti-malarial medicines in public and private sector outlets in six malaria-endemic countries. Malar J. 2011 Oct 31;10:326. PMID:22039838

Odhiambo FO, Hamel MJ, Williamson J, Lindblade K, ter Kuile FO, Peterson E, Otieno P, Kariuki S, Vulule J, Slutsker L, Newman RD. Intermittent preventive treatment in infants for the prevention of malaria in rural Western kenya: a randomized, double-blind placebo-controlled trial. PLoS One. 2010 Apr 2;5(4):e10016. PMID:20368815

Oehme R, Hartelt K, Backe H, Brockmann S, Kimmig P. Foci of tick-borne diseases in southwest Germany. Int J Med Microbiol. 2002 Jun;291 Suppl 33:22-9. PMID:12141751

Oesterholt MJ, Alifrangis M, Sutherland CJ, Omar SA, Sawa P, Howitt C, Gouagna LC, Sauerwein RW, Bousema T. Submicroscopic gametocytes and the transmission of antifolate-resistant Plasmodium falciparum in Western Kenya. PLoS One. 2009;4(2):e4364. Epub 2009 Feb 5. PMID:19194499

Ogutu B, Tiono AB, Makanga M, Premji Z, Gbadoé AD, Ubben D, Marrast AC, Gaye O. Treatment of asymptomatic carriers with artemether-lumefantrine: an opportunity to reduce the burden of malaria? Malar J. 2010 Jan 22;9:30. PMID:20096111

Ogutu BR, Baiden R, Diallo D, Smith PG, Binka FN. Sustainable development of a GCP-compliant clinical trials platform in Africa: the malaria clinical trials alliance perspective. Malar J. 2010 Apr 20;9:103. PMID:20406478

Ohgitani T, Okabe T, Sasaki N. [Studies on immunity to Babesia gibsoni in dogs immunostimulation by Bordetella bronchiseptica]. [Article in Japanese]. Nihon Saikingaku Zasshi. 1990 Jul;45(4):785-95. PMID:2232161

Ohrt C, Willingmyre GD, Lee P, Knirsch C, Milhous W. Assessment of azithromycin in combination with other antimalarial drugs against Plasmodium falciparum in vitro. Antimicrob Agents Chemother. 2002 Aug;46(8):2518-24. PMID:12121927

Ojeda JJ, Orozco L, Flores R, Rojas C, Figueroa JV, Alvarez JA. Validation of an attenuated live vaccine against babesiosis in native cattle in an endemic area. Transbound Emerg Dis. 2010 Apr;57(1-2):84-6. PMID:20537115

Okafor HU, Shu EN, Oguonu T. Therapeutic efficacy and effect on gametocyte carriage of an artemisinin and a non-based combination treatment in children with uncomplicated P. falciparum malaria, living in an area with high-level chloroquine resistance. J Trop Pediatr. 2010 Dec;56(6):398-406. Epub 2010 Feb 8. PMID:20144932

Okamura M, Yokoyama N, Takabatake N, Okubo K, Ikehara Y, Igarashi I. Modification of host erythrocyte membranes by trypsin and chymotrypsin treatments and effects on the in vitro growth of bovine and equine Babesia parasites. J Parasitol. 2007 Feb;93(1):208-11. PMID:17436968

Okeke TA, Uzochukwu BS. Improving childhood malaria treatment and referral practices by training patent medicine vendors in rural south-east Nigeria. Malar J. 2009 Nov 20;8:260. PMID:19930561

Okpako LC, Ajaiyeoba EO. In vitro and in vivo antimalarial studies of Striga hermonthica and Tapinanthus sessilifolius extracts. Afr J Med Med Sci. 2004 Mar;33(1):73-5. PMID:15490799

Okubo K, Yokoyama N, Takabatake N, Okamura M, Igarashi I. Amount of cholesterol in host membrane affects erythrocyte invasion and replication by Babesia bovis. Parasitology. 2007 May;134(Pt 5):625-30. Epub 2006 Dec 6. PMID:17147838

Okumu FO, Moore SJ. Combining indoor residual spraying and insecticide-treated nets for malaria control in Africa: a review of possible outcomes and an outline of suggestions for the future. Malar J. 2011 Jul 28;10:208. PMID:21798053

Oladosu LA, Olufemi BE. Haematology of experimental babesiosis and ehrlichiosis in steroid immunosuppressed horses. Zentralbl Veterinarmed B. 1992 Jul;39(5):345-52. PMID:1519411

Oladosu LA. Effects of intravenous corticosteroid on the pathogenicity of Babesia equi infection of donkeys (Equus asinus). Zentralbl Veterinarmed B. 1988 Aug;35(7):509-14. PMID:3188726

Olajide OA, Ajayi AM, Wright CW. Anti-inflammatory properties of cryptolepine. Phytother Res. 2009 Oct;23(10):1421-5. PMID:19288476

Olajide OA, Heiss EH, Schachner D, Wright CW, Vollmar AM, Dirsch VM. Synthetic cryptolepine inhibits DNA binding of NF-kappaB. Bioorg Med Chem. 2007 Jan 1;15(1):43-9. Epub 2006 Oct 24. PMID:17064915

Olayemi IK, Ande AT, Chita S, Ibemesi G, Ayanwale VA, Odeyemi OM. Insecticide susceptibility profile of the principal malaria vector, Anopheles gambiae s.l. (Diptera: Culicidae), in north-central Nigeria. J Vector Borne Dis. 2011 Jun;48(2):109-12. PMID:21715735

Oleson CV, Sivalingam JJ, O'Neill BJ, Staas WE Jr. Transverse myelitis secondary to coexistent Lyme disease and babesiosis. J Spinal Cord Med. 2003 Summer;26(2):168-71. PMID:12828297

Oldfield E. Targeting isoprenoid biosynthesis for drug discovery: bench to bedside. Acc Chem Res. 2010 Sep 21;43(9):1216-26. PMID:20560544

Oliveira AB, Dolabela MF, Braga FC, Jácome RL, Varotti FP, Póvoa MM. Plant-derived antimalarial agents: new leads and efficient phythomedicines. Part I. Alkaloids. An Acad Bras Cienc. 2009 Dec;81(4):715-40. PMID:19893898

Oliveira JB, Hernández-Gamboa J, Jiménez-Alfaro C, Zeledón R, Blandón M, Urbina A. First report of Trypanosoma vivax infection in dairy cattle from Costa Rica. Vet Parasitol. 2009 Jul 7;163(1-2):136-9. Epub 2009 Apr 5. PMID:19414224

Oliveira TM, Furuta PI, de Carvalho D, Machado RZ. A study of cross-reactivity in serum samples from dogs positive for Leishmania sp., Babesia canis and Ehrlichia canis in enzyme-linked immunosorbent assay and indirect fluorescent antibody test. Rev Bras Parasitol Vet. 2008 Jan-Mar;17(1):7-11. PMID:18554433

Olivieri NF, Pakbaz Z, Vichinsky E. Hb E/beta-thalassaemia: a common & clinically diverse disorder. Indian J Med Res. 2011 Oct;134:522-31. PMID:22089616

Olugbile S, Habel C, Servis C, Spertini F, Verdini A, Corradin G. Malaria vaccines - The long synthetic peptide approach: Technical and conceptual advancements. Curr Opin Mol Ther. 2010 Feb;12(1):64-76. PMID:20140818

Oluwafemi AJ, Okanla EO, Camps P, Muñoz-Torrerob D, Mackey ZB, Chiang PK, Seville S, Wright CW. Evaluation of cryptolepine and huperzine derivatives as lead compounds towards new agents for the treatment of human African trypanosomiasis. Nat Prod Commun. 2009 Feb;4(2):193-8. PMID:19370921

Omar MS, Collins WE, Contacos PG. Gametocytocidal and sporontocidal effects of antimalarial drugs on malaria parasites. I. Effect of single and multiple doses of primaquine on Plasmodium cynomolgi. Exp Parasitol. 1973 Oct;34(2):229-41. PMID:4200769

Omar MS, Collins WE. Studies on the antimalarial effects of RC-12 and WR 14,997 on the development of Plasmodium cynomolgi in mosquitoes and Rhesus monkeys. Am J Trop Med Hyg. 1974 May;23(3):339-49. PMID:4207342

Omar MS, Gwadz RW, Miller LH. Incorporation of nucleic acid precursors by Plasmodium cynomolgi in Anopheles balabacensis. Tropenmed Parasitol. 1975 Sep;26(3):303-6. PMID:1189024

Onaku LO, Attama AA, Okore VC, Tijani AY, Ngene AA, Esimone CO. Antagonistic antimalarial properties of pawpaw leaf aqueous extract in combination with artesunic acid in Plasmodium berghei-infected mice. J Vector Borne Dis. 2011 Jun;48(2):96-100. PMID:21715732

Ondo JP, Lekana-Douki JB, Bongui JB, Zang Edou ES, Zatra R, Toure-Ndouo FS, Elomri A, Lebibi J, Seguin E. In vitro antiplasmodial activity and cytotoxicity of extracts and fractions of Vitex madiensis, medicinal plant of Gabon. Trop Med Int Health. 2011 Dec 5. [Epub ahead of print]. PMID:22141406

O'Neill PM, Barton VE, Ward SA. The molecular mechanism of action of artemisinin--the debate continues. Molecules. 2010 Mar 12;15(3):1705-21. PMID:20336009

Ong KR, Stavropoulos C, Inada Y. Babesiosis, asplenia, and AIDS. Lancet. 1990 Jul 14;336(8707):112. PMID:1975291

Onwujekwe O, Hanson K, Uzochukwu B. Do poor people use poor quality providers? Evidence from the treatment of presumptive malaria in Nigeria. Trop Med Int Health. 2011 Sep;16(9):1087-98. Epub 2011 Jun 27. PMID:21702870

Onwujekwe O, Onoka C, Uzochukwu B, Hanson K. Constraints to universal coverage: inequities in health service use and expenditures for different health conditions and providers. Int J Equity Health. 2011 Nov 13;10(1):50. PMID:22078263

Onyamboko MA, Meshnick SR, Fleckenstein L, Koch MA, Atibu J, Lokomba V, Douoguih M, Hemingway-Foday J, Wesche D, Ryder RW, Bose C, Wright LL, Tshefu AK, Capparelli EV. Pharmacokinetics and pharmacodynamics of artesunate and dihydroartemisinin following oral treatment in pregnant women with asymptomatic Plasmodium falciparum infections in Kinshasa DRC. Malar J. 2011 Feb 28;10:49. PMID:21352601

Ooka H, Terkawi MA, Goo YK, Luo Y, Li Y, Yamagishi J, Nishikawa Y, Igarashi I, Xuan X. Babesia microti: molecular and antigenic characterizations of a novel 94-kDa protein (BmP94). Exp Parasitol. 2011 Jan;127(1):287-93. Epub 2010 Jun 25. PMID:20599995

OPTIMALVAC consortium, Cavanagh DR, Dubois PM, Holtel A, Kisser A, Leroy O, Locke E, Moorthy VS, Remarque EJ, Shi YP. Towards validated assays for key immunological outcomes in malaria vaccine development. Vaccine. 2011 Apr 12;29(17):3093-5. Epub 2011 Feb 4. PMID:21296116

Orinda GO, Gale KR, Wright IG, Parrodi F. Bovine babesiosis: failure to induce interferon gamma production in response to Babesia bovis antigens in cattle. Int J Parasitol. 1992 May;22(3):395-8. PMID:1639576

Orinda GO, Waltisbuhl DJ, Young AS, Wright IG. Low doses of natural human interferon alpha inhibit the development of Babesia microti infection in BALB/c mice. Vet Parasitol. 1994 May;53(1-2):53-8. PMID:8091618

Orinda GO, Wright IG, Leatch G, Young AS. Human interferon alpha fails to inhibit the development of Babesia bigemina and Anaplasma marginale infections in cattle. Vet Parasitol. 1993 Mar;47(1-2):149-55. PMID:8493761

Oróstegui-Pinilla D, Rodríguez-Morales AJ. Neonatal Plasmodium vivax malaria. Trop Biomed. 2011 Aug;28(2):339-42. PMID:22041754

Osolodkin DI, Zakharevich NV, Palyulin VA, Danilenko VN, Zefirov NS. Bioinformatic analysis of glycogen synthase kinase 3: human versus parasite kinases. Parasitology. 2011 Feb 24:1-11. [Epub ahead of print]. PMID:21349219

Otranto D, de Caprariis D, Lia RP, Tarallo V, Lorusso V, Testini G, Dantas-Torres F, Latrofa S, Diniz PP, Mencke N, Maggi RG, Breitschwerdt E, Capelli G, Stanneck D. Prevention of endemic canine vector-borne diseases using imidacloprid 10% and permethrin 50% in young dogs: a longitudinal field study. Vet Parasitol. 2010 Sep 20;172(3-4):323-32. Epub 2010 May 25. PMID:20591573

Oueriagli Nabih F, Touhami M, Laffinti A, Abilkacem L. [Mood disorder after malaria prophylaxis with mefloquine (two case reports)]. [Article in French]. Encephale. 2011 Oct;37(5):393-6. 2011 Mar 25. PMID:22032283

Ouwe-Missi-Oukem-Boyer O, Ndouo FS, Ollomo B, Mezui-Me-Ndong J, Noulin F, Lachard I, Ndong-Atome GR, Makuwa M, Roques P, Branger M, Preux PM, Mazier D, Bisser S. Hepatitis C virus infection may lead to slower emergence of P. falciparum in blood. PLoS One. 2011 Jan 10;6(1):e16034. PMID:21249226

Overdulve JP, Antonisse HW. Measurement of the effect of low temperature on protozoa by titration. II. Titration of Babesia rodhaini, using prepatent period and survival time, before and after storage at minus 76 degree C. Exp Parasitol. 1970 Apr;27(2):323-41. PMID:5446635

Oyelade J, Ewejobi I, Brors B, Eils R, Adebiyi E. Computational identification of signalling pathways in Plasmodium falciparum. Infect Genet Evol. 2011 Jun;11(4):755-64. Epub 2010 Nov 26. PMID:21112415

Oz HS, Hughes WT. Acute fulminating babesiosis in hamsters infected with Babesia microti. Int J Parasitol. 1996 Jun;26(6):667-70. PMID:8875313

Padte NN, Li X, Tsuji M, Vasan S. Clinical development of a novel CD1d-binding NKT cell ligand as a vaccine adjuvant. Clin Immunol. 2011 Aug;140(2):142-51. Epub 2010 Dec 24. PMID:21185784

Paglia MG, Vairo F, Bevilacqua N, Ghirga P, Narciso P, Severini C, Nicastri E. Molecular diagnosis and species identification of imported malaria in returning travellers in Italy. Diagn Microbiol Infect Dis. 2011 Nov 10. [Epub ahead of print]. PMID:22078908

Palacios Fraire S. Analysis of the principal problems impeding normal development of malaria eradication programs. Bull Pan Am Health Organ. 1975;9(4):283-94. PMID:1240013

Palacpac NM, Arisue N, Tougan T, Ishii KJ, Horii T. Plasmodium falciparum serine repeat antigen 5 (SE36) as a malaria vaccine candidate. Vaccine. 2011 Aug 11;29(35):5837-45. Epub 2011 Jun 28. PMID:21718740

Palmer DA, Buening GM, Carson CA. Cryopreservation of Babesia bovis for in vitro cultivation. Parasitology. 1982 Jun;84(Pt 3):567-72. PMID:7099713

Palmer GH, McElwain TF. Molecular basis for vaccine development against anaplasmosis and babesiosis. Vet Parasitol. 1995 Mar;57(1-3):233-53. PMID:7597787

Pancewicz S, Moniuszko A, Bieniarz E, Puciło K, Grygorczuk S, Zajkowska J, Czupryna P, Kondrusik M, Swierzbińska-Pijanowska R. Anti-Babesia microti antibodies in foresters highly exposed to tick bites in Poland. Scand J Infect Dis. 2011 Mar;43(3):197-201. Epub 2010 Dec 9. PMID:21142620

Pande M, Dubey VK, Jagannadham MV. Crystallization and preliminary X-ray analysis of cryptolepain, a novel glycosylated serine protease from Cryptolepis buchanani. Acta Crystallogr Sect F Struct Biol Cryst Commun. 2007 Feb 1;63(Pt 2):74-7. Epub 2007 Jan 17. PMID:17277443

Pande M, Dubey VK, Sahu V, Jagannadham MV. Conformational plasticity of cryptolepain: accumulation of partially unfolded states in denaturants induced equilibrium unfolding. J Biotechnol. 2007 Sep 30;131(4):404-17. Epub 2007 Aug 7. PMID:17825936

Pande M, Dubey VK, Yadav SC, Jagannadham MV. A novel serine protease cryptolepain from Cryptolepis buchanani: purification and biochemical characterization. J Agric Food Chem. 2006 Dec 27;54(26):10141-50. PMID:17177552

Pandey JP, Morais CG, Fontes CJ, Braga EM. Immunoglobulin GM 3 23 5,13,14 phenotype is strongly associated with IgG1 antibody responses to Plasmodium vivax vaccine candidate antigens PvMSP1-19 and PvAMA-1. Malar J. 2010 Aug 9;9:229. PMID:20696056

Pantaleo A, Ferru E, Carta F, Mannu F, Giribaldi G, Vono R, Lepedda AJ, Pippia P, Turrini F. Analysis of changes in tyrosine and serine phosphorylation of red cell membrane proteins induced by P. falciparum growth. Proteomics. 2010 Oct;10(19):3469-79. PMID:20799346

Pantaleo A, Ferru E, Vono R, Giribaldi G, Lobina O, Nepveu F, Ibrahim H, Nallet JP, Carta F, Mannu F, Pippia P, Campanella E, Low PS, Turrini F. New antimalarial indolone-N-oxides, generating radical species, destabilize the host cell membrane at early stages of Plasmodium falciparum growth: role of band 3 tyrosine phosphorylation. Free Radic Biol Med. 2011 Nov 15. [Epub ahead of print]. PMID:22142474

Pantanowitz L, Aufranc S 3rd, Monahan-Earley R, Dvorak A, Telford SR 3rd. Transfusion medicine illustrated. Morphologic hallmarks of Babesia. Transfusion. 2002 Nov;42(11):1389. PMID:12421208

Pantanowitz L, Telford SR 3rd, Cannon ME. The impact of babesiosis on transfusion medicine. Transfus Med Rev. 2002 Apr;16(2):131-43. PMID:11941575

Papireddy K, Smilkstein M, Kelly JX, Shweta, Salem SM, Alhamadsheh M, Haynes SW, Challis GL, Reynolds KA. Antimalarial activity of natural and synthetic prodiginines. J Med Chem. 2011 Aug 11;54(15):5296-306. Epub 2011 Jul 8. PMID:21736388

Parikh R, Amole I, Tarpley M, Gbadero D, Davidson M, Vermund SH. Cost comparison of microscopy vs. empiric treatment for malaria in Southwestern Nigeria: a prospective study. Malar J. 2010 Dec 22;9:371. PMID:21176228

Parise ÉV, Araújo GC, Castro JG, Berdarrain FP. Epidemiological profile of malaria in the state of Tocantins, Brazil, from 2003 to 2008. Rev Inst Med Trop Sao Paulo. 2011 Jun;53(3):141-7. PMID:21755236

Pastrana-Mena R, Dinglasan RR, Franke-Fayard B, Vega-Rodríguez J, Fuentes-Caraballo M, Baerga-Ortiz A, Coppens I, Jacobs-Lorena M, Janse CJ, Serrano AE. Glutathione reductase-null malaria parasites have normal blood stage growth but arrest during development in the mosquito. J Biol Chem. 2010 Aug 27;285(35):27045-56. Epub 2010 Jun 23. PMID:20573956

Pasvol G, Weatherall DJ, Wilson RJ, Smith DH, Gilles HM. Fetal haemoglobin and malaria. Lancet. 1976 Jun 12;1(7972):1269-72. PMID:73695

Patarroyo JH, Prates AA, Tavares CA, Mafra CL, Vargas MI. Exoantigens of an attenuated strain of Babesia bovis used as a vaccine against bovine babesiosis. Vet Parasitol. 1995 Oct;59(3-4):189-99. PMID:8533277

Patarroyo ME, Cifuentes G, Pirajján C, Moreno-Vranich A, Vanegas M. Atomic evidence that modification of H-bonds established with amino acids critical for host-cell binding induces sterile immunity against malaria. Biochem Biophys Res Commun. 2010 Apr 9;394(3):529-35. Epub 2010 Mar 4. PMID:20206601

Pates HV, Line JD, Keto AJ, Miller JE. Personal protection against mosquitoes in Dar es Salaam, Tanzania, by using a kerosene oil lamp to vaporize transfluthrin. Med Vet Entomol. 2002 Sep;16(3):277-84. PMID:12243228

Patouillard E, Conteh L, Webster J, Kweku M, Chandramohan D, Greenwood B. Coverage, adherence and costs of intermittent preventive treatment of malaria in children employing different delivery strategies in Jasikan, Ghana. PLoS One. 2011;6(11):e24871. Epub 2011 Nov 3. PMID:22073137

Patterson D, Vilensky JA, Robertson WM, Berger J. Treatment and diagnostic accuracy of neurosyphilis at Boston City Hospital's Neurological Unit, 1930-1979. J Neurol Sci. 2011 Nov 29. [Epub ahead of print]. PMID:22129939

Paul JH, Seaforth CE, Tikasingh T. Eryngium foetidum L.: a review. Fitoterapia. 2011 Apr;82(3):302-8. Epub 2010 Nov 6. PMID:21062639

Paulo A, Duarte A, Gomes ET. In vitro antibacterial screening of Cryptolepis sanguinolenta alkaloids. J Ethnopharmacol. 1994 Oct;44(2):127-30. PMID:7853864

Paulo A, Gomes ET, Steele J, Warhurst DC, Houghton PJ. Antiplasmodial activity of Cryptolepis sanguinolenta alkaloids from leaves and roots. Planta Med. 2000 Feb;66(1):30-4. PMID:10705730

Paulo A, Jimeno ML, Gomes ET, Houghton PJ. Steroidal alkaloids from Cryptolepis obtusa. Phytochemistry. 2000 Feb;53(3):417-22. PMID:10703068

Paulo A, Pimentel M, Viegas S, Pires I, Duarte A, Cabrita J, Gomes ET. Cryptolepis sanguinolenta activity against diarrhoeal bacteria. J Ethnopharmacol. 1994 Oct;44(2):73-7. PMID:7853867

Payne RC, Osorio O, Ybañez A. Tick-borne diseases of cattle in Paraguay. II. Immunisation against anaplasmosis and babesiosis. Trop Anim Health Prod. 1990 May;22(2):101-8. PMID:2196724

Payne RC. Cryopreservation of bovine blood infected with Babesia major for use in the indirect fluorescent antibody test. Res Vet Sci. 1978 May;24(3):375. PMID:353926

Pays JF. [A mosquito net for everyone in 2010].[Article in French]. Bull Soc Pathol Exot. 2010 Oct;103(4):223-9. Epub 2010 Jul 20. PMID:20652477

Pearce GW, Gooden EL, Johnson DR. Specifications of the International Cooperation Administration for DDT water-dispersible powder for use in malaria control programmes. Bull World Health Organ. 1959;20:913-20. PMID:14431217

Pearson CD, McLean SA, Tetley K, Phillips RS. Induction of secondary antibody responses to Plasmodium chabaudi in vitro. Clin Exp Immunol. 1983 Apr;52(1):121-8. PMID:6861369

Peirce MA, Norton CC, Donnelly J. The preservation of Cytoecetes phagocytophila in liquid nitrogen. Res Vet Sci. 1974 May;16(3):393-4. PMID:4855005

Pell C, Straus L, Andrew EV, Meñaca A, Pool R. Social and cultural factors affecting uptake of interventions for malaria in pregnancy in Africa: a systematic review of the qualitative research. PLoS One. 2011;6(7):e22452. Epub 2011 Jul 20. PMID:21799859

Pena AC, Penacho N, Mancio-Silva L, Neres R, Seixas JD, Fernandes AC, Romão CC, Mota MM, Bernardes GJ, Pamplona A. A novel Carbon Monoxide-Releasing Molecule (CO-RM) fully protects mice from Severe Malaria Antimicrob Agents Chemother. 2011 Dec 12. [Epub ahead of print]. PMID:22155828

Pendse S, Bilyk JR, Lee MS. The ticking time bomb. Surv Ophthalmol. 2006 May-Jun;51(3):274-9. PMID:16644367

Penna-Coutinho J, Cortopassi WA, Oliveira AA, França TC, Krettli AU. Antimalarial activity of potential inhibitors of Plasmodium falciparum lactate dehydrogenase enzyme selected by docking studies. PLoS One. 2011;6(7):e21237. Epub 2011 Jul 14. PMID:21779323

Penzhorn BL, Lewis BD, de Waal DT, López Rebollar LM. Sterilisation of Babesia canis infections by imidocarb alone or in combination with diminazene. J S Afr Vet Assoc. 1995 Sep;66(3):157-9. PMID:8596187

Penzhorn BL. Why is Southern African canine babesiosis so virulent? An evolutionary perspective. Parasit Vectors. 2011 Apr 13;4:51. PMID:21489239

Perdrizet GA, Olson NH, Krause PJ, Banever GT, Spielman A, Cable RG. Babesiosis in a renal transplant recipient acquired through blood transfusion. Transplantation. 2000 Jul 15;70(1):205-8. PMID:10919602

Peregrine AS. Chemotherapy and delivery systems: haemoparasites. Vet Parasitol. 1994 Aug;54(1-3):223-48. PMID:7846852

Pereira EA, Ishikawa EA, Fontes CJ. Adherence to Plasmodium vivax malaria treatment in the Brazilian Amazon Region. Malar J. 2011 Dec 13;10(1):355. [Epub ahead of print]. PMID:22165853

Perić M, Fajdetić A, Rupčić R, Alihodzic S, Ziher D, Bukvić Krajačić M, Smith KS, Ivezić Schönfeld Z, Padovan J, Landek G, Jelić D, Hutinec A, Mesić M, Ager A, Ellis WY, Milhous WK, Ohrt C, Spaventi R. Antimalarial Activity of 9a-N Substituted 15-Membered Azalides with Improved In Vitro and In Vivo Activity over Azithromycin. J Med Chem. 2011 Dec 12. [Epub ahead of print]. PMID:22148880

Perkins HA, Busch MP. Transfusion-associated infections: 50 years of relentless challenges and remarkable progress. Transfusion. 2010 Oct;50(10):2080-99. PMID:20738828

Perlaza BL, Sauzet JP, Brahimi K, BenMohamed L, Druilhe P. Interferon-γ, a valuable surrogate marker of Plasmodium falciparum pre-erythrocytic stages protective immunity. Malar J. 2011 Feb 8;10(1):27. PMID:21303495

Permin A, Yelifari L, Bloch P, Steenhard N, Hansen NP, Nansen P. Parasites in cross-bred pigs in the Upper East region of Ghana. Vet Parasitol. 1999 Nov;87(1):63-71. PMID:10628701

Perret PC. [The travelling child: recommendations].[Article in Spanish]. Rev Chilena Infectol. 2011 Apr;28(2):153-6. Epub 2011 May 5. PMID:21720694

Persing DH, Conrad PA. Babesiosis: new insights from phylogenetic analysis. Infect Agents Dis. 1995 Dec;4(4):182-95. PMID:8665084

Peters W, Bafort J, Ramkaran AE. The chemotherapy of rodent malaria. XI. Cyclically transmitted, chloroquine-resistant variants of the Keyberg 173 strain of Plasmodium berghei. Ann Trop Med Parasitol. 1970 Mar;64(1):41-51. PMID:5485709

Peters W, Porter M. The chemotherapy of rodent malaria, XXVI. The potential value of WR 122,455 (a 9-phenanthrenemethanol) against drug-resistant malaria parasites. Ann Trop Med Parasitol. 1976 Sep;70(3):271-81. PMID:788658

Peters W, Robinson BL, Milhous WK. The chemotherapy of rodent malaria. LI. Studies on a new 8-aminoquinoline, WR 238,605. Ann Trop Med Parasitol. 1993 Dec;87(6):547-52. PMID:8122915

Peters W, Stewart LB, Robinson BL. The chemotherapy of rodent malaria. LXI. Drug combinations to impede the selection of drug resistance, part 4: the potential role of 8-aminoquinolines. Ann Trop Med Parasitol. 2003 Apr;97(3):221-36. PMID:12803854

Peters W. Partial inhibition by mepacrine of the development of sulphonamide resistance in Plasmodium berghei. Nature. 1969 Aug 23;223(5208):858-9. PMID:5799037

Peters W. Prevention of drug resistance in rodent malaria by the use of drug mixtures. Bull World Health Organ. 1974;51(4):379-83. PMID:4619060

Peters W. Recent advances in antimalarial chemotherapy and drug resistance. Adv Parasitol. 1974;12:69-114. PMID:4217563

Peters W. The chemotherapy of rodent malaria. II. Host-parasite relationships. 2. The relationship between chloroquine sensitivity and the age of the host cell. Ann Trop Med Parasitol. 1968 Jun;62(2):246-61. PMID:5751426

Peters W. The chemotherapy of rodent malaria. X. Dynamics of drug resistance. II. Acquisition and loss of chloroquine resistance in Plasmodium berghei observed by continuous bioassay. Ann Trop Med Parasitol. 1970 Mar;64(1):25-40. PMID:5485708

Peters W. The chemotherapy of rodent malaria. XVII. Dynamics of drug resistance. 3. Influence of drug combinations on the development of resistance to chloroquine in P. berghei. Ann Trop Med Parasitol. 1973 Jun;67(2):143-54. PMID:4578935

Peters W. The evolution of tafenoquine--antimalarial for a new millennium? J R Soc Med. 1999 Jul;92(7):345-52. PMID:10615272

Petersen E. Malaria chemoprophylaxis: when should we use it and what are the options? Expert Rev Anti Infect Ther. 2004 Feb;2(1):119-32. PMID:15482177

Phillips MA, Rathod PK. Plasmodium dihydroorotate dehydrogenase: a promising target for novel anti-malarial chemotherapy. Infect Disord Drug Targets. 2010 Jun;10(3):226-39. PMID:20334617

Phillips RS, Wakelin D. Trichuris muris: effect of concurrent infections with rodent piroplasms on immune expulsion from mice. Exp Parasitol. 1976 Feb;39(1):95-100. PMID:1253888

Phillips RS. Antigenic variation in Babesia rodhaini demonstrated by immunization with irradiated parasites. Parasitology. 1971 Oct;63(2):315-22. PMID:5002030

Phillips RS. Evidence that piroplasms can undergo antigenic variation. Nature. 1971 Jun 4;231(5301):323. PMID:4930987

Phillips RS. Immunity of rats and mice following injection with 60Co irradiated Babesia rodhaini infected red cells. Parasitology. 1971 Apr;62(2):221-31. PMID:4995421

Phillips RS. Resistance of mice and rats to Babesia rodhaini challenge after inoculation with irradiated B. rodhaini infected red cells. Trans R Soc Trop Med Hyg. 1970;64(4):470. PMID:4991940

Phillips RS. Resistance of mice and rats to challenge by Babesia rodhaini after inoculation with irradiated red cells infected with B. rodhaini. Nature. 1970 Sep 19;227(5264):1255. PMID:4989140

Phiri HT, Bridges DJ, Glover SJ, van Mourik JA, de Laat B, M'baya B, Taylor TE, Seydel KB, Molyneux ME, Faragher EB, Craig AG, Bunn JE. Elevated plasma von Willebrand factor and propeptide levels in malawian children with malaria. PLoS One. 2011;6(11):e25626. Epub 2011 Nov 17. PMID:22125593

Phiri K, Esan M, van Hensbroek MB, Khairallah C, Faragher B, Ter Kuile FO. Intermittent preventive therapy for malaria with monthly artemether-lumefantrine for the post-discharge management of severe anaemia in children aged 4-59 months in southern Malawi: a multicentre, randomised, placebo-controlled trial. Lancet Infect Dis. 2011 Dec 13. [Epub ahead of print]. PMID:22172305

Phompradit P, Kuesap J, Chaijaroenkul W, Rueangweerayut R, Hongkaew Y, Yamnuan R, Na-Bangchang K. Prevalence and distribution of glucose-6-phosphate dehydrogenase (G6PD) variants in Thai and Burmese populations in malaria endemic areas of Thailand. Malar J. 2011 Dec 15;10(1):368. [Epub ahead of print]. PMID:22171972

Phyo AP, Lwin KM, Price RN, Ashley EA, Russell B, Sriprawat K, Lindegardh N, Singhasivanon P, White NJ, Nosten F. Dihydroartemisinin-piperaquine versus chloroquine in the treatment of Plasmodium vivax malaria in Thailand: a randomized controlled trial. Clin Infect Dis. 2011 Nov;53(10):977-84. PMID:22002979

Piedade R, Gil JP. The pharmacogenetics of antimalaria artemisinin combination therapy. Expert Opin Drug Metab Toxicol. 2011 Oct;7(10):1185-200. Epub 2011 Sep 8. PMID:21899476

Pierce MA, Ellis RD, Martin LB, Malkin E, Tierney E, Miura K, Fay MP, Marjason J, Elliott SL, Mullen GE, Rausch K, Zhu D, Long CA, Miller LH. Phase 1 safety and immunogenicity trial of the Plasmodium falciparum blood-stage malaria vaccine AMA1-C1/ISA 720 in Australian adults. Vaccine. 2010 Mar 2;28(10):2236-42. Epub 2010 Jan 4. PMID:20051276

Pinder M, Moorthy VS, Akanmori BD, Genton B, Brown GV. MALVAC 2009: progress and challenges in development of whole organism malaria vaccines for endemic countries, 3-4 June 2009, Dakar, Senegal. Vaccine. 2010 Jul 5;28(30):4695-702. Epub 2010 May 14. PMID:20470799

Pinto AC, Chaves FC, dos Santos PA, Nunez CV, Tadei WP, Pohlit AM. Piper peltatum: biomass and 4-nerolidylcatechol production. Planta Med. 2010 Sep;76(13):1473-6. Epub 2010 Mar 1. PMID:20195961

Pinzon-Charry A, McPhun V, Kienzle V, Hirunpetcharat C, Engwerda C, McCarthy J, Good MF. Low doses of killed parasite in CpG elicit vigorous CD4+ T cell responses against blood-stage malaria in mice. J Clin Invest. 2010 Aug 2;120(8):2967-78. Epub 2010 Jul 12. PMID:20628205

Pipano E, Alekceev E, Galker F, Fish L, Samish M, Shkap V. Immunity against Boophilus annulatus induced by the Bm86 (Tick-GARD) vaccine. Exp Appl Acarol. 2003;29(1-2):141-9. PMID:14580066

Pipano E, Jeruham I, Frank M. Pentamidine in chemoimmunisation of cattle against Babesia bigemina infection. Trop Anim Health Prod. 1979 Feb;11(1):13-6. PMID:442205

Pipano E, Krigel Y, Markovics A, Rubinstein E, Frank M. Mitigation of the response of Friesian calves to live Babesia bovis vaccine by treatment with long acting oxytetracycline. Vet Rec. 1985 Oct 19;117(16):413-4. PMID:4071930

Pipano E, Markovics A, Kriegel Y, Frank M, Fish L. Use of long-acting oxytetracycline in the immunisation of cattle against Babesia bovis and B bigemina. Res Vet Sci. 1987 Jul;43(1):64-6. PMID:3628985

Pipano E, Shkap V, Kriegel Y, Leibovitz B, Savitsky I, Fish L. Babesia bovis and B. bigemina: Persistence of infection in friesian cows following vaccination with live antibabesial vaccines. Vet J. 2002 Jul;164(1):64-8. PMID:12359486

Pipano E. Immunization against intracellular blood protozoans of cattle. Prog Clin Biol Res. 1980;47:301-14. PMID:6782586

Pipano E. Vaccines against hemoparasitic diseases in Israel with special reference to quality assurance. Trop Anim Health Prod. 1997 Nov;29(4 Suppl):86S-90S. PMID:9512751

Pitasawat B, Champakaew D, Choochote W, Jitpakdi A, Chaithong U, Kanjanapothi D, Rattanachanpichai E, Tippawangkosol P, Riyong D, Tuetun B, Chaiyasit D. Aromatic plant-derived essential oil: an alternative larvicide for mosquito control. Fitoterapia. 2007 Apr;78(3):205-10. Epub 2007 Feb 6. PMID:17337133

Ploemen IH, Prudêncio M, Douradinha BG, Ramesar J, Fonager J, van Gemert GJ, Luty AJ, Hermsen CC, Sauerwein RW, Baptista FG, Mota MM, Waters AP, Que I, Lowik CW, Khan SM, Janse CJ, Franke-Fayard BM. Visualisation and quantitative analysis of the rodent malaria liver stage by real time imaging. PLoS One. 2009 Nov 18;4(11):e7881. PMID:19924309

Pohlit AM, Lopes NP, Gama RA, Tadei WP, Neto VF. Patent literature on mosquito repellent inventions which contain plant essential oils--a review. Planta Med. 2011 Apr;77(6):598-617. Epub 2011 Feb 15. PMID:21328177

Pohlit AM, Rezende AR, Lopes Baldin EL, Lopes NP, Neto VF. Plant extracts, isolated phytochemicals, and plant-derived agents which are lethal to arthropod vectors of human tropical diseases--a review. Planta Med. 2011 Apr;77(6):618-30. Epub 2011 Mar 22. PMID:21432748

Ponsa N, Sattabongkot J, Kittayapong P, Eikarat N, Coleman RE. Transmission-blocking activity of tafenoquine (WR-238605) and artelinic acid against naturally circulating strains of Plasmodium vivax in Thailand. Am J Trop Med Hyg. 2003 Nov;69(5):542-7. PMID:14695093

Ponsar F, Van Herp M, Zachariah R, Gerard S, Philips M, Jouquet G. Abolishing user fees for children and pregnant women trebled uptake of malaria-related interventions in Kangaba, Mali. Health Policy Plan. 2011 Nov;26 Suppl 2:ii72-83. PMID:22027922

Popovsky MA, Lindberg LE, Syrek AL, Page PL. Prevalence of Babesia antibody in a selected blood donor population. Transfusion. 1988 Jan-Feb;28(1):59-61. PMID:3341068

Popovsky MA. Transfusion-transmitted babesiosis. Transfusion. 1991 May;31(4):296-8. PMID:2020992

Porter KA, Cole SR, Eron JJ Jr, Zheng Y, Hughes MD, Lockman S, Poole C, Skinner-Adams TS, Hosseinipour M, Shaffer D, D'Amico R, Sawe FK, Siika A, Stringer E, Currier JS, Chipato T, Salata R, McCarthy JS, Meshnick SR. HIV-1 protease inhibitors and clinical malaria: A secondary analysis of ACTG A5208. Antimicrob Agents Chemother. 2011 Nov 28. [Epub ahead of print]. PMID:22123685

Posnett ES, Fehrsen J, De Waal DT, Ambrosio RE. Detection of Babesia equi in infected horses and carrier animals using a DNA probe. Vet Parasitol. 1991 Jul;39(1-2):19-32. PMID:1897117

Posnett ES, Metaferia E, Wiliamson S, Brown CG, Canning EU. In vitro cultivation of an African strain of Babesia bigemina, its characterisation and infectivity in cattle. Parasitol Res. 1998;84(4):302-9. PMID:9569096

Potgieter FT, Van Vuuren AS. The transmission of Babesia bovis using frozen infective material obtained from Boophilus microplus larvae. Onderstepoort J Vet Res. 1974 Jun;41(2):79-80. PMID:4449642

Potgieter FT. Chemotherapy of Babesia felis infection: efficacy of certain drugs. J S Afr Vet Assoc. 1981 Dec;52(4):289-93. PMID:7341778

Powell RD, Berglund EM. Effects of chloroquine upon the maturation of asexual erythrocytic forms of Plasmodium vivax in vitro. Am J Trop Med Hyg. 1974 Nov;23(6):1007-14. PMID:4611251

Powell RD. Development of new antimalarial drugs. Am J Trop Med Hyg. 1972 Sep;21(5):744-8. PMID:4561522

Powell VI, Grima K. Exchange transfusion for malaria and Babesia infection. Transfus Med Rev. 2002 Jul;16(3):239-50. PMID:12075561

Prabhu P, Patravale V. Novel Targets for Malaria Therapy. Curr Drug Targets. 2011 Jul 14. [Epub ahead of print]. PMID:21756223

Pradines B, Bertaux L, Pomares C, Delaunay P, Marty P. Reduced in vitro susceptibility to artemisinin derivatives associated with multi-resistance in a traveller returning from South-East Asia. Malar J. 2011 Sep 18;10:268. PMID:21923936

Pradines B, Briolant S, Henry M, Oeuvray C, Baret E, Amalvict R, Didillon E, Rogier C. Absence of association between pyronaridine in vitro responses and polymorphisms in genes involved in quinoline resistance in Plasmodium falciparum. Malar J. 2010 Nov 25;9:339. PMID:21108786

Pradines B, Mamfoumbi MM, Tall A, Sokhna C, Koeck JL, Fusai T, Mosnier J, Czarnecki E, Spiegel A, Trape JF, Kombila M, Rogier C. In vitro activity of tafenoquine against the asexual blood stages of Plasmodium falciparum isolates from Gabon, Senegal, and Djibouti. Antimicrob Agents Chemother. 2006 Sep;50(9):3225-6. PMID:16940138

Prasad K, Winter J, Bhat UM, Acharya RV, Prabhu GK. Image Analysis Approach for Development of a Decision Support System for Detection of Malaria Parasites in Thin Blood Smear Images. J Digit Imaging. 2011 Dec 7. [Epub ahead of print]. PMID:22146834

Prato M, Giribaldi G. Matrix Metalloproteinase-9 and Haemozoin: Wedding Rings for Human Host and Plasmodium falciparum Parasite in Complicated Malaria. J Trop Med. 2011;2011:628435. Epub 2011 May 26. PMID:21760809

Precigout E, Delbecq S, Vallet A, Carcy B, Camillieri S, Hadj-Kaddour K, Kleuskens J, Schetters T, Gorenflot A. Association between sequence polymorphism in an epitope of Babesia divergens Bd37 exoantigen and protection induced by passive transfer. Int J Parasitol. 2004 Apr;34(5):585-93. PMID:15064123

Precigout E, Gorenflot A, Valentin A, Bissuel G, Carcy B, Brasseur P, Moreau Y, Schrevel J. Analysis of immune responses of different hosts to Babesia divergens isolates from different geographic areas and capacity of culture-derived exoantigens to induce efficient cross-protection. Infect Immun. 1991 Aug;59(8):2799-805. PMID:1713201

Premaratna R, Galappaththy G, Chandrasena N, Fernando R, Nawasiwatte T, de Silva NR, de Silva HJ. What clinicians who practice in countries reaching malaria elimination should be aware of: lessons learnt from recent experience in Sri Lanka. Malar J. 2011 Oct 14;10:302. PMID:21999636

Prendergast A, Walker AS, Mulenga V, Chintu C, Gibb DM. Improved growth and anemia in HIV-infected African children taking cotrimoxazole prophylaxis. Clin Infect Dis. 2011 Apr 1;52(7):953-6. PMID:21427404

Price JE, Dolan TT. A comparison of the efficacy of imidocarb dipropionate and tetracycline hydrochloride in the treatment of canine ehrlichiosis. Vet Rec. 1980 Sep 20;107(12):275-7. PMID:7210420

Price RN, Douglas NM, Anstey NM, von Seidlein L. Plasmodium vivax treatments: what are we looking for? Curr Opin Infect Dis. 2011 Dec;24(6):578-85. PMID:21986614

Priest JW, Kwon JP, Montgomery JM, Bern C, Moss DM, Freeman AR, Jones CC, Arrowood MJ, Won KY, Lammie PJ, Gilman RH, Mead JR. Cloning and characterization of the acidic ribosomal protein P2 of Cryptosporidium parvum, a new 17-kilodalton antigen. Clin Vaccine Immunol. 2010 Jun;17(6):954-65. Epub 2010 Apr 21. PMID:20410328

Prince HE, Lapé-Nixon M, Patel H, Yeh C. Comparison of the Babesia duncani (WA1) IgG detection rates among clinical sera submitted to a reference laboratory for WA1 IgG testing and blood donor specimens from diverse geographic areas of the United States. Clin Vaccine Immunol. 2010 Nov;17(11):1729-33. Epub 2010 Sep 22. PMID:20861326

Prusty D, Dar A, Priya R, Sharma A, Dana S, Choudhury NR, Rao NS, Dhar SK. Single-stranded DNA binding protein from human malarial parasite Plasmodium falciparum is encoded in the nucleus and targeted to the apicoplast. Nucleic Acids Res. 2010 Nov;38(20):7037-53. Epub 2010 Jun 22. PMID:20571080

Pruthi RK, Marshall WF, Wiltsie JC, Persing DH. Human babesiosis. Mayo Clin Proc. 1995 Sep;70(9):853-62. PMID:7643639

Przyjemski CJ. Was babesiosis transmitted by transfusion? N Engl J Med. 1981 Mar 19;304(12):733. PMID:7193287

Pudney M, Gray JS. Therapeutic efficacy of atovaquone against the bovine intraerythrocytic parasite, Babesia divergens. J Parasitol. 1997 Apr;83(2):307-10. PMID:9105316

Purfield AE, Tidwell RR, Meshnick SR. Interactions of DB75, a novel antimalarial agent, with other antimalarial drugs in vitro. Antimicrob Agents Chemother. 2008 Jun;52(6):2253-5. Epub 2008 Mar 24. PMID:18362196

Puri SK, Dutta GP. Blood schizontocidal activity of WR 238605 (Tafenoquine) against Plasmodium cynomolgi and Plasmodium fragile infections in rhesus monkeys. Acta Trop. 2003 Apr;86(1):35-40. PMID:12711101

Purnell RE, Brocklesby DW. Babesia divergens in splenectomised calves: immunogenicity of lyophilised plasma from an infected animal. Res Vet Sci. 1977 Sep;23(2):255-6. PMID:928989

Purnell RE, Gunter TD, Schroder J. Development of a prophylactic regime using long-acting tetracycline for the control of redwater and heartwater in susceptible cattle moved into an endemic area. Trop Anim Health Prod. 1989 Feb;21(1):11-9. PMID:2711456

Purnell RE, Lewis D, Brocklesby DW, Taylor SM. Bovine babesiosis: steps towards an irradiated vaccine. J S Afr Vet Assoc. 1979 Dec;50(4):339-44. PMID:553975

Purnell RE, Lewis D, Young ER. Investigations on the prophylactic effect of treatment with imidocarb diproprionate on Babesia divergens infections in splenectomized calves. Br Vet J. 1980 Sep-Oct;136(5):452-6. PMID:7225772

Purnell RE, Lewis D, Young ER. Quinuronium sulphate for the treatment of Babesia divergens infections of splenectomised calves. Vet Rec. 1981 Jun 20;108(25):538-9. PMID:7269188

Purvis AC. Immunodepression in Babesia microti infections. Parasitology. 1977 Oct;75(2):197-205. PMID:337221

Pussard E, Merzouk M, Barennes H. Increased uptake of quinine into the brain by inhibition of P-glycoprotein. Eur J Pharm Sci. 2007 Oct;32(2):123-7. Epub 2007 Jul 10. PMID:17698330

Qi C, Zhou D, Liu J, Cheng Z, Zhang L, Wang L, Wang Z, Yang D, Wang S, Chai T. Detection of Babesia divergens using molecular methods in anemic patients in Shandong Province, China. Parasitol Res. 2011 Jul;109(1):241-5. Epub 2011 Apr 19. PMID:21503639

Qi WJ, Fang Q. [Progress of research on DNA vaccines against parasitosis].[Article in Chinese]. Zhongguo Xue Xi Chong Bing Fang Zhi Za Zhi. 2011 Jun;23(3):340-4. PMID:22164511

Quashie NB, Duah NO, Abuaku B, Koram KA. The in-vitro susceptibilities of Ghanaian Plasmodium falciparum to antimalarial drugs. Ann Trop Med Parasitol. 2007 Jul;101(5):391-8. PMID:17550644

Queener SF, Dean RA, Bartlett MS, Milhous WK, Berman JD, Ellis WY, Smith JW. Efficacy of intermittent dosage of 8-aminoquinolines for therapy or prophylaxis of Pneumocystis pneumonia in rats. J Infect Dis. 1992 Apr;165(4):764-8. PMID:1532406

Quelhas D, Jiménez A, Quintó L, Serra-Casas E, Mayor A, Cisteró P, Puyol L, Wilson DW, Richards JS, Nhampossa T, Macete E, Aide P, Mandomando I, Sanz S, Aponte JJ, Alonso PL, Beeson JG, Menéndez C, Dobaño C. IgG against Plasmodium falciparum variant surface antigens and growth inhibitory antibodies in Mozambican children receiving intermittent preventive treatment with sulfadoxine-pyrimethamine. Immunobiology. 2011 Jul;216(7):793-802. Epub 2010 Dec 25. PMID:21257227

Queryriaux B, Texier G, Ollivier L, Galoisy-Guibal L, Michel R, Meynard JB, Decam C, Verret C, Pommier de Santi V, Spiegel A, Boutin JP, Migliani R, Deparis X. Plasmodium vivax Malaria among military personnel, French Guiana, 1998-2008. Emerg Infect Dis. 2011 Jul;17(7):1280-2. PMID:21762587

Quintão-Silva MG, Melo MN, Ribeiro MF. Comparison of duplex PCR and microscopic techniques for the identification of Babesia bigemina and Babesia bovis in engorged female ticks of Boophilus microplus. Zoonoses Public Health. 2007;54(3-4):147-51. PMID:17456146

Rabinovich SA. [Experimental investigation of the antimalarial drug haloquine. 3. Investigation of the possibility to restrain the development of chemoresistance to chloridine (daraprim) by combined administration of chloridine with haloquine].[Article in Russian]. Med Parazitol (Mosk). 1965 Jul-Aug;34(4):434-9. PMID:5871367

Radford AJ, Van Leeuwen H, Christian SH. Social aspects in the changing epidemiology of malaria in the highlands of New Guinea. Ann Trop Med Parasitol. 1976 Mar;70(1):11-23. PMID:1267506

Raether W, Seidenath H. Survival of Aegyptianella pullorum, Anaplasma marginale and various parasitic protozoa following prolonged storage in liquid nitrogen. Z Parasitenkd. 1977 Aug 25;53(1):41-6. PMID:919686

Rafaj RB, Matijatko V, Kis I, Kucer N, Zivicnjak T, Lemo N, Zvorc Z, Brkljacić M, Mrljak V. Alterations in some blood coagulation parameters in naturally occurring cases of canine babesiosis. Acta Vet Hung. 2009 Jun;57(2):295-304. PMID:19584042

Raghavendra K, Barik TK, Reddy BP, Sharma P, Dash AP. Malaria vector control: from past to future. Parasitol Res. 2011 Apr;108(4):757-79. Epub 2011 Jan 13. PMID:21229263

Rah JH, Depee S, Kraemer K, Steiger G, Bloem MW, Spiegel P, Wilkinson C, Bilukha O. Program experience with micronutrient powders and current evidence. J Nutr. 2012 Jan;142(1):191S-6S. Epub 2011 Nov 30. PMID:22131547

Rahmatullah M, Mollik AH, Rahman S, Hasan N, Agarwala B, Jahan R. A medicinal plant study of the Santal tribe in Rangpur district, Bangladesh. J Altern Complement Med. 2010 Apr;16(4):419-25. PMID:20423211

Raiesi A, Nikpour F, Ansari-Moghaddam A, Ranjbar M, Rakhshani F, Mohammadi M, Haghdost A, Taghizadeh-Asl R, Sakeni M, Safari R, Saffari M. Baseline results of the first malaria indicator survey in Iran at the health facility level. Malar J. 2011 Oct 27;10:319. PMID:22029447

Raiten DJ, Namasté S, Brabin B. Considerations for the safe and effective use of iron interventions in areas of malaria burden - executive summary. Int J Vitam Nutr Res. 2011 Jan;81(1):57-71. PMID:22002219

Rajatileka S, Burhani J, Ranson H. Mosquito age and susceptibility to insecticides. Trans R Soc Trop Med Hyg. 2011 May;105(5):247-53. Epub 2011 Feb 26. PMID:21353689

Rajgor DD, Gogtay NJ, Kadam VS, Kamtekar KD, Dalvi SS, Chogle AR, Aigal U, Bichile LS, Kain KC, Kshirsagar NA. Efficacy of a 14-day primaquine regimen in preventing relapses in patients with Plasmodium vivax malaria in Mumbai, India. Trans R Soc Trop Med Hyg. 2003 Jul-Aug;97(4):438-40. PMID:15259476

Raju M, Salazar JC, Leopold H, Krause PJ. Atovaquone and azithromycin treatment for babesiosis in an infant. Pediatr Infect Dis J. 2007 Feb;26(2):181-3. PMID:17259886

Rakotomanana F, Ratovonjato J, Randremanana RV, Randrianasolo L, Raherinjafy R, Rudant JP, Richard V. Geographical and environmental approaches to urban malaria in Antananarivo (Madagascar). BMC Infect Dis. 2010 Jun 16;10:173. PMID:20553598

Raman J, Little F, Roper C, Kleinschmidt I, Cassam Y, Maharaj R, Barnes KI. Five years of large-scale dhfr and dhps mutation surveillance following the phased implementation of artesunate plus sulfadoxine-pyrimethamine in Maputo Province, Southern Mozambique. Am J Trop Med Hyg. 2010 May;82(5):788-94. PMID:20439956

Raman J, Mauff K, Muianga P, Mussa A, Maharaj R, Barnes KI. Five years of antimalarial resistance marker surveillance in Gaza Province, Mozambique, following artemisinin-based combination therapy roll out. PLoS One. 2011;6(10):e25992. Epub 2011 Oct 14. PMID:22022487

Ramazani A, Sardari S, Zakeri S, Vaziri B. In vitro antiplasmodial and phytochemical study of five Artemisia species from Iran and in vivo activity of two species. Parasitol Res. 2010 Aug;107(3):593-9. Epub 2010 May 18. PMID:20480374

Ramharter M, Noedl H, Thimasarn K, Wiedermann G, Wernsdorfer G, Wernsdorfer WH. In vitro activity of tafenoquine alone and in combination with artemisinin against Plasmodium falciparum. Am J Trop Med Hyg. 2002 Jul;67(1):39-43. PMID:12363062

Ramharter M, Walochnik J, Lagler H, Winkler S, Wernsdorfer WH, Stoiser B, Graninger W. Clinical and molecular characterization of a near fatal case of human babesiosis in Austria. J Travel Med. 2010 Nov-Dec;17(6):416-8. PMID:21050324

Ramos Júnior WM, Sardinha JF, Costa MR, Santana MS, Alecrim MG, Lacerda MV. Clinical aspects of hemolysis in patients with P. vivax malaria treated with primaquine, in the Brazilian Amazon. Braz J Infect Dis. 2010 Jul-Aug;14(4):410-2. PMID:20963329

Ranatunga P, Wanduragala L. Reactions and haematology in imported Jersey cattle premunized in Ceylon. Br Vet J. 1972 Jan;128(1):9-18. PMID:5062160

Ranjbar-Bahadori S, Eckert B, Omidian Z, Shirazi NS, Shayan P. Babesia ovis as the main causative agent of sheep babesiosis in Iran. Parasitol Res. 2012 Apr;110(4):1531-6. PMID:21975684

Rank RG, Weidanz WP, Bondi A. Nonsterilizing immunity in avian malaria: an antibody-independent phenomenon. Proc Soc Exp Biol Med. 1976 Feb;151(2):257-9. PMID:1082596

Ranque S. The treatment of babesiosis. N Engl J Med. 2001 Mar 8;344(10):773-4. PMID:11236790

Raoult D, Soulayrol L, Toga B, Dumon H, Casanova P. Babesiosis, pentamidine, and cotrimoxazole. Ann Intern Med. 1987 Dec;107(6):944. PMID:3500663

Rashid HB, Chaudhry M, Rashid H, Pervez K, Khan MA, Mahmood AK. Comparative efficacy of diminazene diaceturate and diminazene aceturate for the treatment of babesiosis in horses. Trop Anim Health Prod. 2008 Aug;40(6):463-7. Epub 2007 Dec 15. PMID:18575975

Rashina MG, Sarikian SIa. [On the development of a network of special institutions for the control of malaria and other parasitic diseases in the USSR].[Article in Russian]. Med Parazitol (Mosk). 1970 Mar-Apr;39(2):132-8. PMID:5473684

Rathore S, Sinha D, Asad M, Böttcher T, Afrin F, Chauhan VS, Gupta D, Sieber SA, Mohmmed A. A cyanobacterial serine protease of Plasmodium falciparum is targeted to the apicoplast and plays an important role in its growth and development. Mol Microbiol. 2010 Jun 10. [Epub ahead of print]. PMID:20545854

Rauwald HW, Kober M, Mutschler E, Lambrecht G. Cryptolepis sanguinolenta: antimuscarinic properties of cryptolepine and the alkaloid fraction at M1, M2 and M3 receptors. Planta Med. 1992 Dec;58(6):486-8. PMID:1484884

Ravaoarisoa E, Zamanka H, Fusai T, Bellalou J, Bedouelle H, Mercereau-Puijalon O, Fandeur T. ecombinant antibodies specific for the Plasmodium falciparum histidine-rich protein 2. MAbs. 2010 Jul 22;2(4). [Epub ahead of print]. PMID:20581462

Ravikumar S, Inbaneson SJ, Suganthi P, Gnanadesigan M. In vitro antiplasmodial activity of ethanolic extracts of mangrove plants from South East coast of India against chloroquine-sensitive Plasmodium falciparum. Parasitol Res. 2011 Apr;108(4):873-8. Epub 2010 Oct 27. PMID:20978786

Ravikumar S, Inbaneson SJ, Suganthi P, Venkatesan M, Ramu A. Mangrove plants as a source of lead compounds for the development of new antiplasmodial drugs from South East coast of India. Parasitol Res. 2011 Jun;108(6):1405-10. Epub 2010 Dec 1. PMID:21120528

Ravikumar S, Ramanathan G, Inbaneson SJ, Ramu A. Antiplasmodial activity of two marine polyherbal preparations from Chaetomorpha antennina and Aegiceras corniculatum against Plasmodium falciparum. Parasitol Res. 2011 Jan;108(1):107-13. Epub 2010 Sep 16. PMID:20844892

Read AF, Day T, Huijben S. The evolution of drug resistance and the curious orthodoxy of aggressive chemotherapy. Proc Natl Acad Sci U S A. 2011 Jun 28;108 Suppl 2:10871-7. Epub 2011 Jun 20. PMID:21690376

Rech A, Bittar CM, de Castro CG, Azevedo KR, dos Santos RP, Machado AR, Schwartsmann G, Goldani L, Brunetto AL. Asymptomatic babesiosis in a child with hepatoblastoma. J Pediatr Hematol Oncol. 2004 Mar;26(3):213. PMID:15125618

Redmond AM, Doolan DL. The Australasian contribution to malaria vaccine development. Parasite Immunol. 2010 Aug;32(8):607.-22. PMID:20626816

Rees P, Schoeman JP. Plasma insulin concentrations in hypoglycaemic dogs with Babesia canis rossi infection. Vet Parasitol. 2008 Mar 25;152(1-2):60-6. Epub 2007 Nov 22. PMID:18164550

Reesink HW. European strategies against the parasite transfusion risk. Transfus Clin Biol. 2005 Feb;12(1):1-4. PMID:15814284

Regassa A, Penzhorn BL, Bryson NR. Progression towards endemic stability to bovine babesiosis in cattle introduced onto a game ranch. Onderstepoort J Vet Res. 2004 Dec;71(4):333-6. PMID:15732461

Reine NJ. Infection and blood transfusion: a guide to donor screening. Clin Tech Small Anim Pract. 2004 May;19(2):68-74. PMID:15179926

Reis C, Cote M, Paul RE, Bonnet S. Questing ticks in suburban forest are infected by at least six tick-borne pathogens. Vector Borne Zoonotic Dis. 2011 Jul;11(7):907-16. Epub 2010 Dec 15. PMID:21158500

Reis PA, Comim CM, Hermani F, Silva B, Barichello T, Portella AC, Gomes FC, Sab IM, Frutuoso VS, Oliveira MF, Bozza PT, Bozza FA, Dal-Pizzol F, Zimmerman GA, Quevedo J, Castro-Faria-Neto HC. Cognitive dysfunction is sustained after rescue therapy in experimental cerebral malaria, and is reduced by additive antioxidant therapy. PLoS Pathog. 2010 Jun 24;6(6):e1000963. PMID:20585569

Reis RC, Melo DR, Perinotto WM, Bittencourt VR. [In vitro pathogenicity of fungic formulation on nymphs and adults of Rhipicephalus sanguineus (Latreile, 1806) (Acari:Ixodidae)].[Article in Portuguese]. Rev Bras Parasitol Vet. 2005 Jul-Sep;14(3):101-5. PMID:16229753

Reis SP, Maddineni S, Rozenblit G, Allen D. Spontaneous splenic rupture secondary to Babesia microti infection: treatment with splenic artery embolization. J Vasc Interv Radiol. 2011 May;22(5):732-4. PMID:21514529

Repetto EC, Traverso A, Giacomazzi CG. Possible clinical failure of artemether-lumefantrine in an italian traveler with uncomplicated falciparum malaria. Mediterr J Hematol Infect Dis. 2011;3(1):e2011041. Epub 2011 Oct 1. PMID:22084655

Resch S, Korenromp E, Stover J, Blakley M, Krubiner C, Thorien K, Hecht R, Atun R. Economic returns to investment in AIDS treatment in low and middle income countries. PLoS One. 2011;6(10):e25310. Epub 2011 Oct 5. PMID:21998648

Restrepo-Pineda E, Arango E, Maestre A, Do Rosário VE, Cravo P. Studies on antimalarial drug susceptibility in Colombia, in relation to Pfmdr1 and Pfcrt. Parasitology. 2008 Apr;135(5):547-53. PMID:18426617

Rey JL. [Public health policy in developing countries and international relations].[Article in French]. Med Trop (Mars). 2011 Apr;71(2):109-10. PMID:21695864

Reyes-Sandoval A, Wyllie DH, Bauza K, Milicic A, Forbes EK, Rollier CS, Hill AV. CD8+ T effector memory cells protect against liver-stage malaria. J Immunol. 2011 Aug 1;187(3):1347-57. Epub 2011 Jun 29. PMID:21715686

Richard D, Bartfai R, Volz J, Ralph SA, Muller S, Stunnenberg HG, Cowman AF. A genome-wide chromatin-associated nuclear peroxiredoxin from the malaria parasite Plasmodium falciparum. J Biol Chem. 2011 Apr 1;286(13):11746-55. Epub 2011 Jan 31. PMID:21282103

Richards JS, Stanisic DI, Fowkes FJ, Tavul L, Dabod E, Thompson JK, Kumar S, Chitnis CE, Narum DL, Michon P, Siba PM, Cowman AF, Mueller I, Beeson JG. Association between naturally acquired antibodies to erythrocyte-binding antigens of Plasmodium falciparum and protection from malaria and high-density parasitemia. Clin Infect Dis. 2010 Oct 15;51(8):e50-60. PMID:20843207

Richier E, Biagini GA, Wein S, Boudou F, Bray PG, Ward SA, Precigout E, Calas M, Dubremetz JF, Vial HJ. Potent antihematozoan activity of novel bisthiazolium drug T16: evidence for inhibition of phosphatidylcholine metabolism in erythrocytes infected with Babesia and Plasmodium spp. Antimicrob Agents Chemother. 2006 Oct;50(10):3381-8. PMID:17005821

Ridley DB, Sánchez AC. Introduction of European priority review vouchers to encourage development of new medicines for neglected diseases. Lancet. 2010 Sep 11;376(9744):922-7. PMID:20833303

Rieckmann KH, Trenholme GM, Williams RL, Carson PE, Frischer H, Desjardins RE. Prophylactic activity of mefloquine hydrochloride (WR 142490) in drug-resistant malaria. Bull World Health Organ. 1974;51(4):375-7. PMID:4619059

Rijken MJ, McGready R, Jullien V, Tarning J, Lindegardh N, Phyo AP, Win AK, His P, Cammas M, Singhasivanon P, White NJ, Nosten F. Pharmacokinetics of amodiaquine and desethylamodiaquine in pregnant and postpartum women with Plasmodium vivax malaria. Antimicrob Agents Chemother. 2011 Sep;55(9):4338-42. Epub 2011 Jun 27. PMID:21709098

Rikhotso BO, Stoltsz WH, Bryson NR, Sommerville JE. The impact of 2 dipping systems on endemic stability to bovine babesiosis and anaplasmosis in cattle in 4 communally grazed areas in Limpopo Province, South Africa. J S Afr Vet Assoc. 2005 Dec;76(4):217-23. PMID:16642719

Ríos L, Alvarez G, Blair S. Serological and parasitological study and report of the first case of human babesiosis in Colombia. Rev Soc Bras Med Trop. 2003 Jul-Aug;36(4):493-8. Epub 2003 Aug 13. PMID:12937727

Rizal A, Beard J, Patwari A. Acute respiratory infection Boston university's collaborative research work in the last decade. Indian Pediatr. 2010 Jan;47(1):19-24. PMID:20139473

Roberts JA, Tracey-Patte PD. Babesia rodhaini: a study of the effects of immune serum. Int J Parasitol. 1975 Dec;5(6):577-81. PMID:1201890

Roberts JA. Some quantitative aspects of the adoptive transfer of immunity to Plasmodium berghei with immune spleen cells. J Protozool. 1971 Aug;18(3):437-40. PMID:5132318

Roberts MC, Groenendyk S. Splenectomy in the horse. Aust Vet J. 1978 Apr;54(4):196-7. PMID:687278

Roca MG, Charle P, Jimenez S, Nunez M. A new malaria protocol in a Congolese refugee camp in West Tanzania. Glob Public Health. 2011;6(4):398-406. PMID:21308578

Rodrigues LA, Henriques G, Borges ST, Hunt P, Sanchez CP, Martinelli A, Cravo P. Experimental evolution of resistance to artemisinin combination therapy results in amplification of the mdr1 gene in a rodent malaria parasite. PLoS One. 2010 Jul 15;5(7):e11593. PMID:20657645

Rodriguez RI, Trees AJ. In vitro responsiveness of Babesia bovis to imidocarb dipropionate and the selection of a drug-adapted line. Vet Parasitol. 1996 Mar;62(1-2):35-41. PMID:8638391

Rodríguez SD, Palmer GH, McElwain TF, McGuire TC, Ruef BJ, Chitko-McKown MG, Brown WC. CD4+ T-helper lymphocyte responses against Babesia bigemina rhoptry-associated protein I. Infect Immun. 1996 Jun;64(6):2079-87. PMID:8675310

Rodríguez-Vivas RI, Quiñones-Avila FJ, Ramírez-Cruz GT, Cruz D, Wagner G. [Isolation of a field strain of Babesia bigemina (Piroplasma: Babesiidae) and establishment of in vitro culture for antigen production].[Article in Spanish]. Rev Biol Trop. 2007 Mar;55(1):127-33. PMID:18457120

Roederer MW, McLeod H, Juliano JJ. Can pharmacogenomics improve malaria drug policy? Bull World Health Organ. 2011 Nov 1;89(11):838-45. Epub 2011 Sep 1. PMID:22084530

Roersch CM. Piper umbellatum L.: a comparative cross-cultural analysis of its medicinal uses and an ethnopharmacological evaluation. J Ethnopharmacol. 2010 Oct 5;131(3):522-37. Epub 2010 Aug 1. PMID:20678569

Rogers RJ. Serum opsonins and the passive transfer of protection in Babesia rodhaini infections of rats. Int J Parasitol. 1974 Apr;4(2):197-201. PMID:4822486

Rogers RJ. The acquired resistance to Babesia argentina of cattle exposed to light infestation with cattle tick (Boophilus microplus). Aust Vet J. 1971 Jun;47(6):237-41. PMID:5106905

Rogers WO, Sem R, Tero T, Chim P, Lim P, Muth S, Socheat D, Ariey F, Wongsrichanalai C. Failure of artesunate-mefloquine combination therapy for uncomplicated Plasmodium falciparum malaria in southern Cambodia. Malar J. 2009 Jan 12;8:10. PMID:19138388

Rogerson SJ, Wijesinghe RS, Meshnick SR. Host immunity as a determinant of treatment outcome in Plasmodium falciparum malaria. Lancet Infect Dis. 2010 Jan;10(1):51-9. PMID:20129149

Röhrig E, Hamel D, Pfister K. Retrospective evaluation of laboratory data on canine vector-borne infections from the years 2004-2008. Berl Munch Tierarztl Wochenschr. 2011 Sep-Oct;124(9-10):411-8. PMID:21950219

Rojas C, Figueroa JV, Alvarado A, Mejia P, Mosqueda JJ, Falcon A, Vega CA, Alvarez A. Bovine babesiosis live vaccine production: use of gamma irradiation on the substrate. Ann N Y Acad Sci. 2006 Oct;1081:405-16. PMID:17135544

Rojas Ruiz FA, García-Sánchez RN, Estupiñan SV, Gómez-Barrio A, Torres Amado DF, Pérez-Solórzano BM, Nogal-Ruiz JJ, Martínez-Fernández AR, Kouznetsov VV. Synthesis and antimalarial activity of new heterocyclic hybrids based on chloroquine and thiazolidinone scaffolds. Bioorg Med Chem. 2011 Aug 1;19(15):4562-73. Epub 2011 Jun 15. PMID:21723734

Rollo IM. Antiplasmodial efficacy of 2,4--diaminopyrimidine0sylfonamide combinations, especially against chloroquine-resistant malaria. Can Med Assoc J. 1975 Jun 14;112(13 Spec No):50-3. PMID:805650

Römsing S, Lindegardh N, Bergqvist Y. Determination of tafenoquine in dried blood spots and plasma using LC and fluorescence detection. Bioanalysis. 2011 Aug;3(16):1847-53. PMID:21877894

Rosa FW. International aspects of perinatal mortality. Clin Obstet Gynecol. 1970 Mar;13(1):57-78. PMID:5430770

Rosenblatt JE. Antiparasitic agents. Mayo Clin Proc. 1999 Nov;74(11):1161-75. PMID:10560606

Rosenblatt JE. Laboratory diagnosis of infections due to blood and tissue parasites. Clin Infect Dis. 2009 Oct 1;49(7):1103-8. PMID:19691431

Rosenthal PJ. Lessons from sickle cell disease in the treatment and control of malaria. N Engl J Med. 2011 Jun 30;364(26):2549-51. PMID:21714653

Rosner F, Zarrabi MH, Benach JL, Habicht GS. Babesiosis in splenectomized adults. Review of 22 reported cases. Am J Med. 1984 Apr;76(4):696-701. PMID:6424470

Rosowsky A, Huang PC, Papathanasopoulos N, Modest EJ. Quinazolines. 12. 1,3-Diaminobenzo(f)quinazolines containing long-chain alkyl or chloro substituents on the central ring. Synthesis and biological evaluation as candidate antifolate and antimalarial agents. J Med Chem. 1974 Nov;17(11):1217-22. PMID:4606974

Rottmann M, McNamara C, Yeung BK, Lee MC, Zou B, Russell B, Seitz P, Plouffe DM, Dharia NV, Tan J, Cohen SB, Spencer KR, González-Páez GE, Lakshminarayana SB, Goh A, Suwanarusk R, Jegla T, Schmitt EK, Beck HP, Brun R, Nosten F, Renia L, Dartois V, Keller TH, Fidock DA, Winzeler EA, Diagana TT. Spiroindolones, a potent compound class for the treatment of malaria. Science. 2010 Sep 3;329(5996):1175-80. PMID:20813948

Rousset JJ, Couzineau P, Baufine-Ducrocq H. [Plasmodium ovale (Stephens 1922)].[Article in French]. Ann Parasitol Hum Comp. 1969 May-Jun;44(3):273-328. PMID:4905936

Rowe AK, Rowe SY, Holloway KA, Ivanovska V, Muhe L, Lambrechts T. Does shortening the training on Integrated Management of Childhood Illness guidelines reduce its effectiveness? A systematic review. Health Policy Plan. 2011 Apr 23. [Epub ahead of print]. PMID:21515912

Rowin KS, Tanowitz HB, Wittner M. Therapy of experimental babesiosis. Ann Intern Med. 1982 Oct;97(4):556-8. PMID:7125412

Ruebush MJ, Hanson WL. Transfer of immunity to Babesia microti of human origin using T lymphocytes in mice. Cell Immunol. 1980 Jul 1;52(2):255-65. PMID:6969120

Ruebush MJ, Steel LK, Kennedy DA. Prostaglandin-mediated suppression of delayed-type hypersensitivity to infected erythrocytes during Babesia microti infection in mice. Cell Immunol. 1986 Apr 1;98(2):300-10. PMID:2944617

Ruebush MJ, Troutman EH, Kennedy DA. Delayed-type hypersensitivity to Babesia microti-infected erythrocytes in mice. Cell Immunol. 1986 Apr 1;98(2):289-99. PMID:3757050

Ruef BJ, Tuo W, Rodriguez SD, Roussel AJ, Chitko-McKown CG, Palmer GH, McElwain TF, Canals A, Zarlenga DS, Gasbarre LC, Brown WC. Immunization with Babesia bigemina rhoptry-associated protein 1 induces a type 1 cytokine response. J Interferon Cytokine Res. 1997 Jan;17(1):45-54. PMID:9041471

Ruff MD, Fowler JL, Fernau RC, Matsuda K. Action of certain antiprotozoal compounds against Babesia gibsoni in dogs. Am J Vet Res. 1973 May;34(5):641-5. PMID:4703508

Rulisa S, Gatarayiha JP, Kabarisa T, Ndayisaba G. Comparison of different artemisinin-based combinations for the treatment of Plasmodium falciparum malaria in children in Kigali, Rwanda, an area of resistance to sulfadoxine-pyrimethamine: artesunate plus sulfadoxine/pyrimethamine versus artesunate plus sulfamethoxypyrazine/pyrimethamine. Am J Trop Med Hyg. 2007 Oct;77(4):612-6. PMID:17978058

Ruocco V, Ruocco E, Schwartz RA, Janniger CK. Kaposi sarcoma and quinine: a potentially overlooked triggering factor in millions of Africans. J Am Acad Dermatol. 2011 Feb;64(2):434-6. PMID:21238829

Russell BM, Udomsangpetch R, Rieckmann KH, Kotecka BM, Coleman RE, Sattabongkot J. Simple in vitro assay for determining the sensitivity of Plasmodium vivax isolates from fresh human blood to antimalarials in areas where P. vivax is endemic. Antimicrob Agents Chemother. 2003 Jan;47(1):170-3. PMID:12499187.

Ryan R, Krause PJ, Radolf J, Freeman K, Spielman A, Lenz R, Levin A. Diagnosis of babesiosis using an immunoblot serologic test. Clin Diagn Lab Immunol. 2001 Nov;8(6):1177-80. PMID:11687460

Sá JM, Chong JL, Wellems TE. Malaria drug resistance: new observations and developments. Essays Biochem. 2011;51:137-60. PMID:22023447

Sá MR. Studies of avian malaria and Brazil in the international scientific context (1907-1945). [Article in English, Portuguese]. Hist Cienc Saude Manguinhos. 2011 Jun 1;18(2):499-518. PMID:21779696

Sabin LL, Rizal A, Brooks MI, Singh MP, Tuchman J, Wylie BJ, Joyce KM, Yeboah-Antwi K, Singh N, Hamer DH. Attitudes, knowledge, and practices regarding malaria prevention and treatment among pregnant women in Eastern India. Am J Trop Med Hyg. 2010 Jun;82(6):1010-6. PMID:20519593

Sabio y García JV, Farber M, Carrica M, Cravero S, Macedo GC, Bigi F, Oliveira SC, Rossetti O, Campos E. Expression of Babesia bovis rhoptry-associated protein 1 (RAP1) in Brucella abortus S19. Microbes Infect. 2008 May;10(6):635-41. Epub 2008 Feb 23. PMID:18462974

Sachs JD. Millennium development goals at 10. Sci Am. 2010 Jun;302(6):30. PMID:20521476

Saeki H, Ishii T. Effect of silica treatment on resistance to Babesia rodhaini infection in immunized mice. Vet Parasitol. 1996 Feb;61(3-4):201-10. PMID:8720558

Saeki H, Ishii T. Studies on route of immunization with a mixture of killed parasites and adjuvants against Babesia rodhaini infection in mice. Nihon Juigaku Zasshi. 1989 Dec;51(6):1173-8. PMID:2601229

Sahgal G, Ramanathan S, Sasidharan S, Mordi MN, Ismail S, Mansor SM. Brine shrimp lethality and acute oral toxicity studies on Swietenia mahagoni (Linn.) Jacq. seed methanolic extract. Pharmacognosy Res. 2010 Jul;2(4):215-20. PMID:21808570

Sahu SS, Gunasekaran K, Vanamail P, Jambulingam P. Seasonal prevalence & resting behaviour of Anopheles minimus Theobald & An. fluviatilis James (Diptera: Culicidae) in east-central India. Indian J Med Res. 2011 Jun;133(6):655-61. PMID:21727666

Saidel-Odes L, Riesenberg K, Schlaeffer F, Smolyakov R, Kafka M, Borer A. Eritrean and Sudanese migrants presenting with malaria in Israel. Travel Med Infect Dis. 2011 Nov;9(6):303-5. Epub 2011 Oct 28. PMID:22037052

Saito-Ito A, Dantrakool A, Kawai A, Yano Y, Takada N. [Babesiosis]. [Article in Japanese]. Nihon Rinsho. 2003 Feb;61 Suppl 2:623-8. PMID:12722292

Saitoito A, Rai SK, He S, Kohsaki M, Tsuji M, Ishihara C. [First demonstration of Babesia parasitizing in human in Japan]. [Article in Japanese]. Kansenshogaku Zasshi. 1999 Nov;73(11):1163-4. PMID:10624098

Saito-Ito A, Tsuji M, Wei Q, He S, Matsui T, Kohsaki M, Arai S, Kamiyama T, Hioki K, Ishihara C. Transfusion-acquired, autochthonous human babesiosis in Japan: isolation of Babesia microti-like parasites with hu-RBC-SCID mice. J Clin Microbiol. 2000 Dec;38(12):4511-6. PMID:11101588

Sakuma M, Setoguchi A, Endo Y. Possible emergence of drug-resistant variants of Babesia gibsoni in clinical cases treated with atovaquone and azithromycin. J Vet Intern Med. 2009 May-Jun;23(3):493-8. PMID:19645835

Salcedo-Amaya AM, Hoeijmakers WA, Bártfai R, Stunnenberg HG. Malaria: could its unusual epigenome be the weak spot? Int J Biochem Cell Biol. 2010 Jun;42(6):781-4. Epub 2010 Mar 18. PMID:20303414

Saleh JA, Yusuph H, Zailani SB, Aji B. Malaria vaccine: the pros and cons. Niger J Med. 2010 Jan-Mar;19(1):8-13. PMID:20232750

Salem GH, Liu X, Johnsrude JD, Dame JB, Roman Reddy G. Development and evaluation of an extra chromosomal DNA-based PCR test for diagnosing bovine babesiosis. Mol Cell Probes. 1999 Apr;13(2):107-13. PMID:10208801

Salih DA, Ali AM, Liu Z, Bakheit MA, Taha KM, El Imam AH, Kullmann B, El Hussein AM, Ahmed JS, Seitzer U. Development of a loop-mediated isothermal amplification method for detection of Theileria lestoquardi. Parasitol Res. 2011 Jul 9. [Epub ahead of print]. PMID:21744022

Salwati E, Minigo G, Woodberry T, Piera KA, de Silva HD, Kenangalem E, Tjitra E, Coppel RL, Price RN, Anstey NM, Plebanski M. Differential cellular recognition of antigens during acute Plasmodium falciparum and Plasmodium vivax malaria. J Infect Dis. 2011 Apr 15;203(8):1192-9. PMID:21451007

Samb B, Desai N, Nishtar S, Mendis S, Bekedam H, Wright A, Hsu J, Martiniuk A, Celletti F, Patel K, Adshead F, McKee M, Evans T, Alwan A, Etienne C. Prevention and management of chronic disease: a litmus test for health-systems strengthening in low-income and middle-income countries. Lancet. 2010 Nov 20;376(9754):1785-97. Epub 2010 Nov 10. PMID:21074253

Sambo LG, Kirigia JM. Africa's health: could the private sector accelerate the progress towards health MDGs? Int Arch Med. 2011 Nov 25;4(1):39. [Epub ahead of print]. PMID:22118626

Sambo LG, Ki-Zerbo G, Kirigia JM. Malaria control in the African Region: perceptions and viewspoints on proceedings of the Africa Leaders Malaria Alliance (ALMA). BMC Proc. 2011 Jun 13;5 Suppl 5:S3. PMID:21810213

Sambri V, Marangoni A, Storni E, Cavrini F, Moroni A, Sparacino M, Cevenini R. [Tick borne zoonosis: selected clinical and diagnostic aspects].[Article in Italian]. Parassitologia. 2004 Jun;46(1-2):109-13. PMID:15305697

Sam-Wobo SO, Agbeyangi OA, Ekpo UF, Akinloye OA, Mafiana CF, Adeleke MA. Rectal Artesunates, Their Utilization, and Parental Perception in the Management of Malaria in Children from Abeokuta, Southwestern Nigeria. Vector Borne Zoonotic Dis. 2011 Oct 24. [Epub ahead of print]. PMID:22022814

Sam-Wobo SO, Akinboroye T, Anosike JC, Adewale B. Knowledge and practices on malaria treatment measures among pregnant women in Abeokuta, Nigeria. Tanzan J Health Res. 2008 Oct;10(4):226-31. PMID:19402584

Sandler SG, Yu H, Rassai N. Risks of blood transfusion and their prevention. Clin Adv Hematol Oncol. 2003 May;1(5):307-13. PMID:16224428

Sannusi A, Aliu YO. Field observations on adult zebu bulls immunised against anaplasmosis by infection and treatment plus integrated tick control. Trop Anim Health Prod. 1986 Feb;18(1):13-20. PMID:3705174

Santoro F, Bernal J, Capron A. Complement activation by parasites. A review. Acta Trop. 1979 Mar;36(1):5-14. PMID:35934

Santos F, Coppede JS, Pereira AL, Oliveira LP, Roberto PG, Benedetti RB, Zucoloto LB, Lucas F, Sobreira L, Marins M. Molecular evaluation of the incidence of Ehrlichia canis, Anaplasma platys and Babesia spp. in dogs from Ribeirão Preto, Brazil. Vet J. 2009 Jan;179(1):145-8. Epub 2007 Oct 24. PMID:17920967

Santos MN, Nogueira PM, Dias FB, Valle D, Moreira LA. Fitness aspects of transgenic Aedes fluviatilis mosquitoes expressing a Plasmodium-blocking molecule. Transgenic Res. 2010 Dec;19(6):1129-35. Epub 2010 Feb 13. PMID:20155397

Santos-Magalhães NS, Mosqueira VC. Nanotechnology applied to the treatment of malaria. Adv Drug Deliv Rev. 2010 Mar 18;62(4-5):560-75. Epub 2009 Nov 13. PMID:19914313

Saraiva VB, de Souza Silva L, Ferreira-DaSilva CT, da Silva-Filho JL, Teixeira-Ferreira A, Perales J, Souza MC, Henriques MG, Caruso-Neves C, de Sá Pinheiro AA. Impairment of the Plasmodium falciparum erythrocytic cycle induced by angiotensin peptides. PLoS One. 2011 Feb 18;6(2):e17174. PMID:21364758

Saralamba S, Pan-Ngum W, Maude RJ, Lee SJ, Tarning J, Lindegårdh N, Chotivanich K, Nosten F, Day NP, Socheat D, White NJ, Dondorp AM, White LJ. Intrahost modeling of artemisinin resistance in Plasmodium falciparum. Proc Natl Acad Sci U S A. 2011 Jan 4;108(1):397-402. Epub 2010 Dec 20. PMID:21173254

Sarr SO, Perrotey S, Fall I, Ennahar S, Zhao M, Diop YM, Candolfi E, Marchioni E. Icacina senegalensis (Icacinaceae), traditionally used for the treatment of malaria, inhibits in vitro Plasmodium falciparum growth without host cell toxicity. Malar J. 2011 Apr 11;10:85. PMID:21481272

Saslis-Lagoudakis CH, Klitgaard BB, Forest F, Francis L, Savolainen V, Williamson EM, Hawkins JA. The use of phylogeny to interpret cross-cultural patterns in plant use and guide medicinal plant discovery: an example from Pterocarpus (Leguminosae). PLoS One. 2011;6(7):e22275. Epub 2011 Jul 18. PMID:21789247

Sato M, Hori Z, Hirose T, Suzuki N. Immune effect of toxoplasma lysate antigen (TLA) on cattle against Theileria sergenti infection. Nihon Juigaku Zasshi. 1985 Dec;47(6):921-9. PMID:4094277

Sato M, Igarashi I, Saito A, Hirose T, Suzuki N. Protection against Babesia infection in beagles immunized with Toxoplasma lysate antigen. Nihon Juigaku Zasshi. 1990 Feb;52(1):155-8. PMID:2179608

Sauerwein RW, Bijker EM, Richie TL. Empowering malaria vaccination by drug administration. Curr Opin Immunol. 2010 Jun;22(3):367-73. Epub 2010 Apr 29. PMID:20434895

Sauerwein RW, Roestenberg M, Moorthy VS. Experimental human challenge infections can accelerate clinical malaria vaccine development. Nat Rev Immunol. 2011 Jan;11(1):57-64. PMID:21179119

Sawczuk M. [Cattle babesiosis]. [Article in Polish]. Wiad Parazytol. 2007;53(2):73-9. PMID:17912800

Sawer IK, Berry MI, Brown MW, Ford JL. The effect of cryptolepine on the morphology and survival of Escherichia coli, Candida albicans and Saccharomyces cerevisiae. J Appl Bacteriol. 1995 Sep;79(3):314-21. PMID:7592125

Schaarschmidt D, Trächsel M, Achermann R, Hartelt K, Oehme R, Müller W. [Importance of PCR for the diagnostics of canine babesiosis]. [Article in German]. Schweiz Arch Tierheilkd. 2006 Dec;148(12):633-40. PMID:17263080

Schaller JL, Burkland GA, Langhoff PJ. Are various Babesia species a missed cause for hypereosinophilia? A follow-up on the first reported case of imatinib mesylate for idiopathic hypereosinophilia. MedGenMed. 2007 Feb 27;9(1):38. PMID:17435644

Scharf BA, Fricke RF, Baskin SI. Comparison of methemoglobin formers in protection against the toxic effects of cyanide. Gen Pharmacol. 1992 Jan;23(1):19-25. PMID:1592224

Schetters T. Vaccination against canine babesiosis. Trends Parasitol. 2005 Apr;21(4):179-84. PMID:15780840

Schetters T. Vaccine development from a commercial point of view. Vet Parasitol. 1995 Mar;57(1-3):267-75. PMID:7597789

Schetters TH, Kleuskens J, Scholtes N, Bos HJ. Strain variation limits protective activity of vaccines based on soluble Babesia canis antigens. Parasite Immunol. 1995 Apr;17(4):215-8. PMID:7542765

Schetters TP, Eling WM. Can Babesia infections be used as a model for cerebral malaria? Parasitol Today. 1999 Dec;15(12):492-7. PMID:10557150

Schetters TP, Kleuskens J, Carcy B, Gorenflot A, Vermeulen A. Vaccination against large Babesia species from dogs. Parassitologia. 2007 May;49 Suppl 1:13-7. PMID:17691601

Schetters TP, Kleuskens J, Scholtes N, Bos HJ. Vaccination of dogs against Babesia canis infection using parasite antigens from in vitro culture. Parasite Immunol. 1992 May;14(3):295-305. PMID:1625906

Schetters TP, Kleuskens J, Scholtes N, Gorenflot A. Parasite localization and dissemination in the Babesia-infected host. Ann Trop Med Parasitol. 1998 Jun;92(4):513-9. PMID:9683902

Schetters TP, Kleuskens JA, Scholtes NC, Gorenflot A, Moubri K, Vermeulen AN. Vaccination of dogs against heterologous Babesia canis infection using antigens from culture supernatants. Vet Parasitol. 2001 Sep 12;100(1-2):75-86. PMID:11522408

Schetters TP, Kleuskens JA, Scholtes NC, Pasman JW, Bos HJ. Vaccination of dogs against Babesia canis infection using antigens from culture supernatants with emphasis on clinical babesiosis. Vet Parasitol. 1994 Apr;52(3-4):219-33. PMID:8073606

Schetters TP, Kleuskens JA, Scholtes NC, Pasman JW, Goovaerts D. Vaccination of dogs against Babesia canis infection. Vet Parasitol. 1997 Dec 15;73(1-2):35-41. PMID:9477490

Schetters TP, Kleuskens JA, Scholtes NC, van de Crommert J, Krijnen E, Moubri K, Gorenflot A, Vermeulen AN. Onset and duration of immunity against Babesia canis infection in dogs vaccinated with antigens from culture supernatants. Vet Parasitol. 2006 May 31;138(1-2):140-6. Epub 2006 Feb 28. PMID:16504401

Schetters TP, Moubri K, Cooke BM. Comparison of Babesia rossi and Babesia canis isolates with emphasis on effects of vaccination with soluble parasite antigens: a review. J S Afr Vet Assoc. 2009 Jun;80(2):75-8. PMID:19831266

Schetters TP, Moubri K, Précigout E, Kleuskens J, Scholtes NC, Gorenflot A. Different Babesia canis isolates, different diseases. Parasitology. 1997 Nov;115 (Pt 5):485-93. PMID:9368899

Schetters TP, Scholtes NC, Kleuskens JA, Bos HJ. Not peripheral parasitaemia but the level of soluble parasite antigen in plasma correlates with vaccine efficacy against Babesia canis. Parasite Immunol. 1996 Jan;18(1):1-6. PMID:9223150

Schetters TP, Strydom T, Crafford D, Kleuskens JA, van de Crommert J, Vermeulen AN. Immunity against Babesia rossi infection in dogs vaccinated with antigens from culture supernatants. Vet Parasitol. 2007 Mar 15;144(1-2):10-9. Epub 2006 Oct 23. PMID:17056181

Schindler R, Wokatsch R, Schröder G. [Immunity and serological reactions against Babesia canis in dogs after infection with living parasites and after immunization with a soluble antigen].[Article in German]. Z Tropenmed Parasitol. 1966 Jul;17(2):226-40. PMID:4969377

Schlitzer M. [New malaria drugs: screening against the entire parasite or target-based – which is the right path?].[Article in German]. Pharm Unserer Zeit. 2011 May;40(3):190-1. PMID:21698606

Schmidt M, Sun H, Rogne P, Scriba GK, Griesinger C, Kuhn LT, Reinscheid UM. Determining the absolute configuration of (+)-mefloquine HCl, the side effect reducing enantiomer of the antimalaria drug Lariam. J Am Chem Soc. 2011 Dec 7. [Epub ahead of print]. PMID:22148194

Schoeler GB, Manweiler SA, Wikel SK. Ixodes scapularis: effects of repeated infestations with pathogen-free nymphs on macrophage and T lymphocyte cytokine responses of BALB/c and C3H/HeN mice. Exp Parasitol. 1999 Aug;92(4):239-48. PMID:10425152

Schoeman JP, Herrtage ME. Adrenal response to the low dose ACTH stimulation test and the cortisol-to-adrenocorticotrophic hormone ratio in canine babesiosis. Vet Parasitol. 2008 Jul 4;154(3-4):205-13. Epub 2008 Apr 7. PMID:18468798

Schoeman JP, Herrtage ME. The response of the pituitary-adrenal and pituitary-thyroidal axes to the plasma glucose perturbations in Babesia canis rossi babesiosis. J S Afr Vet Assoc. 2007 Dec;78(4):215-20. PMID:18507221

Schoeman JP, Rees P, Herrtage ME. Endocrine predictors of mortality in canine babesiosis caused by Babesia canis rossi. Vet Parasitol. 2007 Sep 1;148(2):75-82. Epub 2007 Jul 5. PMID:17614201

Schoeman JP. Canine babesiosis. Onderstepoort J Vet Res. 2009 Mar;76(1):59-66. PMID:19967929

Schoepflin S, Marfurt J, Goroti M, Baisor M, Mueller I, Felger I. Heterogeneous distribution of Plasmodium falciparum drug resistance haplotypes in subsets of the host population. Malar J. 2008 May 6;7:78. PMID:18460212

Schreiber A, Härter G, Schubert A, Bunjes D, Mertens T, Michel D. Antiviral treatment of cytomegalovirus infection and resistant strains. Expert Opin Pharmacother. 2009 Feb;10(2):191-209. PMID:19236193

Schrével J, Millerioux V, Sinou V, Frappier F, Santus R, Grellier P. New trends in chemotherapy on human and animal blood parasites. Parasitol Res. 1996;82(3):283-4. PMID:8801568

Schuck DC, Ribeiro RY, Nery AA, Ulrich H, Garcia CR. Flow cytometry as a tool for analyzing changes in Plasmodium falciparum cell cycle following treatment with indol compounds. Cytometry A. 2011 Nov;79(11):959-64. Epub 2011 Aug 30. PMID:22015733

Schwenk RJ, Richie TL. Protective immunity to pre-erythrocytic stage malaria. Trends Parasitol. 2011 Jul;27(7):306-14. Epub 2011 Mar 23. PMID:21435951

Schwint ON, Ueti MW, Palmer GH, Kappmeyer LS, Hines MT, Cordes RT, Knowles DP, Scoles GA. Imidocarb dipropionate clears persistent Babesia caballi infection with elimination of transmission potential. Antimicrob Agents Chemother. 2009 Oct;53(10):4327-32. Epub 2009 Jul 20. PMID:19620328

Seale A, Bains A, Avrett S. Partnership, sex, and marginalization: Moving the Global Fund sexual orientation and gender identities agenda. Health Hum Rights. 2010 Jun 15;12(1):123-35. PMID:20930259

Seboxa T, Mao P, Pinchouk N, Anbessie J, Alemu H, Diro E. Artemether-Lumefantrin (Coartem) and artesunate with sulfadoxine-pyrimethamine therapeutic efficacy in the treatment of uncomplicated malaria at Gilgel Gibe II (GGII) South-Western Ethiopia. Ethiop Med J. 2010 Oct;48(4):285-91. PMID:21280430

Sedaghat MM, Dehkordi AS, Khanavi M, Abai MR, Mohtarami F, Vatandoost H. Chemical composition and larvicidal activity of essential oil of Cupressus arizonica E.L. Greene against malaria vector Anopheles stephensi Liston (Diptera: Culicidae). Pharmacognosy Res. 2011 Apr;3(2):135-9. PMID:21772758

Seinen W, Stegmann T, Kuil H. Complement does not play a role in promoting Babesia rodhaini infections in Balb/C mice. Z Parasitenkd. 1982;68(3):249-57. PMID:6218704

Sellers EL, Ross DA, Green AD. Improvements in compliance with medical force protection measures by simplification of the anti-malarial chemoprophylaxis regime. J R Army Med Corps. 2011 Jun;157(2):156-9. PMID:21805765

Semel ME, Tavakkolizadeh A, Gates JD. Babesiosis in the immediate postoperative period after splenectomy for trauma. Surg Infect (Larchmt). 2009 Dec;10(6):553-6. PMID:19622029

Sengaloundeth S, Green MD, Fernández FM, Manolin O, Phommavong K, Insixiengmay V, Hampton CY, Nyadong L, Mildenhall DC, Hostetler D, Khounsaknalath L, Vongsack L, Phompida S, Vanisaveth V, Syhakhang L, Newton PN. A stratified random survey of the proportion of poor quality oral artesunate sold at medicine outlets in the Lao PDR - implications for therapeutic failure and drug resistance. Malar J. 2009 Jul 28;8:172. PMID:19638225

Senthil Nathan S. The use of Eucalyptus tereticornis Sm. (Myrtaceae) oil (leaf extract) as a natural larvicidal agent against the malaria vector Anopheles stephensi Liston (Diptera: Culicidae). Bioresour Technol. 2007 Jul;98(9):1856-60. Epub 2006 Sep 25. PMID:16997545

Serghides L. The Case for the Use of PPARγ Agonists as an Adjunctive Therapy for Cerebral Malaria. PPAR Res. 2012;2012:513865. Epub 2011 Jun 9. PMID:21772838

Serghides L, Kim H, Lu Z, Kain DC, Miller C, Francis RC, Liles WC, Zapol WM, Kain KC. Inhaled nitric oxide reduces endothelial activation and parasite accumulation in the brain, and enhances survival in experimental cerebral malaria. PLoS One. 2011;6(11):e27714. Epub 2011 Nov 16. PMID:22110737

Sergiev VP, Litvinov SK. [Russian experience with international health cooperation at early stages of its development].[Article in Russian]. Vestn Ross Akad Med Nauk. 2010;(11):11-5. PMID:21309153

Sertel S, Eichhorn T, Sieber S, Sauer A, Weiss J, Plinkert PK, Efferth T. Factors determining sensitivity or resistance of tumor cell lines towards artesunate. Chem Biol Interact. 2010 Apr 15;185(1):42-52. Epub 2010 Feb 6. PMID:20144594

Sertel S, Eichhorn T, Simon CH, Plinkert PK, Johnson SW, Efferth T. Pharmacogenomic identification of c-Myc/Max-regulated genes associated with cytotoxicity of artesunate towards human colon, ovarian and lung cancer cell lines. Molecules. 2010 Apr 22;15(4):2886-910. PMID:20428086

Seshadri P, Dev AV, Viggeswarpu S, Sathyendra S, Peter JV. Acute pancreatitis and subdural haematoma in a patient with severe falciparum malaria: case report and review of literature. Malar J. 2008 May 30;7:97. PMID:18510778

Sethi S, Alcid D, Kesarwala H, Tolan RW Jr. Probable congenital babesiosis in infant, new jersey, USA. Emerg Infect Dis. 2009 May;15(5):788-91. PMID:19402971

Setty S, Khalil Z, Schori P, Azar M, Ferrieri P. Babesiosis. Two atypical cases from Minnesota and a review. Am J Clin Pathol. 2003 Oct;120(4):554-9. PMID:14560566

Sevene E, González R, Menéndez C. Current knowledge and challenges of antimalarial drugs for treatment and prevention in pregnancy. Expert Opin Pharmacother. 2010 Jun;11(8):1277-93. PMID:20408744

Sevinc F, Turgut K, Sevinc M, Ekici OD, Coskun A, Koc Y, Erol M, Ica A. Therapeutic and prophylactic efficacy of imidocarb dipropionate on experimental Babesia ovis infection of lambs. Vet Parasitol. 2007 Oct 21;149(1-2):65-71. Epub 2007 Aug 20. PMID:17709209

Shah F, Mukherjee P, Desai P, Avery M. Computational approaches for the discovery of cysteine protease inhibitors against malaria and SARS. Curr Comput Aided Drug Des. 2010 Mar;6(1):1-23. PMID:20370692

Shah M, Kariuki S, Vanden Eng J, Blackstock AJ, Garner K, Gatei W, Gimnig JE, Lindblade K, Terlouw D, Ter Kuile F, Hawley WA, Phillips-Howard P, Nahlen B, Walker E, Hamel MJ, Slutsker L, Shi YP. Effect of Transmission Reduction by Insecticide-Treated Bednets (ITNs) on Antimalarial Drug Resistance in Western Kenya. PLoS One. 2011;6(11):e26746. Epub 2011 Nov 11. PMID:22096496

Shah NK, Alker AP, Sem R, Susanti AI, Muth S, Maguire JD, Duong S, Ariey F, Meshnick SR, Wongsrichanalai C. Molecular surveillance for multidrug-resistant Plasmodium falciparum, Cambodia. Emerg Infect Dis. 2008 Oct;14(10):1637-40. PMID:18826834

Shah NK, Dhillon GP, Dash AP, Arora U, Meshnick SR, Valecha N. Antimalarial drug resistance of Plasmodium falciparum in India: changes over time and space. Lancet Infect Dis. 2011 Jan;11(1):57-64. PMID:21183147

Shaio MF, Yang KD. Response of babesiosis to a combined regimen of quinine and azithromycin. Trans R Soc Trop Med Hyg. 1997 Mar-Apr;91(2):214-5. PMID:9196774

Shanks GD, Edstein MD. Modern malaria chemoprophylaxis. Drugs. 2005;65(15):2091-110. PMID:16225366

Shanks GD, Kain KC, Keystone JS. Malaria chemoprophylaxis in the age of drug resistance. II. Drugs that may be available in the future. Clin Infect Dis. 2001 Aug 1;33(3):381-5. Epub 2001 Jul 5. PMID:11438908

Shanks GD, Oloo AJ, Aleman GM, Ohrt C, Klotz FW, Braitman D, Horton J, Brueckner R. A new primaquine analogue, tafenoquine (WR 238605), for prophylaxis against Plasmodium falciparum malaria. Clin Infect Dis. 2001 Dec 15;33(12):1968-74. Epub 2001 Nov 7. PMID:11700577

Shapira MY, Resnick IB, Chou S, Neumann AU, Lurain NS, Stamminger T, Caplan O, Saleh N, Efferth T, Marschall M, Wolf DG. Artesunate as a potent antiviral agent in a patient with late drug-resistant cytomegalovirus infection after hematopoietic stem cell transplantation. Clin Infect Dis. 2008 May 1;46(9):1455-7. PMID:18419454

Sharma SK, Jalees S, Kumar K, Rahman SJ. Knowledge, attitude and beliefs about malaria in a tribal area of Bastar district (Madhya Pradesh). Indian J Public Health. 1993 Oct-Dec;37(4):129-32. PMID:8077001

Sharma SP, Bansal GC. Chemoprophylaxis with diminazene aceturate in experimental Babesia bigemina infection in cattle. Res Vet Sci. 1984 Jul;37(1):126-7. PMID:6473911

Sharma VP. Battling the malaria iceberg with chloroquine in India. Malar J. 2007 Aug 7;6:105. PMID:17683630

Shehory-Rubin Z. [Dr. Sarah Ben Ami Solodar: a pioneer in the fight against malaria in the moshavot in the Upper Galilee].[Article in Hebrew]. Harefuah. 2010 Sep;149(9):609-13, 618. PMID:21302479

Shepard CC, Walker LL, Van Landingham M, Redus MA. Kinetic testing of drugs against Mycobacterium leprae in mice. Activity of cephaloridine, rifampin, streptovaricin, vadrine, and viomycin. Am J Trop Med Hyg. 1971 Jul;20(4):616-20. PMID:4398128

Sherr VT. Human babesiosis--an unrecorded reality. Absence of formal registry undermines its detection, diagnosis and treatment, suggesting need for immediate mandatory reporting. Med Hypotheses. 2004;63(4):609-15. PMID:15325004

Shewchuk T, O'Connell KA, Goodman C, Hanson K, Chapman S, Chavasse D. The ACTwatch project: methods to describe anti-malarial markets in seven countries. Malar J. 2011 Oct 31;10:325. PMID:22039780

Shiff C, Thuma P, Sullivan D, Mharakurwa S. Designing a sustainable strategy for malaria control? Malar J. 2011 Aug 3;10:220. PMID:21812949

Shih CM, Wang CC. Ability of azithromycin in combination with quinine for the elimination of babesial infection in humans. Am J Trop Med Hyg. 1998 Oct;59(4):509-12. PMID:9790419

Shimada T, Shikano S, Hashiguchi R, Matsuki N, Ono K. Effects of depletion of T cell subpopulations on the course of infection and anti-parasite delayed type hypersensitivity response in mice infected with Babesia microti and Babesia rodhaini. J Vet Med Sci. 1996 Apr;58(4):343-7. PMID:8741267

Shipitcina NK. [Main results of the study of malaria vectors and development of control measures for them in the Soviet Union for the past 50 years].[Article in Russian]. Med Parazitol (Mosk). 1967 Sep-Oct;36(5):525-32. PMID:4886730

Shiraki H, Kozar MP, Melendez V, Hudson TH, Ohrt C, Magill AJ, Lin AJ. Antimalarial activity of novel 5-aryl-8-aminoquinoline derivatives. J Med Chem. 2011 Jan 13;54(1):131-42. Epub 2010 Dec 8. PMID:21141892

Shittu I, Emmanuel A, Nok AJ. Antimalaria Effect of the Ethanolic Stem Bark Extracts of Ficus platyphylla Del. J Parasitol Res. 2011;2011:618209. Epub 2011 Nov 24. PMID:22174991

Shkap V, de Vos AJ, Zweygarth E, Jongejan F. Attenuated vaccines for tropical theileriosis, babesiosis and heartwater: the continuing necessity. Trends Parasitol. 2007 Sep;23(9):420-6. Epub 2007 Jul 25. PMID:17656155

Shkap V, Leibovitz B, Krigel Y, Hammerschlag J, Marcovics A, Fish L, Molad T, Savitsky I, Mazuz M. Vaccination of older Bos taurus bulls against bovine babesiosis. Vet Parasitol. 2005 May 15;129(3-4):235-42. PMID:15845278

Shkap V, Pipano E, McElwain TF, Herzberg U, Krigel Y, Fish L, Palmer GH. Cross-protective immunity induced by Babesia bovis clones with antigenically unrelated variable merozoite surface antigens. Vet Immunol Immunopathol. 1994 Jun;41(3-4):367-74. PMID:7941314

Shkap V, Rasulov I, Abdurasulov S, Fish L, Leibovitz B, Krigel Y, Molad T, Mazuz ML, Savitsky I. Babesia bigemina: attenuation of an Uzbek isolate for immunization of cattle with live calf- or culture-derived parasites. Vet Parasitol. 2007 May 31;146(3-4):221-6. Epub 2007 Mar 26. PMID:17368728

Shoemaker JP, McAllister RG Jr, Selby JB, Hoffman RV Jr. Effect of hypothyroidism on parasitemia and survival in rodent malaria. Am J Med Sci. 1974 Nov;268(5):281-5. PMID:4617503

Shoemaker JP. Plasmodium berghei: possible role of thyroxine in growth and metabolism. Exp Parasitol. 1974 Oct;36(2):261-4. PMID:4606914

Shoemaker RC, Hudnell HK, House DE, Van Kempen A, Pakes GE; COL40155 Study Team. Atovaquone plus cholestyramine in patients coinfected with Babesia microti and Borrelia burgdorferi refractory to other treatment. Adv Ther. 2006 Jan-Feb;23(1):1-11. PMID:16644602

Shukla RK, Tiwari A. Carbohydrate molecules: an expanding horizon in drug delivery and biomedicine. Crit Rev Ther Drug Carrier Syst. 2011;28(3):255-92. PMID:21663577

Shulman IA, Appleman MD. Transmission of parasitic and bacterial infections through blood transfusion within the U.S. Crit Rev Clin Lab Sci. 1991;28(5-6):447-59. PMID:1772589

Shulman IA. Parasitic infections and their impact on blood donor selection and testing. Arch Pathol Lab Med. 1994 Apr;118(4):366-70. PMID:8166586

Shute PG, Maryon M. Some observations on true latency and long-term relapses in P. vivax malaria. Arch Roum Pathol Exp Microbiol. 1968 Dec;27(4):893-8. PMID:4393171

Sibinovic KH, Milar R, Ristic M, Cox HW. In vivo and in vitro effects of serum antigens of babesial infection and their antibodies on parasitized and normal erythrocytes. Ann Trop Med Parasitol. 1969 Sep;63(3):327-36. PMID:4906995

Sibinovic KH, Sibinovic S, Ristic M, Cox HW. Immunogenic properties of babesial serum antigens. J Parasitol. 1967 Dec;53(6):1121-9. PMID:4169599

Sicuri E, Biao P, Hutton G, Tediosi F, Menendez C, Lell B, Kremsner P, Conteh L, Grobusch MP. Cost-effectiveness of intermittent preventive treatment of malaria in infants (IPTi) for averting anaemia in Gabon: a comparison between intention to treat and according to protocol analyses. Malar J. 2011 Oct 17;10:305. PMID:22004614

Sicuri E, Davy C, Marinelli M, Oa O, Ome M, Siba P, Conteh L, Mueller I. The economic cost to households of childhood malaria in Papua New Guinea: a focus on intra-country variation. Health Policy Plan. 2011 Jun 22. [Epub ahead of print]. PMID:21697246

Sieber S, Gdynia G, Roth W, Bonavida B, Efferth T. Combination treatment of malignant B cells using the anti-CD20 antibody rituximab and the anti-malarial artesunate. Int J Oncol. 2009 Jul;35(1):149-58. PMID:19513562

Sikulu M, Dowell KM, Hugo LE, Wirtz RA, Michel K, Peiris KH, Moore S, Killeen GF, Dowell FE. Evaluating RNAlater® as a preservative for using near-infrared spectroscopy to predict Anopheles gambiae age and species. Malar J. 2011 Jul 8;10:186. PMID:21740582

Silva O, Duarte A, Cabrita J, Pimentel M, Diniz A, Gomes E. Antimicrobial activity of Guinea-Bissau traditional remedies. J Ethnopharmacol. 1996 Jan;50(1):55-9. PMID:8778508

Silver KL, Zhong K, Leke RG, Taylor DW, Kain KC. Dysregulation of angiopoietins is associated with placental malaria and low birth weight. PLoS One. 2010 Mar 1;5(3):e9481. PMID:20208992

Simba DO, Kakoko D, Tomson G, Premji Z, Petzold M, Mahindi M, Gustafsson LL. Adherence to artemether/lumefantrine treatment in children under real-life situations in rural Tanzania. Trans R Soc Trop Med Hyg. 2012 Jan;106(1):3-9. Epub 2011 Nov 17. PMID:22099005

Simonsen KA, Harwell JI, Lainwala S. Clinical presentation and treatment of transfusion-associated babesiosis in premature infants. Pediatrics. 2011 Oct;128(4):e1019-24. Epub 2011 Sep 2. PMID:21890833

Simpson JA, Jamsen KM, Price RN, White NJ, Lindegardh N, Tarning J, Duffull SB. Towards optimal design of anti-malarial pharmacokinetic studies. Malar J. 2009 Aug 6;8:189. PMID:19656413

Simpson KN, Baran RW, Kirbach SE, Dietz B. Economics of Switching to Second-Line Antiretroviral Therapy with Lopinavir/Ritonavir in Africa: Estimates Based on DART Trial Results and Costs for Uganda and Kenya. Value Health. 2011 Dec;14(8):1048-54. Epub 2011 Nov 6. PMID:22152173

Sinclair D, Gogtay N, Brand F, Olliaro P. Artemisinin-based combination therapy for treating uncomplicated Plasmodium vivax malaria. Cochrane Database Syst Rev. 2011 Jul 6;(7):CD008492. PMID:21735431

Singh RK, Dhiman RC, Mittal PK, Dua VK. Susceptibility status of dengue vectors against various insecticides in Koderma (Jharkhand), India. J Vector Borne Dis. 2011 Jun;48(2):116-8. PMID:21715737

Singh Y, Sawyer LS, Pinkoski LS, Dupuis KW, Hsu JC, Lin L, Corash L. Photochemical treatment of plasma with amotosalen and long-wavelength ultraviolet light inactivates pathogens while retaining coagulation function. Transfusion. 2006 Jul;46(7):1168-77. PMID:16836564

Sinou V, Malaika LT, Taudon N, Lwango R, Alegre SS, Bertaux L, Sugnaux F, Parzy D, Benakis A. Pharmacokinetics and pharmacodynamics of a new ACT formulation: Artesunate/Amodiaquine (TRIMALACT) following oral administration in African malaria patients. Eur J Drug Metab Pharmacokinet. 2009 Jul-Sep;34(3-4):133-42. PMID:20166428

Siński E, Welc-Faleciak R, Pogłód R. Babesia spp. infections transmitted through blood transfusion. Wiad Parazytol. 2011;57(2):77-81. PMID:21682090

Sipos W, Schmoll F, Bagó Z, Hobbiger A, Wodak E. [Isoimmune haemolytic icterus in neonatal calves as a consequence of vaccination against piroplasmosis].[Article in German]. Berl Munch Tierarztl Wochenschr. 2002 May-Jun;115(5-6):167-72. PMID:12058589

Siraskar B, Ballal A, Bobbala D, Föller M, Lang F. Effect of amphotericin B on parasitemia and survival of plasmodium berghei-infected mice. Cell Physiol Biochem. 2010;26(3):347-54. Epub 2010 Aug 24. PMID:20798519

Sirima SB, Gansané A. Artesunate-amodiaquine for the treatment of uncomplicated malaria. Expert Opin Investig Drugs. 2007 Jul;16(7):1079-85. PMID:17594191

Sirivichayakul C, Sabchareon A, Pengsaa K, Thaiarporn I, Chaivisuth A, Na-Bangchang K, Wisetsing P, Chanthavanich P, Pojjaroen-Anant C. Comparative study of the effectiveness and pharmacokinetics of two rectal artesunate/oral mefloquine combination regimens for the treatment of uncomplicated childhood falciparum malaria. Ann Trop Paediatr. 2007 Mar;27(1):17-24. PMID:17469728

Siswantoro H, Russell B, Ratcliff A, Prasetyorini B, Chalfein F, Marfurt J, Kenangalem E, Wuwung M, Piera KA, Ebsworth EP, Anstey NM, Tjitra E, Price RN. In vivo and in vitro efficacy of chloroquine against Plasmodium malariae and P. ovale in Papua, Indonesia. Antimicrob Agents Chemother. 2011 Jan;55(1):197-202. Epub 2010 Oct 11. PMID:20937779

Skotarczak B, Cichocka A. Isolation and amplification by polymerase chain reaction DNA of Babesia microti and Babesia divergens in ticks in Poland. Ann Agric Environ Med. 2001;8(2):187-9. PMID:11748876

Skotarczak B, Sawczuk M. [Occurrence of Babesia microti in ticks Ixodes ricinus on selected areas of western Pomerania].[Article in Polish]. Wiad Parazytol. 2003;49(3):273-80. PMID:16889031

Skotarczak B. [Babesiosis of human and domestic dog; ethiology, pathogenesis, diagnostics].[Article in Polish]. Wiad Parazytol. 2007;53(4):271-80. PMID:18441872

Slovut DP, Benedetti E, Matas AJ. Babesiosis and hemophagocytic syndrome in an asplenic renal transplant recipient. Transplantation. 1996 Aug 27;62(4):537-9. PMID:8781622

Small PM. Tuberculosis: a new vision for the 21st century. Kekkaku. 2009 Nov;84(11):721-6. PMID:19999594

Smith LA, Wright-Kanuth MS. Transfusion-transmitted parasites. Clin Lab Sci. 2003 Fall;16(4):239-45, 251. PMID:14626442

Smith N, Obala A, Simiyu C, Menya D, Khwa-Otsyula B, O'Meara WP. Accessibility, availability and affordability of anti-malarials in a rural district in Kenya after implementation of a national subsidy scheme. Malar J. 2011 Oct 26;10:316. PMID:22029829

Smith RD, Carpenter J, Cabrera A, Gravely SM, Erp EE, Osorno M, Ristic M. Bovine babesiosis: vaccination against tick-borne challenge exposure with culture-derived Babesia bovis immunogens. Am J Vet Res. 1979 Dec;40(12):1678-82. PMID:230765

Smith RD, James MA, Ristic M, Aikawa M, Vega y Murguia CA. Bovine babesiosis: protection of cattle with culture-derived soluble Babesia bovis antigen. Science. 1981 Apr 17;212(4492):335-8. PMID:7209532

Smith RD. Babesia bovis: computer simulation of the relationship between the tick vector, parasite, and bovine host. Exp Parasitol. 1983 Aug;56(1):27-40. PMID:6873224

Smith RP, Evans AT, Popovsky M, Mills L, Spielman A. Transfusion-acquired babesiosis and failure of antibiotic treatment. JAMA. 1986 Nov 21;256(19):2726-7. PMID:3773183

Smith TA, Chitnis N, Briët OJ, Tanner M. Uses of mosquito-stage transmission-blocking vaccines against Plasmodium falciparum. Trends Parasitol. 2011 May;27(5):190-6. Epub 2011 Feb 1. PMID:21277257

Snow M. Babesiosis: another tick-borne disease. Nursing. 2009 Jun;39(6):55. PMID:19474614

Snow RW, Okiro EA, Gething PW, Atun R, Hay SI. Equity and adequacy of international donor assistance for global malaria control: an analysis of populations at risk and external funding commitments. Lancet. 2010 Oct 23;376(9750):1409-16. PMID:20889199

Snyder EL, Dodd RY. Reducing the risk of blood transfusion. Hematology Am Soc Hematol Educ Program. 2001:433-42. PMID:11722997

Snyman HW. Malaria symposium--opening address. S Afr Med J. 1974 May 25;48(25):1075-7. PMID:4602109

Sodeman TM, Contacos PG, Collins WE, Smith CS, Jumper JR. Studies on the prophylactic and radical curative activity of RC-12 against Plasmodium cynomolgi in Macaca mulatta. Bull World Health Organ. 1972;47(3):425-8. PMID:4631044

Soerono M, Badawi AS, Muir DA, Soedono A, Siran M. Observations on doubly resistant Anopheles aconitus Dönitz in Java, Indonesia, and on its amenability to treatment with malathion. Bull World Health Organ. 1965;33(4):453-9. PMID:5294991

Soh PN, Witkowski B, Olagnier D, Nicolau ML, Garcia-Alvarez MC, Berry A, Benoit-Vical F. In vitro and in vivo properties of ellagic acid in malaria treatment. Antimicrob Agents Chemother. 2009 Mar;53(3):1100-6. Epub 2008 Nov 17. PMID:19015354

Sokhna C, Cissé B, Bâ el H, Milligan P, Hallett R, Sutherland C, Gaye O, Boulanger D, Simondon K, Simondon F, Targett G, Lines J, Greenwood B, Trape JF. A trial of the efficacy, safety and impact on drug resistance of four drug regimens for seasonal intermittent preventive treatment for malaria in Senegalese children. PLoS One. 2008 Jan 23;3(1):e1471. PMID:18213379

Solano-Gallego L, Baneth G. Babesiosis in dogs and cats--expanding parasitological and clinical spectra. Vet Parasitol. 2011 Sep 8;181(1):48-60. Epub 2011 Apr 19. PMID:21571435

Solari MA, Nari A, Cardozo H. Impact of Babesia bovis and Babesia bigemina on the production of beef cattle in Uruguay. Mem Inst Oswaldo Cruz. 1992;87 Suppl 3:143-9. PMID:1343684

Solomon VR, Lee H. Chloroquine and its analogs: a new promise of an old drug for effective and safe cancer therapies. Eur J Pharmacol. 2009 Dec 25;625(1-3):220-33. Epub 2009 Oct 15. PMID:19836374

Soltys MA. A review of studies on immunization against protozoan diseases of animals. Z Tropenmed Parasitol. 1973 Sep;24(3):309-22. PMID:4598206

Soomro S, Langenberg T, Mahringer A, Konkimalla VB, Horwedel C, Holenya P, Brand A, Cetin C, Fricker G, Dewerchin M, Carmeliet P, Conway EM, Jansen H, Efferth T. Design of novel artemisinin-like derivatives with cytotoxic and anti-angiogenic properties. J Cell Mol Med. 2011 May;15(5):1122-35. Epub 2010 Jul 12. PMID:20629994

Sowunmi A, Akinrinola IA, Gbotosho GO, Okuboyejo TM, Happi CT. A Simple Dose Regimen of Artesunate and Amodiaquine Based on Arm Span- or Age Range for Childhood Falciparum Malaria: A Preliminary Evaluation. J Trop Pediatr. 2011 Nov 3. [Epub ahead of print]. PMID:22052702

Sowunmi A, Gbotosho GO, Happi CT, Fateye BA. Factors contributing to anaemia after uncomplicated Plasmodiumfalciparum malaria in children. Acta Trop. 2010 Feb;113(2):155-61. Epub 2009 Oct 27. PMID:19874795

Spadafora C, Gerena L, Kopydlowski KM. Comparison of the in vitro invasive capabilities of Plasmodium falciparum schizonts isolated by Percoll gradient or using magnetic based separation. Malar J. 2011 Apr 18;10:96. PMID:21501476

Spaete J, Patrozou E, Rich JD, Sweeney JD. Red cell exchange transfusion for babesiosis in Rhode Island. J Clin Apher. 2009;24(3):97-105. PMID:19291782

Specos MM, García JJ, Tornesello J, Marino P, Vecchia MD, Tesoriero MV, Hermida LG. Microencapsulated citronella oil for mosquito repellent finishing of cotton textiles. Trans R Soc Trop Med Hyg. 2010 Oct;104(10):653-8. Epub 2010 Jul 31. PMID:20673937

Speeckaert MM, Speeckaert R, Delanghe JR. Biological and clinical aspects of soluble transferrin receptor. Crit Rev Clin Lab Sci. 2010 Dec;47(5-6):213-28. PMID:21391831

Spicer N, Bogdan D, Brugha R, Harmer A, Murzalieva G, Semigina T. 'It's risky to walk in the city with syringes': understanding access to HIV/AIDS services for injecting drug users in the former Soviet Union countries of Ukraine and Kyrgyzstan. Global Health. 2011 Jul 13;7:22. PMID:21752236

Spry C, van Schalkwyk DA, Strauss E, Saliba KJ. Pantothenate utilization by Plasmodium as a target for antimalarial chemotherapy. Infect Disord Drug Targets. 2010 Jun;10(3):200-16. PMID:20334619

Squires JM, Ferreira JF, Lindsay DS, Zajac AM. Effects of artemisinin and Artemisia extracts on Haemonchus contortus in gerbils (Meriones unguiculatus). Vet Parasitol. 2011 Jan 10;175(1-2):103-8. Epub 2010 Sep 16. PMID:20943323

Sréter T, Kálmán D, Sréterné Lancz Z, Széll Z, Egyed L. [Babesia microti and Anaplasma phagocytophilum: two emerging zoonotic pathogens in Europe and Hungary].[Article in Hungarian]. Orv Hetil. 2005 Mar 27;146(13):595-600. PMID:15856623

Sréter T, Sréterné Lancz Z, Széll Z, Egyed L. [Rickettsia helvetica: an emerging tick-borne pathogen in Hungary and Europe].[Article in Hungarian]. Orv Hetil. 2005 Dec 11;146(50):2547-52. PMID:16440500

Sridaran S, McClintock SK, Syphard LM, Herman KM, Barnwell JW, Udhayakumar V. Anti-folate drug resistance in Africa: meta-analysis of reported dihydrofolate reductase (dhfr) and dihydropteroate synthase (dhps) mutant genotype frequencies in African Plasmodium falciparum parasite populations. Malar J. 2010 Aug 30;9:247. PMID:20799995

Sserugga JN, Jonsson NN, Bock RE, More SJ. Serological evidence of exposure to tick fever organisms in young cattle on Queensland dairy farms. Aust Vet J. 2003 Mar;81(3):147-52. PMID:15080428

Staines HM, Croft SL, Horrocks PD. Developing novel strategies to prevent parasitic infections. Expert Rev Anti Infect Ther. 2011 Jul;9(7):783-5. PMID:21810050

Stańczak J, Myjak P, Bajer A, Siński E, Wedrychowicz H, Majewska AC, Gołab E, Budak A. [Usefulness of the molecular techniques for detecting and/or identifing of parasites and fungi in humans and animals or pathogens transmitted by ticks. Part III].[Article in Polish]. Wiad Parazytol. 2001;47(3):465-75. PMID:16894762

Standfast NF, Bock RE, Wiecek MM, deVos AJ, Jorgensen WK, Kingston TG. Overcoming constraints to meeting increased demand for Babesia bigemina vaccine in Australia. Vet Parasitol. 2003 Jul 29;115(3):213-22. PMID:12935736

Standfast NF, Jorgensen WK. Comparison of the infectivity of Babesia bovis, Babesia bigemina and Anaplasma centrale for cattle after cryopreservation in either dimethylsulphoxide (DMSO) or polyvinylpyrrolidone (PVP). Aust Vet J. 1997 Jan;75(1):62-3. PMID:9034504

Steele JH. Veterinary public health in the United States, 1776 to 1976. J Am Vet Med Assoc. 1976 Jul 1;169(1):74-82. PMID:776913

Stegeman JR, Birkenheuer AJ, Kruger JM, Breitschwerdt EB. Transfusion-associated Babesia gibsoni infection in a dog. J Am Vet Med Assoc. 2003 Apr 1;222(7):959-63, 952. PMID:12685786

Steinhardt LC, Magill AJ, Arguin PM. Review: malaria chemoprophylaxis for travelers to latin america. Am J Trop Med Hyg. 2011 Dec;85(6):1015-24. PMID:22144437

Steinhaus RK, Baskin SI, Clark JH, Kirby SD. Formation of methemoglobin and metmyoglobin using 8-aminoquinoline derivatives or sodium nitrite and subsequent reaction with cyanide. J Appl Toxicol. 1990 Oct;10(5):345-51. PMID:2254586

Steketee RW, Slutsker L. Targeting of intermittent preventive treatment for malaria. Lancet Infect Dis. 2011 Dec 13. [Epub ahead of print]. PMID:22172304

Stell JG, Wheelhouse RT, Wright CW. Metabolism of cryptolepine and 2-fluorocryptolepine by aldehyde oxidase. J Pharm Pharmacol. 2012 Feb;64(2):237-43. Epub 2011 Nov 18. PMID:22221099

Stephens R, Langhorne J. Effector memory Th1 CD4 T cells are maintained in a mouse model of chronic malaria. PLoS Pathog. 2010 Nov 24;6(11):e1001208. PMID:21124875

Stewart NP, de Vos AJ, Shiels I. Elimination of Theileria buffeli infections from cattle by concurrent treatment with primaquine phosphate and halofuginone lactate. Trop Anim Health Prod. 1990 May;22(2):109-15. PMID:2115212

Stowell CP, Gelfand JA, Shepard JA, Kratz A. Case records of the Massachusetts General Hospital. Case 17-2007. A 25-year-old woman with relapsing fevers and recent onset of dyspnea. N Engl J Med. 2007 May 31;356(22):2313-9. PMID:17538091

Stramer SL, Hollinger FB, Katz LM, Kleinman S, Metzel PS, Gregory KR, Dodd RY. Emerging infectious disease agents and their potential threat to transfusion safety. Transfusion. 2009 Aug;49 Suppl 2:1S-29S. PMID:19686562

Stresman GH. Beyond temperature and precipitation: ecological risk factors that modify malaria transmission. Acta Trop. 2010 Dec;116(3):167-72. Epub 2010 Aug 17. PMID:20727338

Stricker RB, Johnson L. Lyme disease: the next decade. Infect Drug Resist. 2011;4:1-9. Epub 2011 Jan 7. PMID:21694904

Stricker RB, Lautin A, Burrascano JJ. Lyme disease: point/counterpoint. Expert Rev Anti Infect Ther. 2005 Apr;3(2):155-65. PMID:15918774

Stricker RB, Lautin A, Burrascano JJ. Lyme disease: the quest for magic bullets. Chemotherapy. 2006;52(2):53-9. Epub 2006 Feb 22. PMID:16498239.

Stricker RB. Counterpoint: long-term antibiotic therapy improves persistent symptoms associated with lyme disease. Clin Infect Dis. 2007 Jul 15;45(2):149-57. Epub 2007 Jun 5. PMID:17578772

Suarez CE, McElwain TF. Transfection systems for Babesia bovis: a review of methods for the transient and stable expression of exogenous genes. Vet Parasitol. 2010 Feb 10;167(2-4):205-15. Epub 2009 Sep 19. PMID:19819628

Suarez CE, Noh S. Emerging perspectives in the research of bovine babesiosis and anaplasmosis. Vet Parasitol. 2011 Aug 4;180(1-2):109-25. Epub 2011 May 27. PMID:21684084

Suarez-Mutis MC, de Souza PP, Freitas LF, Miranda ES, Campos MR, Osorio-de-Castro CG. Pharmaceutical services for endemic situations in the Brazilian Amazon: organization of services and prescribing practices for Plasmodium vivax and Plasmodium falciparum non-complicated malaria in high-risk municipalities. . Malar J. 2011 Nov 3;10(1):335. [Epub ahead of print]. PMID:22050832

Subeki, Matsuura H, Yamasaki M, Yamato O, Maede Y, Katakura K, Suzuki M, Trimurningsih, Chairul, Yoshihara T. Effects of Central Kalimantan plant extracts on intraerythrocytic Babesia gibsoni in culture. J Vet Med Sci. 2004 Jul;66(7):871-4. PMID:15297762

Subeki, Nomura S, Matsuura H, Yamasaki M, Yamato O, Maede Y, Katakura K, Suzuki M, Trimurningsih, Chairul, Yoshihara T. Anti-babesial activity of some central kalimantan plant extracts and active oligostilbenoids from Shorea balangeran. Planta Med. 2005 May;71(5):420-3. PMID:15931579

Sudomo M, Arianti Y, Wahid I, Safruddin D, Pedersen EM, Charlwood JD. Towards eradication: three years after the tsunami of 2004, has malaria transmission been eliminated from the island of Simeulue? Trans R Soc Trop Med Hyg. 2010 Dec;104(12):777-81. Epub 2010 Oct 16. PMID:20952042

Sun T, Tenenbaum MJ, Greenspan J, Teichberg S, Wang RT, Degnan T, Kaplan MH. Morphologic and clinical observations in human infection with Babesia microti. J Infect Dis. 1983 Aug;148(2):239-48. PMID:6684141

Sundaram GS, Venkatesh C, Syam Kumar UK, Ila H, Junjappa H. A concise formal synthesis of alkaloid cryptotackiene and substituted 6H-indolo[2,3-b]quinolines. J Org Chem. 2004 Aug 20;69(17):5760-2. PMID:15307753

Sutherland CJ, Babiker H, Mackinnon MJ, Ranford-Cartwright L, El Sayed BB. Rational deployment of antimalarial drugs in Africa: should first-line combination drugs be reserved for paediatric malaria cases? Parasitology. 2011 Oct;138(12):1459-68. Epub 2011 Aug 3. PMID:21810298

Suwanarusk R, Chavchich M, Russell B, Jaidee A, Chalfein F, Barends M, Prasetyorini B, Kenangalem E, Piera KA, Lek-Uthai U, Anstey NM, Tjitra E, Nosten F, Cheng Q, Price RN. Amplification of pvmdr1 associated with multidrug-resistant Plasmodium vivax. J Infect Dis. 2008 Nov 15;198(10):1558-64. PMID:18808339

Suwandittakul N, Chaijaroenkul W, Harnyuttanakorn P, Mungthin M, Na Bangchang K. Drug resistance and in vitro susceptibility of Plasmodium falciparum in Thailand during 1988-2003. Korean J Parasitol. 2009 Jun;47(2):139-44. Epub 2009 May 27. PMID:19488420

Suzuki K, Wakabayashi H, Takahashi M, Fukushima K, Yabuki A, Endo Y. A Possible treatment strategy and clinical factors to estimate the treatment response in Bebesia gibsoni infection. J Vet Med Sci. 2007 May;69(5):563-8. PMID:17551236

Swai ES, French NP, Beauchamp G, Fitzpatrick JL, Bryant MJ, Kambarage D, Ogden NH. A longitudinal study of sero-conversion to tick-borne pathogens in smallholder dairy youngstock in Tanzania. Vet Parasitol. 2005 Jul 15;131(1-2):129-37. PMID:15936149

Swampillai AL, Salomoni P, Short SC. The Role of Autophagy in Clinical Practice. Clin Oncol (R Coll Radiol). 2011 Oct 26. [Epub ahead of print]. PMID:22032864

Sykes A, Hendriksen I, Mtove G, Mandea V, Mrema H, Rutta B, Mapunda E, Manjurano A, Amos B, Reyburn H, Whitty CJ. Azithromycin plus artesunate versus artemether-lumefantrine for treatment of uncomplicated malaria in Tanzanian children: a randomized, controlled trial. Clin Infect Dis. 2009 Oct 15;49(8):1195-201. PMID:19769536

Taboada J, Merchant SR. Babesiosis of companion animals and man. Vet Clin North Am Small Anim Pract. 1991 Jan;21(1):103-23. PMID:2014615

Tachibana M, Wu Y, Iriko H, Muratova O, MacDonald NJ, Sattabongkot J, Takeo S, Otsuki H, Torii M, Tsuboi T. N-terminal prodomain of Pfs230 synthesized using a cell-free system is sufficient to induce complement-dependent malaria transmission-blocking activity. Clin Vaccine Immunol. 2011 Aug;18(8):1343-50. Epub 2011 Jun 29. PMID:21715579

Tagbor H, Bruce J, Agbo M, Greenwood B, Chandramohan D. Intermittent screening and treatment versus intermittent preventive treatment of malaria in pregnancy: a randomised controlled non-inferiority trial. PLoS One. 2010 Dec 28;5(12):e14425. PMID:21203389

Tagliaferri L, Prunotto G, Hakizimana J, Rios WP, Pelucchi C, Principi N, Esposito S. Knowledge of Malaria Among Women of Burundi and its Impact on the Incidence of the Disease. J Trop Pediatr. 2011 Oct 11. [Epub ahead of print]. PMID:21990107

Tahar R, Vivas L, Basco L, Thompson E, Ibrahim H, Boyer J, Nepveu F. Indolone-N-oxide derivatives: in vitro activity against fresh clinical isolates of Plasmodium falciparum, stage specificity and in vitro interactions with established antimalarial drugs. J Antimicrob Chemother. 2011 Nov;66(11):2566-72. Epub 2011 Aug 22. PMID:21862474

Taiwo B, Lee C, Venkat D, Tambar S, Sutton SH. Can tumor necrosis factor alpha blockade predispose to severe babesiosis? Arthritis Rheum. 2007 Feb 15;57(1):179-81. PMID:17266091

Tajima T, Zhi N, Lin Q, Rikihisa Y, Horowitz HW, Ralfalli J, Wormser GP, Hechemy KE. Comparison of two recombinant major outer membrane proteins of the human granulocytic ehrlichiosis agent for use in an enzyme-linked immunosorbent assay. Clin Diagn Lab Immunol. 2000 Jul;7(4):652-7. PMID:10882667

Takabatake N, Okamura M, Yokoyama N, Okubo K, Ikehara Y, Igarashi I. Involvement of a host erythrocyte sialic acid content in Babesia bovis infection. J Vet Med Sci. 2007 Oct;69(10):999-1004. PMID:17984585

Takahashi M, Omata Y, Oikawa H, Claveria F, Igarashi I, Saito A, Suzuki N. Protective immune response of Isospora felis-infected mice against Babesia microti infection. J Vet Med Sci. 1993 Aug;55(4):587-90. PMID:8399737

Takala SL, Coulibaly D, Thera MA, Batchelor AH, Cummings MP, Escalante AA, Ouattara A, Traoré K, Niangaly A, Djimdé AA, Doumbo OK, Plowe CV. Extreme polymorphism in a vaccine antigen and risk of clinical malaria: implications for vaccine development. Sci Transl Med. 2009 Oct 14;1(2):2ra5. PMID:20165550

Talour K, Karam A, Dreux N, Lemasson G, Gilbert D, Abasq C, Misery L. Incipiens linear IgA disease with IgA antibodies directed against 200-kDa epidermal antigens. Eur J Dermatol. 2011 May-Jun;21(3):411-2. PMID:21515442

Tambrallo LJ, Buening GM, McLaughlin RM. The effect of neutrophils, tumor necrosis factor, and granulocyte macrophage/colony stimulating factor on Babesia bovis and Babesia bigemina in culture. Vet Parasitol. 1992 Jul;43(3-4):177-88. PMID:1413450

Tammemagi L. Iron-dextran in the treatment of anaemia associated with bovine babesiosis. Aust Vet J. 1966 Jul;42(7):260-1. PMID:4961184

Tan TM, Goh KL, Binh LN, Ting RC, Kara UA. Identification of a Plasmodium berghei antigen sharing common features with P. falciparum and P. chabaudi parasitophorous-vacuole membrane antigens. Parasitol Res. 1996;82(2):130-35. PMID:8825207

Tanne JH. Trial shows vaccine halves malaria episodes in children in Africa. BMJ. 2011 Oct 20;343:d6832. PMID:22016456

Tapas S, Kumar A, Dhindwal S, Preeti, Kumar P. Structural analysis of chorismate synthase from Plasmodium falciparum: a novel target for antimalaria drug discovery. Int J Biol Macromol. 2011 Nov 1;49(4):767-77. Epub 2011 Jul 27. PMID:21801743

Taraskina LA. [The development of public health in the Democratic Republic of Vietnam].[Article in Russian]. Sov Zdravookhr. 1968;27(3):80-2. PMID:5675744

Tarello W. Cutaneous lesions in dogs with Dirofilaria (Nochtiella) repens infestation and concurrent tick-borne transmitted diseases. Vet Dermatol. 2002 Oct;13(5):267-74. PMID:12358611

Tarello W. Dermatitis associated with Dirofilaria (Nochtiella) repens microfilariae in dogs from central Italy. Acta Vet Hung. 2002;50(1):63-78. PMID:12061238

Tarello W. Dermatitis associated with Dirofilaria repens microfilariae in three dogs in Saudi Arabia. J Small Anim Pract. 2003 Mar;44(3):132-4. PMID:12653329

Tarello W. Effective imidocarb dipropionate therapy for Babesia shortti in falcons. Vet Rec. 2006 Feb 18;158(7):239-40. PMID:16489163

Targett G. Malaria elimination: how far can we go without a vaccine? Clin Med. 2011 Oct;11(5):422-3. PMID:22034696

Tatem AJ, Smith DL. International population movements and regional Plasmodium falciparum malaria elimination strategies. Proc Natl Acad Sci U S A. 2010 Jul 6;107(27):12222-7. Epub 2010 Jun 21. PMID:20566870

Taylor CA, Moreira C, Murray MJ. A retrospective study of malaria in pediatric oncology patients in Senegal. J Pediatr Hematol Oncol. 2011 Jul;33(5):325-9. PMID:21694554

Taylor DA. Profile: Ogobara Doumbo. Mali researcher shows how to reverse brain drain. Science. 2011 Jun 24;332(6037):1498-9. PMID:21700851

Taylor RJ, McHardy N. Preliminary observations on the combined use of imidocarb and Babesia blood vaccine in cattle. J S Afr Vet Assoc. 1979 Dec;50(4):326-9. PMID:553972

Taylor SM, Elliott CT, Kenny J. Babesia divergens: sequential exposure to heterologous tick-borne challenge of cattle immunized with a fraction of parasitized erythrocytes. J Comp Pathol. 1986 Jan;96(1):101-7. PMID:3944282

Taylor SM, Elliott CT, Kenny J. Inhibition of Babesia divergens in cattle by oxytetracycline. Vet Rec. 1986 Jan 25;118(4):98-102. PMID:3952967

Taylor SM, Elliott CT, Kenny J. Isolation of antigenic proteins from erythrocytes parasitised with Babesia divergens and a comparison of their immunising potential. Vet Parasitol. 1986 Jun;21(2):99-105. PMID:3739209

Taylor SM, Kenny J, Mallon T, Elliott CT. The immunization of cattle against Babesia divergens with fractions of parasitized erythrocytes. Vet Parasitol. 1984 Nov;16(3-4):235-42. PMID:6542721

Taylor SM, Kenny J, Mallon T. The effect of route of administration of a Babesia divergens inactivated vaccine on protection against homologous challenge. J Comp Pathol. 1983 Jul;93(3):423-8. PMID:6886086

Taylor SM, Kenny J, Purnell RE, Lewis D. Exposure of cattle immunised against redwater to tick challenge in the field: challenge by a homologous strain of B divergens. Vet Rec. 1980 Feb 23;106(8):167-70. PMID:7361409

Taylor SM, Kenny J, Purnell RE, Lewis D. Exposure of cattle immunised against redwater to tick-induced challenge in the field: challenge by a heterologous strain of Babesia divergens. Vet Rec. 1980 Apr 26;106(17):385-7. PMID:7434497

Taylor SM, van Eijk AM, Hand CC, Mwandagalirwa K, Messina JP, Tshefu AK, Atua B, Emch M, Muwonga J, Meshnick SR, Ter Kuile FO. Quantification of the burden and consequences of pregnancy-associated malaria in the Democratic Republic of the Congo. J Infect Dis. 2011 Dec;204(11):1762-71. Epub 2011 Oct 11. PMID:21990422

Taylor WM, Simpson CF, Martin FG. Certain aspects of toxicity of an amicarbalide formulation to ponies. Am J Vet Res. 1972 Mar;33(3):533-41. PMID:5014461

Tchoumbougnang F, Zollo PH, Dagne E, Mekonnen Y. In vivo antimalarial activity of essential oils from Cymbopogon citratus and Ocimum gratissimum on mice infected with Plasmodium berghei. Planta Med. 2005 Jan;71(1):20-3. PMID:15678368

Tekete MM, Toure S, Fredericks A, Beavogui AH, Sangare CP, Evans A, Smith P, Maiga H, Traore ZI, Doumbo OK, Barnes KI, Djimde AA. Effects of amodiaquine and artesunate on sulphadoxine-pyrimethamine pharmacokinetic parameters in children under five in Mali. Malar J. 2011 Sep 21;10:275. PMID:21936885

Tekwani BL, Walker LA. 8-Aminoquinolines: future role as antiprotozoal drugs. Curr Opin Infect Dis. 2006 Dec;19(6):623-31. PMID:17075340

Tempesta MS. The clinical efficacy of cryptolepis sanguinolenta in the treatment of malaria. Ghana Med J. 2010 Mar;44(1):1-2. PMID:21326982

ten Hagen TL, Sulzer AJ, Kidd MR, Lal AA, Hunter RL. Role of adjuvants in the modulation of antibody isotype, specificity, and induction of protection by whole blood-stage Plasmodium yoelii vaccines. J Immunol. 1993 Dec 15;151(12):7077-85. PMID:8258712

Tepongning RN, Lucantoni L, Nasuti CC, Dori GU, Yerbanga SR, Lupidi G, Marini C, Rossi G, Esposito F, Habluetzel A. Potential of a Khaya ivorensis -Alstonia boonei extract combination as antimalarial prophylactic remedy. J Ethnopharmacol. 2011 Sep 1;137(1):743-51. Epub 2011 Jun 30. PMID:21742022

Terkawi MA, Aboge G, Jia H, Goo YK, Ooka H, Yamagishi J, Nishikawa Y, Yokoyama N, Igarashi I, Kawazu SI, Fujisaki K, Xuan X. Molecular and immunological characterization of Babesia gibsoni and Babesia microti heat shock protein-70. Parasite Immunol. 2009 Jun;31(6):328-40. PMID:19493212

Terkawi MA, Jia H, Zhou J, Lee EG, Igarashi I, Fujisaki K, Nishikawa Y, Xuan X. Babesia gibsoni ribosomal phosphoprotein P0 induces cross-protective immunity against B. microti infection in mice. Vaccine. 2007 Mar 1;25(11):2027-35. Epub 2006 Dec 8. PMID:17229504

Terkawi MA, Zhang G, Jia H, Aboge G, Goo YK, Nishikawa Y, Yokoyama N, Igarashi I, Kawazu SI, Fujisaki K, Xuan X. C3 contributes to the cross-protective immunity induced by Babesia gibsoni phosphoriboprotein P0 against a lethal B. rodhaini infection. Parasite Immunol. 2008 Jun-Jul;30(6-7):365-70. PMID:18533933

Terry MC, Heames RM. Antimalarial chemoprophylaxis in a deployed Naval Unit. J R Nav Med Serv. 2011;97(2):59-61. PMID:22013637

Terzian LA, Stahler N, Dawkins AT Jr. The sporogonous of Plasmodium vivax in Anopheles mosquitoes as a system for evaluating the prophylactic and curative capabilities of potential antimalarial compounds. Exp Parasitol. 1968 Aug;23(1):56-66. PMID:4876903

Tetzlaff CL, Carlomagno MA, McMurray DN. Reduced dietary protein content suppresses infection with Babesia microti. Med Microbiol Immunol. 1988;177(6):305-15. PMID:3216813

Tetzlaff CL, Rice-Ficht AC, Woods VM, Brown WC. Induction of proliferative responses of T cells from Babesia bovis-immune cattle with a recombinant 77-kilodalton merozoite protein (Bb-1). Infect Immun. 1992 Feb;60(2):644-52. PMID:1730498

Teuscher F, Gatton ML, Chen N, Peters J, Kyle DE, Cheng Q. Artemisinin-induced dormancy in plasmodium falciparum: duration, recovery rates, and implications in treatment failure. J Infect Dis. 2010 Nov 1;202(9):1362-8. PMID:20863228

Tewari AK, Sharma NN, Rao JR, Mishra AK, Das SK. Effect of Mycobacterium phlei on the development of immunity to Babesia bigemina. Vet Parasitol. 1996 Apr;62(3-4):223-30. PMID:8686168

Tewari K, Flynn BJ, Boscardin SB, Kastenmueller K, Salazar AM, Anderson CA, Soundarapandian V, Ahumada A, Keler T, Hoffman SL, Nussenzweig MC, Steinman RM, Seder RA. Poly(I:C) is an effective adjuvant for antibody and multi-functional CD4+ T cell responses to Plasmodium falciparum circumsporozoite protein (CSP) and αDEC-CSP in non human primates. Vaccine. 2010 Oct 21;28(45):7256-66. Epub 2010 Sep 21. PMID:20846528

Thanaketpaisarn O, Waiwut P, Sakurai H, Saiki I. Artesunate enhances TRAIL-induced apoptosis in human cervical carcinoma cells through inhibition of the NF-κB and PI3K/Akt signaling pathways. Int J Oncol. 2011 Jul;39(1):279-85. Epub 2011 Apr 28. PMID:21537836

Thanh NV, Toan TQ, Cowman AF, Casey GJ, Phuc BQ, Tien NT, Hung NM, Biggs BA. Monitoring for Plasmodium falciparum drug resistance to artemisinin and artesunate in Binh Phuoc Province, Vietnam: 1998-2009. Malar J. 2010 Jun 24;9:181. PMID:20573274

Thanh NX, Trung TN, Phong NC, Thien NX, Dai B, Shanks GD, Chavchich M, Edstein MD. Open label randomized comparison of dihydroartemisinin-piperaquine and artesunate-amodiaquine for the treatment of uncomplicated Plasmodium falciparum malaria in central Vietnam. Trop Med Int Health. 2009 May;14(5):504-11. Epub 2009 Mar 19. PMID:19320869

Thelot FL. [HIV/AIDS in South Africa and Haiti: the failure of epidemic governance and achievement of the MDGs].[Article in French]. Sante. 2009 Jul-Sep;19(3):121-32. PMID:20185388

Theron M, Hesketh RL, Subramanian S, Rayner JC. An adaptable two-color flow cytometric assay to quantitate the invasion of erythrocytes by Plasmodium falciparum parasites. Cytometry A. 2010 Nov;77(11):1067-74. PMID:20872885

Thomford JW, Conrad PA, Boyce WM, Holman PJ, Jessup DA. Isolation and in vitro cultivation of Babesia parasites from free-ranging desert bighorn sheep (Ovis canadensis nelsoni) and mule deer (Odocoileus hemionus) in California. J Parasitol. 1993 Feb;79(1):77-84. PMID:8437062

Thompson C, Spielman A, Krause PJ. Coinfecting deer-associated zoonoses: Lyme disease, babesiosis, and ehrlichiosis. Clin Infect Dis. 2001 Sep 1;33(5):676-85. Epub 2001 Aug 6. PMID:11486290

Thompson JH. Gametocytemia in falciparum malaria. JAMA. 1971 Jun 14;216(11):1866. PMID:4931429

Thompson KC, Todorovic RA, Mateus G, Adams LG. Methods to improve the health of cattle in the tropics: immunisation and chemoprophylaxis against haemoparasitic infections. Trop Anim Health Prod. 1978 May;10(2):75-81. PMID:664017

Thomsen TT, Ishengoma DS, Mmbando BP, Lusingu JP, Vestergaard LS, Theander TG, Lemnge MM, Bygbjerg IC, Alifrangis M. Prevalence of Single Nucleotide Polymorphisms in the Plasmodium falciparum Multidrug Resistance Gene (Pfmdr-1) in Korogwe District in Tanzania Before and After Introduction of Artemisinin-Based Combination Therapy. Am J Trop Med Hyg. 2011 Dec;85(6):979-83. PMID:22144430

Thoongsuwan S, Cox HW, Patrick RA. Serologic specificity of immunoconglutinin associated with infectious anemia of rats and its role in nonspecific acquired resistance. J Parasitol. 1978 Dec;64(6):1060-6. PMID:739300

Thoongsuwan S, Cox HW. Antigenic variants of the haemosporidian parasite, Babesia rodhaini, selected by in vitro treatment with immune globulin. Ann Trop Med Parasitol. 1973 Dec;67(4):373-85. PMID:4132544

Thwing JI, Odero CO, Odhiambo FO, Otieno KO, Kariuki S, Ord R, Roper C, McMorrow M, Vulule J, Slutsker L, Newman RD, Hamel MJ, Desai M. In-vivo efficacy of amodiaquine-artesunate in children with uncomplicated Plasmodium falciparum malaria in western Kenya. Trop Med Int Health. 2009 Mar;14(3):294-300. Epub 2009 Jan 28. PMID:19187521

Tian LG, Cheng GJ, Wang FF, Guo J, Cai YC, Wang TP, Chen JX, Zhou XN. [Efficacy of tribendimdine in treatment of hookworm infection]. [Article in Chinese]. Zhongguo Xue Xi Chong Bing Fang Zhi Za Zhi. 2011 Apr;23(2):202-3. PMID:22164629

Tilley L, Dixon MW, Kirk K. The Plasmodium falciparum-infected red blood cell. Int J Biochem Cell Biol. 2011 Jun;43(6):839-42. Epub 2011 Mar 31. PMID:21458590

Timms P, Barry DN, Gill AC, Sharp PJ, de Vos AJ. Failure of a recombinant Babesia bovis antigen to protect cattle against heterologous strain challenge. Res Vet Sci. 1988 Sep;45(2):267-9. PMID:3194602

Timms P, Dalgliesh RJ, Barry DN, Dimmock CK, Rodwell BJ. Babesia bovis: comparison of culture-derived parasites, non-living antigen and conventional vaccine in the protection of cattle against heterologous challenge. Aust Vet J. 1983 Mar;60(3):75-7. PMID:6347164

Timms P, Rodwell BJ, Barry DN. Development of a Babesia rodhaini mouse assay for quality control of the serum component of a bovine babesiosis vaccine. Res Vet Sci. 1983 Nov;35(3):331-3. PMID:6665317

Timms P, Stewart NP, Dalgliesh RJ. Comparison of tick and blood challenge for assessing immunity to Babesia bovis. Aust Vet J. 1983 Aug;60(8):257-9. PMID:6639533

Timms P, Stewart NP. Growth of Babesia bovis parasites in stationary and suspension cultures and their use in experimental vaccination of cattle. Res Vet Sci. 1989 Nov;47(3):309-14. PMID:2595088

Timms P. Development of babesial vaccines. Trans R Soc Trop Med Hyg. 1989;83 Suppl:73-9. PMID:2696164

Timofeev BA, Bolotin IM, Stepanova LP, Bogdanov AA Jr, Georgiu K, Malyshev SN, Petrovsky VV, Klibanov AL, Torchilin VP. Liposomal diamidine (imidocarb): preparation and animal studies. J Microencapsul. 1994 Nov-Dec;11(6):627-32. PMID:7884627

Timofeev BA, Bolotin IM, Stepanova LP, Bogdanov AA, Georgiu Kh, Malyshev SN, Petrovskiĭ, Klibanov AL, Torchilin VP. [A liposomal form of diamidine: reduced toxicity].[Article in Russian]. Antibiot Khimioter. 1991 Sep;36(9):34-6. PMID:1781710

Tine RC, Faye B, Ndour CT, Ndiaye JL, Ndiaye M, Bassene C, Magnussen P, Bygbjerg IC, Sylla K, Ndour JD, Gaye O. Impact of combining intermittent preventive treatment with home management of malaria in children less than 10 years in a rural area of Senegal: a cluster randomized trial. Malar J. 2011 Dec 13;10(1):358. [Epub ahead of print].PMID:22166001

Tinto H, Guekoun L, Zongo I, Guiguemdé RT, D'Alessandro U, Ouédraogo JB. Chloroquine-resistance molecular markers (Pfcrt T76 and Pfmdr-1 Y86) and amodiaquine resistance in Burkina Faso. Trop Med Int Health. 2008 Feb;13(2):238-40. PMID:18304270

Tiono AB, Dicko A, Ndububa DA, Agbenyega T, Pitmang S, Awobusuyi J, Pamba A, Duparc S, Goh LE, Harrell E, Carter N, Ward SA, Greenwood B, Winstanley PA. Chlorproguanil-dapsone-artesunate versus chlorproguanil-dapsone: a randomized, double-blind, phase III trial in African children, adolescents, and adults with uncomplicated Plasmodium falciparum malaria. Am J Trop Med Hyg. 2009 Dec;81(6):969-78. PMID:19996424

Tipke M, Diallo S, Coulibaly B, Störzinger D, Hoppe-Tichy T, Sie A, Müller O. Substandard anti-malarial drugs in Burkina Faso. Malar J. 2008 May 27;7:95. PMID:18505584

Titanji VP, Zofou D, Ngemenya MN. The antimalarial potential of medicinal plants used for the treatment of malaria in Cameroonian folk medicine. Afr J Tradit Complement Altern Med. 2008 Apr 10;5(3):302-21. PMID:20161952

Tiwari S, Ghosh SK, Mittal PK, Dash AP. Effectiveness of a new granular formulation of biolarvicide Bacillus thuringiensis Var. israelensis against larvae of malaria vectors in India. Vector Borne Zoonotic Dis. 2011 Jan;11(1):69-75. Epub 2010 May 22. PMID:20491582

Tjornehoj K, Lawrence JA, Whiteland AP, Kafuwa PT. Field observations on the duration of immunity in cattle after vaccination against Anaplasma and Babesia species. Onderstepoort J Vet Res. 1996 Mar;63(1):1-5. PMID:8848296

Tobler WD Jr, Cotton D, Lepore T, Agarwal S, Mahoney EJ. Case Report: Successful non-operative management of spontaneous splenic rupture in a patient with babesiosis. World J Emerg Surg. 2011 Jan 20;6:4. PMID:21251311

Todorovic R, Gonzalez E, Lopez G. Immunization against anaplasmosis and babesiosis. Part II. Evaluation of cryo-preserved vaccines using different doses and routes of inoculation. Tropenmed Parasitol. 1978 Jun;29(2):210-4. PMID:675843

Todorovic RA, Gonzalez EF, Adams LG. Babesia bigemina, Babesia argentina, and Anaplasma marginale: Coinfectious immunity in bovines. Exp Parasitol. 1975 Apr;37(2):179-92. PMID:1123013

Todorovic RA, Gonzalez EF, Adams LG. Bovine babesiosis: sterile immunity to Babesia bigemina and Babesia argentina infections. Trop Anim Health Prod. 1973 Nov;5(4):234-45. PMID:4807692

Todorovic RA, Gonzalez EF, Garcia O. Immunization against anaplasmosis and babesiosis. Part III. Evaluation of immunization under field conditions in the Cauca River Valley. Tropenmed Parasitol. 1979 Mar;30(1):43-52. PMID:442200.

Todorovic RA, Vizcaino OG, Gonzalez EF, Adams LG. Chemoprophylaxis (Imidocarb) against Babesia bigemina and Babesia argentina infections. Am J Vet Res. 1973 Sep;34(9):1153-61. PMID:4747036

Todorovic RA. Bovine babesiasis: its diagnosis and control. Am J Vet Res. 1974 Aug;35(8):1045-52. PMID:4850812

Toh SQ, Glanfield A, Gobert GN, Jones MK. Heme and blood-feeding parasites: friends or foes? Parasit Vectors. 2010 Nov 18;3:108. PMID:21087517

Tokmalaev AK, Khodzhaeva NM. [Role of cytokines in the clinical course of tropical malaria in children].[Article in Russian]. Med Parazitol (Mosk). 2011 Apr-Jun;(2):28-30. PMID:21797063

Tomillero A, Moral MA. Gateways to clinical trials. Methods Find Exp Clin Pharmacol. 2010 Jun;32(5):331-88. PMID:20664824

Tona L, Kambu K, Ngimbi N, Cimanga K, Vlietinck AJ. Antiamoebic and phytochemical screening of some Congolese medicinal plants. J Ethnopharmacol. 1998 May;61(1):57-65. PMID:9687082

Tona L, Ngimbi NP, Tsakala M, Mesia K, Cimanga K, Apers S, De Bruyne T, Pieters L, Totté J, Vlietinck AJ. Antimalarial activity of 20 crude extracts from nine African medicinal plants used in Kinshasa, Congo. J Ethnopharmacol. 1999 Dec 15;68(1-3):193-203. PMID:10624878

Tonhosolo R, Gabriel HB, Matsumura MY, Cabral FJ, Yamamoto MM, D'Alexandri FL, Sussmann RA, Belmonte R, Peres VJ, Crick DC, Wunderlich G, Kimura EA, Katzin AM. Intraerythrocytic stages of Plasmodium falciparum biosynthesize menaquinone. FEBS Lett. 2010 Dec 1;584(23):4761-8. Epub 2010 Oct 29. PMID:21036171

Tonnetti L, Eder AF, Dy B, Kennedy J, Pisciotto P, Benjamin RJ, Leiby DA. Transfusion-transmitted Babesia microti identified through hemovigilance. Transfusion. 2009 Dec;49(12):2557-63. Epub 2009 Jul 16. PMID:19624607

Tonnetti L, Proctor MC, Reddy HL, Goodrich RP, Leiby DA. Evaluation of the Mirasol pathogen [corrected] reduction technology system against Babesia microti in apheresis platelets and plasma. Transfusion. 2010 May;50(5):1019-27. Epub 2009 Dec 18. PMID:20030791

Topolovec J, Puntarić D, Antolović-Pozgain A, Vuković D, Topolovec Z, Milas J, Drusko-Barisić V, Venus M. Serologically detected "new" tick-borne zoonoses in eastern Croatia. Croat Med J. 2003 Oct;44(5):626-9. PMID:14515426

Torina A, Caracappa S. Anaplasmosis in cattle in Italy. Vet Res Commun. 2007 Aug;31 Suppl 1:73-8. PMID:17682850

Torina A, Vicente J, Alongi A, Scimeca S, Turlá R, Nicosia S, Di Marco V, Caracappa S, de la Fuente J. Observed prevalence of tick-borne pathogens in domestic animals in Sicily, Italy during 2003-2005. Zoonoses Public Health. 2007;54(1):8-15. PMID:17359441

Torrentino-Madamet M, Desplans J, Travaillé C, James Y, Parzy D. Microaerophilic respiratory metabolism of Plasmodium falciparum mitochondrion as a drug target. Curr Mol Med. 2010 Feb;10(1):29-46. PMID:20205678

Torres-Vélez FJ, Nace EK, Won KY, Bartlett J, Eberhard M, Guarner J. Development of an immunohistochemical assay for the detection of babesiosis in formalin-fixed, paraffin-embedded tissue samples. Am J Clin Pathol. 2003 Dec;120(6):833-8. PMID:14671971

Totino PR, Daniel-Ribeiro CT, Ferreira-da-Cruz Mde F. Refractoriness of eryptotic red blood cells to Plasmodium falciparum infection: a putative host defense mechanism limiting parasitaemia. PLoS One. 2011;6(10):e26575. Epub 2011 Oct 21. PMID:22031840

Touré AO, Koné LP, Jambou R, Konan TD, Demba S, Beugre GE, Koné M. [In vitro susceptibility of P. falciparum isolates from Abidjan (Côte d'Ivoire) to quinine, artesunate and chloroquine].[Article in French]. Sante. 2008 Jan-Mar;18(1):43-7. PMID:18684691

Tozan Y, Klein EY, Darley S, Panicker R, Laxminarayan R, Breman JG. Prereferral rectal artesunate for treatment of severe childhood malaria: a cost-effectiveness analysis. Lancet. 2010 Dec 4;376(9756):1910-5. Epub 2010 Nov 29. PMID:21122910

Trape JF, Tall A, Diagne N, Ndiath O, Ly AB, Faye J, Dieye-Ba F, Roucher C, Bouganali C, Badiane A, Sarr FD, Mazenot C, Touré-Baldé A, Raoult D, Druilhe P, Mercereau-Puijalon O, Rogier C, Sokhna C. Malaria morbidity and pyrethroid resistance after the introduction of insecticide-treated bednets and artemisinin-based combination therapies: a longitudinal study. Lancet Infect Dis. 2011 Dec;11(12):925-32. Epub 2011 Aug 17. PMID:21856232

Trenholme KR, Brown CL, Skinner-Adams TS, Stack C, Lowther J, To J, Robinson MW, Donnelly SM, Dalton JP, Gardiner DL. Aminopeptidases of malaria parasites: new targets for chemotherapy. Infect Disord Drug Targets. 2010 Jun;10(3):217-25. PMID:20334618

Trigg PI, Gutteridge WE, Williamson J. The effects of cordycepin on malaria parasites. Trans R Soc Trop Med Hyg. 1971;65(4):514-20. PMID:4999656

Trigg PI. Drug use and design in the nineties. Acta Leiden. 1991;60(1):147-56. PMID:1820704

Trigg PI. Parasite cultivation in relation to research on the chemotherapy of malaria. Bull World Health Organ. 1976;53(4):399-406. PMID:1086733

Tripathi AK, Prajapati V, Ahmad A, Aggarwal KK, Khanuja SP. Piperitenone oxide as toxic, repellent, and reproduction retardant toward malarial vector Anopheles stephensi (Diptera: Anophelinae). J Med Entomol. 2004 Jul;41(4):691-8. PMID:15311462

Tripathi R, Khanna M, Dwivedi AK. Efficacy of novel oral formulations of α/β arteether against multidrug-resistant malaria in mice. Chemotherapy. 2010;56(3):178-83. Epub 2010 May 21. PMID:20501998

Tripathi R, Pandey SK, Rizvi A. Clarithromycin, a cytochrome P450 inhibitor, can reverse mefloquine resistance in Plasmodium yoelii nigeriensis- infected Swiss mice. Parasitology. 2011 Aug;138(9):1069-76. Epub 2011 Jul 15. PMID:21756423

Trongtokit Y, Rongsriyam Y, Komalamisra N, Krisadaphong P, Apiwathnasorn C. Laboratory and field trial of developing medicinal local Thai plant products against four species of mosquito vectors. Southeast Asian J Trop Med Public Health. 2004 Jun;35(2):325-33. PMID:15691131

Trotta M, Carli E, Novari G, Furlanello T, Solano-Gallego L. Clinicopathological findings, molecular detection and characterization of Babesia gibsoni infection in a sick dog from Italy. Vet Parasitol. 2009 Nov 12;165(3-4):318-22. Epub 2009 Jul 21. PMID:19679397

Trumpfheller C, Longhi MP, Caskey M, Idoyaga J, Bozzacco L, Keler T, Schlesinger SJ, Steinman RM. Dendritic cell-targeted protein vaccines: a novel approach to induce T cell immunity. J Intern Med. 2011 Nov 29. [Epub ahead of print]. PMID:22126373

Tsabang N, Fokou PV, Tchokouaha LR, Noguem B, Bakarnga-Via I, Nguepi MS, Nkongmeneck BA, Boyom FF. Ethnopharmacological survey of Annonaceae medicinal plants used to treat malaria in four areas of Cameroon. J Ethnopharmacol. 2012 Jan 6;139(1):171-80. Epub 2011 Nov 4. PMID:22079831

Tschan S, Mordmüller B, Kun JF. Threonine peptidases as drug targets against malaria. Expert Opin Ther Targets. 2011 Apr;15(4):365-78. Epub 2011 Feb 1. PMID:21281254

Tsogoeva SB. Recent progress in the development of synthetic hybrids of natural or unnatural bioactive compounds for medicinal chemistry. Mini Rev Med Chem. 2010 Aug;10(9):773-93. PMID:20105118

Tsuji M, Terada Y, Arai S, Okada H, Ishihara C. Use of the Bo-RBC-SCID mouse model for isolation of a Babesia parasite from grazing calves in Japan. Exp Parasitol. 1995 Dec;81(4):512-8. PMID:8542992

Tsuji N, Miyoshi T, Battsetseg B, Matsuo T, Xuan X, Fujisaki K. A cysteine protease is critical for Babesia spp. transmission in Haemaphysalis ticks. PLoS Pathog. 2008 May 16;4(5):e1000062. PMID:18483546

Tsuzuki A, Khamlome B, Kawada H, Eto H, Phompida S, Takagi M. The efficacy and physical condition of olyset insecticide-treated nets after 5 years use in rural Lao PDR. Southeast Asian J Trop Med Public Health. 2011 Mar;42(2):268-73. PMID:21710846

Tuliaganov KS. [Status and perspectives of development of therapeutic services in Uzbekistan].[Article in Russian]. Ter Arkh. 1974;46(6):98-101. PMID:4279462

Tuo W, Estes DM, Brown WC. Comparative effects of interleukin-12 and interleukin-4 on cytokine responses by antigen-stimulated memory CD4+ T cells of cattle: IL-12 enhances IFN-gamma production, whereas IL-4 has marginal effects on cytokine expression. J Interferon Cytokine Res. 1999 Jul;19(7):741-9. PMID:10454344

Tynan A, Atkinson JA, Toaliu H, Taleo G, Fitzgerald L, Whittaker M, Riley I, Schubert M, Vallely A. Community participation for malaria elimination in Tafea Province, Vanuatu: part II. Social and cultural aspects of treatment-seeking behaviour. Malar J. 2011 Jul 26;10:204. PMID:21787434

Ucakacon P, Achan J, Kutyabami P, Odoi A, Kalyango Nj. Prescribing practices for malaria in a rural Ugandan hospital: evaluation of a new malaria treatment policy. Afr Health Sci. 2011 Aug;11 Suppl 1:S53-9. PMID:22135645

Uguen C, Girard L, Brasseur P, Leblay R. .[Human babesiosis in 1997].[Article in French]. Rev Med Interne. 1997;18(12):945-51. PMID:9499998

Uhnoo I, Cars O, Christensson D, Nyström-Rosander C. First documented case of human babesiosis in Sweden. Scand J Infect Dis. 1992;24(4):541-7. PMID:1411322

Uilenberg G, Franssen FF, Perié NM, Spanjer AA. Three groups of Babesia canis distinguished and a proposal for nomenclature. Vet Q. 1989 Jan;11(1):33-40. PMID:2655263

Uilenberg G, Schreuder BE, Silayo RS, Mpangala C. Studies on Theileriidae (Sporozoa) in Tanzania. IV. A field trial on immunization against East Coast fever (Theileria parva infection of cattle). Tropenmed Parasitol. 1976 Sep;27(3):329-36. PMID:982549

Uilenberg G, Verdiesen PA, Zwart D. Imidocarb: a chemoprophylactic experiment with Babesia canis. Vet Q. 1981 Jul;3(3):118-23. PMID:7268745

Uilenberg G. [Notes on bovine babesiosis and anaplasmosis in Madagascar. VI. Artificial premunization].[Article in French]. Rev Elev Med Vet Pays Trop. 1971;24(1):23-35. PMID:5106007

Uilenberg G. [Studies in the field of tick-borne blood parasites].[Article in Dutch]. Tijdschr Diergeneeskd. 1987 Oct 15;112(20):1163-71. PMID:3672475

Ukaga CN, Nwoke BE, Onyeka PI, Anosike JC, Udujih OS, Udujih OG, Obilor RC, Nwachukwu MI. The use of herbs in malaria treatment in parts of Imo State, Nigeria. Tanzan Health Res Bull. 2006 Sep;8(3):183-5. PMID:18254512

Ungar-Waron H, Paz R, Shkap V, Bin H, Pipano E. IgM rheumatoid factor in cattle immunized against babesiosis. Zentralbl Veterinarmed B. 1991 Sep;38(7):492-6. PMID:1776376

Urgaonkar S, Cortese JF, Barker RH, Cromwell M, Serrano AE, Wirth DF, Clardy J, Mazitschek R. A concise silylamine approach to 2-amino-3-hydroxy-indoles with potent in vivo antimalaria activity. Org Lett. 2010 Sep 17;12(18):3998-4001. PMID:20718474

Uriel A, Lewthwaite P. Malaria therapy in HIV: drug interactions between nevirapine and quinine. Int J STD AIDS. 2011 Dec;22(12):768. PMID:22174067

Ushe TC, Palmer GH, Sotomayor L, Figueroa JV, Buening GM, Perryman LE, McElwain TF. Antibody response to a Babesia bigemina rhoptry-associated protein 1 surface-exposed and neutralization-sensitive epitope in immune cattle. Infect Immun. 1994 Dec;62(12):5698-701. PMID:7525490

Uzochukwu BS, Obikeze EN, Onwujekwe OE, Onoka CA, Griffiths UK. Cost-effectiveness analysis of rapid diagnostic test, microscopy and syndromic approach in the diagnosis of malaria in Nigeria: implications for scaling-up deployment of ACT. Malar J. 2009 Nov 23;8:265. PMID:19930666

Uzoka FM, Obot O, Barker K, Osuji J. An experimental comparison of fuzzy logic and analytic hierarchy process for medical decision support systems. Comput Methods Programs Biomed. 2011 Jul;103(1):10-27. Epub 2010 Jul 15. PMID:20633949

Valbonesi M, Bruni R. Clinical application of therapeutic erythrocytapheresis (TEA). Transfus Sci. 2000 Jun;22(3):183-94. PMID:10831921

Valderramos SG, Scanfeld D, Uhlemann AC, Fidock DA, Krishna S. Investigations into the role of the Plasmodium falciparum SERCA (PfATP6) L263E mutation in artemisinin action and resistance. Antimicrob Agents Chemother. 2010 Sep;54(9):3842-52. Epub 2010 Jun 21. PMID:20566762

Vale N, Moreira R, Gomes P. Primaquine revisited six decades after its discovery. Eur J Med Chem. 2009 Mar;44(3):937-53. Epub 2008 Sep 11. PMID:18930565

Valecha N, Looareesuwan S, Martensson A, Abdulla SM, Krudsood S, Tangpukdee N, Mohanty S, Mishra SK, Tyagi PK, Sharma SK, Moehrle J, Gautam A, Roy A, Paliwal JK, Kothari M, Saha N, Dash AP, Björkman A. Arterolane, a new synthetic trioxolane for treatment of uncomplicated Plasmodium falciparum malaria: a phase II, multicenter, randomized, dose-finding clinical trial. Clin Infect Dis. 2010 Sep 15;51(6):684-91. PMID:20687837

Valentin A, Precigout E, L'Hostis M, Carcy B, Gorenflot A, Schrevel J. Cellular and humoral immune responses induced in cattle by vaccination with Babesia divergens culture-derived exoantigens correlate with protection. Infect Immun. 1993 Feb;61(2):734-41. PMID:8423099

Van Bortel W, Trung HD, Hoi le X, Van Ham N, Van Chut N, Luu ND, Roelants P, Denis L, Speybroeck N, D'Alessandro U, Coosemans M. Malaria transmission and vector behaviour in a forested malaria focus in central Vietnam and the implications for vector control. Malar J. 2010 Dec 23;9:373. PMID:21182774

Van de Maele I, Savary-Bataille K, Gielen I, Daminet S. An unusual form of canine babesiosis. Can Vet J. 2008 Mar;49(3):283-6. PMID:18390102

Van den Bossche P, Mudenge D. The effect of short-interval deltamethrin applications to control tsetse on the seroprevalence of babesiosis in cattle. Trop Anim Health Prod. 1999 Aug;31(4):215-22. PMID:10504101

Van den Steen PE, Geurts N, Deroost K, Van Aelst I, Verhenne S, Heremans H, Van Damme J, Opdenakker G. Immunopathology and dexamethasone therapy in a new model for malaria-associated acute respiratory distress syndrome. Am J Respir Crit Care Med. 2010 May 1;181(9):957-68. Epub 2010 Jan 21. PMID:20093644

van Duivenvoorde LM, Voorberg-van der Wel A, van der Werff NM, Braskamp G, Remarque EJ, Kondova I, Kocken CH, Thomas AW. Suppression of Plasmodium cynomolgi in rhesus macaques by coinfection with Babesia microti. Infect Immun. 2010 Mar;78(3):1032-9. Epub 2010 Jan 4. PMID:20048045

van Eijk AM, Terlouw DJ. Azithromycin for treating uncomplicated malaria. Cochrane Database Syst Rev. 2011 Feb 16;(2):CD006688. PMID:21328286

van Heerden J. Diamidine poisoning in a dog. J S Afr Vet Assoc. 1981 Dec;52(4):338-9. PMID:7341787

Van Miert S, Hostyn S, Maes BU, Cimanga K, Brun R, Kaiser M, Mátyus P, Dommisse R, Lemière G, Vlietinck A, Pieters L. Isoneocryptolepine, a synthetic indoloquinoline alkaloid, as an antiplasmodial lead compound. J Nat Prod. 2005 May;68(5):674-7. PMID:15921407

Van Miert S, Jonckers T, Cimanga K, Maes L, Maes B, Lemière G, Dommisse R, Vlietinck A, Pieters L. In vitro inhibition of beta-haematin formation, DNA interactions, antiplasmodial activity, and cytotoxicity of synthetic neocryptolepine derivatives. Exp Parasitol. 2004 Nov-Dec;108(3-4):163-8. PMID:15582513

Van Niekerk CJ, Zweygarth E. In vitro cultivation of Babesia occultans. Onderstepoort J Vet Res. 1996 Sep;63(3):259-61. PMID:8917864

Van Noorden R. Demand for malaria drug soars. Nature. 2010 Aug 5;466(7307):672-3. PMID:20686539

Van Solingen RM, Evans J. Lyme disease. Curr Opin Rheumatol. 2001 Jul;13(4):293-9. PMID:11555731

van Vugt M, van Beest A, Sicuri E, van Tulder M, Grobusch MP. Malaria treatment and prophylaxis in endemic and nonendemic countries: evidence on strategies and their cost-effectiveness. Future Microbiol. 2011 Dec;6:1485-500. PMID:22122444

van Wolfswinkel ME, Hesselink DA, Zietse R, Hoorn EJ, van Genderen PJ. Hyponatraemia in imported malaria is common and associated with disease severity. Malar J. 2010 May 25;9:140. PMID:20497587

Vanderberg JP. Inactivity of rodent malaria anti-sporozoite antibodies against exoerythrocytic forms. Am J Trop Med Hyg. 1973 Sep;22(5):573-7. PMID:4580967

Vane JR. The fight against rheumatism: from willow bark to COX-1 sparing drugs. J Physiol Pharmacol. 2000 Dec;51(4 Pt 1):573-86. PMID:11192932

Vannier E, Gewurz BE, Krause PJ. Human babesiosis. Infect Dis Clin North Am. 2008 Sep;22(3):469-88, viii-ix. PMID:18755385

Vannier E, Krause PJ. Update on babesiosis. Interdiscip Perspect Infect Dis. 2009;2009:984568. Epub 2009 Aug 27. PMID:19727410

Vargas S, Ndjoko Ioset K, Hay AE, Ioset JR, Wittlin S, Hostettmann K. Screening medicinal plants for the detection of novel antimalarial products applying the inhibition of β-hematin formation. J Pharm Biomed Anal. 2011 Dec 15;56(5):880-6. Epub 2011 Jul 5. PMID:21872416

Vásquez AM, Sanín F, Alvarez LG, Tobón A, Ríos A, Blair S. [Therapeutic efficacy of a regimen of artesunate-mefloquine-primaquine treatment for Plasmodium falciparum malaria and treatment effects on gametocytic development].[Article in Spanish]. Biomedica. 2009 Jun;29(2):307-19. PMID:20128355

Vega CA, Buening GM, Rodriguez SD, Carson CA, McLaughlin K. Cryopreservation of Babesia bigemina for in vitro cultivation. Am J Vet Res. 1985 Feb;46(2):421-3. PMID:3922260

Vercammen F, De Deken R, Maes L. Prophylactic activity of imidocarb against experimental infection with Babesia canis. Vet Parasitol. 1996 Jun;63(3-4):195-8. PMID:8966987

Verma G, Dua VK, Agarwal DD, Atul PK. Anti-malarial activity of Holarrhena antidysenterica and Viola canescens, plants traditionally used against malaria in the Garhwal region of north-west Himalaya. Malar J. 2011 Feb 2;10:20. PMID:21288335

Ververis K, Karagiannis TC. Potential non-oncological applications of histone deacetylase inhibitors. Am J Transl Res. 2011;3(5):454-67. Epub 2011 Oct 10. PMID:22046487

Vial HJ, Gorenflot A. Chemotherapy against babesiosis. Vet Parasitol. 2006 May 31;138(1-2):147-60. Epub 2006 Feb 28. PMID:16504402

Vicente E, Duchowicz PR, Ortiz Edel V, Monge A, Castro EA. Exploring 3-arylquinoxaline-2-carbonitrile 1,4-di-N-oxides activities against neglected diseases with QSAR. Chem Biol Drug Des. 2010 Jul;76(1):59-69. Epub 2010 May 11. PMID:20492446

Vinayak S, Alam MT, Sem R, Shah NK, Susanti AI, Lim P, Muth S, Maguire JD, Rogers WO, Fandeur T, Barnwell JW, Escalante AA, Wongsrichanalai C, Ariey F, Meshnick SR, Udhayakumar V. Multiple genetic backgrounds of the amplified Plasmodium falciparum multidrug resistance (pfmdr1) gene and selective sweep of 184F mutation in Cambodia. J Infect Dis. 2010 May 15;201(10):1551-60. PMID:20367478

Vincke IH. The effects of pyrimethamine and sulphormethoxine on the pre-erythrocytic and sporogonous cycle of Plasmodium berghei berghei. Ann Soc Belges Med Trop Parasitol Mycol. 1970;50(3):339-58. PMID:5514572

Vivas L, Rattray L, Stewart L, Bongard E, Robinson BL, Peters W, Croft SL. Anti-malarial efficacy of pyronaridine and artesunate in combination in vitro and in vivo. Acta Trop. 2008 Mar;105(3):222-8. Epub 2007 Dec 23. PMID:18279817

Vivas L, Rattray L, Stewart LB, Robinson BL, Fugmann B, Haynes RK, Peters W, Croft SL. Antimalarial efficacy and drug interactions of the novel semi-synthetic endoperoxide artemisone in vitro and in vivo. J Antimicrob Chemother. 2007 Apr;59(4):658-65. Epub 2007 Mar 2. PMID:17337512

Vizcaino O, Corrier DE, Terry MK, Carson CA, Lee AJ, Kuttler KL, Ristic M, Treviño GS. Comparison of three methods of immunization against bovine anaplasmosis: evaluation of protection afforded against field challenge exposure. Am J Vet Res. 1980 Jul;41(7):1066-8. PMID:7436100

Vogel G, Roberts L. Malaria. Vaccine trial meets modest expectations, buoys hopes. Science. 2011 Oct 21;334(6054):298-9. PMID:22021827

Vogel G. The 'do unto others' malaria vaccine. Science. 2010 May 14;328(5980):847-8. PMID:20466919

Vollnberg A, Prajakwong S, Sirichaisinthop J, Wiedermann G, Wernsdorfer G, Wernsdorfer WH. In-vitro interaction of tafenoquine and chloroquine in Plasmodium falciparum from northwestern Thailand. Wien Klin Wochenschr. 2003;115 Suppl 3:28-32. PMID:15508777

Vreden SG, van den Broek MF, Oettinger MC, Verhave JP, Meuwissen JH, Sauerwein RW. Cytokines inhibit the development of liver schizonts of the malaria parasite Plasmodium berghei in vivo. Eur J Immunol. 1992 Sep;22(9):2271-5. PMID:1516619

Vulchovski Ia. [Comparative test of the efficacy of babesicidal agents]. [Article in Bulgarian]. Vet Med Nauki. 1977;14(3):79-87.PMID:906312

Vyas JM, Telford SR, Robbins GK. Treatment of refractory Babesia microti infection with atovaquone-proguanil in an HIV-infected patient: case report. Clin Infect Dis. 2007 Dec 15;45(12):1588-90. PMID:18190320

Waage J, Banerji R, Campbell O, Chirwa E, Collender G, Dieltiens V, Dorward A, Godfrey-Faussett P, Hanvoravongchai P, Kingdon G, Little A, Mills A, Mulholland K, Mwinga A, North A, Patcharanarumol W, Poulton C, Tangcharoensathien V, Unterhalter E. The Millennium Development Goals: a cross-sectoral analysis and principles for goal setting after 2015 Lancet and London International Development Centre Commission. Lancet. 2010 Sep 18;376(9745):991-1023. PMID:20833426

Waki S, Suzuki M. Development and decline of antiplasmodial indirect fluorescent antibodies in mice infected with Plasmodium berghei (NK65) and treated with drugs. Bull World Health Organ. 1974;50(6):521-6. PMID: 4617640.

Waldron SJ, Jorgensen WK. Transmission of Babesia spp by the cattle tick (Boophilus microplus) to cattle treated with injectable or pour-on formulations of ivermectin and moxidectin. Aust Vet J. 1999 Oct;77(10):657-9. PMID:10590793

Wallce AL, Harris A, Allen JP. Reiter treponeme. A review of the literature. Bull World Health Organ. 1967;36 Suppl:1-103. PMID:4865377

Walker AS, Ford D, Gilks CF, Munderi P, Ssali F, Reid A, Katabira E, Grosskurth H, Mugyenyi P, Hakim J, Darbyshire JH, Gibb DM, Babiker AG. Daily co-trimoxazole prophylaxis in severely immunosuppressed HIV-infected adults in Africa started on combination antiretroviral therapy: an observational analysis of the DART cohort. Lancet. 2010 Apr 10;375(9722):1278-86. Epub 2010 Mar 27. PMID:20347483

Walsh DS, Eamsila C, Sasiprapha T, Sangkharomya S, Khaewsathien P, Supakalin P, Tang DB, Jarasrumgsichol P, Cherdchu C, Edstein MD, Rieckmann KH, Brewer TG. Efficacy of monthly tafenoquine for prophylaxis of Plasmodium vivax and multidrug-resistant P. falciparum malaria. J Infect Dis. 2004 Oct 15;190(8):1456-63. Epub 2004 Sep 20. PMID:15378438

Walsh DS, Looareesuwan S, Wilairatana P, Heppner DG Jr, Tang DB, Brewer TG, Chokejindachai W, Viriyavejakul P, Kyle DE, Milhous WK, Schuster BG, Horton J, Braitman DJ, Brueckner RP. Randomized dose-ranging study of the safety and efficacy of WR 238605 (Tafenoquine) in the prevention of relapse of Plasmodium vivax malaria in Thailand. J Infect Dis. 1999 Oct;180(4):1282-7. PMID:10479159

Walsh DS, Wilairatana P, Tang DB, Heppner DG Jr, Brewer TG, Krudsood S, Silachamroon U, Phumratanaprapin W, Siriyanonda D, Looareesuwan S. Randomized trial of 3-dose regimens of tafenoquine (WR238605) versus low-dose primaquine for preventing Plasmodium vivax malaria relapse. Clin Infect Dis. 2004 Oct 15;39(8):1095-103. Epub 2004 Sep 24. PMID:15486831

Waltisbuhl DJ, Goodger BV, Wright IG, Mirre GB, Commins MA. Babesia bovis: vaccination studies with three groups of high molecular weight antigens from lysate of infected erythrocytes. Parasitol Res. 1987;73(4):319-23. PMID:3303020

Wang C, Ahluwalia SK, Li Y, Gao D, Poudel A, Chowdhury E, Boudreaux MK, Kaltenboeck B. Frequency and therapy monitoring of canine Babesia spp. infection by high-resolution melting curve quantitative FRET-PCR. Vet Parasitol. 2010 Feb 26;168(1-2):11-8. Epub 2009 Oct 28. PMID:19931290

Wang HZ, He YX, Yang CJ, Zhou W, Zou CG. Hepcidin Is Regulated during Blood-Stage Malaria and Plays a Protective Role in Malaria Infection. J Immunol. 2011 Dec 15;187(12):6410-6. Epub 2011 Nov 14. PMID:22084434

Wang TJ, Liang MH, Sangha O, Phillips CB, Lew RA, Wright EA, Berardi V, Fossel AH, Shadick NA. Coexposure to Borrelia burgdorferi and Babesia microti does not worsen the long-term outcome of lyme disease. Clin Infect Dis. 2000 Nov;31(5):1149-54. Epub 2000 Nov 6. PMID:11073744

Wang W, Gallant JN, Katz SI, Dolloff NG, Smith CD, Abdulghani J, Allen JE, Dicker DT, Hong B, Navaraj A, El-Deiry WS. Quinacrine sensitizes hepatocellular carcinoma cells to TRAIL and chemotherapeutic agents. Cancer Biol Ther. 2011 Aug 1;12(3):229-38. Epub 2011 Aug 1. PMID:21725212

Wangchuk P, Keller PA, Pyne SG, Taweechotipatr M, Tonsomboon A, Rattanajak R, Kamchonwongpaisan S. Evaluation of an ethnopharmacologically selected Bhutanese medicinal plants for their major classes of phytochemicals and biological activities. J Ethnopharmacol. 2011 Sep 1;137(1):730-42. Epub 2011 Jun 28. PMID:21741462

Wanjohi JM, Ngeranwa JN, Rumberia RM, Muraguri GR, Mbogo SK. Immunization of cattle against East Coast fever using Theileria parva (Marikebuni) and relaxation of tick control in North Rift, Kenya. Onderstepoort J Vet Res. 2001 Sep;68(3):217-23. PMID:11769354

Ward RA. The influence of Ronald Ropss upon the early development of malaria vector control procedures in the United States Army. J Trop Med Hyg. 1973 Aug;76(8):207-9. PMID:4582106

Warhurst DC, Folwell RO. Measurement of the growth rate of the erythrocytic stages of Plasmodium berghei and comparisons of the potency of inocula after various treatments. Ann Trop Med Parasitol. 1968 Sep;62(3):349-60. PMID:5714962

Watts G. Lost in translation. BMJ. 2011 Nov 2;343:d7047. PMID:22049526

Webb EL, Mawa PA, Ndibazza J, Kizito D, Namatovu A, Kyosiimire-Lugemwa J, Nanteza B, Nampijja M, Muhangi L, Woodburn PW, Akurut H, Mpairwe H, Akello M, Lyadda N, Bukusuba J, Kihembo M, Kizza M, Kizindo R, Nabulime J, Ameke C, Namujju PB, Tweyongyere R, Muwanga M, Whitworth JA, Elliott AM. Effect of single-dose anthelmintic treatment during pregnancy on an infant's response to immunisation and on susceptibility to infectious diseases in infancy: a randomised, double-blind, placebo-controlled trial. Lancet. 2011 Jan 1;377(9759):52-62. Epub 2010 Dec 20. PMID:21176950

Webert KE, Cserti CM, Hannon J, Lin Y, Pavenski K, Pendergrast JM, Blajchman MA. Proceedings of a Consensus Conference: pathogen inactivation-making decisions about new technologies. Transfus Med Rev. 2008 Jan;22(1):1-34. PMID:18063190

Wei Q, Tsuji M, Zamoto A, Kohsaki M, Matsui T, Shiota T, Telford SR 3rd, Ishihara C. Human babesiosis in Japan: isolation of Babesia microti-like parasites from an asymptomatic transfusion donor and from a rodent from an area where babesiosis is endemic. J Clin Microbiol. 2001 Jun;39(6):2178-83. PMID:11376054

Weilgama DJ, Jorgensen WK, Dalgliesh RJ, Navaratne M, Weerasinghe C. Comparison between Sri Lankan and Australian strains of Babesia bovis in the vaccination of imported cattle in Sri Lanka. Trop Anim Health Prod. 1989 May;21(2):141-5. PMID:2665254

Wein S, Maynadier M, Tran Van Ba C, Cerdan R, Peyrottes S, Fraisse L, Vial H. Reliability of antimalarial sensitivity tests depends on drug mechanisms of action. J Clin Microbiol. 2010 May;48(5):1651-60. Epub 2010 Mar 10. PMID:20220159

Weinberg GA. Laboratory diagnosis of ehrlichiosis and babesiosis. Pediatr Infect Dis J. 2001 Apr;20(4):435-7. PMID:11332670

Weiss LM, Wittner M, Tanowitz HB. The treatment of babesiosis. N Engl J Med. 2001 Mar 8;344(10):773. PMID:11236789

Weiss LM, Wittner M, Wasserman S, Oz HS, Retsema J, Tanowitz HB. Efficacy of azithromycin for treating Babesia microti infection in the hamster model. J Infect Dis. 1993 Nov;168(5):1289-92. PMID:8228366

Weiss LM. Babesiosis in humans: a treatment review. Expert Opin Pharmacother. 2002 Aug;3(8):1109-15. PMID:12150690

Welc-Faleciak R, Rodo A, Siński E, Bajer A. Babesia canis and other tick-borne infections in dogs in Central Poland. Vet Parasitol. 2009 Dec 23;166(3-4):191-8. Epub 2009 Sep 26. PMID: 19837515

Weld ED, Eimer KM, Saharia K, Orenstein A, Hess JR. Transfusion medicine illustrated. The expanding range and severity of babesiosis. Transfusion. 2010 Feb;50(2):290-1. PMID:20233358

Wells TN, Poll EM. When is enough enough? The need for a robust pipeline of high-quality antimalarials. Discov Med. 2010 May;9(48):389-98. PMID:20515606

Wells TN. Microbiology. Is the tide turning for new malaria medicines? Science. 2010 Sep 3;329(5996):1153-4. PMID:20813940

Wells TN. Natural products as starting points for future anti-malarial therapies: going back to our roots? Malar J. 2011 Mar 15;10 Suppl 1:S3. [Epub ahead of print]. PMID:21411014

Wen W. China: a new medicine born of tradition. UNESCO Cour. 1979 Jul;7:25-7. PMID:12309932

Wendel Neto S. Current concepts on the transmission of bacteria and parasites by blood components. Sao Paulo Med J. 1995 Nov-Dec;113(6):1036-52. PMID:8731290

Wendel S, Leiby DA. Parasitic infections in the blood supply: assessing and countering the threat. Dev Biol (Basel). 2007;127:17-41. PMID:17486879

Wendel S. Current concepts on transmission of bacteria and parasites by blood components. Vox Sang. 1994;67 Suppl 3:161-74. PMID:7975485

Were PS, Kinyanjui P, Gicheru MM, Mwangi E, Ozwara HS. Prophylactic and curative activities of extracts from Warburgia ugandensis Sprague (Canellaceae) and Zanthoxylum usambarense (Engl.) Kokwaro (Rutaceae) against Plasmodium knowlesi and Plasmodium berghei. J Ethnopharmacol. 2010 Jul 6;130(1):158-62. Epub 2010 Apr 29. PMID:20435133

Wernsdorfer WH. Global challenges of changing epidemiological patterns of malaria. Acta Trop. 2011 Jul 19. [Epub ahead of print]. PMID:21784053

Whegang SY, Tahar R, Foumane VN, Soula G, Gwét H, Thalabard JC, Basco LK. Efficacy of non-artemisinin- and artemisinin-based combination therapies for uncomplicated falciparum malaria in Cameroon. Malar J. 2010 Feb 19;9:56. PMID:20170477

White DJ, Talarico J, Chang HG, Birkhead GS, Heimberger T, Morse DL. Human babesiosis in New York State: Review of 139 hospitalized cases and analysis of prognostic factors. Arch Intern Med. 1998 Oct 26;158(19):2149-54. PMID:9801183

White MT, Conteh L, Cibulskis R, Ghani AC. Costs and cost-effectiveness of malaria control interventions - a systematic review. Malar J. 2011 Nov 3;10:337. PMID:22050911

White MT, Griffin JT, Churcher TS, Ferguson NM, Basáñez MG, Ghani AC. Modelling the impact of vector control interventions on Anopheles gambiae population dynamics. Parasit Vectors. 2011 Jul 28;4:153. PMID:21798055

White NJ. A vaccine for malaria. N Engl J Med. 2011 Nov 17;365(20):1926-7. Epub 2011 Oct 18. PMID:22007716

White NJ. Determinants of relapse periodicity in Plasmodium vivax malaria. Malar J. 2011 Oct 11;10:297. PMID:21989376

Whitty CJ. The RTS,S malaria vaccine. BMJ. 2011 Oct 27;343:d6986. PMID:22034149

Wiesner J, Ortmann R, Jomaa H, Schlitzer M. New antimalarial drugs. Angew Chem Int Ed Engl. 2003 Nov 10;42(43):5274-93. PMID:14613157

Wiesner J, Reichenberg A, Heinrich S, Schlitzer M, Jomaa H. The plastid-like organelle of apicomplexan parasites as drug target. Curr Pharm Des. 2008;14(9):855-71. PMID:18473835

Wijaya A, Wulansari R, Ano H, Inokuma H, Makimura S. Therapeutic effect of clindamycin and tetracycline on Babesia rodhaini infection in mouse model. J Vet Med Sci. 2000 Aug;62(8):835-9. PMID:10993180

Wijesinghe RS, Atkinson JA, Bobogare A, Wini L, Whittaker M. Exploring provider and community responses to the new malaria diagnostic and treatment regime in Solomon Islands. Malar J. 2011 Jan 10;10:3. PMID:21219614

Willadsen P, Kemp DH, Cobon GS, Wright IG. Successful vaccination against Boophilus microplus and Babesia bovis using recombinant antigens. Mem Inst Oswaldo Cruz. 1992;87 Suppl 3:289-94. PMID:1343705

Willadsen P, Kemp DH. Novel vaccination for control of the Babesia vector, Boophilus microplus. Trans R Soc Trop Med Hyg. 1989;83 Suppl:107. PMID:2623756

Willadsen P. Vaccines, genetics and chemicals in tick control: the Australian experience. Trop Anim Health Prod. 1997 Nov;29(4 Suppl):91S-94S. PMID:9512752

Willcox M, Benoit-Vical F, Fowler D, Bourdy G, Burford G, Giani S, Graziose R, Houghton P, Randrianarivelojosia M, Rasoanaivo P. Do ethnobotanical and laboratory data predict clinical safety and efficacy of anti-malarial plants? Malar J. 2011 Mar 15;10 Suppl 1:S7. [Epub ahead of print]. PMID:21411018

Willcox M. Improved traditional phytomedicines in current use for the clinical treatment of malaria. Planta Med. 2011 Apr;77(6):662-71. Epub 2011 Jan 3. PMID:21204042

Willcox ML, Graz B, Diakite C, Falquet J, Dackouo F, Sidibe O, Giani S, Diallo D. Is parasite clearance clinically important after malaria treatment in a high transmission area? A 3-month follow-up of home-based management with herbal medicine or ACT. Trans R Soc Trop Med Hyg. 2011 Jan;105(1):23-31. Epub 2010 Nov 5. PMID:21056445

Willerson D Jr, Rieckmann KH, Carson PE, Frischer H. Effects of minocycline against chloroquine-resistant falciparum malaria. Am J Trop Med Hyg. 1972 Nov;21(6):857-62. PMID:4564446

William T, Menon J, Rajahram G, Chan L, Ma G, Donaldson S, Khoo S, Frederick C, Jelip J, Anstey NM, Yeo TW. Severe Plasmodium knowlesi malaria in a tertiary care hospital, Sabah, Malaysia. Emerg Infect Dis. 2011 Jul;17(7):1248-55. PMID:21762579

Williams SL, de Oliveira CA, Vazquez H, McCammon JA. From Zn to Mn: the study of novel manganese-binding groups in the search for new drugs against tuberculosis. Chem Biol Drug Des. 2011 Feb;77(2):117-23. PMID:21266015

Wilson AL; IPTc Taskforce. A systematic review and meta-analysis of the efficacy and safety of intermittent preventive treatment of malaria in children (IPTc). PLoS One. 2011 Feb 14;6(2):e16976. PMID:21340029

Wilson ML, Walker ED, Mzilahowa T, Mathanga DP, Taylor TE. Malaria elimination in Malawi: Research needs in highly endemic, poverty-stricken contexts. Acta Trop. 2011 Nov 15. [Epub ahead of print]. PMID:22100546

Wilson NO, Ceesay FK, Obed SA, Adjei AA, Gyasi RK, Rodney P, Ndjakani Y, Anderson WA, Lucchi NW, Stiles JK. Intermittent preventive treatment with sulfadoxine-pyrimethamine against malaria and anemia in pregnant women. Am J Trop Med Hyg. 2011 Jul;85(1):12-21. PMID:21734118

Winger CM, Canning EU, Culverhouse JD. A monoclonal antibody-derived antigen of Babesia divergens: characterization and investigation of its ability to protect gerbils against virulent homologous challenge. Parasitology. 1989 Dec;99 Pt 3:341-8. PMID:2608311

Winger CM, Canning EU, Culverhouse JD. A strain of Babesia divergens, attenuated after long term culture. Res Vet Sci. 1989 Jan;46(1):110-3. PMID:2922498

Winger CM, Canning EU, Culverhouse JD. A strain of Babesia divergens, attenuated after long term culture. Res Vet Sci. 1989 Jan;46(1):110-3. PMID:2922498

Winger CM, Canning EU, Culverhouse JD. Induction of protective immunity to Babesia divergens in Mongolian gerbils, Meriones unguiculatus, using culture-derived immunogens. Vet Parasitol. 1987 Dec;26(1-2):43-53. PMID:3439004

Winter G, Chen Q, Wahlgren M. Meeting report: the molecular background of severe and complicated malaria. Mol Biochem Parasitol. 2004 Mar;134(1):37-41. PMID:14747141

Winter R, Kelly JX, Smilkstein MJ, Hinrichs D, Koop DR, Riscoe MK. Optimization of endochin-like quinolones for antimalarial activity. Exp Parasitol. 2011 Feb;127(2):545-51. Epub 2010 Oct 30. PMID:21040724

Winterburn TJ, Phylip LH, Bur D, Wyatt DM, Berry C, Kay J. N-terminal extension of the yeast IA3 aspartic proteinase inhibitor relaxes the strict intrinsic selectivity. FEBS J. 2007 Jul;274(14):3685-94. Epub 2007 Jul 2. PMID:17608726

Wiseman V, McElroy B, Conteh L, Stevens W. Malaria prevention in The Gambia: patterns of expenditure and determinants of demand at the household level. Trop Med Int Health. 2006 Apr;11(4):419-31. PMID:16553925

Wiśniewski M, Zak DJ. [Achievements and perspectives of research into development of a vaccine against malaria].[Article in Polish]. Wiad Parazytol. 2010;56(2):133-40. PMID:20707297

Witkowski B, Lelièvre J, Barragán MJ, Laurent V, Su XZ, Berry A, Benoit-Vical F. Increased tolerance to artemisinin in Plasmodium falciparum is mediated by a quiescence mechanism. Antimicrob Agents Chemother. 2010 May;54(5):1872-7. Epub 2010 Feb 16. PMID:20160056

Wittlin S, Ekland E, Craft JC, Lotharius J, Bathurst I, Fidock DA, Fernandes P. In Vitro and In Vivo Activity of Solithromycin (CEM-101) Against Plasmodium Species. Antimicrob Agents Chemother. 2011 Nov 14. [Epub ahead of print]. PMID:22083475

Wittner M, Lederman J, Tanowitz HB, Rosenbaum GS, Weiss LM. Atovaquone in the treatment of Babesia microti infections in hamsters. Am J Trop Med Hyg. 1996 Aug;55(2):219-22. PMID:8780464

Wittner M, Rowin KS, Tanowitz HB, Hobbs JF, Saltzman S, Wenz B, Hirsch R, Chisholm E, Healy GR. Successful chemotherapy of transfusion babesiosis. Ann Intern Med. 1982 May;96(5):601-4. PMID:7200341

Wodecka B, Rymaszewska A, Sawczuk M, Skotarczak B. Detectability of tick-borne agents DNA in the blood of dogs, undergoing treatment for borreliosis. Ann Agric Environ Med. 2009 Jun;16(1):9-14. PMID:19572472

Wohlfarth C, Efferth T. Natural products as promising drug candidates for the treatment of hepatitis B and C. Acta Pharmacol Sin. 2009 Jan;30(1):25-30. Epub 2008 Dec 8. PMID:19060918

Wójcik-Fatla A, Cisak E, Chmielewska-Badora J, Zwoliński J, Buczek A, Dutkiewicz J. Prevalence of Babesia microti in Ixodes ricinus ticks from Lublin region (eastern Poland). Ann Agric Environ Med. 2006;13(2):319-22. PMID:17196008

Wong WS, Chung JY, Wong KF. Images in haematology. Human babesiosis. Br J Haematol. 2008 Feb;140(4):364. Epub 2007 Nov 27. PMID:18042268

Wongsrichanalai C, Meshnick SR. Declining artesunate-mefloquine efficacy against falciparum malaria on the Cambodia-Thailand border. Emerg Infect Dis. 2008 May;14(5):716-9. PMID:18439351

Wongsrichanalai C, Varma JK, Juliano JJ, Kimerling ME, MacArthur JR. Extensive drug resistance in malaria and tuberculosis. Emerg Infect Dis. 2010 Jul;16(7):1063-7. MID:20587175

Wood PR, Clark IA. Genetic control of Propionibacterium acnes-induced protection of mice against Babesia microti. Infect Immun. 1982 Jan;35(1):52-7. PMID:7054129

Wormser GP, Lombardo G, Silverblatt F, El Khoury MY, Prasad A, Yelon JA, Sanda A, Karim S, Coku L, Savino JA. Babesiosis as a cause of fever in patients undergoing a splenectomy. Am Surg. 2011 Mar;77(3):345-7. PMID:21375849

Wormser GP, Prasad A, Neuhaus E, Joshi S, Nowakowski J, Nelson J, Mittleman A, Aguero-Rosenfeld M, Topal J, Krause PJ. Emergence of resistance to azithromycin-atovaquone in immunocompromised patients with Babesia microti infection. Clin Infect Dis. 2010 Feb 1;50(3):381-6. PMID:20047477

Wrenger C, Müller IB, Schifferdecker AJ, Jain R, Jordanova R, Groves MR. Specific inhibition of the aspartate aminotransferase of Plasmodium falciparum. J Mol Biol. 2011 Jan 28;405(4):956-71. Epub 2010 Nov 16. PMID:21087616

Wright CW. Recent developments in naturally derived antimalarials: cryptolepine analogues. J Pharm Pharmacol. 2007 Jun;59(6):899-904. PMID:17637183

Wright CW. Recent developments in research on terrestrial plants used for the treatment of malaria. Nat Prod Rep. 2010 Jul;27(7):961-8. Epub 2010 Jun 8. PMID:20532364

Wright IG, Casu R, Commins MA, Dalrymple BP, Gale KR, Goodger BV, Riddles PW, Waltisbuhl DJ, Abetz I, Berrie DA, et al. The development of a recombinant Babesia vaccine. Vet Parasitol. 1992 Sep;44(1-2):3-13. PMID:1441189

Wright IG, Goodger BV, Leatch G, Aylward JH, Rode-Bramanis K, Waltisbuhl DJ. Protection of Babesia bigemina-immune animals against subsequent challenge with virulent Babesia bovis. Infect Immun. 1987 Feb;55(2):364-8. PMID:3542832

Wright IG, Goodger BV, Rode-Bramanis K, Mattick JS, Mahoney DF, Waltisbuhl DJ. The characterisation of an esterase derived from Babesia bovis and its use as a vaccine. Z Parasitenkd. 1983;69(6):703-14. PMID:6419487

Wright IG, Mirre GB, Rode-Bramanis K, Chamberlain M, Goodger BV, Waltisbuhl DJ. Protective vaccination against virulent Babesia bovis with a low-molecular-weight antigen. Infect Immun. 1985 Apr;48(1):109-13. PMID:3980077

Wright IG, White M, Tracey-Patte PD, Donaldson RA, Goodger BV, Waltisbuhl DJ, Mahoney DF. Babesia bovis: isolation of a protective antigen by using monoclonal antibodies. Infect Immun. 1983 Jul;41(1):244-50. PMID:6345394

Wu T, Wu S, Yin Q, Dai H, Li S, Dong F, Chen B, Fang H. [Biosynthesis of amorpha-4,11-diene, a precursor of the antimalarial agent artemisinin, in Escherichia coli through introducing mevalonate pathway].[Article in Chinese]. Sheng Wu Gong Cheng Xue Bao. 2011 Jul;27(7):1040-8. PMID:22016988

Wudhikarn K, Perry EH, Kemperman M, Jensen KA, Kline SE. Transfusion-transmitted babesiosis in an immunocompromised patient: a case report and review. Am J Med. 2011 Sep;124(9):800-5. Epub 2011 Jun 16. PMID:21683324

Wurtz N, Chapus C, Desplans J, Parzy D. cAMP-dependent protein kinase from Plasmodium falciparum: an update. Parasitology. 2011 Jan;138(1):1-25. Epub 2010 Jul 21. PMID:20663247

Wylie BJ, Hashmi AH, Singh N, Singh MP, Tuchman J, Hussain M, Sabin L, Yeboah-Antwi K, Banerjee C, Brooks MI, Desai M, Udhayakumar V, Macleod WB, Dash AP, Hamer DH. Availability and utilization of malaria prevention strategies in pregnancy in eastern India. BMC Public Health. 2010 Sep 17;10:557. PMID:20849590

Xiao SH, Keiser J, Chen MG, Tanner M, Utzinger J. Research and development of antischistosomal drugs in the People's Republic of China a 60-year review. Adv Parasitol. 2010;73:231-95. PMID:20627145

Xiao SH, Sun J, Xue J, Du XL, Zhang HB. Ultrastructural alterations of juvenile Schistosoma japonicum harbored in mice following mefloquine administration. Parasitol Res. 2011 Jul 13. [Epub ahead of print]. PMID:21750873

Xu WC, Shen JG, Jiang JQ. Phytochemical and biological studies of the plants from the genus Daphne. Chem Biodivers. 2011 Jul;8(7):1215-33. PMID:21766444

Xu X, Oliveira F, Chang BW, Collin N, Gomes R, Teixeira C, Reynoso D, My Pham V, Elnaiem DE, Kamhawi S, Ribeiro JM, Valenzuela JG, Andersen JF. Structure and function of a "yellow" protein from saliva of the sand fly Lutzomyia longipalpis that confers protective immunity against Leishmania major infection. J Biol Chem. 2011 Sep 16;286(37):32383-93. Epub 2011 Jul 27. PMID:21795673

Xue J, Zhan B, Guo J, He N, Qiang HQ, Hotez P, Xiao SH. Acquired hookworm immunity in the golden hamster (Mesocricetus auratus) elicited by living Necator americanus third-stage infective larvae. Exp Parasitol. 2012 Jan;130(1):6-12. Epub 2011 Oct 21. PMID:22024448

Xue RD. Introduction to symposium on mosquitoes and plants. J Am Mosq Control Assoc. 2008 Mar;24(1):134-7. PMID:18437828

Yabsley MJ, Davidson WR, Stallknecht DE, Varela AS, Swift PK, Devos JC Jr, Dubay SA. Evidence of tick-borne organisms in mule deer (Odocoileus hemionus) from the western United States. Vector Borne Zoonotic Dis. 2005 Winter;5(4):351-62. PMID:16417431

Yabsley MJ, Romines J, Nettles VF. Detection of Babesia and Anaplasma species in rabbits from Texas and Georgia, USA. Vector Borne Zoonotic Dis. 2006 Spring;6(1):7-13. PMID:16584322

Yadav S, Mittal PK, Saxena PN, Singh RK. Effect of synergist piperonyl butoxide (PBO) on the toxicity of some essential oils against mosquito larvae. J Commun Dis. 2009 Mar;41(1):33-8. PMID:19886173

Yadav S, Mittal PK, Saxena PN, Singh RK. Effect of synergist piperonyl butoxide (PBO) on the toxicity of some essential oils against mosquito larvae. J Commun Dis. 2008 Dec;40(4):263-8. PMID:19579718

Yadouleton A, Martin T, Padonou G, Chandre F, Asidi A, Djogbenou L, Dabiré R, Aïkpon R, Boko M, Glitho I, Akogbeto M. Cotton pest management practices and the selection of pyrethroid resistance in Anopheles gambiae population in northern Benin. Parasit Vectors. 2011 Apr 13;4:60. PMID:21489266

Yamasaki M, Hwang SJ, Ohta H, Yamato O, Maede Y, Takiguchi M. Flow cytometry to evaluate the level of Babesia gibsoni parasitemia in vivo and in vitro by using the fluorescent nucleic acid stain SYTO16. Jpn J Vet Res. 2008 Feb;55(4):129-36. PMID:18380154

Yamasaki M, Tajima M, Yamato O, Hwang SJ, Ohta H, Maede Y. Heat shock response of Babesia gibsoni heat shock protein 70. J Parasitol. 2008 Feb;94(1):119-24. PMID:18372630

Yao B, Zhao J, Ma L, Liu Z. Studies on the pathogenicity of Babesia bovis in water buffaloes after cryopreservation and resuscitation. Trop Anim Health Prod. 1997 Nov;29(4 Suppl):40S-42S. PMID:9512744

Yardley V, Gamarro F, Croft SL. Antileishmanial and antitrypanosomal activities of the 8-aminoquinoline tafenoquine. Antimicrob Agents Chemother. 2010 Dec;54(12):5356-8. Epub 2010 Sep 13. PMID:20837750

Yavo W, Faye B, Kuete T, Djohan V, Oga SA, Kassi RR, Diatta M, Ama MV, Tine R, Ndiaye JL, Evi JB, Same-Ekobo A, Faye O, Koné M. Multicentric assessment of the efficacy and tolerability of dihydroartemisinin-piperaquine compared to artemether-lumefantrine in the treatment of uncomplicated Plasmodium falciparum malaria in sub-Saharan Africa. Malar J. 2011 Jul 20;10:198. PMID:21774826

Ye VM, Bhatia SK. Metabolic engineering for the production of clinically important molecules: Omega-3 fatty acids, artemisinin, and taxol. Biotechnol J. 2011 Oct 21. [Epub ahead of print]. PMID:22021189

Yeates C. Sitamaquine (GlaxoSmithKline/Walter Reed Army Institute). Curr Opin Investig Drugs. 2002 Oct;3(10):1446-52. PMID:12431016

Yeboah-Antwi K, Pilingana P, Macleod WB, Semrau K, Siazeele K, Kalesha P, Hamainza B, Seidenberg P, Mazimba A, Sabin L, Kamholz K, Thea DM, Hamer DH. Community case management of fever due to malaria and pneumonia in children under five in Zambia: a cluster randomized controlled trial. PLoS Med. 2010 Sep 21;7(9):e1000340. PMID:20877714

Yeshiwondim AK, Tekle AH, Dengela DO, Yohannes AM, Teklehaimanot A. Therapeutic efficacy of chloroquine and chloroquine plus primaquine for the treatment of Plasmodium vivax in Ethiopia. Acta Trop. 2010 Feb;113(2):105-13. Epub 2009 Oct 14. PMID:19835832

Yeung S, Van Damme W, Socheat D, White NJ, Mills A. Access to artemisinin combination therapy for malaria in remote areas of Cambodia. Malar J. 2008 May 29;7:96. PMID:18510724

Yewhalaw D, Wassie F, Steurbaut W, Spanoghe P, Van Bortel W, Denis L, Tessema DA, Getachew Y, Coosemans M, Duchateau L, Speybroeck N. Multiple insecticide resistance: an impediment to insecticide-based malaria vector control program. PLoS One. 2011 Jan 12;6(1):e16066. PMID:21264325

Yin H, Luo J. Ticks of small ruminants in China. Parasitol Res. 2007 Sep;101 Suppl 2:S187-9. PMID:17823826

Yoeli M, Most H. Sporozoite-induced infections of Plasmodium berghei administered by the oral route. Science. 1971 Sep 10;173(4001):1031-2. PMID:5098964

Yoeli M. [The development of malaria research before and since Ronald Ross].[Article in German]. Munch Med Wochenschr. 1973 Feb 2;115(5):151-8. PMID:4633457

Yoeli M. Landmarks in malaria research (a review). Acta Trop. 1974;31(4):321-8. PMID:4141222

Yokoyama N, Bork S, Nishisaka M, Hirata H, Matsuo T, Inoue N, Xuan X, Suzuki H, Sugimoto C, Igarashi I. Roles of the Maltese cross form in the development of parasitemia and protection against Babesia microti infection in mice. Infect Immun. 2003 Jan;71(1):411-7. PMID:12496191

Yokoyama N, Okamura M, Igarashi I. Erythrocyte invasion by Babesia parasites: current advances in the elucidation of the molecular interactions between the protozoan ligands and host receptors in the invasion stage. Vet Parasitol. 2006 May 31;138(1-2):22-32. Epub 2006 Feb 28. PMID:16504403

Yoshida S, Araki H, Yokomine T. Baculovirus-based nasal drop vaccine confers complete protection against malaria by natural boosting of vaccine-induced antibodies in mice. Infect Immun. 2010 Feb;78(2):595-602. Epub 2009 Nov 9. PMID:19901059

Yoshinari NH, Abrão MG, Bonoldi VL, Soares CO, Madruga CR, Scofield A, Massard CL, da Fonseca AH. Coexistence of antibodies to tick-borne agents of babesiosis and Lyme borreliosis in patients from Cotia county, State of São Paulo, Brazil. Mem Inst Oswaldo Cruz. 2003 Apr;98(3):311-8. Epub 2003 Jul 18. PMID:12886408

Young AS, Cox FE. The effect of betamethasone on Babesia microti and B. rodhaini infections in rodents. Parasitology. 1971 Dec;63(3):447-53. PMID:4945066

Young AS, Groocock CM, Kariuki DP. Integrated control of ticks and tick-borne diseases of cattle in Africa. Parasitology. 1988 Apr;96 (Pt 2):403-32. PMID:3287285

Young AS, Mutugi JJ, Kariuki DP, Lampard D, Maritim AC, Ngumi PN, Linyonyi A, Leitch BL, Ndungu SG, Lesan AC, et al. Immunisation of cattle against theileriosis in Nakuru District of Kenya by infection and treatment and the introduction of unconventional tick control. Vet Parasitol. 1992 May;42(3-4):225-40. PMID: 1496782

Young C, Krause PJ. The problem of transfusion-transmitted babesiosis. Transfusion. 2009 Dec;49(12):2548-50. PMID:20163687

Yu DH, Li YH, Yoon JS, Lee JH, Lee MJ, Yu IJ, Chae JS, Park JH. Ehrlichia chaffeensis infection in dogs in South Korea. Vector Borne Zoonotic Dis. 2008 Jun;8(3):355-8. PMID:18399775

Yu ZX, Li JX, Yang CQ, Hu WL, Wang LJ, Chen XY. The Jasmonate-Responsive AP2/ERF Transcription Factors AaERF1 and AaERF2 Positively Regulate Artemisinin Biosynthesis in Artemisia annua L. Mol Plant. 2011 Nov 20. [Epub ahead of print]. PMID:22104293

Yuan D, Bassie L, Sabalza M, Miralpeix B, Dashevskaya S, Farre G, Rivera SM, Banakar R, Bai C, Sanahuja G, Arjó G, Avilla E, Zorrilla-López U, Ugidos-Damboriena N, López A, Almacellas D, Zhu C, Capell T, Hahne G, Twyman RM, Christou P. The potential impact of plant biotechnology on the Millennium Development Goals. Plant Cell Rep. 2011 Mar;30(3):249-65. Epub 2011 Jan 20. PMID:21249369

Yuan J, Cheng KC, Johnson RL, Huang R, Pattaradilokrat S, Liu A, Guha R, Fidock DA, Inglese J, Wellems TE, Austin CP, Su XZ. Chemical genomic profiling for antimalarial therapies, response signatures, and molecular targets. Science. 2011 Aug 5;333(6043):724-9. PMID:21817045

Yukich J, D'Acremont V, Kahama J, Swai N, Lengeler C. Cost savings with rapid diagnostic tests for malaria in low-transmission areas: evidence from Dar es Salaam, Tanzania. Am J Trop Med Hyg. 2010 Jul;83(1):61-8. PMID:20595479

Yunker CE, Kuttler KL, Johnson LW. Attenuation of Babesia bovis by in vitro cultivation. Vet Parasitol. 1987 Apr;24(1-2):7-13. PMID:3590611

Yusuf RU, Omar SA, Ngure RM. The effect of point mutations in dihydrofolate reductase genes and multidrug resistance gene 1-86 on treatment of falciparum malaria in Sudan. J Infect Dev Ctries. 2010 Mar 8;4(2):61-9. PMID:20212335

Zakeri S, Farahani MS, Afsharpad M, Salehi M, Raeisi A, Djadid ND. High prevalence of the 437G mutation associated with sulfadoxine resistance among Plasmodium falciparum clinical isolates from Iran, three years after the introduction of sulfadoxine-pyrimethamine. Int J Infect Dis. 2010 Sep;14 Suppl 3:e123-8. PMID:20399698

Zaman J, Shahbazi A, Asgharzadeh M. Plasmodium vivax dhfr mutations among isolates from malarious areas of Iran. Korean J Parasitol. 2011 Jun;49(2):125-31. Epub 2011 Jun 14. PMID:21738267

Zambelli AB, Leisewitz AL. A prospective, randomized comparison of Oxyglobin (HB-200) and packed red blood cell transfusion for canine babesiosis. J Vet Emerg Crit Care (San Antonio). 2009 Feb;19(1):102-12. PMID:19691591

Zamoto A, Tsuji M, Kawabuchi T, Wei Q, Asakawa M, Ishihara C. U.S.-type Babesia microti isolated from small wild mammals in Eastern Hokkaido, Japan. J Vet Med Sci. 2004 Aug;66(8):919-26. PMID:15353841

Zamoto A, Tsuji M, Wei Q, Cho SH, Shin EH, Kim TS, Leonova GN, Hagiwara K, Asakawa M, Kariwa H, Takashima I, Ishihara C. Epizootiologic survey for Babesia microti among small wild mammals in northeastern Eurasia and a geographic diversity in the beta-tubulin gene sequences. J Vet Med Sci. 2004 Jul;66(7):785-92. PMID:15297749

Zaugg JL, Lane VM. Efficacy of buparvaquone as a therapeutic and clearing agent of Babesia equi of European origin in horses. Am J Vet Res. 1992 Aug;53(8):1396-9. PMID:1510317

Zhang B, Watts KM, Hodge D, Kemp LM, Hunstad DA, Hicks LM, Odom AR. A second target of the antimalarial and antibacterial agent fosmidomycin revealed by cellular metabolic profiling. Biochemistry. 2011 May 3;50(17):3570-7. Epub 2011 Apr 11. PMID:21438569

Zhang L, Sathunuru R, Caridha D, Pybus B, O'Neil MT, Kozar MP, Lin AJ. Antimalarial activities of new guanidylimidazole and guanidylimidazoline derivatives. J Med Chem. 2011 Oct 13;54(19):6634-46. Epub 2011 Sep 2. PMID:21848332

Zhang W, Xu D, Niu Z, Yin K, Liu P, Chen L. Isolation and characterization of Pseudomonas sp. DX7 capable of degrading sulfadoxine. Biodegradation. 2011 Nov 25. [Epub ahead of print]. PMID:22116408

Zhang Y, Guiguemde WA, Sigal M, Zhu F, Connelly MC, Nwaka S, Guy RK. Synthesis and structure-activity relationships of antimalarial 4-oxo-3-carboxyl quinolones. Bioorg Med Chem. 2010 Apr 1;18(7):2756-66. Epub 2010 Feb 11. PMID:20206533

Zhao JL, Liu ZL, Yao BA, Ma LH. Culture-derived Babesia orientalis exoantigens used as a vaccine against buffalo babesiosis. Parasitol Res. 2002 May;88(13 Suppl 1):S38-40. PMID:12051606

Zhao Y, Jiang W, Li B, Yao Q, Dong J, Cen Y, Pan X, Li J, Zheng J, Pang X, Zhou H. Artesunate enhances radiosensitivity of human non-small cell lung cancer A549 cells via increasing NO production to induce cell cycle arrest at G2/M phase. Int Immunopharmacol. 2011 Dec;11(12):2039-46. Epub 2011 Sep 9. PMID:21907831

Zhao Y, Love KR, Hall SW, Beardell FV. A fatal case of transfusion-transmitted babesiosis in the State of Delaware. Transfusion. 2009 Dec;49(12):2583-7. Epub 2009 Nov 9. PMID:19906041

Zhou J, Zhang G, Nishikawa Y, Fujisaki K, Xuan X. A 38-kDa protein from Babesia gibsoni and its antibody response in an experimentally infected dog. Vet Parasitol. 2006 Nov 5;141(3-4):345-8. Epub 2006 Jul 3. PMID:16815635

Zhu AY, Zhou Y, Khan S, Deitsch KW, Hao Q, Lin H. Plasmodium falciparum Sir2A Preferentially Hydrolyzes Medium and Long Chain Fatty Acyl Lysine. ACS Chem Biol. 2011 Oct 21. [Epub ahead of print]. PMID:21992006

Zhu H, Zhou CS, Liao YK, Bai YY. [Pharmacognostic identification of Cryptolepis buchanaii].[Article in Chinese]. Zhongguo Zhong Yao Za Zhi. 2004 Jul;29(7):634-6. PMID:15503764

Zhu J, Lin S. [Investigation on folk medicine and health care of She ethnic group in Zhejiang province].[Article in Chinese]. Zhonghua Yi Shi Za Zhi. 2002 Oct;32(4):195-9. PMID:12639431

Zhu L, Tian Y. Chemical composition and larvicidal activity of Blumea densiflora essential oils against Anopheles anthropophagus: a malarial vector mosquito. Parasitol Res. 2011 Nov;109(5):1417-22. Epub 2011 May 10. PMID:21556689

Zhu L, Tian YJ. Chemical composition and larvicidal effects of essential oil of Blumea martiniana against Anopheles anthropophagus. Asian Pac J Trop Med. 2011 May;4(5):371-4. Epub 2011 Jun 22. PMID:21771679

Zintl A, Skerrett HE, Gray JS, Brophy PO, Mulcahy G. Babesia divergens (Phylum Apicomplexa) in vitro growth in the presence of calf serum. Vet Parasitol. 2004 Jun 21;122(2):127-30. PMID:15177717

Zintl A, Westbrook C, Skerrett HE, Gray JS, Mulcahy G. Chymotrypsin and neuraminidase treatment inhibits host cell invasion by Babesia divergens (Phylum Apicomplexa). Parasitology. 2002 Jul;125(Pt 1):45-50. PMID:12166519

Zivkovic D, Seinen W, Kuil H, Albers-van Bemmel CM, Speksnijder JE. Immunity to Babesia in mice. I. Adoptive transfer of immunity to Babesia rodhaini with immune spleen cells and the effect of irradiation on the protection of immune mice. Vet Immunol Immunopathol. 1984 Mar;5(4):343-57. PMID:6730310

Zivkovic D, Speksnijder JE, Kuil H, Seinen W. Immunity to Babesia in mice. II. Cross protection between various Babesia and Plasmodium species and its relevance to the nature of Babesia immunity. Vet Immunol Immunopathol. 1984 Mar;5(4):359-68. PMID:6730311

Zivkovic Z, Torina A, Mitra R, Alongi A, Scimeca S, Kocan KM, Galindo RC, Almazán C, Blouin EF, Villar M, Nijhof AM, Mani R, La Barbera G, Caracappa S, Jongejan F, de la Fuente J. Subolesin expression in response to pathogen infection in ticks. BMC Immunol. 2010 Feb 19;11:7. PMID:20170494

Zobba R, Parpaglia ML, Spezzigu A, Pittau M, Alberti A. First molecular identification and phylogeny of a Babesia sp. from a symptomatic sow (Sus scrofa Linnaeus 1758). J Clin Microbiol. 2011 Jun;49(6):2321-4. Epub 2011 Apr 13. PMID:21490184

Zofou D, Kengne AB, Tene M, Ngemenya MN, Tane P, Titanji VP. In vitro antiplasmodial activity and cytotoxicity of crude extracts and compounds from the stem bark of Kigelia africana (Lam.) Benth (Bignoniaceae). Parasitol Res. 2011 Jun;108(6):1383-90. Epub 2011 Apr 13. PMID:21487780

Zong S, Kron MW, Epp C, Engler T, Bujard H, Kochanek S, Kreppel F. ΔE1 and high-capacity adenoviral vectors expressing full-length codon-optimized merozoite surface protein 1 for vaccination against Plasmodium falciparum. J Gene Med. 2011 Nov 16. [Epub ahead of print]. PMID:22095915

Zsila F, Visy J, Mády G, Fitos I. Selective plasma protein binding of antimalarial drugs to alpha1-acid glycoprotein. Bioorg Med Chem. 2008 Apr 1;16(7):3759-72. Epub 2008 Feb 2. PMID:18289858

Zweygarth E, Ahmed JS, Rehbein G. The effect of halofuginone, Wellcome 993 C, oxytetracycline, and diminazene diaceturate on Babesia equi-infected lymphoblastoid cell cultures. J Parasitol. 1984 Aug;70(4):542-4. PMID:6502356

Zweygarth E, Just MC, de Waal DT. Continuous in vitro cultivation of erythrocytic stages of Babesia equi. Parasitol Res. 1995;81(4):355-8. PMID:7624296

Zweygarth E, Van Niekerk C, Just MC, De Waal DT. In vitro cultivation of a Babesia sp. from cattle in South Africa. Onderstepoort J Vet Res. 1995 Jun;62(2):139-42. PMID:8600438

The Definitive Collection of Academic References on Lyme Disease and the Pathology of Borrelia

Introduction — Lyme Disease

I have been studying tick infections full-time for many years. While we have learned many things about Bartonella, Babesia and Lyme disease, we still have many issues that limit application of effective care throughout the world.

Further, the number of true experts on Borrrelia, and who have read most of the publications in English print, is possibly under a hundred individuals.

Finally, Borrelia has huge impacts in human biochemistry, hormones, sleep, sleep quality, personality, insight, hatred, agitation, rigidity, sadness, body sensations, tissue and organs.

The references that follow are a small sample of materials related to this infection.

This book is written for individuals who have a master's degree, a Ph.D. or M.D. in the medical sciences. It is also only for those doing research on these infections. If you are not trained at least at the master's level in mammalian related science, this text is not for you.

Aberer E, Fingerle V, Wutte N, Fink-Puches R, Cerroni L. Within European margins. Lancet. 2011 Jan 8;377(9760):178. PMID:21215884

Abul-Kasim K. Neuroborreliosis with enhancement of the third, fifth, sixth, and twelfth cranial nerves. Acta Neurol Belg. 2010 Jun;110(2):215. PMID:20873460

Adamaszek M, Heinrich A, Rang A, Langner S, Khaw AV. Cerebral sinuvenous thrombosis associated with Lyme neuroborreliosis. J Neurol. 2010 Mar;257(3):481-3. Epub 2009 Nov 26. PMID:19941147

Adham FK, El-Samie-Abd EM, Gabre RM, El Hussein H. Detection of tick blood parasites in Egypt using PCR assay II- Borrelia burgdorferi sensu lato. J Egypt Soc Parasitol. 2010 Dec;40(3):553-64. PMID:21268526

Adusumilli S, Booth CJ, Anguita J, Fikrig E. Passage through Ixodes scapularis ticks enhances the virulence of a weakly pathogenic isolate of Borrelia burgdorferi. Infect Immun. 2010 Jan;78(1):138-44. Epub 2009 Oct 12. PMID:19822652

Agarwal R, Sze G. Neuro-lyme disease: MR imaging findings. Radiology. 2009 Oct;253(1):167-73. Epub 2009 Jul 8. PMID:19587309

Alcalde-Encinas MD, Peñalver-González E, Pavia AR, Tornel Sánchez G. [Diagnostic utility of serology to B. burgdorferi in Cartagena].[Article in Spanish]. Rev Clin Esp. 2010 Jun;210(6):314. PMID:20434146

Alonso S, Márquez FJ, Solano-Gallego L. Borrelia burgdorferi Serosurvey in Wild Deer in England and Wales. Vector Borne Zoonotic Dis. 2012 Mar 26. [Epub ahead of print]. PMID:22448654

Al-Robaiy S, Dihazi H, Kacza J, Seeger J, Schiller J, Huster D, Knauer J, Straubinger RK. Metamorphosis of Borrelia burgdorferi organisms--RNA, lipid and protein composition in context with the spirochetes' shape. J Basic Microbiol. 2010 Dec;50 Suppl 1:S5-17. PMID:20967786

Al-Sharif B, Hall MC. Lyme disease testing in children in an endemic area. WMJ. 2011 Oct;110(5):228-33; quiz 247. PMID:22164580

ALSUntangled Group. ALSUntangled update 1: investigating a bug (Lyme Disease) and a drug (Iplex) on behalf of people with ALS. Amyotroph Lateral Scler. 2009 Aug;10(4):248-50. PMID:19701824

Andersen CL. [Picture of the month: erythema migrans].[Article in Danish]. Ugeskr Laeger. 2011 Feb 21;173(8):590. PMID:21333263

Andres C, Ziai M, Bruckbauer H, Ring J, Hofmann H. Acrodermatitis chronica atrophicans in two children. Int J Dermatol. 2010 Feb;49(2):180-3. PMID:20465643

Ang CW, Notermans DW, Hommes M, Simoons-Smit AM, Herremans T. Large differences between test strategies for the detection of anti-Borrelia antibodies are revealed by comparing eight ELISAs and five immunoblots. Eur J Clin Microbiol Infect Dis. 2011 Aug;30(8):1027-32. Epub 2011 Jan 27. PMID:21271270

Angel TE, Luft BJ, Yang X, Nicora CD, Camp DG 2nd, Jacobs JM, Smith RD. Proteome analysis of Borrelia burgdorferi response to environmental change. PLoS One. 2010 Nov 2;5(11):e13800. PMID:21072190

Angelakis E, Billeter SA, Breitschwerdt EB, Chomel BB, Raoult D. Potential for tick-borne bartonelloses. Emerg Infect Dis. 2010 Mar;16(3):385-91. PMID:20202411

Antonara S, Ristow L, Coburn J. Adhesion mechanisms of Borrelia burgdorferi. Adv Exp Med Biol. 2011;715:35-49. PMID:21557056

Antonara S, Ristow L, McCarthy J, Coburn J. Effect of Borrelia burgdorferi OspC at the site of inoculation in mouse skin. Infect Immun. 2010 Nov;78(11):4723-33. Epub 2010 Aug 9. PMID:20696825

Arnez M, Avsic-Zupanc T. Tick-borne encephalitis in children: an update on epidemiology and diagnosis. Expert Rev Anti Infect Ther. 2009 Dec;7(10):1251-60. PMID:19968516

Arnež M, Ružić-Sabljić E. Borrelia burgdorferi sensu lato bacteremia in Slovenian children with solitary and multiple erythema migrans. Pediatr Infect Dis J. 2011 Nov;30(11):988-90. PMID:21709599

Arnez M, Ruzić-Sabljić E. Lyme borreliosis and acute peripheral facial palsy in Slovenian children. Pediatr Infect Dis J. 2010 Feb;29(2):182-4. PMID:19952981

Asadipooya K, Dehghanian A, Omrani GH, Abbasi F. Short-course treatment in neurobrucellosis: a study in Iran. Neurol India. 2011 Jan-Feb;59(1):101-3. PMID:21339673

Aslan M, Kasapcopur O, Yasar H, Polat E, Saribas S, Cakan H, Dirican A, Torun MM, Arısoy N, Kocazeybek B. Do infections trigger juvenile idiopathic arthritis? Rheumatol Int. 2011 Feb;31(2):215-20. Epub 2009 Dec 13. PMID:20012631

Ates L, Hanssen-Hübner C, Norris DE, Richter D, Kraiczy P, Hunfeld KP. Comparison of in vitro activities of tigecycline, doxycycline, and tetracycline against the spirochete Borrelia burgdorferi. Ticks Tick Borne Dis. 2010 Mar;1(1):30-4. Epub 2010 Jan 7. PMID:21771509

Atkinson S, Ayers A. The potential of the internet for alternative caring practices for health. Anthropol Med. 2010 Apr;17(1):75-86. PMID:20419518

Aucott J, Morrison C, Munoz B, Rowe PC, Schwarzwalder A, West SK. Diagnostic challenges of early Lyme disease: lessons from a community case series. BMC Infect Dis. 2009 Jun 1;9:79. PMID:19486523

Augsten R, Pfister W, Königsdörffer E. [Acute posterior multifocal placoid pigment epitheliopathy (APMPPE) and borreliosis].[Article in German]. Klin Monbl Augenheilkd. 2009 Jun;226(6):512-3. Epub 2009 Jun 8. PMID:19507106

Aupee O, Almeras D, Le Garlantezec P, Bohand X. [Doxycycline]. [Article in French]. Med Trop (Mars). 2009 Dec;69(6):556-8. PMID:20099667

Auwaerter PG, Bakken JS, Dattwyler RJ, Dumler JS, Halperin JJ, McSweegan E, Nadelman RB, O'Connell S, Shapiro ED, Sood SK, Steere AC, Weinstein A, Wormser GP. Antiscience and ethical concerns associated with advocacy of Lyme disease. Lancet Infect Dis. 2011 Sep;11(9):713-9. PMID:21867956

Auwaerter PG, Bakken JS, Dattwyler RJ, Dumler JS, Halperin JJ, McSweegan E, Nadelman RB, O'Connell S, Sood SK, Weinstein A, Wormser GP. Scientific evidence and best patient care practices should guide the ethics of Lyme disease activism. J Med Ethics. 2011 Feb;37(2):68-73. Epub 2010 Nov 21. PMID:21097940

Babu K, Murthy PR. Neuroretinitis as a manifestation of Lyme disease in South India: a case report. Ocul Immunol Inflamm. 2010 Apr;18(2):97-8. PMID:20370334

Babu V, Sukumarannair S, Saul Z. Pancytopenia in a patient with Lyme disease. Infection. 2010 Aug;38(4):339-40. Epub 2010 Apr 1. PMID:20358248

Bachmann M, Horn K, Rudloff I, Goren I, Holdener M, Christen U, Darsow N, Hunfeld KP, Koehl U, Kind P, Pfeilschifter J, Kraiczy P, Mühl H. Early production of IL-22 but not IL-17 by peripheral blood mononuclear cells exposed to live Borrelia burgdorferi: the role of monocytes and interleukin-1. PLoS Pathog. 2010 Oct 14;6(10):e1001144. PMID:20976193

Bacino L, Gazzarata M, Siri G, Cordone S, Bellotti P. [Complete atrioventricular block as the first clinical manifestation of a tick bite (Lyme disease)].[Article in Italian]. G Ital Cardiol (Rome). 2011 Mar;12(3):214-6. PMID:21560478

Baggs EM, Stack SH, Finney-Crawley JR, Simon NP. Peromyscus maniculatus, a possible reservoir host of Borrelia garinii from the Gannet Islands off Newfoundland and Labrador. J Parasitol. 2011 Oct;97(5):792-4. Epub 2011 Mar 17. PMID:21506809

Baker PJ. Chronic Lyme disease: in defense of the scientific enterprise. FASEB J. 2010 Nov;24(11):4175-7. Epub 2010 Jul 14. PMID:20631327

Baker PJ. The pain of "chronic Lyme disease": moving the discourse in a different direction. FASEB J. 2012 Jan;26(1):11-2. Epub 2011 Sep 7. PMID:21900506

Balátová P, Kurzová Z, Hulínská D. [Serology of Lyme borreliosis and human granulocytic ehrlichiosis in 2005-2010].[Article in Czech]. Epidemiol Mikrobiol Imunol. 2011 Jun;60(2):74-6. PMID:21838175

Balicer RD, Mimouni D, Bar-Zeev Y, Levine H, Davidovitch N, Ankol OH, Zarka SS. Post exposure prophylaxis of tick-borne relapsing fever. Eur J Clin Microbiol Infect Dis. 2010 Mar;29(3):253-8. Epub 2009 Dec 13. PMID:20012878

Baneth G, Bourdeau P, Bourdoiseau G, Bowman D, Breitschwerdt E, Capelli G, Cardoso L, Dantas-Torres F, Day M, Dedet JP, Dobler G, Ferrer L, Irwin P, Kempf V, Kohn B, Lappin M, Little S, Maggi R, Miro G, Naucke T, Oliva G, Otranto D, Penzhorn B, Pfeffer M, Roura X, Sainz A, Shaw S, Shin S, Solano-Gallego L, Straubinger R, Traub R, Trees A, Truyen U, Demonceau T, Fitzgerald R, Gatti D, Hostetler J, Kilmer B, Krieger K, Mencke N, Mendao C, Mottier L, Pachnicke S, Rees B, Siebert S, Stanneck D, Tarancon Mingote M, von Simson C, Weston S. Vector-Borne Diseases - constant challenge for practicing veterinarians: recommendations from the CVBD World Forum. Parasit Vectors. 2012 Mar 20;5(1):55. [Epub ahead of print]. PMID:22433172

Banik S, Terekhova D, Iyer R, Pappas CJ, Caimano MJ, Radolf JD, Schwartz I. BB0844, an RpoS-regulated protein, is dispensable for Borrelia burgdorferi infectivity and maintenance in the mouse-tick infectious cycle. Infect Immun. 2011 Mar;79(3):1208-17. Epub 2010 Dec 20. PMID:21173312

Baranova NS, Spirin NN, Shipova EG, Stepanov IO. [Lesions of nervous systems in remote stages of Lyme borreliosis].[Article in Russian]. Zh Nevrol Psikhiatr Im S S Korsakova. 2010;110(2):90- PMID:20607922

Barber RM, Li Q, Diniz PP, Porter BF, Breitschwerdt EB, Claiborne MK, Birkenheuer AJ, Levine JM, Levine GJ, Chandler K, Kenny P, Nghiem P, Wei S, Greene CE, Kent M, Platt SR, Greer K, Schatzberg SJ. Evaluation of brain tissue or cerebrospinal fluid with broadly reactive polymerase chain reaction for Ehrlichia, Anaplasma, spotted fever group Rickettsia, Bartonella, and Borrelia species in canine neurological diseases (109 cases). J Vet Intern Med. 2010 Mar-Apr;24(2):372-8. PMID:20102497

Barbour AG, Bunikis J, Travinsky B, Hoen AG, Diuk-Wasser MA, Fish D, Tsao JI. Niche partitioning of Borrelia burgdorferi and Borrelia miyamotoi in the same tick vector and mammalian reservoir species. Am J Trop Med Hyg. 2009 Dec;81(6):1120-31. PMID:19996447

Barbour AG, Travinsky B. Evolution and distribution of the ospC Gene, a transferable serotype determinant of Borrelia burgdorferi. MBio. 2010 Sep 28;1(4). pii: e00153-10. PMID:20877579

Bárcena-Uribarri I, Thein M, Sacher A, Bunikis I, Bonde M, Bergström S, Benz R. P66 porins are present in both Lyme disease and relapsing fever spirochetes: a comparison of the biophysical properties of P66 porins from six Borrelia species. Biochim Biophys Acta. 2010 Jun;1798(6):1197-203. Epub 2010 Feb 25. PMID:20188698

Barthold SW, Hodzic E, Imai DM, Feng S, Yang X, Luft BJ. Ineffectiveness of tigecycline against persistent Borrelia burgdorferi. Antimicrob Agents Chemother. 2010 Feb;54(2):643-51. Epub 2009 Dec 7. PMID:19995919

Bartosik K, Lachowska-Kotowska P, Szymańska J, Pabis A, Buczek A. Lyme borreliosis in south-eastern Poland: relationships with environmental factors and medical attention standards. Ann Agric Environ Med. 2011 Jun;18(1):131-7. PMID:21736278

Baumann M, Birnbacher R, Koch J, Strobl R, Rostásy K. Uncommon manifestations of neuroborreliosis in children. Eur J Paediatr Neurol. 2010 May;14(3):274-7. Epub 2009 Sep 12. PMID:19748808

Baumgartner JD, Christin L. [2011 news in infections diseases: selected readings].[Article in French]. Rev Med Suisse. 2012 Jan 11;8(323):32-5. PMID:22303737

Bazovska S, Durovska J, Derdakova M, Taragelova V, Pancak J, Zaborska M, Traubner P. The genospecies B. burgdorferi s.l., isolated from ticks and from neurological patients with suspected Lyme borreliosis. Neuro Endocrinol Lett. 2011;32(4):491-5. PMID:21876490

Bazovská S, Durovská J, Pancák J, Záborská M, Derdáková M. [Lyme borreliosis and demyelinating disease of the central nervous system]. [Article in Czech]. Epidemiol Mikrobiol Imunol. 2011 Feb;60(1):45-7. PMID:21542236

Becker AM, Blevins JS, Tomson FL, Eitson JL, Medeiros JJ, Yarovinsky F, Norgard MV, van Oers NS. Invariant NKT cell development requires a full complement of functional CD3 zeta immunoreceptor tyrosine-based activation motifs. J Immunol. 2010 Jun 15;184(12):6822-32. Epub 2010 May 14. PMID:20483726

Belloni B, Andres C, Ring J, Hofmann H. [5-yr-old with borrelial lymphocytoma].[Article in German]. MMW Fortschr Med. 2011 Mar 10;153(10):40. PMID:21644358

Benedix F, Geyer A, Röcken M, Biedermann T. Butterfly rash in a young boy: a quiz. Acta Derm Venereol. 2010;90(1):109-11. PMID:20107747

Benoit VM, Fischer JR, Lin YP, Parveen N, Leong JM. Allelic variation of the Lyme disease spirochete adhesin DbpA influences spirochetal binding to decorin, dermatan sulfate, and mammalian cells. Infect Immun. 2011 Sep;79(9):3501-9. Epub 2011 Jun 27. PMID:21708995

Benoit VM, Petrich A, Alugupalli KR, Marty-Roix R, Moter A, Leong JM, Boyartchuk VL. Genetic control of the innate immune response to Borrelia hermsii influences the course of relapsing fever in inbred strains of mice. Infect Immun. 2010 Feb;78(2):586-94. Epub 2009 Dec 7. PMID:19995898

Berende A, Oosting M, Kullberg BJ, Netea MG, Joosten LA. Activation of innate host defense mechanisms by Borrelia. Eur Cytokine Netw. 2010 Mar;21(1):7-18. Review. PMID:20146985

Berger RE, McGillicuddy DC. Lyme carditis. Intern Emerg Med. 2009 Oct;4(5):419-21. Epub 2009 Jul 21. PMID:19626420

Bergler-Czop B, Lis-Swiety A, Brzezińska-Wcisło L. Scleroderma linearis: hemiatrophia faciei progressiva (Parry-Romberg syndrom) without any changes in CNS and linear scleroderma "en coup de sabre" with CNS tumor. BMC Neurol. 2009 Jul 27;9:39. PMID:19635150

Berrada ZL, Telford SR 3rd. Burden of tick-borne infections on American companion animals. Top Companion Anim Med. 2009 Nov;24(4):175-81. PMID:19945085

Berton M, Nojavan H, Bens G, Estève E. [Localized inflammatory alopecia of the scalp: An unusual presentation of tularemia].[Article in French]. Ann Dermatol Venereol. 2012 Apr;139(4):273-6. Epub 2012 Feb 23. PMID:22482480

Bestor A, Stewart PE, Jewett MW, Sarkar A, Tilly K, Rosa PA. Use of the Cre-lox recombination system to investigate the lp54 gene requirement in the infectious cycle of Borrelia burgdorferi. Infect Immun. 2010 Jun;78(6):2397-407. Epub 2010 Mar 15. PMID:20231410

Bhate C, Schwartz RA. Lyme disease: Part I. Advances and perspectives. J Am Acad Dermatol. 2011 Apr;64(4):619-36; quiz 637-8. PMID:21414493

Bhate C, Schwartz RA. Lyme disease: Part II. Management and prevention. J Am Acad Dermatol. 2011 Apr;64(4):639-53; quiz 654, 653. PMID:21414494

Bhattacharya D, Bensaci M, Luker KE, Luker G, Wisdom S, Telford SR, Hu LT. Development of a baited oral vaccine for use in reservoir-targeted strategies against Lyme disease. Vaccine. 2011 Oct 13;29(44):7818-25. Epub 2011 Aug 2. PMID:21816190

Bhattacharya IS, Dweck M, Francis M. Lyme carditis: a reversible cause of complete atrioventricular block. J R Coll Physicians Edinb. 2010 Jun;40(2):121-2. PMID:21125053

Bhide MR, Escudero R, Camafeita E, Gil H, Jado I, Anda P. Complement factor H binding by different Lyme disease and relapsing fever Borrelia in animals and human. BMC Res Notes. 2009 Jul 15;2:134. PMID:19604355

Biesiada G, Czepiel J, Leśniak M, Garlicki A, Mach T. [The analysis of epidemiology, clinical symptoms, serological tests in the course of borreliosis].[Article in Polish]. Przegl Lek. 2010;67(3):181-3. PMID:20687381

Bigi S, Aebi C, Nauer C, Bigler S, Steinlin M. Acute transverse myelitis in Lyme neuroborreliosis. Infection. 2010 Oct;38(5):413-6. Epub 2010 May 27. PMID:20505978

Bilski B. Occurrence of cases of borreliosis certified as an occupational disease in the province of Wielkopolska (Poland). Ann Agric Environ Med. 2009 Dec;16(2):211-7. PMID:20047253

Binder SC, Telschow A, Meyer-Hermann M. Population Dynamics of Borrelia burgdorferi in Lyme Disease. Front Microbiol. 2012;3:104. Epub 2012 Mar 22. PMID:22470370

Bischoff A. [Positive anti-Borrelia antibody test: still not confirmation of borreliosis].[Article in German]. MMW Fortschr Med. 2011 Apr 7;153(14):14. PMID:21966862

Blaho VA, Buczynski MW, Brown CR, Dennis EA. Lipidomic analysis of dynamic eicosanoid responses during the induction and resolution of Lyme arthritis. J Biol Chem. 2009 Aug 7;284(32):21599-612. Epub 2009 Jun 1. PMID:19487688

Blaho VA, Buczynski MW, Dennis EA, Brown CR. Cyclooxygenase-1 orchestrates germinal center formation and antibody class-switch via regulation of IL-17. J Immunol. 2009 Nov 1;183(9):5644-53. PMID:19843949

Blaho VA, Zhang Y, Hughes-Hanks JM, Brown CR. 5-Lipoxygenase-deficient mice infected with Borrelia burgdorferi develop persistent arthritis. J Immunol. 2011 Mar 1;186(5):3076-84. Epub 2011 Jan 26. PMID:21270404

Blanc F, Ballonzoli L, Marcel C, De Martino S, Jaulhac B, de Seze J. Lyme optic neuritis. J Neurol Sci. 2010 Aug 15;295(1-2):117-9. Epub 2010 Jun 8. PMID:20621802

Blanc F. [Epidemiology of Lyme borreliosis and neuroborreliosis in France].[Article in French]. Rev Neurol (Paris). 2009 Aug-Sep;165(8-9):694-701. Epub 2009 May 17. PMID:19447458

Boggs SR, Cunnion KM, Raafat RH. Ceftriaxone-induced hemolysis in a child with Lyme arthritis: a case for antimicrobial stewardship. Pediatrics. 2011 Nov;128(5):e1289-92. Epub 2011 Oct 3. PMID:21969285

Bolotin EI, Burukhina EG. [Ecology and epidemiology of tick-borne infections in the Primorsky Krai].[Article in Russian]. Parazitologiia. 2009 Sep-Oct;43(5):418-27. PMID:19957909

Bonin S, Tothova SM, Barbazza R, Brunetti D, Stanta G, Trevisan G. Evidence of multiple infectious agents in mycosis fungoides lesions. Exp Mol Pathol. 2010 Aug;89(1):46-50. Epub 2010 May 12. PMID:20470773

Bonnet N, Guis S, Drancourt M, Brouqui P, Berbis P. Borreliosis in a patient treated with anti-TNFα therapy: first case. J Eur Acad Dermatol Venereol. 2011 Mar;25(3):367-8. PMID:20524947

Bouchard C, Beauchamp G, Nguon S, Trudel L, Milord F, Lindsay LR, Bélanger D, Ogden NH. Associations between Ixodes scapularis ticks and small mammal hosts in a newly endemic zone in southeastern Canada: implications for Borrelia burgdorferi transmission. Ticks Tick Borne Dis. 2011 Dec;2(4):183-90. Epub 2011 Nov 10. PMID:22108010

Bourré-Tessier J, Milord F, Pineau C, Vinet E. Indigenous Lyme disease in Quebec. J Rheumatol. 2011 Jan;38(1):183. PMID:21196590

Branda JA, Aguero-Rosenfeld ME, Ferraro MJ, Johnson BJ, Wormser GP, Steere AC. 2-tiered antibody testing for early and late Lyme disease using only an immunoglobulin G blot with the addition of a VlsE band as the second-tier test. Clin Infect Dis. 2010 Jan 1;50(1):20-6. PMID:19947857

Branda JA, Linskey K, Kim YA, Steere AC, Ferraro MJ. Two-tiered antibody testing for Lyme disease with use of 2 enzyme immunoassays, a whole-cell sonicate enzyme immunoassay followed by a VlsE C6 peptide enzyme immunoassay. Clin Infect Dis. 2011 Sep;53(6):541-7. PMID:21865190

Brandenburg AH, van Dam AP, Schellekens J. Problems in comparing test strategies for detection of anti-Borrelia antibodies. Eur J Clin Microbiol Infect Dis. 2011 Aug;30(8):1033-4; author reply 1035-7. Epub 2011 Apr 12. PMID:21484251

Brattig NW, Tenner-Racz K, Korten S, Hoerauf A, Büttner DW. Immunohistology of ectopic secondary lymph follicles in subcutaneous nodules from patients with hyperreactive onchocerciasis (sowda). Parasitol Res. 2010 Aug;107(3):657-66. Epub 2010 Jun 4. PMID:20524133

Brei B, Brownstein JS, George JE, Pound JM, Miller JA, Daniels TJ, Falco RC, Stafford KC 3rd, Schulze TL, Mather TN, Carroll JF, Fish D. Evaluation of the United States Department Of Agriculture Northeast Area-wide Tick Control Project by meta-analysis. Vector Borne Zoonotic Dis. 2009 Aug;9(4):423-30. PMID:19650737

Bremell D, Hagberg L. Clinical characteristics and cerebrospinal fluid parameters in patients with peripheral facial palsy caused by Lyme neuroborreliosis compared with facial palsy of unknown origin (Bell's palsy). BMC Infect Dis. 2011 Aug 10;11:215. PMID:21831262

Bremell D, Säll C, Gisslén M, Hagberg L. Lyme neuroborreliosis in HIV-1 positive men successfully treated with oral doxycycline: a case series and literature review. J Med Case Reports. 2011 Sep 19;5:465. PMID:21929779

Briffotaux J, Kobryn K. Preventing broken Borrelia telomeres: ResT couples dual hairpin telomere formation with product release. J Biol Chem. 2010 Dec 24;285(52):41010-8. Epub 2010 Oct 14. PMID:20952394

Brinkerhoff RJ, Folsom-O'Keefe CM, Streby HM, Bent SJ, Tsao K, Diuk-Wasser MA. Regional variation in immature Ixodes scapularis parasitism on North American songbirds: implications for transmission of the Lyme pathogen, Borrelia burgdorferi. J Med Entomol. 2011 Mar;48(2):422-8. PMID:21485384

Brissette CA, Bykowski T, Cooley AE, Bowman A, Stevenson B. Borrelia burgdorferi RevA antigen binds host fibronectin. Infect Immun. 2009 Jul;77(7):2802-12. Epub 2009 Apr 27. PMID:19398540

Brissette CA, Rossmann E, Bowman A, Cooley AE, Riley SP, Hunfeld KP, Bechtel M, Kraiczy P, Stevenson B. The borrelial fibronectin-binding protein RevA is an early antigen of human Lyme disease. Clin Vaccine Immunol. 2010 Feb;17(2):274-80. Epub 2009 Dec 23. PMID:20032216

Brisson D, Baxamusa N, Schwartz I, Wormser GP. Biodiversity of Borrelia burgdorferi strains in tissues of Lyme disease patients. PLoS One. 2011;6(8):e22926. Epub 2011 Aug 4. PMID:21829670

Brisson D, Vandermause MF, Meece JK, Reed KD, Dykhuizen DE. Evolution of northeastern and midwestern Borrelia burgdorferi, United States. Emerg Infect Dis. 2010 Jun;16(6):911-7. PMID:20507740

British Infection Association. The epidemiology, prevention, investigation and treatment of Lyme borreliosis in United Kingdom patients: a position statement by the British Infection Association. J Infect. 2011 May;62(5):329-38. Epub 2011 Mar 21. PMID:21421007

Broekhuijsen-van Henten DM, Braun KP, Wolfs TF. Clinical presentation of childhood neuroborreliosis; neurological examination may be normal. Arch Dis Child. 2010 Nov;95(11):910-4. Epub 2010 Jun 28. PMID:20584849

Bröker M. Following a tick bite: double infections by tick-borne encephalitis virus and the spirochete borrelia and other potential multiple infections. Zoonoses Public Health. 2012 May;59(3):176-80. Epub 2011 Aug 18. PMID:21848518

Brorson Ø, Brorson SH, Scythes J, MacAllister J, Wier A, Margulis L. Destruction of spirochete Borrelia burgdorferi round-body propagules (RBs) by the antibiotic tigecycline. Proc Natl Acad Sci U S A. 2009 Nov 3;106(44):18656-61. Epub 2009 Oct 20. PMID:19843691

Brorson Ø. [Borrelia burgdorferi--a unique bacterium].[Article in Norwegian]. Tidsskr Nor Laegeforen. 2009 Oct 22;129(20):2114-7. PMID:19855450

Brueckner-Schmutterer K, Baleanu D, Bergua A. [Intermediate uveitis as the "first symptom" of multiple sclerosis].[Article in German]. Klin Monbl Augenheilkd. 2010 Jan;227(1):73-5. Epub 2010 Jan 20. PMID:20091454

Brunner J, Herrmann M, Metzler M, Gaipl U, Reuter G, Haas JP. Oligoclonal expansion of T cells in persistent oligoarticular juvenile idiopathic arthritis. Clin Exp Rheumatol. 2010 Jul-Aug;28(4):592-3. Epub 2010 Aug 31. PMID:20659414

Brunner J, Moschovakis G, Prelog M, Walder G, Wuerzner R, Zimmerhackl LB. Lyme neuroborreliosis: aetiology and diagnosis of facial palsy in children from Tyrol. Klin Padiatr. 2010 Sep;222(5):302-7. Epub 2010 May 7. PMID:20455197

Brunner JL, Cheney L, Keesing F, Killilea M, Logiudice K, Previtali A, Ostfeld RS. Molting success of Ixodes scapularis varies among individual blood meal hosts and species. J Med Entomol. 2011 Jul;48(4):860-6. PMID:21845946

Buchwald F, Abul-Kasim K, Tham J, Hansen BU. Fatal course of cerebral vasculitis induced by neuroborreliosis. Neurol India. 2010 Jan-Feb;58(1):139-41. PMID:20228487

Buczek A, Rudek A, Bartosik K, Szymanska J, Wojcik-Fatla A. Seroepidemiological study of Lyme borreliosis among forestry workers in southern Poland. Ann Agric Environ Med. 2009 Dec;16(2):257-61. PMID:20047259

Bulut C, Tufan ZK, Altun S, Altinel E, Kinikli S, Demiröz AP. [An overlooked disease of tick bites: Lyme disease].[Article in Turkish]. Mikrobiyol Bul. 2009 Jul;43(3):487-92. PMID:19795626

Burbelo PD, Bren KE, Ching KH, Coleman A, Yang X, Kariu T, Iadarola MJ, Pal U. Antibody profiling of Borrelia burgdorferi infection in horses. Clin Vaccine Immunol. 2011 Sep;18(9):1562-7. Epub 2011 Jul 20. PMID:21775514

Burbelo PD, Issa AT, Ching KH, Cohen JI, Iadarola MJ, Marques A. Rapid, simple, quantitative, and highly sensitive antibody detection for lyme disease. Clin Vaccine Immunol. 2010 Jun;17(6):904-9. Epub 2010 Apr 14. PMID:20392886

Burgasova OA, Uskov AN, Grichenko NE, Tseneva GIa. [Features of cytokine levels in serum of patients with tick-borne borreliosis with different clinical signs].[Article in Russian]. Zh Mikrobiol Epidemiol Immunobiol. 2010 May-Jun;(3):67-71. PMID:20734722

Burman M, Nguyen HL, Murthy V, Sen Gupta P, Davies C, Wragg A, Peterson D, Chowdhury TA. Severe orthostatic hypotension in a diabetic patient may not be due to diabetic autonomic neuropathy. Clin Med. 2011 Jun;11(3):290-1. PMID:21902089

Burns LH, Adams CA, Riley SP, Jutras BL, Bowman A, Chenail AM, Cooley AE, Haselhorst LA, Moore AM, Babb K, Fried MG, Stevenson B. BpaB, a novel protein encoded by the Lyme disease spirochete's cp32 prophages, binds to erp Operator 2 DNA. Nucleic Acids Res. 2010 Sep;38(16):5443-55. Epub 2010 Apr 26. PMID:20421207

Busson L, Reynders M, Van den Wijngaert S, Dahma H, Decolvenaer M, Vasseur L, Vandenberg O. Evaluation of commercial screening tests and blot assays for the diagnosis of Lyme borreliosis. Diagn Microbiol Infect Dis. 2012 May 4. [Epub ahead of print]. PMID:22560168

Caimano MJ, Kenedy MR, Kairu T, Desrosiers DC, Harman M, Dunham-Ems S, Akins DR, Pal U, Radolf JD. The hybrid histidine kinase Hk1 is part of a two-component system that is essential for survival of Borrelia burgdorferi in feeding Ixodes scapularis ticks. Infect Immun. 2011 Aug;79(8):3117-30. Epub 2011 May 23. PMID:21606185

Cairns V. Post-Lyme disease symptoms. Am J Med. 2010 Aug;123(8):e21; author reply e23. PMID:20670705

Calderaro A, Montecchini S, Gorrini C, Piccolo G, Chezzi C, Dettori G. Presence of anti-Borrelia burgdorferi antibodies and Borrelia burgdorferi sensu lato DNA in samples of subjects in an area of the Northern Italy in the period 2002-2008. Diagn Microbiol Infect Dis. 2011 Aug;70(4):455-60. Epub 2011 Mar 11. PMID:21397424

Cameron D. Obstacles to trials of chronic Lyme disease in actual practice. Minerva Med. 2009 Oct;100(5):435-6. PMID:19910896

Cameron DJ. Insufficient evidence to deny antibiotic treatment to chronic Lyme disease patients. Med Hypotheses. 2009 Jun;72(6):688-91. Epub 2009 Mar 5. PMID:19268485

Capelli G, Ravagnan S, Montarsi F, Ciocchetta S, Cazzin S, Porcellato E, Babiker AM, Cassini R, Salviato A, Cattoli G, Otranto D. Occurrence and identification of risk areas of Ixodes ricinus-borne pathogens: a cost-effectiveness analysis in north-eastern Italy. Parasit Vectors. 2012 Mar 27;5:61. PMID:22452970

Cardoso L, Mendao C, Madeira de Carvalho L. Prevalence of Dirofilaria immitis, Ehrlichia canis, Borrelia burgdorferi sensu lato, Anaplasma spp. and Leishmania infantum in apparently healthy and CVBD-suspect dogs in Portugal – a national serological study. Parasit Vectors. 2012 Mar 27;5(1):62. [Epub ahead of print]. PMID:22452990

Carpi G, Cagnacci F, Wittekindt NE, Zhao F, Qi J, Tomsho LP, Drautz DI, Rizzoli A, Schuster SC. Metagenomic profile of the bacterial communities associated with Ixodes ricinus ticks. PLoS One. 2011;6(10):e25604. Epub 2011 Oct 13. PMID:22022422

Carrade D, Foley J, Sullivan M, Foley CW, Sykes JE. Spatial distribution of seroprevalence for Anaplasma phagocytophilum, Borrelia burgdorferi, Ehrlichia canis, and Dirofilaria immitis in dogs in Washington, Oregon, and California. Vet Clin Pathol. 2011 Sep;40(3):293-302. Epub 2011 Aug 9. PMID:21827514

Carroll JF, Hill DE, Allen PC, Young KW, Miramontes E, Kramer M, Pound JM, Miller JA, George JE. The impact of 4-Poster deer self-treatment devices at three locations in Maryland. Vector Borne Zoonotic Dis. 2009 Aug;9(4):407-16. PMID:19650735

Carroll JF, Pound JM, Miller JA, Kramer M. Sustained control of Gibson Island, Maryland, populations of Ixodes scapularis and Amblyomma americanum (Acari: Ixodidae) by community-administered 4-Poster deer self-treatment bait stations. Vector Borne Zoonotic Dis. 2009 Aug;9(4):417-21. PMID:19650736

Casjens SR, Fraser-Liggett CM, Mongodin EF, Qiu WG, Dunn JJ, Luft BJ, Schutzer SE. Whole genome sequence of an unusual Borrelia burgdorferi sensu lato isolate. J Bacteriol. 2011 Mar;193(6):1489-90. Epub 2011 Jan 7. PMID:21217002

Casjens SR, Mongodin EF, Qiu WG, Dunn JJ, Luft BJ, Fraser-Liggett CM, Schutzer SE. Whole-genome sequences of two Borrelia afzelii and two Borrelia garinii Lyme disease agent isolates. J Bacteriol. 2011 Dec;193(24):6995-6. PMID:22123755

Casjens SR, Mongodin EF, Qiu WG, Luft BJ, Schutzer SE, Gilcrease EB, Huang WM, Vujadinovic M, Aron JK, Vargas LC, Freeman S, Radune D, Weidman JF, Dimitrov GI, Khouri HM, Sosa JE, Halpin RA, Dunn JJ, Fraser CM. Genome stability of Lyme disease spirochetes: comparative genomics of Borrelia burgdorferi plasmids. PLoS One. 2012;7(3):e33280. Epub 2012 Mar 14. PMID:22432010

Casselli T, Tourand Y, Bankhead T. Altered Murine Tissue Colonization by Borrelia burgdorferi following Targeted Deletion of Linear Plasmid 17-Carried Genes. Infect Immun. 2012 May;80(5):1773-82. Epub 2012 Feb 21. PMID:22354033

Cekanac R, Pavlovic N, Gledovic Z, Grgurevic A, Stajkovic N, Lepsanovic Z, Ristanovic E. Prevalence of Borrelia burgdorferi in Ixodes ricinus ticks in Belgrade area. Vector Borne Zoonotic Dis. 2010 Jun;10(5):447-52. PMID:20017716

Centers for Disease Control and Prevention (CDC). Tickborne relapsing fever in a mother and newborn child--Colorado, 2011. MMWR Morb Mortal Wkly Rep. 2012 Mar 16;61(10):174-6. PMID:22419050

Cerar D, Cerar T, Ruzić-Sabljić E, Wormser GP, Strle F. Subjective symptoms after treatment of early Lyme disease. Am J Med. 2010 Jan;123(1):79-86. PMID:20102996

Cerar T, Ogrinc K, Strle F, Ruzić-Sabljić E. Humoral immune responses in patients with Lyme neuroborreliosis. Clin Vaccine Immunol. 2010 Apr;17(4):645-50. Epub 2010 Feb 17. PMID:20164248

Cerny R, Rozsypal H, Kozner P, Machala L. Bilateral Holmes-Adie syndrome as an early manifestation of the HIV neuropathy. Neurol Sci. 2010 Oct;31(5):661-3. Epub 2010 Jun 22. PMID:20567990

Chaconas G, Kobryn K. Structure, function, and evolution of linear replicons in Borrelia. Annu Rev Microbiol. 2010;64:185-202. PMID:20536352

Chaconas G. CSM murray award lecture - functional studies of the Lyme disease spirochete - from molecules to mice. Can J Microbiol. 2012 Mar;58(3):236-48. Epub 2012 Feb 17. PMID:22339274

Chambert T, Staszewski V, Lobato E, Choquet R, Carrie C, McCoy KD, Tveraa T, Boulinier T. Exposure of black-legged kittiwakes to Lyme disease spirochetes: dynamics of the immune status of adult hosts and effects on their survival. J Anim Ecol. 2012 Mar 19. [Epub ahead of print]. PMID:22428953

Chan K, Casjens S, Parveen N. Detection of established virulence genes and plasmids to differentiate Borrelia burgdorferi strains. Infect Immun. 2012 Apr;80(4):1519-29. Epub 2012 Jan 30. PMID:22290150

Chandra A, Latov N, Wormser GP, Marques AR, Alaedini A. Epitope mapping of antibodies to VlsE protein of Borrelia burgdorferi in post-Lyme disease syndrome. Clin Immunol. 2011 Oct;141(1):103-10. Epub 2011 Jul 2. PMID:21778118

Chandra A, Wormser GP, Klempner MS, Trevino RP, Crow MK, Latov N, Alaedini A. Anti-neural antibody reactivity in patients with a history of Lyme borreliosis and persistent symptoms. Brain Behav Immun. 2010 Aug;24(6):1018-24. Epub 2010 Mar 18. PMID:20227484

Chandra A, Wormser GP, Marques AR, Latov N, Alaedini A. Anti-Borrelia burgdorferi antibody profile in post-Lyme disease syndrome. Clin Vaccine Immunol. 2011 May;18(5):767-71. Epub 2011 Mar 16. PMID:21411605

Chandrashekar R, Mainville CA, Beall MJ, O'Connor T, Eberts MD, Alleman AR, Gaunt SD, Breitschwerdt EB. Performance of a commercially available in-clinic ELISA for the detection of antibodies against Anaplasma phagocytophilum, Ehrlichia canis, and Borrelia burgdorferi and Dirofilaria immitis antigen in dogs. Am J Vet Res. 2010 Dec;71(12):1443-50. PMID:21117995

Chang BL, Shih CM, Ro LS, Huang CC, Lyu RK, Chen RS, Lee JD, Chao LL, Kuo HC. Acute neuroborreliosis with involvement of the central nervous system. J Neurol Sci. 2010 Aug 15;295(1-2):10-5. Epub 2010 Jun 18. PMID:20561635

Chang CM, Landgren O, Koshiol J, Björkholm M, Löve TJ, Kristinsson SY. Borrelia and subsequent risk of solid tumors and hematologic malignancies in Sweden. Int J Cancer. 2012 Feb 9. [Epub ahead of print]. PMID:22322900

Chao LL, Chen YJ, Shih CM. First detection and molecular identification of Borrelia garinii isolated from human skin in Taiwan. J Med Microbiol. 2010 Feb;59(Pt 2):254-7. Epub 2009 Nov 12. PMID:19910482

Chao LL, Chen YJ, Shih CM. First isolation and molecular identification of Borrelia burgdorferi sensu stricto and Borrelia afzelii from skin biopsies of patients in Taiwan. Int J Infect Dis. 2011 Mar;15(3):e182-7. Epub 2010 Dec 13. PMID:21147012

Check JH, Cohen R. Sympathetic neural hyperalgesia edema syndrome, a frequent cause of pelvic pain in women, mistaken for Lyme disease with chronic fatigue. Clin Exp Obstet Gynecol. 2011;38(4):412-3. PMID:22268288

Chen S, Kumru OS, Zückert WR. Determination of Borrelia surface lipoprotein anchor topology by surface proteolysis. J Bacteriol. 2011 Nov;193(22):6379-83. Epub 2011 Sep 9. PMID:21908659

Chen S, Zückert WR. Probing the Borrelia burgdorferi surface lipoprotein secretion pathway using a conditionally folding protein domain. J Bacteriol. 2011 Dec;193(23):6724-32. Epub 2011 Sep 30. PMID:21965569

Childs JE. Low tech versus high tech approaches for vector-borne disease control. Vector Borne Zoonotic Dis. 2009 Aug;9(4):355-6. PMID:19650728

Chmelar J, Calvo E, Pedra JH, Francischetti IM, Kotsyfakis M. Tick salivary secretion as a source of antihemostatics. J Proteomics. 2012 Apr 27. [Epub ahead of print]. PMID:22564820

Chmielewski T, Andrzejewski K, Maczka I, Fiecek B, Radlińska M, Tylewska-Wierzbanowska S. [Ticks infected with bacteria pathogenic to humans in municipal parks in Warsaw].[Article in Polish]. Przegl Epidemiol. 2011;65(4):577-81. PMID:22390042

Chmielewski T, Tylewska-Wierzbanowska S. Interactions between Borrelia burgdorferi and mouse fibroblasts. Pol J Microbiol. 2010;59(3):157-60. PMID:21033577

Chojnowska S, Kępka A, Szajda SD, Waszkiewicz N, Bierć M, Zwierz K. Exoglycosidase markers of diseases. Biochem Soc Trans. 2011 Jan;39(1):406-9. PMID:21265813

Chrubasik C, Jacobson R. Re: tick bites in a Lyme borreliosis highly endemic area in Switzerland. Int J Med Microbiol. 2012 Jan;302(1):61-2. Epub 2011 Sep 9. PMID:21907617

Cohn KA, Thompson AD, Shah SS, Hines EM, Lyons TW, Welsh EJ, Nigrovic LE. Validation of a clinical prediction rule to distinguish Lyme meningitis from aseptic meningitis. Pediatrics. 2012 Jan;129(1):e46-53. Epub 2011 Dec 19. PMID:22184651

Coipan EC, Vladimirescu AF. First report of lyme disease spirochetes in ticks from Romania (Sibiu County). Exp Appl Acarol. 2010 Oct;52(2):193-7. Epub 2010 Mar 16. PMID:20232115

Coipan EC, Vladimirescu AF. Ixodes ricinus ticks (Acari: Ixodidae): vectors for Lyme disease spirochetes in Romania. Exp Appl Acarol. 2011 Jul;54(3):293-300. Epub 2011 Mar 24. PMID:21431930

Coleman AS, Pal U. BBK07, a dominant in vivo antigen of Borrelia burgdorferi, is a potential marker for serodiagnosis of Lyme disease. Clin Vaccine Immunol. 2009 Nov;16(11):1569-75. Epub 2009 Sep 23. PMID:19776192

Coleman AS, Rossmann E, Yang X, Song H, Lamichhane CM, Iyer R, Schwartz I, Pal U. BBK07 immunodominant peptides as serodiagnostic markers of Lyme disease. Clin Vaccine Immunol. 2011 Mar;18(3):406-13. Epub 2010 Dec 22. PMID:21177911

Coleman JL, Katona LI, Kuhlow C, Toledo A, Okan NA, Tokarz R, Benach JL. Evidence that two ATP-dependent (Lon) proteases in Borrelia burgdorferi serve different functions. PLoS Pathog. 2009 Nov;5(11):e1000676. Epub 2009 Nov 26. PMID:19956677

Colin de Verdiere N, Hamane S, Assous MV, Sertour N, Ferquel E, Cornet M. Tickborne relapsing fever caused by Borrelia persica, Uzbekistan and Tajikistan. Emerg Infect Dis. 2011 Jul;17(7):1325-7. PMID:21762608

Colombo MJ, Abraham D, Shibuya A, Alugupalli KR. B1b lymphocyte-derived antibodies control Borrelia hermsii independent of Fcα/μ receptor and in the absence of host cell contact. Immunol Res. 2011 Dec;51(2-3):249-56. PMID:22139824

Colombo MJ, Sun G, Alugupalli KR. T-cell-independent immune responses do not require CXC ligand 13-mediated B1 cell migration. Infect Immun. 2010 Sep;78(9):3950-6. Epub 2010 Jun 28. PMID:20584971

Colović N, Bumbasirević L, Palibrk V, Vidović A, Colović M. [Neuroborreliosis in patient with aplastic anaemia secondary to therapy with ticlopidine].[Article in Serbian]. Srp Arh Celok Lek. 2010 Sep-Oct;138(9-10):632-4. PMID:21180094

Comstedt P, Asokliene L, Eliasson I, Olsen B, Wallensten A, Bunikis J, Bergström S. Complex population structure of Lyme borreliosis group spirochete Borrelia garinii in subarctic Eurasia. PLoS One. 2009 Jun 9;4(6):e5841. PMID:19513109

Connally NP, Durante AJ, Yousey-Hindes KM, Meek JI, Nelson RS, Heimer R. Peridomestic Lyme disease prevention: results of a population-based case-control study. Am J Prev Med. 2009 Sep;37(3):201-6. PMID:19595558

Cordonnier P, Iltis C, Martinez C, Blaison G, Martinot M. [Neuroborreliosis after an early Lyme disease treated by azithromycin]. [Article in French]. Med Mal Infect. 2010 Aug;40(8):493-5. Epub 2009 Nov 28. PMID:19945810

Cornell KA, Primus S, Martinez JA, Parveen N. Assessment of methylthioadenosine/S-adenosylhomocysteine nucleosidases of Borrelia burgdorferi as targets for novel antimicrobials using a novel high-throughput method. J Antimicrob Chemother. 2009 Jun;63(6):1163-72. Epub 2009 Apr 17. PMID:19376840

Coulon CL, Landin D. Lyme disease as an underlying cause of supraspinatus tendinopathy in an overhead athlete. Phys Ther. 2012 May;92(5):740-7. Epub 2012 Jan 12. PMID:22247404

Coumou J, Hovius JW. [Lyme disease].[Article in Dutch]. Ned Tijdschr Tandheelkd. 2011 Jun;118(6):310-6. PMID:21761794

Coumou J, van der Poll T, Speelman P, Hovius JW. Tired of Lyme borreliosis. Lyme borreliosis in the Netherlands. Neth J Med. 2011 Mar;69(3):101-11. PMID:21444934

Couper D, Margos G, Kurtenbach K, Turton S. Prevalence of Borrelia infection in ticks from wildlife in south-west England. Vet Rec. 2010 Dec 25;167(26):1012-4. PMID:21262733

Couto CG, Lorentzen L, Beall MJ, Shields J, Bertolone N, Couto JI, Couto KM, Nash S, Slack J, Kvitko H, Westendorf N, Marin L, Iazbik MC, Vicario FC, Sanz P, Ruano R. Serological study of selected vector-borne diseases in shelter dogs in central Spain using point-of-care assays. Vector Borne Zoonotic Dis. 2010 Nov;10(9):885-8. Epub 2010 Apr 26. PMID:20420531

Cromley RG, Cromley EK. Choropleth map legend design for visualizing community health disparities. Int J Health Geogr. 2009 Sep 24;8:52. PMID:19778435

Crowder CD, Matthews HE, Schutzer S, Rounds MA, Luft BJ, Nolte O, Campbell SR, Phillipson CA, Li F, Sampath R, Ecker DJ, Eshoo MW. Genotypic variation and mixtures of Lyme Borrelia in Ixodes ticks from North America and Europe. PLoS One. 2010 May 14;5(5):e10650. PMID:20498837

Crowder CD, Rounds MA, Phillipson CA, Picuri JM, Matthews HE, Halverson J, Schutzer SE, Ecker DJ, Eshoo MW. Extraction of total nucleic acids from ticks for the detection of bacterial and viral pathogens. J Med Entomol. 2010 Jan;47(1):89-94. PMID:20180313

Cullen E. Lyme disease and climate change. Ir Med J. 2010 Apr;103(4):101-2. PMID:20486310

Cutler S. Spirochaetes: past lessons to future directions. Clin Microbiol Infect. 2011 Apr;17(4):481-3. PMID:21414080

Cutler SJ, Bonilla EM, Singh RJ. Population structure of East African relapsing fever Borrelia spp. Emerg Infect Dis. 2010 Jul;16(7):1076-80. PMID:20587177

Cutler SJ, Rinky IJ, Bonilla EM. Does RecA have a role in Borrelia recurrentis? Clin Microbiol Infect. 2011 Feb;17(2):195-7. PMID:20456459

Cutler SJ. Relapsing fever--a forgotten disease revealed. J Appl Microbiol. 2010 Apr;108(4):1115-22. Epub 2009 Oct 20. PMID:19886891

Czell D, Rodic B, Imoberdorf R. [Neuroborreliosis--a disease with many faces].[Article in German]. Praxis (Bern 1994). 2011 May 11;100(10):607-12. PMID:21563099

Czupryna P, Moniuszko A, Czeczuga A, Pancewicz S, Zajkowska J. Ultrasonographic evaluation of knee joints in patients with Lyme disease. Int J Infect Dis. 2012 Apr;16(4):e252-5. Epub 2012 Jan 31. PMID:22300957

Dai J, Narasimhan S, Zhang L, Liu L, Wang P, Fikrig E. Tick histamine release factor is critical for Ixodes scapularis engorgement and transmission of the lyme disease agent. PLoS Pathog. 2010 Nov 24;6(11):e1001205. PMID:21124826

Dai J, Wang P, Adusumilli S, Booth CJ, Narasimhan S, Anguita J, Fikrig E. Antibodies against a tick protein, Salp15, protect mice from the Lyme disease agent. Cell Host Microbe. 2009 Nov 19;6(5):482-92. PMID:19917502

Daniels TJ, Falco RC, McHugh EE, Vellozzi J, Boccia T, Denicola AJ, Pound JM, Miller JA, George JE, Fish D. Acaricidal treatment of white-tailed deer to control Ixodes scapularis (Acari: Ixodidae) in a New York Lyme disease-endemic community. Vector Borne Zoonotic Dis. 2009 Aug;9(4):381-7. PMID:19650732

Dattwyler RJ. A commentary on the treatment of early lyme disease. Clin Infect Dis. 2010 Feb 15;50(4):521-2. PMID:20070236

Day MJ. One health: the importance of companion animal vector-borne diseases. Parasit Vectors. 2011 Apr 13;4:49. PMID:21489237

Day MJ. The immunopathology of canine vector-borne diseases. Parasit Vectors. 2011 Apr 13;4:48. PMID:21489234

de Carvalho IL, Zeidner N, Ullmann A, Hojgaard A, Amaro F, Zé-Zé L, Alves MJ, de Sousa R, Piesman J, Núncio MS. Molecular characterization of a new isolate of Borrelia lusitaniae derived from Apodemus sylvaticus in Portugal. Vector Borne Zoonotic Dis. 2010 Jun;10(5):531-4. PMID:19725761

D'Elios MM, Codolo G, de Bernard M. Reply to letter by Nardelli and Schell commenting on the pathogenesis of Lyme arthritis. Arthritis Rheum. 2009 Jul;60(7):2205. PMID:19565494

Derler AM, Eisendle K, Baltaci M, Obermoser G, Zelger B. High prevalence of 'Borrelia-like' organisms in skin biopsies of sarcoidosis patients from Western Austria. J Cutan Pathol. 2009 Dec;36(12):1262-8. PMID:19469874

Desenclos JC, Laporte A, Brouqui P. [Louse-borne infections in humans].[Article in French]. Med Mal Infect. 2011 Jun;41(6):295-300. Epub 2011 Mar 30. PMID:21450425

Dessau RB, Bangsborg JM, Ejlertsen T, Skarphedinsson S, Schønheyder HC. Utilization of serology for the diagnosis of suspected Lyme borreliosis in Denmark: survey of patients seen in general practice. BMC Infect Dis. 2010 Nov 1;10:317. PMID:21040576

Dessau RB, Ejlertsen T, Hilden J. Simultaneous use of serum IgG and IgM for risk scoring of suspected early Lyme borreliosis: graphical and bivariate analyses. APMIS. 2010 Apr;118(4):313-23. PMID:20402677

Di Renzi S, Martini A, Binazzi A, Marinaccio A, Vonesch N, D'Amico W, Moro T, Fiorentini C, Ciufolini MG, Visca P, Tomao P. Risk of acquiring tick-borne infections in forestry workers from Lazio, Italy. Eur J Clin Microbiol Infect Dis. 2010 Dec;29(12):1579-81. Epub 2010 Aug 18. PMID:20714765

Diaz JH. Endemic tickborne infectious diseases in Louisiana and the Gulf South. J La State Med Soc. 2009 Nov-Dec;161(6):325-6, 328, 330-1 passim. PMID:20108827

DiCarlo EF, Kahn LB. Inflammatory diseases of the bones and joints. Semin Diagn Pathol. 2011 Feb;28(1):53-64. PMID:21675377

Dickinson GS, Alugupalli KR. Deciphering the role of Toll-like receptors in humoral responses to Borreliae. Front Biosci (Schol Ed). 2012 Jan 1;4:699-712. PMID:22202086

Dickinson GS, Piccone H, Sun G, Lien E, Gatto L, Alugupalli KR. Toll-like receptor 2 deficiency results in impaired antibody responses and septic shock during Borrelia hermsii infection. Infect Immun. 2010 Nov;78(11):4579-88. Epub 2010 Aug 9. PMID:20696824

Dieterich R, Hammerschmidt C, Richter D, Skerka C, Wallich R, Matuschka FR, Zipfel PF, Kraiczy P. Inadequate binding of immune regulator factor H is associated with sensitivity of Borrelia lusitaniae to human complement. Infect Immun. 2010 Nov;78(11):4467-76. Epub 2010 Sep 7. PMID:20823202

Dietrich F, Schmidgen T, Maggi RG, Richter D, Matuschka FR, Vonthein R, Breitschwerdt EB, Kempf VA. Prevalence of Bartonella henselae and Borrelia burgdorferi sensu lato DNA in ixodes ricinus ticks in Europe. Appl Environ Microbiol. 2010 Mar;76(5):1395-8. Epub 2010 Jan 8. PMID:20061459

Dillon R, O'Connell S, Wright S. Lyme disease in the U.K.: clinical and laboratory features and response to treatment. Clin Med. 2010 Oct;10(5):454-7. PMID:21117376

Diuk-Wasser MA, Hoen AG, Cislo P, Brinkerhoff R, Hamer SA, Rowland M, Cortinas R, Vourc'h G, Melton F, Hickling GJ, Tsao JI, Bunikis J, Barbour AG, Kitron U, Piesman J, Fish D. Human risk of infection with Borrelia burgdorferi, the Lyme disease agent, in eastern United States. Am J Trop Med Hyg. 2012 Feb;86(2):320-7. PMID:22302869

Djukic M, Schmidt-Samoa C, Lange P, Spreer A, Neubieser K, Eiffert H, Nau R, Schmidt H. Cerebrospinal fluid findings in adults with acute Lyme neuroborreliosis. J Neurol. 2012 Apr;259(4):630-6. Epub 2011 Sep 6. PMID:21898139

Djukic M, Schmidt-Samoa C, Nau R, von Steinbüchel N, Eiffert H, Schmidt H. The diagnostic spectrum in patients with suspected chronic Lyme neuroborreliosis--the experience from one year of a university hospital's Lyme neuroborreliosis outpatients clinic. Eur J Neurol. 2011 Apr;18(4):547-55. Epub 2010 Oct 27. PMID:20977545

Dlouhý P, Honegr K, Krbková L, Pícha D, Rohačová H, Štruncová V. [Lyme borreliosis. Recommendations for diagnosis, therapy and prevention].[Article in Czech]. Klin Mikrobiol Infekc Lek. 2011 Aug;17(4):144-9. PMID:22213854.

Dobler G, Rieg S. [Tick-borne infections].[Article in German]. Dtsch Med Wochenschr. 2011 Jun;136(22):1175-9. Epub 2011 May 24. PMID:21611923

Dolan MC, Jordan RA, Schulze TL, Schulze CJ, Manning MC, Ruffolo D, Schmidt JP, Piesman J, Karchesy JJ. Ability of two natural products, nootkatone and carvacrol, to suppress Ixodes scapularis and Amblyomma americanum (Acari:Ixodidae) in a Lyme disease endemic area of New Jersey. J Econ Entomol. 2009 Dec;102(6):2316-24. PMID:20069863

Dolan MC, Schulze TL, Jordan RA, Dietrich G, Schulze CJ, Hojgaard A, Ullmann AJ, Sackal C, Zeidner NS, Piesman J. Elimination of Borrelia burgdorferi and Anaplasma phagocytophilum in rodent reservoirs and Ixodes scapularis ticks using a doxycycline hyclate-laden bait. Am J Trop Med Hyg. 2011 Dec;85(6):1114-20. PMID:22144454

Dombrowski C, Kan W, Motaleb MA, Charon NW, Goldstein RE, Wolgemuth CW. The elastic basis for the shape of Borrelia burgdorferi. Biophys J. 2009 Jun 3;96(11):4409-17. PMID:19486665

Donta ST. Subjective symptoms after treatment of Lyme disease. Am J Med. 2010 Aug;123(8):e29; author reply e31. PMID:20670709

Douglas TA, Tamburro D, Fredolini C, Espina BH, Lepene BS, Ilag L, Espina V, Petricoin EF 3rd, Liotta LA, Luchini A. The use of hydrogel microparticles to sequester and concentrate bacterial antigens in a urine test for Lyme disease. Biomaterials. 2011 Feb;32(4):1157-66. Epub 2010 Oct 28. PMID:21035184

Dourmishev LA, Gergovska MJ, Nikolova KK, Balabanova MB. Erythema annulare centrifugum in a patient operated on for breast carcinoma. Acta Dermatovenerol Croat. 2010 Dec;18(4):264-6. PMID:21251444

Drecktrah D, Douglas JM, Samuels DS. Use of rpsL as a Counterselectable Marker in Borrelia burgdorferi. Appl Environ Microbiol. 2010 Feb;76(3):985-7. Epub 2009 Dec 4. PMID:19966024

Dresser AR, Hardy PO, Chaconas G. Investigation of the genes involved in antigenic switching at the vlsE locus in Borrelia burgdorferi: an essential role for the RuvAB branch migrase. PLoS Pathog. 2009 Dec;5(12):e1000680. Epub 2009 Dec 4. PMID:19997508

Dryden M, Hodgkins E. Parasites 100-vector-borne diseases in pets: the stealth health threat. Compend Contin Educ Vet. 2010;32(6):E1-4. PMID:20949426

Dubrey SW, Mehta PA, O'Connell S. Lyme disease and the heart in the UK. Br J Hosp Med (Lond). 2011 Nov;72(11):621-2, 624-5. PMID:22083002

Dulebohn DP, Bestor A, Rego RO, Stewart PE, Rosa PA. Borrelia burgdorferi linear plasmid 38 is dispensable for completion of the mouse-tick infectious cycle. Infect Immun. 2011 Sep;79(9):3510-7. Epub 2011 Jun 27. PMID:21708994

Duncan CJ, Carle G, Seaton RA. Tick bite and early Lyme borreliosis. BMJ. 2012 May 14;344:e3124. PMID:22586232

Dunham-Ems SM, Caimano MJ, Pal U, Wolgemuth CW, Eggers CH, Balic A, Radolf JD. Live imaging reveals a biphasic mode of dissemination of Borrelia burgdorferi within ticks. J Clin Invest. 2009 Dec;119(12):3652-65. Epub 2009 Nov 16. PMID:19920352

Durovska J, Bazovska S, Ondrisova M, Pancak J. Our experience with examination of antibodies against antigens of Borrelia burgdorferi in patients with suspected lyme disease. Bratisl Lek Listy. 2010;111(3):153-5. PMID:20437826

Durovska J, Bazovska S, Pancak J, Zaborska M, Derdakova M, Traubner P. Infection with B. burgdorferi s.l., and the CNS demyelinating disease. A case report. Neuro Endocrinol Lett. 2011;32(4):411-4. PMID:21876503

Dutkiewicz J, Cisak E, Sroka J, Wójcik-Fatla A, Zając V. Biological agents as occupational hazards - selected issues. Ann Agric Environ Med. 2011 Dec;18(2):286-93. PMID:22216801

Dyachenko V, Pantchev N, Balzer HJ, Meyersen A, Straubinger RK. First case of Anaplasma platys infection in a dog from Croatia. Parasit Vectors. 2012 Mar 9;5:49. PMID:22401583

Earl TJ. Cardiac manifestations of Lyme disease. Med Health R I. 2010 Nov;93(11):339-41. PMID:21155514

Earnhart CG, Rhodes DV, Marconi RT. Disulfide-mediated oligomer formation in Borrelia burgdorferi outer surface protein C, a critical virulence factor and potential Lyme disease vaccine candidate. Clin Vaccine Immunol. 2011 Jun;18(6):901-6. Epub 2011 Apr 27. PMID:21525304

Edson RS, Bundrick JB, Litin SC. Clinical pearls in infectious diseases. Mayo Clin Proc. 2011 Mar;86(3):245-8. PMID:21364116

Eggers CH, Caimano MJ, Malizia RA, Kariu T, Cusack B, Desrosiers DC, Hazlett KR, Claiborne A, Pal U, Radolf JD. The coenzyme A disulphide reductase of Borrelia burgdorferi is important for rapid growth throughout the enzootic cycle and essential for infection of the mammalian host. Mol Microbiol. 2011 Nov;82(3):679-97. Epub 2011 Oct 12. PMID:21923763

Eisen L, Eisen RJ, Mun J, Salkeld DJ, Lane RS. Transmission cycles of Borrelia burgdorferi and B. bissettii in relation to habitat type in northwestern California. J Vector Ecol. 2009 Jun;34(1):81-91. PMID:20514140

Eisen L, Eisen RJ. Using geographic information systems and decision support systems for the prediction, prevention, and control of vector-borne diseases. Annu Rev Entomol. 2011;56:41-61. PMID:20868280

Eisen RJ, Eisen L, Girard YA, Fedorova N, Mun J, Slikas B, Leonhard S, Kitron U, Lane RS. A spatially-explicit model of acarological risk of exposure to Borrelia burgdorferi-infected Ixodes pacificus nymphs in northwestern California based on woodland type, temperature, and water vapor. Ticks Tick Borne Dis. 2010 Mar;1(1):35-43. PMID:20532183

Eisen RJ, Piesman J, Zielinski-Gutierrez E, Eisen L. What do we need to know about disease ecology to prevent Lyme disease in the northeastern United States? J Med Entomol. 2012 Jan;49(1):11-22. PMID:22308766

Ekeberg Ø. Demanding diagnostics--important diagnosis.[Article in English, Norwegian]. Tidsskr Nor Laegeforen. 2012 Mar 6;132(5):539-40. PMID:22398773

Eker HE, Izmirli H, Akin S, Ozyilkan NB, Aribogan A, Arslan G. Meperidine induced seizure in a patient with lyme borreliosis. J Clin Med Res. 2009 Dec;1(5):302-4. Epub 2009 Dec 28. PMID:22481996

Ekner A, Dudek K, Sajkowska Z, Majláthová V, Majláth I, Tryjanowski P. Anaplasmataceae and Borrelia burgdorferi sensu lato in the sand lizard Lacerta agilis and co-infection of these bacteria in hosted Ixodes ricinus ticks. Parasit Vectors. 2011 Sep 20;4:182. PMID:21933412

Elamin M, Alderazi Y, Mullins G, Farrell MA, O'Connell S, Counihan TJ. Perineuritis in acute lyme neuroborreliosis. Muscle Nerve. 2009 Jun;39(6):851-4. PMID:19441045

Elamin M, Monaghan T, Mulllins G, Ali E, Corbett-Feeney G, O'Connell S, Counihan TJ. The clinical spectrum of Lyme neuroborreliosis. Ir Med J. 2010 Feb;103(2):46-9. PMID:20666055

Elbaum-Garfinkle S. Close to home: a history of Yale and Lyme disease. Yale J Biol Med. 2011 Jun;84(2):103-8. PMID:21698040

Embers ME, Barthold SW, Borda JT, Bowers L, Doyle L, Hodzic E, Jacobs MB, Hasenkampf NR, Martin DS, Narasimhan S, Phillippi-Falkenstein KM, Purcell JE, Ratterree MS, Philipp MT. Persistence of Borrelia burgdorferi in rhesus macaques following antibiotic treatment of disseminated infection. PLoS One. 2012;7(1):e29914. Epub 2012 Jan 11. PMID:22253822

Emkey GR, Stone JH. A 46-year-old woman with chin pain and a fainting spell. Arthritis Care Res (Hoboken). 2010 Mar;62(3):434-8. PMID:20391493

Ergünay K, Saygan MB, Aydoğan S, Litzba N, Sener B, Lederer S, Niedrig M, Hasçelik G, Us D. Confirmed exposure to tick-borne encephalitis virus and probable human cases of tick-borne encephalitis in Central/Northern Anatolia, Turkey. Zoonoses Public Health. 2011 May;58(3):220-7. PMID:20604912

Espinoza-León F, Arocha F, Hassanhi M, Arévalo J. [Using the polymerase chain reaction to Borrelia burgdorferi infection in localized scleroderma injure (morphea), in Venezuelan patients].[Article in Spanish]. Invest Clin. 2010 Sep;51(3):381-90. PMID:21305774

Estrada-Peña A, Ayllón N, de la Fuente J. Impact of climate trends on tick-borne pathogen transmission. Front Physiol. 2012;3:64. Epub 2012 Mar 27. PMID:22470348

Evans NJ, Bown K, Timofte D, Simpson VR, Birtles RJ. Fatal borreliosis in bat caused by relapsing fever spirochete, United Kingdom. Emerg Infect Dis. 2009 Aug;15(8):1331-3. PMID:19751613

Evans R, Mavin S, McDonagh S, Chatterton JM, Milner R, Ho-Yen DO. More specific bands in the IgG western blot in sera from Scottish patients with suspected Lyme borreliosis. J Clin Pathol. 2010 Aug;63(8):719-21. Epub 2010 Jun 30. PMID:20595179

Fallon BA, Levin ES, Schweitzer PJ, Hardesty D. Inflammation and central nervous system Lyme disease. Neurobiol Dis. 2010 Mar;37(3):534-41. Epub 2009 Nov 26. PMID:19944760

Fand R. Pruritus in latent Lyme disease. Conn Med. 2009 Aug;73(7):445. PMID:19708331

Fikrig E, Narasimhan S, Neelakanta G, Pal U, Chen M, Flavell R. Toll-like receptors 1 and 2 heterodimers alter Borrelia burgdorferi gene expression in mice and ticks. J Infect Dis. 2009 Oct 15;200(8):1331-40. PMID:19754309

Fine AM, Brownstein JS, Nigrovic LE, Kimia AA, Olson KL, Thompson AD, Mandl KD. Integrating spatial epidemiology into a decision model for evaluation of facial palsy in children. Arch Pediatr Adolesc Med. 2011 Jan;165(1):61-7. PMID:21199982

Fine LM, Earnhart CG, Marconi RT. Genetic transformation of the relapsing fever spirochete Borrelia hermsii: stable integration and expression of green fluorescent protein from linear plasmid 200. J Bacteriol. 2011 Jul;193(13):3241-5. Epub 2011 May 6. PMID:21551306

Fish D, Childs JE. Community-based prevention of Lyme disease and other tick-borne diseases through topical application of acaricide to white-tailed deer: background and rationale. Vector Borne Zoonotic Dis. 2009 Aug;9(4):357-64. PMID:19650729

Fisher JB, Curtis CE. An unexpected case of Lyme disease in a soldier serving in northern Iraq. Mil Med. 2010 May;175(5):367-9. PMID:20486511

Floden AM, Watt JA, Brissette CA. Borrelia burgdorferi enolase is a surface-exposed plasminogen binding protein. PLoS One. 2011;6(11):e27502. Epub 2011 Nov 8. PMID:22087329

Flythe JE, Rueda JF, Riscoe MK, Watnick S. Silicate nephrolithiasis after ingestion of supplements containing silica dioxide. Am J Kidney Dis. 2009 Jul;54(1):127-30. Epub 2008 Dec 19. PMID:19100669

Foley JE, Nieto NC. The ecology of tick-transmitted infections in the redwood chipmunk (Tamias ochrogenys). Ticks Tick Borne Dis. 2011 Jun;2(2):88-93. PMID:21643481

Fomenko NV, Borgoiakov VIu, Panov VV. [Genetic features of Borrelia miyamotoi transmitted by Ixodes persulcatus].[Article in Russian]. Mol Gen Mikrobiol Virusol. 2011;(2):12-7. PMID:21786631

Fomenko NV, Livanova NN, Borgoiakov VIu, Kozlova IV, Shulaĭkina IV, Pukhovskaia NM, Tokarevich KN, Livanov SG, Doroshchenko EK, Ivanov LI. [Detection of Borrelia miyamotoi in ticks Ixodes persulcatus from Russia].[Article in Russian]. Parazitologiia. 2010 May-Jun;44(3):201-11. PMID:20795483

Fossati-Bellani MR, Steele RW. A 4-year-old with a "pirate face". Clin Pediatr (Phila). 2011 Jun;50(6):567-9. Epub 2010 Dec 6. PMID:21138849

Frank DB, Patel AR, Sanchez GR, Shah MJ, Bonney WJ. Junctional tachycardia in a child with Lyme carditis. Pediatr Cardiol. 2011 Jun;32(5):689-91. Epub 2011 Mar 6. PMID:21380716

Franke J, Fritzsch J, Tomaso H, Straube E, Dorn W, Hildebrandt A. Coexistence of pathogens in host-seeking and feeding ticks within a single natural habitat in Central Germany. Appl Environ Microbiol. 2010 Oct;76(20):6829-36. Epub 2010 Aug 20. PMID:20729315

Franke J, Hildebrandt A, Meier F, Straube E, Dorn W. Prevalence of Lyme disease agents and several emerging pathogens in questing ticks from the German Baltic coast. J Med Entomol. 2011 Mar;48(2):441-4. PMID:21485387

Franke J, Meier F, Moldenhauer A, Straube E, Dorn W, Hildebrandt A. Established and emerging pathogens in Ixodes ricinus ticks collected from birds on a conservation island in the Baltic Sea. Med Vet Entomol. 2010 Dec;24(4):425-32. Epub 2010 Sep 26. PMID:20868431

Franke J, Moldenhauer A, Hildebrandt A, Dorn W. Are birds reservoir hosts for Borrelia afzelii? Ticks Tick Borne Dis. 2010 Jun;1(2):109-12. Epub 2010 Mar 24. PMID:21771517

Freedman JC, Rogers EA, Kostick JL, Zhang H, Iyer R, Schwartz I, Marconi RT. Identification and molecular characterization of a cyclic-di-GMP effector protein, PlzA (BB0733): additional evidence for the existence of a functional cyclic-di-GMP regulatory network in the Lyme disease spirochete, Borrelia burgdorferi. FEMS Immunol Med Microbiol. 2010 Mar;58(2):285-94. Epub 2009 Nov 23. PMID:20030712

French JB, Cen Y, Vrablik TL, Xu P, Allen E, Hanna-Rose W, Sauve AA. Characterization of nicotinamidases: steady state kinetic parameters, classwide inhibition by nicotinaldehydes, and catalytic mechanism. Biochemistry. 2010 Dec 14;49(49):10421-39. Epub 2010 Nov 15. PMID:20979384

Fritzen CM, Huang J, Westby K, Freye JD, Dunlap B, Yabsley MJ, Schardein M, Dunn JR, Jones TF, Moncayo AC. Infection prevalences of common tick-borne pathogens in adult lone star ticks (Amblyomma americanum) and American dog ticks (Dermacentor variabilis) in Kentucky. Am J Trop Med Hyg. 2011 Oct;85(4):718-23. PMID:21976578

Fryland L, Wilhelmsson P, Lindgren PE, Nyman D, Ekerfelt C, Forsberg P. Low risk of developing Borrelia burgdorferi infection in the south-east of Sweden after being bitten by a Borrelia burgdorferi-infected tick. Int J Infect Dis. 2011 Mar;15(3):e174-81. Epub 2010 Dec 17. PMID:21168354

Füessl HS. [From tick bite to borreliosis: the dreaded small blood sucker].[Article in German]. MMW Fortschr Med. 2011 Jun 2;153(22):14-7. PMID:21688404

Fühler M, Ottmann KW, Tronnier M. [Cutaneous marginal zone lymphoma (SALT) and infection with Borrelia burgdorferi].[Article in German]. Hautarzt. 2010 Feb;61(2):145-7. PMID:19399378

Füssle HS. [Erythema migrans. Can borrelia be transmitted other than by ticks?].[Article in German]. MMW Fortschr Med. 2011 Sep 29;153(39):22. PMID:21991831

Fukunaga M, Tabuchi N. [Molecular mechanism of the borrelial proteins at interface with host and vector tick interactions].[Article in Japanese]. Nihon Saikingaku Zasshi. 2010 Dec;65(2-4):343-53. PMID:20808056

Gajović O, Todorović Z, Nesić L, Lazić Z. [Lyme borreliosis—diagnostic difficulties in interpreting serological results].[Article in Serbian]. Med Pregl. 2010 Nov-Dec;63(11-12):839-43. PMID:21553464

Galeone M, Colucci R, D'Erme AM, Moretti S, Lotti T. Potential Infectious Etiology of Behçet's Disease. Patholog Res Int. 2012;2012:595380. Epub 2011 Dec 29. PMID:22254152

Galiukov IA, Vasilenko FI, Lapidus MS, Anochin AS. [Early recurrence of neuroborreliosis with a fatal outcome].[Article in Russian]. Arkh Patol. 2010 Mar-Apr;72(2):36-7. PMID:20698315

Gan L, Miller FW. State of the art: what we know about infectious agents and myositis. Curr Opin Rheumatol. 2011 Nov;23(6):585-94. PMID:21885972

García-Soler P, Núñez-Cuadros E, Milano-Manso G, Ruiz Sánchez P. [Severe Jarisch-Herxheimer reaction in tick-borne relapsing fever].[Article in Spanish]. Enferm Infecc Microbiol Clin. 2011 Nov;29(9):710-1. Epub 2011 Jun 30. PMID:21723003

Garment AR, Demopoulos BP. False-positive seroreactivity to Borrelia burgdorferi in a patient with thyroiditis. Int J Infect Dis. 2010 Sep;14 Suppl 3:e373. Epub 2010 Jul 1. PMID:20594886

Garnett JM, Connally NP, Stafford KC 3rd, Cartter ML. Evaluation of deer-targeted interventions on Lyme disease incidence in Connecticut. Public Health Rep. 2011 May-Jun;126(3):446-54. PMID:21553675

Garro AC, Rutman MS, Simonsen K, Jaeger JL, Chapin K, Lockhart G. Prevalence of Lyme meningitis in children with aseptic meningitis in a Lyme disease-endemic region. Pediatr Infect Dis J. 2011 Nov;30(11):990-2. PMID:21909050

Gassner F, van Vliet AJ, Burgers SL, Jacobs F, Verbaarschot P, Hovius EK, Mulder S, Verhulst NO, van Overbeek LS, Takken W. Geographic and temporal variations in population dynamics of Ixodes ricinus and associated Borrelia infections in The Netherlands. Vector Borne Zoonotic Dis. 2011 May;11(5):523-32. Epub 2010 Nov 17. PMID:21083369

Gautam A, Dixit S, Philipp MT, Singh SR, Morici LA, Kaushal D, Dennis VA. Interleukin-10 alters effector functions of multiple genes induced by Borrelia burgdorferi in macrophages to regulate Lyme disease inflammation. Infect Immun. 2011 Dec;79(12):4876-92. Epub 2011 Sep 26. PMID:21947773

Gęca A, Gola J, Dudek S, Jasik K, Muc-Wierzgoń M, Nowakowska-Zajdel E, Niedworok E, Mazurek U. Expression of genes associated with H factor in fibroblasts infected with Borrelia spirochaetes. Scand J Immunol. 2012 Jun 11. [Epub ahead of print]. PMID:22686626

Geng Z, Hou XX, Wan KL, Hao Q. [Isolation and identification of Borrelia burgdorferi sensu lato from ticks in six provinces in China.].[Article in Chinese]. Zhonghua Liu Xing Bing Xue Za Zhi. 2010 Dec;31(12):1346-1348. PMID:21223661

Gerber B, Eichenberger S, Haug K, Wittenbrink MM, Reusch CE. Association of urine protein excretion and infection with Borrelia burgdorferi sensu lato in Bernese Mountain dogs. Vet J. 2009 Dec;182(3):487-8. Epub 2008 Oct 17. PMID:18930416

Gerber B, Eichenberger S, Haug K, Wittenbrink MM. [The dilemma with Lyme borreliosis in the dog with particular consideration of "Lyme nephritis"].[Article in German]. Schweiz Arch Tierheilkd. 2009 Oct;151(10):479-83. PMID:19780008

Gerber B, Eichenberger S, Joller-Jemelka HI, Wittenbrink MM, Reusch CE. Complement C3 in Bernese Mountain dogs. Vet Clin Pathol. 2010 Jun;39(2):164-8. Epub 2009 Dec 8. PMID:20003027

Gerber B, Haug K, Eichenberger S, Reusch CE, Wittenbrink MM. Comparison of a rapid immunoassay for antibodies to the C6 antigen with conventional tests for antibodies to Borrelia burgdorferi in dogs in Europe. Vet Rec. 2009 Nov 14;165(20):594-7. PMID:19915191

Gern L, Douet V, López Z, Rais O, Cadenas FM. Diversity of Borrelia genospecies in Ixodes ricinus ticks in a Lyme borreliosis endemic area in Switzerland identified by using new probes for reverse line blotting. Ticks Tick Borne Dis. 2010 Mar;1(1):23-9. Epub 2009 Dec 16. PMID:21771508

Gern L, Lienhard R, Péter O. [Diseases and pathogenic agents transmitted by ticks in Switzerland].[Article in French]. Rev Med Suisse. 2010 Oct 13;6(266):1906-9. PMID:21089555

Gerritzen A, Brandt S. Serodiagnosis of Lyme borreliosis with bead based immunoassays using multiplex technology. Methods. 2012 Mar 3. [Epub ahead of print]. PMID:22406491

Gershon A. Unproven therapies don't belong in Lyme disease guidelines. South Med J. 2009 Oct;102(10):1088-9; author reply 1089-91. PMID:19738539

Gerth-Kahlert C, Wermund TK. [Optic neuritis].[Article in German]. Klin Monbl Augenheilkd. 2011 May;228(5):425-31. Epub 2011 Mar 11. PMID:21400403

Gesslbauer B, Poljak A, Handwerker C, Schüler W, Schwendenwein D, Weber C, Lundberg U, Meinke A, Kungl AJ. Comparative membrane proteome analysis of three Borrelia species. Proteomics. 2012 Mar;12(6):845-58. PMID:22539435

Gheorghiev C, De Montleau F, Defuentes G. [Alcohol and epilepsy: a case report between alcohol withdrawal seizures and neuroborreliosis]. [Article in French]. Encephale. 2011 Jun;37(3):231-7. Epub 2010 Dec 3. PMID:21703439

Gilbert L. Altitudinal patterns of tick and host abundance: a potential role for climate change in regulating tick-borne diseases? Oecologia. 2010 Jan;162(1):217-25. Epub 2009 Aug 15. PMID:19685082

Gilmore RD Jr, Howison RR, Dietrich G, Patton TG, Clifton DR, Carroll JA. The bba64 gene of Borrelia burgdorferi, the Lyme disease agent, is critical for mammalian infection via tick bite transmission. Proc Natl Acad Sci U S A. 2010 Apr 20;107(16):7515-20. Epub 2010 Apr 5. PMID:20368453

Girard YA, Fedorova N, Lane RS. Genetic diversity of Borrelia burgdorferi and detection of B. bissettii-like DNA in serum of north-coastal California residents. J Clin Microbiol. 2011 Mar;49(3):945-54. Epub 2010 Dec 22. PMID:21177909

Girard YA, Travinsky B, Schotthoefer A, Fedorova N, Eisen RJ, Eisen L, Barbour AG, Lane RS. Population structure of the lyme borreliosis spirochete Borrelia burgdorferi in the western black-legged tick (Ixodes pacificus) in Northern California. Appl Environ Microbiol. 2009 Nov;75(22):7243-52. Epub 2009 Sep 25. PMID:19783741

Girschick HJ, Morbach H, Tappe D. Treatment of Lyme borreliosis. Arthritis Res Ther. 2009;11(6):258. Epub 2009 Dec 17. PMID:20067594

Glotzbecker MP, Kocher MS, Sundel RP, Shore BJ, Spencer SA, Kasser JR. Primary lyme arthritis of the pediatric hip. J Pediatr Orthop. 2011 Oct-Nov;31(7):787-90. PMID:21926878

Goldberg EM, Rotondo KM. Complete antrioventricular block due to Lyme reinfection in a six year-old boy. Med Health R I. 2010 May;93(5):158-60. PMID:20533727

Gómez-Díaz E, Boulinier T, Sertour N, Cornet M, Ferquel E, McCoy KD. Genetic structure of marine Borrelia garinii and population admixture with the terrestrial cycle of Lyme borreliosis. Environ Microbiol. 2011 Sep;13(9):2453-67. Epub 2011 Jun 8. PMID:21651685

Gorson KC, Kolb DA, Marks DS, Hayes MT, Baquis GD. Acute brachial diplegia due to Lyme disease. Neurologist. 2011 Jan;17(1):24-7. PMID:21192188

Gouveia EA, Alves MF, Mantovani E, Oyafuso LK, Bonoldi VL, Yoshinari NH. Profile of patients with Baggio-Yoshinari Syndrome admitted at "Instituto de Infectologia Emilio Ribas". Rev Inst Med Trop Sao Paulo. 2010 Nov-Dec;52(6):297-303. PMID:21225212

Graham J, Stockley K, Goldman RD. Tick-borne illnesses: a CME update. Pediatr Emerg Care. 2011 Feb;27(2):141-7; quiz 148-50. PMID:21293226

Greco TP Jr, Conti-Kelly AM, Greco TP. Antiphospholipid antibodies in patients with purported 'chronic Lyme disease'. Lupus. 2011 Nov;20(13):1372-7. Epub 2011 Jul 5. PMID:21729977

Greengarten PJ, Tuininga AR, Morath SU, Falco RC, Norelus H, Daniels TJ. Occurrence of soil- and tick-borne fungi and related virulence tests for pathogenicity to Ixodes scapularis (Acari: Ixodidae). J Med Entomol. 2011 Mar;48(2):337-44. PMID:21485371

Grisold W, Vass A. Antibiotic responsive demyelinating neuropathy related to Lyme disease. Neurology. 2010 Mar 16;74(11):935; author reply 935. PMID:20231674

Groshong AM, Gibbons NE, Yang XF, Blevins JS. Rrp2, a prokaryotic enhancer-like binding protein, is essential for viability of Borrelia burgdorferi. J Bacteriol. 2012 Apr 27. [Epub ahead of print]. PMID:22544267

Grygorczuk S, Osada J, Swierzbińska R, Zajkowska J, Kondrusik M, Pancewicz S, Dąbrowska M. Expression of Fas receptor on human T lymphocytes under stimulation with Borrelia burgdorferi sensu lato - preliminary results. Adv Med Sci. 2010;55(2):228-34. PMID:20639186

Grzeszczuk A, Puzanowska B, Zirako S. Anaplasma phagocytophilum infection in patients with early Lyme borreliosis, erythema migrans, in north-eastern Poland. Clin Microbiol Infect. 2009 Dec;15 Suppl 2:17-8. Epub 2009 Apr 3. PMID:19374650

Güneş T, Poyraz O, Ataş M, Alim A. [Seroprevalence of tick-borne encephalitis virus (TBEV) among the residents of rural areas in Sinop, central Black-Sea region, Turkey].[Article in Turkish]. Mikrobiyol Bul. 2010 Oct;44(4):585-91. PMID:21063971

Gueorguiev Penev D, Laurent E, Baron S, Diot E, Bastides F, de Gialluly C, Bernard L, Rusch E. [Lyme borreliosis: census of adult patients hospitalized in Indre-et-Loire (France), from the Hospital Discharge Data (1999-2006)].[Article in French]. Rev Epidemiol Sante Publique. 2010 Oct;58(5):339-47. Epub 2010 Aug 13. PMID:20708866

Guerrier G, Doherty T. Comparison of antibiotic regimens for treating louse-borne relapsing fever: a meta-analysis. Trans R Soc Trop Med Hyg. 2011 Sep;105(9):483-90. Epub 2011 Jul 30. PMID:21803390

Guinda J M, López D LM, Martínez Pérez-Balsa A, Villamil C I, Jove Castelo MJ. [Fast onset cognitive impairment: neuroborreliosis and positive 14-3-3 protein].[Article in Spanish]. Rev Chilena Infectol. 2011 Jun;28(3):274-5. Epub 2011 Jul 14. PMID:21879156

Gulati RK. Doxycycline in children?--the unanswered question. Pediatr Dermatol. 2010 Jul-Aug;27(4):419. PMID:20653877

Guo BP, Teneberg S, Münch R, Terunuma D, Hatano K, Matsuoka K, Angström J, Borén T, Bergström S. Relapsing fever Borrelia binds to neolacto glycans and mediates rosetting of human erythrocytes. Proc Natl Acad Sci U S A. 2009 Nov 17;106(46):19280-5. Epub 2009 Nov 2. PMID:19884498

Guo X, Booth CJ, Paley MA, Wang X, DePonte K, Fikrig E, Narasimhan S, Montgomery RR. Inhibition of neutrophil function by two tick salivary proteins. Infect Immun. 2009 Jun;77(6):2320-9. Epub 2009 Mar 30. PMID:19332533

Gupta PK, Patel R, Bhatti MT. Neuroretinitis secondary to concurrent infection with cat scratch disease and lyme disease. Eye (Lond). 2009 Jul;23(7):1607. Epub 2008 Sep 12. PMID:18791545

Haapasalo K, Suomalainen P, Sukura A, Siikamaki H, Jokiranta TS. Fatal babesiosis in man, Finland, 2004. Emerg Infect Dis. 2010 Jul;16(7):1116-8. PMID:20587183

Haene A, Tröger M. Diffuse hyperintense brainstem lesions in neuroborreliosis. Neurology. 2009 Jul 28;73(4):326. PMID:19636055

Hagen K. [Risk of infections among orienteers].[Article in Norwegian]. Tidsskr Nor Laegeforen. 2009 Jun 25;129(13):1326-8. PMID:19561657.

Haitham E, Gimenez G, Sokhna C, Bilcha KD, Ali J, Barker SC, Cutler SJ, Raoult D, Drancourt M. Multispacer sequence typing relapsing Fever borreliae in Africa. PLoS Negl Trop Dis. 2012 Jun;6(6):e1652. Epub 2012 Jun 5. PMID:22679518

Hakimi R. [Debatable borreliosis diagnosis. Patients stuck with the costs].[Article in German]. MMW Fortschr Med. 2009 Jul 23;151(30-33):7. PMID:19725176

Hallström T, Haupt K, Kraiczy P, Hortschansky P, Wallich R, Skerka C, Zipfel PF. Complement regulator-acquiring surface protein 1 of Borrelia burgdorferi binds to human bone morphogenic protein 2, several extracellular matrix proteins, and plasminogen. J Infect Dis. 2010 Aug 15;202(3):490-8. PMID:20565259

Halperin JJ. A tale of two spirochetes: lyme disease and syphilis. Neurol Clin. 2010 Feb;28(1):277-91. PMID:19932386

Halperin JJ. Nervous system Lyme disease. J R Coll Physicians Edinb. 2010 Sep;40(3):248-55. PMID:21127770

Halperin JJ. Nervous system lyme disease: is there a controversy? Semin Neurol. 2011 Jul;31(3):317-24. Epub 2011 Sep 30. PMID:21964848

Halperin JJ. Neurologic manifestations of lyme disease. Curr Infect Dis Rep. 2011 Aug;13(4):360-6. PMID:21484219

Hamer SA, Hickling GJ, Sidge JL, Rosen ME, Walker ED, Tsao JI. Diverse Borrelia burgdorferi strains in a bird-tick cryptic cycle. Appl Environ Microbiol. 2011 Mar;77(6):1999-2007. Epub 2011 Jan 21. PMID:21257811

Hamer SA, Hickling GJ, Sidge JL, Walker ED, Tsao JI. Synchronous phenology of juvenile Ixodes scapularis, vertebrate host relationships, and associated patterns of Borrelia burgdorferi ribotypes in the midwestern United States. Ticks Tick Borne Dis. 2012 Apr;3(2):65-74. Epub 2012 Jan 31. PMID:22297162

Hamer SA, Tsao JI, Walker ED, Hickling GJ. Invasion of the lyme disease vector Ixodes scapularis: implications for Borrelia burgdorferi endemicity. Ecohealth. 2010 Aug;7(1):47-63. Epub 2010 Mar 13. PMID:20229127

Hansen MG, Christoffersen M, Thuesen LR, Petersen MR, Bojesen AM. Seroprevalence of Borrelia burgdorferi sensu lato and Anaplasma phagocytophilum in Danish horses. Acta Vet Scand. 2010 Jan 18;52:3. PMID:20082693

Hanses F, Audebert FX, Glück T, Salzberger B, Ehrenstein BP. [Suspected borreliosis - what's behind it?].[Article in German]. Dtsch Med Wochenschr. 2011 Aug;136(33):1652-5. Epub 2011 Aug 10. PMID:21833884

Hao Q, Hou X, Geng Z, Wan K. Distribution of Borrelia burgdorferi sensu lato in China. J Clin Microbiol. 2011 Feb;49(2):647-50. Epub 2010 Nov 24. PMID:21106783

Harman MW, Dunham-Ems SM, Caimano MJ, Belperron AA, Bockenstedt LK, Fu HC, Radolf JD, Wolgemuth CW. The heterogeneous motility of the Lyme disease spirochete in gelatin mimics dissemination through tissue. Proc Natl Acad Sci U S A. 2012 Feb 21;109(8):3059-64. Epub 2012 Feb 6. PMID:22315410

Harrison A, Bown KJ, Horak IG. Detection of Anaplasma bovis in an undescribed tick species collected from the eastern rock sengi Elephantulus myurus. J Parasitol. 2011 Dec;97(6):1012-6. Epub 2011 Jun 28. PMID:21711102

Harrison BA, Rayburn WH Jr, Toliver M, Powell EE, Engber BR, Durden LA, Robbins RG, Prendergast BF, Whitt PB. Recent discovery of widespread Ixodes affinis (Acari: Ixodidae) distribution in North Carolina with implications for Lyme disease studies. J Vector Ecol. 2010 Jun;35(1):174-9. PMID:20618664

Hartiala P, Hytönen J, Yrjänäinen H, Honkinen M, Terho P, Söderström M, Penttinen MA, Viljanen MK. TLR2 utilization of Borrelia does not induce p38- and IFN-beta autocrine loop-dependent expression of CD38, resulting in poor migration and weak IL-12 secretion of dendritic cells. J Immunol. 2010 May 15;184(10):5732-42. Epub 2010 Apr 14. PMID:20393136

Hashimoto Y. [Borrelia burgdorferi].[Article in Japanese]. Nihon Rinsho. 2010 Jun;68 Suppl 6:231-3. PMID:20942045

Hassett AL, Radvanski DC, Buyske S, Savage SV, Sigal LH. Psychiatric comorbidity and other psychological factors in patients with "chronic Lyme disease". Am J Med. 2009 Sep;122(9):843-50. PMID:19699380

Hassler D. [A case of suspected borreliosis].[Article in German]. Dtsch Med Wochenschr. 2012 Jan;137(1-2):46. Epub 2011 Dec 16. PMID:22180284

Hastey CJ, Elsner RA, Barthold SW, Baumgarth N. Delays and Diversions Mark the Development of B Cell Responses to Borrelia burgdorferi Infection. J Immunol. 2012 Apr 30. [Epub ahead of print]. PMID:22547698

Haufs MG. Different Symptoms. Dtsch Arztebl Int. 2009 Jul;106(31-32):524; author reply 525. Epub 2009 Aug 3. PMID:19730721

Haven J, Vargas LC, Mongodin EF, Xue V, Hernandez Y, Pagan P, Fraser-Liggett CM, Schutzer SE, Luft BJ, Casjens SR, Qiu WG. Pervasive recombination and sympatric genome diversification driven by frequency-dependent selection in Borrelia burgdorferi, the Lyme disease bacterium. Genetics. 2011 Nov;189(3):951-66. Epub 2011 Sep 2. PMID:21890743

Hawley KL, Olson CM Jr, Iglesias-Pedraz JM, Navasa N, Cervantes JL, Caimano MJ, Izadi H, Ingalls RR, Pal U, Salazar JC, Radolf JD, Anguita J. CD14 cooperates with complement receptor 3 to mediate MyD88-independent phagocytosis of Borrelia burgdorferi. Proc Natl Acad Sci U S A. 2012 Jan 24;109(4):1228-32. Epub 2012 Jan 9. PMID:22232682

Hayes EB. Looking the other way: preventing vector-borne disease among travelers to the United States. Travel Med Infect Dis. 2010 Sep;8(5):277-84. Epub 2010 Sep 9. PMID:20971437

He M, Ouyang Z, Troxell B, Xu H, Moh A, Piesman J, Norgard MV, Gomelsky M, Yang XF. Cyclic di-GMP is essential for the survival of the lyme disease spirochete in ticks. PLoS Pathog. 2011 Jun;7(6):e1002133. Epub 2011 Jun 30. PMID:21738477

Heckler AK, Shmorhun D. Asymptomatic, transient complete heart block in a pediatric patient with Lyme disease. Clin Pediatr (Phila). 2010 Jan;49(1):82-5. Epub 2009 Feb 3. PMID:19190204

Heilpern AJ, Wertheim W, He J, Perides G, Bronson RT, Hu LT. Matrix metalloproteinase 9 plays a key role in lyme arthritis but not in dissemination of Borrelia burgdorferi. Infect Immun. 2009 Jul;77(7):2643-9. Epub 2009 Apr 13. PMID:19364840

Heller JE, Benito-Garcia E, Maher NE, Chibnik LB, Maher CP, Shadick NA. Behavioral and attitudes survey about Lyme disease among a Brazilian population in the endemic area of Martha's Vineyard, Massachusetts. J Immigr Minor Health. 2010 Jun;12(3):377-83. Epub 2008 Sep 16. PMID:18792780

Henningsson AJ, Malmvall BE, Ernerudh J, Matussek A, Forsberg P. Neuroborreliosis--an epidemiological, clinical and healthcare cost study from an endemic area in the south-east of Sweden. Clin Microbiol Infect. 2010 Aug;16(8):1245-51. Epub 2009 Sep 29. PMID:19793326

Henningsson AJ, Tjernberg I, Malmvall BE, Forsberg P, Ernerudh J. Indications of Th1 and Th17 responses in cerebrospinal fluid from patients with Lyme neuroborreliosis: a large retrospective study. J Neuroinflammation. 2011 Apr 20;8:36. PMID:21507218

Henry B, Roth D, Reilly R, MacDougall L, Mak S, Li M, Muhamad M. How big is the Lyme problem? Using novel methods to estimate the true number of Lyme disease cases in British Columbia residents from 1997 to 2008. Vector Borne Zoonotic Dis. 2011 Jul;11(7):863-8. Epub 2011 Mar 17. PMID:21413887

Herman-Giddens ME. RE: Endemic tickborne infectious diseases in Louisiana and the Gulf south. J La State Med Soc. 2009 Nov-Dec; 161(6):325-339. J La State Med Soc. 2010 Mar-Apr;162(2):64; author reply 64-5. PMID:20521734

Hernández-Montfort JA, Awkal M, Martagón-Villamil JA. Looking back at Lyme carditis. Am J Med. 2010 Jun;123(6):e9-e10. PMID:20569746

Herzer P. [45-year-old woman with joint pain and suspected Lyme arthritis].[Article in German]. Dtsch Med Wochenschr. 2009 Sep;134(36):1741-2. Epub 2009 Aug 28. PMID:19718595

Hesse C, Johansson I, Mattsson N, Bremell D, Andreasson U, Halim A, Anckarsäter R, Blennow K, Anckarsäter H, Zetterberg H, Larson G, Hagberg L, Grahn A. The N-terminal domain of α-dystroglycan, released as a 38 kDa protein, is increased in cerebrospinal fluid in patients with Lyme neuroborreliosis. Biochem Biophys Res Commun. 2011 Sep 2;412(3):494-9. Epub 2011 Aug 6. PMID:21843510

Heyman P, Cochez C, Hofhuis A, van der Giessen J, Sprong H, Porter SR, Losson B, Saegerman C, Donoso-Mantke O, Niedrig M, Papa A. A clear and present danger: tick-borne diseases in Europe. Expert Rev Anti Infect Ther. 2010 Jan;8(1):33-50. PMID:20014900

Hilborn ED, Catanzaro DG, Jackson LE. Repeated holdout cross-validation of model to estimate risk of Lyme disease by landscape characteristics. Int J Environ Health Res. 2012;22(1):1-11. Epub 2011 Jun 2. PMID:21644127

Hildebrandt A, Franke J, Schmoock G, Pauliks K, Krämer A, Straube E. Diversity and coexistence of tick-borne pathogens in central Germany. J Med Entomol. 2011 May;48(3):651-5. PMID:21661327

Hildebrandt A, Pauliks K, Sachse S, Straube E. Coexistence of Borrelia spp. and Babesia spp. in Ixodes ricinus ticks in Middle Germany. Vector Borne Zoonotic Dis. 2010 Nov;10(9):831-7. Epub 2010 Apr 26. PMID:20420533

Hildebrandt A, Straube E, Neubauer H, Schmoock G. Coxiella burnetii and coinfections in Ixodes ricinus ticks in Central Germany. Vector Borne Zoonotic Dis. 2011 Aug;11(8):1205-7. Epub 2010 Dec 13. PMID:21142964

Hildenbrand P, Craven DE, Jones R, Nemeskal P. Lyme neuroborreliosis: manifestations of a rapidly emerging zoonosis. AJNR Am J Neuroradiol. 2009 Jun;30(6):1079-87. Epub 2009 Apr 3. PMID:19346313

Hinterseher I, Gäbel G, Corvinus F, Lück C, Saeger HD, Bergert H, Tromp G, Kuivaniemi H. Presence of Borrelia burgdorferi sensu lato antibodies in the serum of patients with abdominal aortic aneurysms. Eur J Clin Microbiol Infect Dis. 2012 May;31(5):781-9. Epub 2011 Aug 13. PMID:21842293

Hird C. Postcards from the edge? J Fam Health Care. 2011 May-Jun;21(3):30-2. PMID:21877394

Ho K, Melanson M, Desai JA. Bell palsy in Lyme disease-endemic regions of Canada: a cautionary case of occult bilateral peripheral facial nerve palsy due to Lyme disease. CJEM. 2012;14(0):1-4. PMID:22480492

Hoen AG, Margos G, Bent SJ, Diuk-Wasser MA, Barbour A, Kurtenbach K, Fish D. Phylogeography of Borrelia burgdorferi in the eastern United States reflects multiple independent Lyme disease emergence events. Proc Natl Acad Sci U S A. 2009 Sep 1;106(35):15013-8. Epub 2009 Aug 14. PMID:19706476

Hoen AG, Rollend LG, Papero MA, Carroll JF, Daniels TJ, Mather TN, Schulze TL, Stafford KC 3rd, Fish D. Effects of tick control by acaricide self-treatment of white-tailed deer on host-seeking tick infection prevalence and entomologic risk for Ixodes scapularis-borne pathogens. Vector Borne Zoonotic Dis. 2009 Aug;9(4):431-8. PMID:19650738

Hofmann H. [The variable spectrum of cutaneous Lyme borreliosis: Diagnosis and therapy].[Article in German]. Hautarzt. 2012 May;63(5):381-9. PMID:22573314

Hojgaard A, Biketov SF, Shtannikov AV, Zeidner NS, Piesman J. Molecular identification of Salp15, a key salivary gland protein in the transmission of lyme disease spirochetes, from Ixodes persulcatus and Ixodes pacificus (Acari: Ixodidae). J Med Entomol. 2009 Nov;46(6):1458-63. PMID:19960697

Holzbauer SM, Kemperman MM, Lynfield R. Death due to community-associated Clostridium difficile in a woman receiving prolonged antibiotic therapy for suspected lyme disease. Clin Infect Dis. 2010 Aug 1;51(3):369-70. PMID:20597684

Hoon-Hanks LL, Morton EA, Lybecker MC, Battisti JM, Samuels DS, Drecktrah D. Borrelia burgdorferi malQ mutants utilize disaccharides and traverse the enzootic cycle. FEMS Immunol Med Microbiol. 2012 Jun 1. [Epub ahead of print]. PMID:22672337

Horká H, Cerná-Kýcková K, Skallová A, Kopecký J. Tick saliva affects both proliferation and distribution of Borrelia burgdorferi spirochetes in mouse organs and increases transmission of spirochetes to ticks. Int J Med Microbiol. 2009 Jun;299(5):373-80. Epub 2009 Jan 15. PMID:19147403

Hospach T, Langendörfer M, Kalle TV, Tewald F, Wirth T, Dannecker GE. Mimicry of lyme arthritis by synovial hemangioma. Rheumatol Int. 2011 Dec;31(12):1639-43. Epub 2009 Dec 16. PMID:20013264

Houck JA, Hojgaard A, Piesman J, Kuchta RD. Low-density microarrays for the detection of Borrelia burgdorferi s.s. (the Lyme disease spirochete) in nymphal Ixodes scapularis. Ticks Tick Borne Dis. 2011 Mar;2(1):27-36. Epub 2010 Nov 27. PMID:21771534

Houtman PM, Jansen TL, Weel J, Grond JK. Borrelial fasciitis: as yet insufficient proof for a distinct entity. Rheumatol Int. 2009 Sep;29(11):1385-8. Epub 2009 Jun 9. PMID:19506881

Hovius JW. Spitting image: tick saliva assists the causative agent of Lyme disease in evading host skin's innate immune response. J Invest Dermatol. 2009 Oct;129(10):2337-9. PMID:19749783

Huegli D, Moret J, Rais O, Moosmann Y, Erard P, Malinverni R, Gern L. Prospective study on the incidence of infection by Borrelia burgdorferi sensu lato after a tick bite in a highly endemic area of Switzerland. Ticks Tick Borne Dis. 2011 Sep;2(3):129-36. Epub 2011 Jul 28. PMID:21890065

Hufschmidt A, Shabarin V, Yakovlev-Leyendecker O, Deppe O, Rauer S. Prevalence of taste disorders in idiopathic and B. burgdorferi-associated facial palsy. J Neurol. 2009 Oct;256(10):1750-2. Epub 2009 Jul 15. PMID:19603242

Hulínská D, Votýpka J, Vanousová D, Hercogová J, Hulínský V, Drevová H, Kurzová Z, Uherková L. Identification of Anaplasma phagocytophilum and Borrelia burgdorferi sensu lato in patients with erythema migrans. Folia Microbiol (Praha). 2009;54(3):246-56. Epub 2009 Aug 2. PMID:19649743

Humphrey PT, Caporale DA, Brisson D. Uncoordinated phylogeography of Borrelia burgdorferi and its tick vector, Ixodes scapularis. Evolution. 2010 Sep;64(9):2653-63. PMID:20394659

Hutschenreuther A, Birkemeyer C, Grötzinger K, Straubinger RK, Rauwald HW. Growth inhibiting activity of volatile oil from Cistus creticus L. against Borrelia burgdorferi s.s. in vitro. Pharmazie. 2010 Apr;65(4):290-5. PMID:20432627

Huttunen P, Lappalainen M, Salo E, Lönnqvist T, Jokela P, Hyypiä T, Peltola H. Differential diagnosis of acute central nervous system infections in children using modern microbiological methods. Acta Paediatr. 2009 Aug;98(8):1300-6. Epub 2009 May 7. PMID:19432824

Hyde JA, Shaw DK, Smith Iii R, Trzeciakowski JP, Skare JT. The BosR regulatory protein of Borrelia burgdorferi interfaces with the RpoS regulatory pathway and modulates both the oxidative stress response and pathogenic properties of the Lyme disease spirochete. Mol Microbiol. 2009 Dec;74(6):1344-55. Epub 2009 Nov 10. PMID:19906179

Hyde JA, Shaw DK, Smith R 3rd, Trzeciakowski JP, Skare JT. Characterization of a conditional bosR mutant in Borrelia burgdorferi. Infect Immun. 2010 Jan;78(1):265-74. Epub 2009 Oct 26. PMID:19858309

Hyde JA, Weening EH, Chang M, Trzeciakowski JP, Höök M, Cirillo JD, Skare JT. Bioluminescent imaging of Borrelia burgdorferi in vivo demonstrates that the fibronectin-binding protein BBK32 is required for optimal infectivity. Mol Microbiol. 2011 Oct;82(1):99-113. Epub 2011 Aug 30. PMID:21854463

Hyde JA, Weening EH, Skare JT. Genetic transformation of Borrelia burgdorferi. Curr Protoc Microbiol. 2011 Feb;Chapter 12:Unit 12C.4. PMID:21400675

Hynote ED, Mervine PC, Stricker RB. Clinical evidence for rapid transmission of Lyme disease following a tickbite. Diagn Microbiol Infect Dis. 2012 Feb;72(2):188-92. Epub 2011 Nov 21. PMID:22104184

Iliopoulou BP, Guerau-de-Arellano M, Huber BT. HLA-DR alleles determine responsiveness to Borrelia burgdorferi antigens in a mouse model of self-perpetuating arthritis. Arthritis Rheum. 2009 Dec;60(12):3831-40. PMID:19950279

Iliopoulou BP, Huber BT. Emergence of chronic Lyme arthritis: putting the breaks on CD28 costimulation. Immunopharmacol Immunotoxicol. 2009 Jun;31(2):180-5. PMID:18792834

Iliopoulou BP, Huber BT. Infectious arthritis and immune dysregulation: lessons from Lyme disease. Curr Opin Rheumatol. 2010 Jul;22(4):451-5. PMID:20375899

Imai DM, Barr BC, Daft B, Bertone JJ, Feng S, Hodzic E, Johnston JM, Olsen KJ, Barthold SW. Lyme neuroborreliosis in 2 horses. Vet Pathol. 2011 Nov;48(6):1151-7. Epub 2011 Feb 1. PMID:21285382

Imirzalioglu C, Hain T, Hossain H, Chakraborty T, Domann E. Erythema caused by a localised skin infection with Arthrobacter mysorens. BMC Infect Dis. 2010 Dec 15;10:352. PMID:21159172

Inoue K, Kabeya H, Fujita H, Makino T, Asano M, Inoue S, Inokuma H, Nogami S, Maruyama S. Serological survey of five zoonoses, scrub typhus, Japanese spotted fever, tularemia, Lyme disease, and Q fever, in feral raccoons (Procyon lotor) in Japan. Vector Borne Zoonotic Dis. 2011 Jan;11(1):15-9. Epub 2010 Jun 16. PMID:20553108

Isogai E, Isogai H, Takahashi K, Kobayashi-Sakamoto M, Okumura K. Antimicrobial activity of three tick defensins and four mammalian cathelicidin-derived synthetic peptides against Lyme disease spirochetes and bacteria isolated from the midgut. Exp Appl Acarol. 2009 Nov;49(3):221-8. Epub 2009 Feb 20. PMID:19229642

Ivanova L, Christova I, Neves V, Aroso M, Meirelles L, Brisson D, Gomes-Solecki M. Comprehensive seroprofiling of sixteen B. burgdorferi OspC: implications for Lyme disease diagnostics design. Clin Immunol. 2009 Sep;132(3):393-400. Epub 2009 Jul 2. PMID:19576856

Jaenson TG, Eisen L, Comstedt P, Mejlon HA, Lindgren E, Bergström S, Olsen B. Risk indicators for the tick Ixodes ricinus and Borrelia burgdorferi sensu lato in Sweden. Med Vet Entomol. 2009 Sep;23(3):226-37. PMID:19712153

Jaenson TG, Jaenson DG, Eisen L, Petersson E, Lindgren E. Changes in the geographical distribution and abundance of the tick Ixodes ricinus during the past 30 years in Sweden. Parasit Vectors. 2012 Jan 10;5:8. PMID:22233771

Jaenson TG, Lindgren E. The range of Ixodes ricinus and the risk of contracting Lyme borreliosis will increase northwards when the vegetation period becomes longer. Ticks Tick Borne Dis. 2011 Mar;2(1):44-9. Epub 2010 Dec 13. PMID:21771536

James FM, Engiles JB, Beech J. Meningitis, cranial neuritis, and radiculoneuritis associated with Borrelia burgdorferi infection in a horse. J Am Vet Med Assoc. 2010 Nov 15;237(10):1180-5. PMID:21073390

Jameson LJ, Medlock JM. Tick surveillance in Great Britain. Vector Borne Zoonotic Dis. 2011 Apr;11(4):403-12. Epub 2010 Sep 17. PMID:20849277

Janols H, Bredberg A, Thuvesson I, Janciauskiene S, Grip O, Wullt M. Lymphocyte and monocyte flow cytometry immunophenotyping as a diagnostic tool in uncharacteristic inflammatory disorders. BMC Infect Dis. 2010 Jul 13;10:205. PMID:20626864

Jenke AC, Stoek LM, Zilbauer M, Wirth S, Borusiak P. Facial palsy: etiology, outcome and management in children. Eur J Paediatr Neurol. 2011 May;15(3):209-13. Epub 2010 Dec 14. PMID:21159531

Jewett MW, Jain S, Linowski AK, Sarkar A, Rosa PA. Molecular characterization of the Borrelia burgdorferi in vivo-essential protein PncA. Microbiology. 2011 Oct;157(Pt 10):2831-40. Epub 2011 Jul 21. PMID:21778210

Jewett MW, Lawrence KA, Bestor A, Byram R, Gherardini F, Rosa PA. GuaA and GuaB are essential for Borrelia burgdorferi survival in the tick-mouse infection cycle. J Bacteriol. 2009 Oct;191(20):6231-41. Epub 2009 Aug 7. PMID:19666713

Jiang S, Gilpin ME, Attia M, Ting YL, Berti PJ. Lyme disease enolpyruvyl-UDP-GlcNAc synthase: fosfomycin-resistant MurA from Borrelia burgdorferi, a fosfomycin-sensitive mutant, and the catalytic role of the active site Asp. Biochemistry. 2011 Mar 29;50(12):2205-12. Epub 2011 Feb 18. PMID:21294548

Jiang Y, Hou XX, Geng Z, Hao Q, Wan KL. Interpretation criteria for standardized Western blot for the predominant species of Borrelia burgdorferi sensu lato in China. Biomed Environ Sci. 2010 Oct;23(5):341-9. PMID:21112481

Jobe DA, Kowalski TJ, Bloemke M, Lovrich SD, Callister SM. Rapid decline of OspC borreliacidal antibodies following treatment of patients with early Lyme disease. Clin Vaccine Immunol. 2011 Jun;18(6):1034-7. Epub 2011 Apr 20. PMID:21508161

John J, Chandran L. Arthritis in children and adolescents. Pediatr Rev. 2011 Nov;32(11):470-9; quiz 480. PMID:22045895

Johnson L, Aylward A, Stricker RB. Healthcare access and burden of care for patients with Lyme disease: a large United States survey. Health Policy. 2011 Sep;102(1):64-71. Epub 2011 Jun 14. PMID:21676482

Johnson L, Stricker RB. Final report of the Lyme disease review panel of the infectious diseases society of america: a pyrrhic victory? Clin Infect Dis. 2010 Nov 1;51(9):1108-9; author reply 1109-1. PMID:20925511

Johnson L, Stricker RB. The Infectious Diseases Society of America Lyme guidelines: a cautionary tale about the development of clinical practice guidelines. Philos Ethics Humanit Med. 2010 Jun 9;5:9. PMID:20529367

Johnson M, Feder HM Jr. Chronic Lyme disease: a survey of Connecticut primary care physicians. J Pediatr. 2010 Dec;157(6):1025-1029.e1-2. Epub 2010 Sep 1. PMID:20813379

Johnson RC, Kodner C, Jarnefeld J, Eck DK, Xu Y. Agents of human anaplasmosis and Lyme disease at Camp Ripley, Minnesota. Vector Borne Zoonotic Dis. 2011 Dec;11(12):1529-34. Epub 2011 Aug 25. PMID:21867420

Jones JD, Albert DA, Thadani V, Rigby WF. Unusual case of a swollen painful toe in a young man. Arthritis Care Res (Hoboken). 2012 Feb;64(2):298-302. PMID:22278969

Jones KL, McHugh GA, Glickstein LJ, Steere AC. Analysis of Borrelia burgdorferi genotypes in patients with Lyme arthritis: High frequency of ribosomal RNA intergenic spacer type 1 strains in antibiotic-refractory arthritis. Arthritis Rheum. 2009 Jul;60(7):2174-82. PMID:19565522

Jones KL, Seward RJ, Ben-Menachem G, Glickstein LJ, Costello CE, Steere AC. Strong IgG antibody responses to Borrelia burgdorferi glycolipids in patients with Lyme arthritis, a late manifestation of the infection. Clin Immunol. 2009 Jul;132(1):93-102. Epub 2009 Apr 2. PMID:19342303

Juricová Z, Hubálek Z. Serologic survey of the wild boar (Sus scrofa) for Borrelia burgdorferi sensu lato. Vector Borne Zoonotic Dis. 2009 Oct;9(5):479-82. PMID:18973452

Jutras BL, Bowman A, Brissette CA, Adams CA, Verma A, Chenail AM, Stevenson B. EbfC (YbaB) is a new type of bacterial nucleoid-associated protein, and a global regulator of gene expression in the Lyme disease spirochete. J Bacteriol. 2012 Apr 27. [Epub ahead of print]. PMID:22544270

Jutras BL, Verma A, Adams CA, Brissette CA, Burns LH, Whetstine CR, Bowman A, Chenail AM, Zückert WR, Stevenson B. BpaB and EbfC DNA-binding proteins regulate production of the Lyme disease spirochete's infection-associated Erp surface proteins. J Bacteriol. 2012 Feb;194(4):778-86. Epub 2011 Dec 9. PMID:22155777

Juvkam KH, Eikeland R. [A man with acutely starting pain in the right hip and thigh].[Article in Norwegian]. Tidsskr Nor Laegeforen. 2011 May 20;131(9-10):959-61. PMID:21606995

Kaiser R, Fingerle V. [Neuroborreliosis].[Article in German]. Nervenarzt. 2009 Oct;80(10):1239-51. PMID:19536517

Kalinova Z, Halanova M, Cislakova L, Sulinova Z, Jarcuska P. Occurrence of IgG antibodies to Anaplasma phagocytophilum in humans suspected of Lyme borreliosis in eastern Slovakia. Ann Agric Environ Med. 2009 Dec;16(2):285-8. PMID:20047263

Kaminsky A. Erythema figuratum.[Article in English, Spanish]. Actas Dermosifiliogr. 2009 Dec;100 Suppl 2:88-109. PMID:20096167

Kanjwal K, Karabin B, Kanjwal Y, Grubb BP. Postural orthostatic tachycardia syndrome following Lyme disease. Cardiol J. 2011;18(1):63-6. PMID:21305487

Karan' LS, Koliasnikova NM, Toporkova MG, Makhneva MA, Nadezhdina MV, Esaulkova AIu, Romanenko VV, Arumova EA, Platonov AE, Maleev VV. [Usage of real time polymerase chain reaction for diagnostics of different tick-borne infections].[Article in Russian]. Zh Mikrobiol Epidemiol Immunobiol. 2010 May-Jun;(3):72-7. PMID:20734723

Karavaev VS, Riabchenko AV, Beklemishev AB. [Enzyme immunoassay-based analysis of OspC recombinant proteins from Borrelia garinii and Borrelia afzelii isolated in West Siberia].[Article in Russian]. Zh Mikrobiol Epidemiol Immunobiol. 2010 Jan-Feb;(1):20-3. PMID:20218339

Karavaev VS, Riabchenko AV, Beklemishev AB. [Immunochemical analysis of recombinant protein FlaA of Western Siberian Borrelia garinii isolate].[Article in Russian]. ZhMikrobiol Epidemiol Immunobiol. 2011 Jul-Aug;(4):66-71. PMID:21913395

Kariu T, Coleman AS, Anderson JF, Pal U. Methods for rapid transfer and localization of lyme disease pathogens within the tick gut. J Vis Exp. 2011 Feb 14;(48). pii: 2544. PMID:21372782

Karlsson J, Andréasson B, Kondori N, Erman E, Riesbeck K, Hogevik H, Wennerås C. Comparative study of immune status to infectious agents in elderly patients with multiple myeloma, Waldenstrom's macroglobulinemia, and monoclonal gammopathy of undetermined significance. Clin Vaccine Immunol. 2011 Jun;18(6):969-77. Epub 2011 Apr 20. PMID:21508164

Karna SL, Sanjuan E, Esteve-Gassent MD, Miller CL, Maruskova M, Seshu J. CsrA modulates levels of lipoproteins and key regulators of gene expression critical for pathogenic mechanisms of Borrelia burgdorferi. Infect Immun. 2011 Feb;79(2):732-44. Epub 2010 Nov 15. PMID:21078860

Karosi T, Rácz T, Szekanecz E, Tóth A, Sziklai I. Recurrent laryngeal nerve paralysis due to subclinical Lyme borreliosis. J Laryngol Otol. 2010 Mar;124(3):336-8. Epub 2009 Sep 10. PMID:19740453

Kash N, Fink-Puches R, Cerroni L. Cutaneous manifestations of B-cell chronic lymphocytic leukemia associated with Borrelia burgdorferi infection showing a marginal zone B-cell lymphoma-like infiltrate. Am J Dermatopathol. 2011 Oct;33(7):712-5. PMID:21946761

Katchanov J, Siebert E, Klingebiel R, Endres M. Infectious vasculopathy of intracranial large- and medium-sized vessels in neurological intensive care unit: a clinico-radiological study. Neurocrit Care. 2010 Jun;12(3):369-74. PMID:20146025

Kawano Y, Shigeto H, Shiraishi Y, Ohyagi Y, Kira J. [Case of Borrelia brainstem encephalitis presenting with severe dysphagia].[Article in Japanese]. Rinsho Shinkeigaku. 2010 Apr;50(4):265-7. PMID:20411811

Keefe LM, Moro MH, Vinasco J, Hill C, Wu CC, Raizman EA. The use of harvested white-tailed deer (Odocoileus virginianus) and geographic information system (GIS) methods to characterize distribution and locate spatial clusters of Borrelia burgdorferi and its vector Ixodes scapularis in Indiana. Vector Borne Zoonotic Dis. 2009 Dec;9(6):671-80. PMID:19272000

Keesing F, Belden LK, Daszak P, Dobson A, Harvell CD, Holt RD, Hudson P, Jolles A, Jones KE, Mitchell CE, Myers SS, Bogich T, Ostfeld RS. Impacts of biodiversity on the emergence and transmission of infectious diseases. Nature. 2010 Dec 2;468(7324):647-52. PMID:21124449

Keesing F, Brunner J, Duerr S, Killilea M, Logiudice K, Schmidt K, Vuong H, Ostfeld RS. Hosts as ecological traps for the vector of Lyme disease. Proc Biol Sci. 2009 Nov 22;276(1675):3911-9. Epub 2009 Aug 19. PMID:19692412

Keller A, Graefen A, Ball M, Matzas M, Boisguerin V, Maixner F, Leidinger P, Backes C, Khairat R, Forster M, Stade B, Franke A, Mayer J, Spangler J, McLaughlin S, Shah M, Lee C, Harkins TT, Sartori A, Moreno-Estrada A, Henn B, Sikora M, Semino O, Chiaroni J, Rootsi S, Myres NM, Cabrera VM, Underhill PA, Bustamante CD, Vigl EE, Samadelli M, Cipollini G, Haas J, Katus H, O'Connor BD, Carlson MR, Meder B, Blin N, Meese E, Pusch CM, Zink A. New insights into the Tyrolean Iceman's origin and phenotype as inferred by whole-genome sequencing. Nat Commun. 2012 Feb 28;3:698. PMID:22426219

Kempf F, De Meeûs T, Vaumourin E, Noel V, Taragel'ová V, Plantard O, Heylen DJ, Eraud C, Chevillon C, McCoy KD. Host races in Ixodes ricinus, the European vector of Lyme borreliosis. Infect Genet Evol. 2011 Dec;11(8):2043-8. Epub 2011 Sep 29. PMID:21983685

Kempf F, McCoy KD, De Meeûs T. Wahlund effects and sex-biased dispersal in Ixodes ricinus, the European vector of Lyme borreliosis: new tools for old data. Infect Genet Evol. 2010 Oct;10(7):989-97. Epub 2010 Jun 19. PMID:20601167

Kenedy MR, Akins DR. The OspE-related proteins inhibit complement deposition and enhance serum resistance of Borrelia burgdorferi, the lyme disease spirochete. Infect Immun. 2011 Apr;79(4):1451-7. Epub 2011 Jan 31. PMID:21282413

Kenedy MR, Lenhart TR, Akins DR. The Role of Borrelia burgdorferi Outer Surface Proteins. FEMS Immunol Med Microbiol. 2012 Apr 28. [Epub ahead of print]. PMID:22540535

Kennedy CE, Azfar RS, Honig PJ. Lyme disease as a cause of acropapular dermatitis of childhood. Pediatr Dermatol. 2009 Sep-Oct;26(5):635-6. PMID:19840337

Kern A, Collin E, Barthel C, Michel C, Jaulhac B, Boulanger N. Tick saliva represses innate immunity and cutaneous inflammation in a murine model of lyme disease. Vector Borne Zoonotic Dis. 2011 Oct;11(10):1343-50. Epub 2011 May 25. PMID:21612525

Kessenich CR. Summer is prime time for Lyme. Nurse Pract. 2011 Aug;36(8):7-8. PMID:21768826

Kesteman T, Rossi C, Bastien P, Brouillard J, Avesani V, Olive N, Martin P, Delmée M. Prevalence and genetic heterogeneity of Borrelia burgdorferi sensu lato in Ixodes ticks in Belgium. Acta Clin Belg. 2010 Sep-Oct;65(5):319-22. PMID:21128558

Kim J, Beldner SJ, Jadonath R, Altman EJ. A safe and cost-effective approach to treating Lyme cardiac disease in an era of health care reform. Pacing Clin Electrophysiol. 2011 Jun;34(6):666-9. Epub 2011 Mar 31. PMID:21453343

Kirmizis D, Chatzidimitriou D. Comment on 'Membranous glomerulonephritis secondary to Borrelia burgdorferi infection presenting as nephrotic syndrome'. Nephrol Dial Transplant. 2010 May;25(5):1723-7. Epub 2010 Feb 9. PMID:20147284

Kiser K. In the Lyme light. Minn Med. 2009 Nov;92(11):10-2. PMID:20069988

Kišová-Vargová L, Mucha R, Cerňanská D, Bhide M. Host-dependent differential expression of factor H binding proteins, their affinity to factor H and complement evasion by Lyme and relapsing fever borreliae. Vet Microbiol. 2011 Mar 24;148(2-4):341-7. PMID:20970929

Kiss T, Cadar D, Krupaci AF, Bordeanu A, Brudaşcă GF, Mihalca AD, Mircean V, Gliga L, Dumitrache MO, Spînu M. Serological reactivity to Borrelia burgdorferi sensu lato in dogs and horses from distinct areas in Romania. Vector Borne Zoonotic Dis. 2011 Sep;11(9):1259-62. Epub 2011 May 25. PMID:21612524

Kitahara R, Simorellis AK, Hata K, Maeno A, Yokoyama S, Koide S, Akasaka K. A delicate interplay of structure, dynamics, and thermodynamics for function: a high pressure NMR study of outer surface protein A. Biophys J. 2012 Feb 22;102(4):916-26. Epub 2012 Feb 21. PMID:22385863

Kjelland V, Stuen S, Skarpaas T, Slettan A. Borrelia burgdorferi sensu lato in Ixodes ricinus ticks collected from migratory birds in Southern Norway. Acta Vet Scand. 2010 Nov 6;52:59. PMID:21054890

Kjelland V, Stuen S, Skarpaas T, Slettan A. Prevalence and genotypes of Borrelia burgdorferi sensu lato infection in Ixodes ricinus ticks in southern Norway. Scand J Infect Dis. 2010 Aug;42(8):579-85. PMID:20429719

Kjelland V, Ytrehus B, Vikørren T, Stuen S, Skarpaas T, Slettan A. Borrelia burgdorferi sensu lato detected in skin of Norwegian mountain hares (Lepus timidus) without signs of dissemination. J Wildl Dis. 2011 Apr;47(2):293-9. PMID:21441181

Klaeger AJ, Herbort CP. Cotton wool spots as possible indicators of retinal vascular pathology in ocular lyme borreliosis. Int Ophthalmol. 2010 Oct;30(5):599-602. Epub 2008 Oct 15. PMID:18854948

Klein M, Pfister HW. [Bacterial infections of the central nervous system].[Article in German]. Nervenarzt. 2010 Feb;81(2):150-61. PMID:20084360

Klempner MS, Halperin JJ, Baker PJ, Shapiro ED, O'Connell S, Fingerle V, Wormser GP. Lyme borreliosis: the challenge of accuracy. Neth J Med. 2012 Jan;70(1):3-5. PMID:22271807

Knap N, Durmisi E, Saksida A, Korva M, Petrovec M, Avsic-Zupanc T. Influence of climatic factors on dynamics of questing Ixodes ricinus ticks in Slovenia. Vet Parasitol. 2009 Oct 14;164(2-4):275-81. Epub 2009 Jun 11. PMID:19560275

Knauer J, Krupka I, Fueldner C, Lehmann J, Straubinger RK. Evaluation of the preventive capacities of a topically applied azithromycin formulation against Lyme borreliosis in a murine model. J Antimicrob Chemother. 2011 Dec;66(12):2814-22. Epub 2011 Sep 15. PMID:21921078

Knopf A, Becker K, Rasch C. [Ambiguous swelling of the earlobe]. [Article in German]. HNO. 2010 Jul;58(7):704-6. PMID:20419446

Koc F, Bozdemir H, Pekoz T, Aksu HS, Ozcan S, Kurdak H. Lyme disease presenting as subacute transverse myelitis. Acta Neurol Belg. 2009 Dec;109(4):326-9. PMID:20120216

Koffi JK, Leighton PA, Pelcat Y, Trudel L, Lindsay LR, Milord F, Ogden NH. Passive surveillance for I. scapularis ticks: enhanced analysis for early detection of emerging Lyme disease risk. J Med Entomol. 2012 Mar;49(2):400-9. PMID:22493860

Kong Y, Akin AR, Francis KP, Zhang N, Troy TL, Xie H, Rao J, Cirillo SL, Cirillo JD. Whole-body imaging of infection using fluorescence. Curr Protoc Microbiol. 2011 May;Chapter 2:Unit 2C.3. PMID:21538304

Konnai S, Yamada S, Imamura S, Nishikado H, Githaka N, Ito T, Takano A, Kawabata H, Murata S, Ohashi K. Identification of TROSPA homologue in Ixodes persulcatus Schulze, the specific vector for human Lyme borreliosis in Japan. Ticks Tick Borne Dis. 2012 Apr;3(2):75-7. Epub 2012 Mar 3. PMID:22445928

Korenberg EI, Anan'ina IuV, Gorelova NB, Savel'eva OV, Kovalevskiĭ IuV, Petrov EM. [Southern taiga combined natural foci of spirochetoses].[Article in Russian]. Zh Mikrobiol Epidemiol Immunobiol. 2011 Sep-Oct;(5):27-30. PMID:22145345

Korenberg ÉI, Nefedova VV, Gorelova NB, Kovalevskiĭ IuV, Fadeeva IA, Golubova DA. [Etiological structure of complex Ixodes tickborne borreliosis natural foci of southern taiga].[Article in Russian]. Vestn Ross Akad Med Nauk. 2011;(10):10-5. PMID:22168033

Korenberg EI, Nefedova VV, Romanenko VN, Gorelova NB. The tick Ixodes pavlovskyi as a host of spirochetes pathogenic for humans and its possible role in the epizootiology and epidemiology of borrelioses. Vector Borne Zoonotic Dis. 2010 Jun;10(5):453-8. PMID:19929222

Kostick JL, Szkotnicki LT, Rogers EA, Bocci P, Raffaelli N, Marconi RT. The diguanylate cyclase, Rrp1, regulates critical steps in the enzootic cycle of the Lyme disease spirochetes. Mol Microbiol. 2011 Jul;81(1):219-31. Epub 2011 Jun 5. PMID:21542866

Kotsyfakis M, Horka H, Salat J, Andersen JF. The crystal structures of two salivary cystatins from the tick Ixodes scapularis and the effect of these inhibitors on the establishment of Borrelia burgdorferi infection in a murine model. Mol Microbiol. 2010 Jul;77(2):456-70. Epub 2010 Jun 1. PMID:20545851

Kowalski TJ, Berth WL, Mathiason MA, Agger WA. Oral antibiotic treatment and long-term outcomes of Lyme facial nerve palsy. Infection. 2011 Jun;39(3):239-45. Epub 2011 Apr 27. PMID:21523405

Kowalski TJ, Tata S, Berth W, Mathiason MA, Agger WA. Antibiotic treatment duration and long-term outcomes of patients with early lyme disease from a lyme disease-hyperendemic area. Clin Infect Dis. 2010 Feb 15;50(4):512-20. PMID:20070237

Kraemer M, Berlit P. Systemic, secondary and infectious causes for cerebral vasculitis: clinical experience with 16 new European cases. Rheumatol Int. 2010 Sep;30(11):1471-6. Epub 2009 Oct 13. PMID:19823835

Krakowetz CN, Lindsay LR, Chilton NB. Genetic diversity in Ixodes scapularis (Acari: Ixodidae) from six established populations in Canada. Ticks Tick Borne Dis. 2011 Sep;2(3):143-50. Epub 2011 Jul 28. PMID:21890067

Kremer S, Holl N, Schmitt E, De Sèze J, Moser T, Dietemann JL. [Imaging of non-traumatic and non-tumoral cord lesions].[Article in French]. J Radiol. 2010 Sep;91(9 Pt 2):969-87. PMID:20814389

Krimer PM, Miller AD, Li Q, Grosenbaugh DA, Susta L, Schatzberg SJ. Molecular and pathological investigations of the central nervous system in Borrelia burgdorferi-infected dogs. J Vet Diagn Invest. 2011 Jul;23(4):757-63. Epub 2011 Jun 13. PMID:21908319

Kristiansen BE, Grude N, Tveten Y, Emmert A. [Laboratory diagnosis of Lyme borreliosis].[Article in Norwegian]. Tidsskr Nor Laegeforen. 2009 Oct 22;129(20):2132-4. PMID:19855455

Krol CG, van der Geer S, Thio HB, Janssen MJ, Jonkers GJ. [Acrodermatitis chronica atrophicans: late manifestation of Lyme borreliosis].[Article in Dutch]. Ned Tijdschr Geneeskd. 2010;154:A2012. PMID:20699042

Kruger D. On target with vector-borne infections: understanding Lyme disease. JAAPA. 2010 May;23(5):22-6. PMID:20480868

Krupka I, Knauer J, Lorentzen L, O'Connor TP, Saucier J, Straubinger RK. Borrelia burgdorferi sensu lato species in Europe induce diverse immune responses against C6 peptides in infected mice. Clin Vaccine Immunol. 2009 Nov;16(11):1546-62. Epub 2009 Sep 2. PMID:19726618

Krupka I, Straubinger RK. Lyme borreliosis in dogs and cats: background, diagnosis, treatment and prevention of infections with Borrelia burgdorferi sensu stricto. Vet Clin North Am Small Anim Pract. 2010 Nov;40(6):1103-19. PMID:20933139

Křupka M, Mašek J, Bartheldyová E, Knötigová PT, Plocková J, Korvasová Z, Skrabalová M, Koudelka S, Kulich P, Zachová K, Czerneková L, Strouhal O, Horynová M, Sebela M, Miller AD, Ledvina M, Raška M, Turánek J. Enhancement of immune response towards non-lipidized Borrelia burgdorferi recombinant OspC antigen by binding onto the surface of metallochelating nanoliposomes with entrapped lipophilic derivatives of norAbuMDP. J Control Release. 2012 Feb 22. [Epub ahead of print]. PMID:22387453

Krupka M, Zachova K, Weigl E, Raska M. Prevention of lyme disease: promising research or sisyphean task? Arch Immunol Ther Exp (Warsz). 2011 Aug;59(4):261-75. Epub 2011 Jun 3. PMID:21633917

Krzyczmanik D, Rybacki M, Wittczak T, Dudek W, Swierczyńska-Machura D, Pałczyński C, Walusiak-Skorupa J. [Coexistence of two occupational infectious diseases in one patient--borreliosis and tick-borne encephalitis--a case report].[Article in Polish]. Med Pr. 2011;62(3):339-44. PMID:21870423

Kubánek M, Sramko M, Berenová D, Hulínská D, Hrbácková H, Malusková J, Lodererová A, Málek I, Kautzner J. Detection of Borrelia burgdorferi sensu lato in endomyocardial biopsy specimens in individuals with recent-onset dilated cardiomyopathy. Eur J Heart Fail. 2012 Feb 29. [Epub ahead of print]. PMID:22379178

Kubicka-Trzaska A, Oleksy P, Karska-Basta I, Romanowska-Dixon B. [Acute posterior multifocal placoid pigment epitheliopathy (APMPPE)--a therapeutic dilemma].[Article in Polish]. Klin Oczna. 2010;112(4-6):127-30. PMID:20825067

Kudryashev M, Cyrklaff M, Alex B, Lemgruber L, Baumeister W, Wallich R, Frischknecht F. Evidence of direct cell-cell fusion in Borrelia by cryogenic electron tomography. Cell Microbiol. 2011 May;13(5):731-41. Epub 2011 Jan 30. PMID:21276171

Kudryashev M, Cyrklaff M, Wallich R, Baumeister W, Frischknecht F. Distinct in situ structures of the Borrelia flagellar motor. J Struct Biol. 2010 Jan;169(1):54-61. Epub 2009 Aug 21. PMID:19699799

Kugeler KJ, Griffith KS, Gould LH, Kochanek K, Delorey MJ, Biggerstaff BJ, Mead PS. A review of death certificates listing Lyme disease as a cause of death in the United States. Clin Infect Dis. 2011 Feb 1;52(3):364-7. Epub 2010 Dec 28. PMID:21189272

Kułakowska A, Zajkowska JM, Ciccarelli NJ, Mroczko B, Drozdowski W, Bucki R. Depletion of plasma gelsolin in patients with tick-borne encephalitis and Lyme neuroborreliosis. Neurodegener Dis. 2011;8(5):375-80. Epub 2011 Mar 10. PMID:21389683

Kullberg BJ, Berende A, van der Meer JW. The challenge of Lyme disease: tired of the Lyme wars. Neth J Med. 2011 Mar;69(3):98-100. PMID:21444933

Kumar M, Kaur S, Kariu T, Yang X, Bossis I, Anderson JF, Pal U. Borrelia burgdorferi BBA52 is a potential target for transmission blocking Lyme disease vaccine. Vaccine. 2011 Nov 8;29(48):9012-9. Epub 2011 Sep 21. PMID:21945261

Kumar M, Yang X, Coleman AS, Pal U. BBA52 facilitates Borrelia burgdorferi transmission from feeding ticks to murine hosts. J Infect Dis. 2010 Apr 1;201(7):1084-95. PMID:20170377

Kumru OS, Schulze RJ, Rodnin MV, Ladokhin AS, Zückert WR. Surface localization determinants of Borrelia OspC/Vsp family lipoproteins. J Bacteriol. 2011 Jun;193(11):2814-25. Epub 2011 Mar 25. PMID:21441503

Kumru OS, Schulze RJ, Slusser JG, Zückert WR. Development and validation of a FACS-based lipoprotein localization screen in the Lyme disease spirochete Borrelia burgdorferi. BMC Microbiol. 2010 Nov 3;10:277. PMID:21047413

Kuo J, Nardelli DT, Warner TF, Callister SM, Schell RF. Interleukin-35 enhances Lyme arthritis in Borrelia-vaccinated and -infected mice. Clin Vaccine Immunol. 2011 Jul;18(7):1125-32. Epub 2011 May 25. PMID:21613457

Kurnatowski P, Warpechowska M, Kurnatowska AJ. Knowledge on Lyme disease among foresters. Int J Occup Med Environ Health. 2011 Mar;24(1):78-93. Epub 2011 Feb 16. PMID:21468905

Kuznetsov AV, Weisenseel P, Flaig MJ, Ruzicka T, Prinz JC. Photoallergic erythroderma due to doxycycline therapy of erythema chronicum migrans. Acta Derm Venereol. 2011 Oct;91(6):734-6. PMID:21681354

Kybicová K, Schánilec P, Hulínská D, Uherková L, Kurzová Z, Spejchalová S. Detection of Anaplasma phagocytophilum and Borrelia burgdorferi sensu lato in dogs in the Czech Republic. Vector Borne Zoonotic Dis. 2009 Dec;9(6):655-61. PMID:19271998

LaDeau SL, Glass GE, Hobbs NT, Latimer A, Ostfeld RS. Data-model fusion to better understand emerging pathogens and improve infectious disease forecasting. Ecol Appl. 2011 Jul;21(5):1443-60. PMID:21830694

LaFleur RL, Callister SM, Dant JC, Jobe DA, Lovrich SD, Warner TF, Wasmoen TL, Schell RF. One-year duration of immunity induced by vaccination with a canine Lyme disease bacterin. Clin Vaccine Immunol. 2010 May;17(5):870-4. Epub 2010 Mar 17. PMID:20237200

LaFrance ME, Pierce JV, Antonara S, Coburn J. The Borrelia burgdorferi integrin ligand P66 affects gene expression by human cells in culture. Infect Immun. 2011 Aug;79(8):3249-61. Epub 2011 May 16. PMID:21576330

Lakos A, Reiczigel J, Solymosi N. The positive predictive value of Borrelia burgdorferi serology in the light of symptoms of patients sent to an outpatient service for tick-borne diseases. Inflamm Res. 2010 Nov;59(11):959-64. Epub 2010 May 13. PMID:20461540

Lakos A, Solymosi N. Maternal Lyme borreliosis and pregnancy outcome. Int J Infect Dis. 2010 Jun;14(6):e494-8. Epub 2009 Nov 18. PMID:19926325

Lalosevic D, Lalosevic V, Stojsic-Milosavljevic A, Stojsic D. Borrelia-like organism in heart capillaries of patient with Lyme-disease seen by electron microscopy. Int J Cardiol. 2010 Dec 3;145(3):e96-8. Epub 2009 Jan 24. PMID:19168240

Lambin EF, Tran A, Vanwambeke SO, Linard C, Soti V. Pathogenic landscapes: interactions between land, people, disease vectors, and their animal hosts. Int J Health Geogr. 2010 Oct 27;9:54. PMID:20979609

Lane RS, Mun J, Peribáñez MA, Fedorova N. Differences in prevalence of Borrelia burgdorferi and Anaplasma spp. infection among host-seeking Dermacentor occidentalis, Ixodes pacificus, and Ornithodoros coriaceus ticks in northwestern California. Ticks Tick Borne Dis. 2010 Dec;1(4):159-67. PMID:21359090

Lane RS, Mun J, Stubbs HA. Horizontal and vertical movements of host-seeking Ixodes pacificus (Acari: Ixodidae) nymphs in a hardwood forest. J Vector Ecol. 2009 Dec;34(2):252-66. PMID:20352083

Lantos PM, Charini WA, Medoff G, Moro MH, Mushatt DM, Parsonnet J, Sanders JW, Baker CJ. Final report of the Lyme disease review panel of the Infectious Diseases Society of America. Clin Infect Dis. 2010 Jul 1;51(1):1-5. PMID:20504239

Lantos PM. Chronic Lyme disease: the controversies and the science. Expert Rev Anti Infect Ther. 2011 Jul;9(7):787-97. PMID:21810051

LaRocca TJ, Crowley JT, Cusack BJ, Pathak P, Benach J, London E, Garcia-Monco JC, Benach JL. Cholesterol lipids of Borrelia burgdorferi form lipid rafts and are required for the bactericidal activity of a complement-independent antibody. Cell Host Microbe. 2010 Oct 21;8(4):331-42. PMID:20951967

Larsson C, Andersson M, Bergström S. Current issues in relapsing fever. Curr Opin Infect Dis. 2009 Oct;22(5):443-9. PMID:19623064

Larsson C, Lundqvist J, van Rooijen N, Bergström S. A novel animal model of Borrelia recurrentis louse-borne relapsing fever borreliosis using immunodeficient mice. PLoS Negl Trop Dis. 2009 Sep 29;3(9):e522. PMID:19787030

Lazarus JJ, McCarter AL, Neifer-Sadhwani K, Wooten RM. ELISA-based measurement of antibody responses and PCR-based detection profiles can distinguish between active infection and early clearance of Borrelia burgdorferi. Clin Dev Immunol. 2012;2012:138069. Epub 2011 Oct 26. PMID:22110528

Lebrun-Frénay C. [Neuroepidemiology. Editorial].[Article in French]. Rev Neurol (Paris). 2009 Aug-Sep;165(8-9):613-4. Epub 2009 Jun 4. PMID:19500812

Lee SH, Vigliotti VS, Vigliotti JS, Jones W, Pappu S. Increased sensitivity and specificity of Borrelia burgdorferi 16S ribosomal DNA detection. Am J Clin Pathol. 2010 Apr;133(4):569-76. PMID:20231610

Lee WY, Moriarty TJ, Wong CH, Zhou H, Strieter RM, van Rooijen N, Chaconas G, Kubes P. An intravascular immune response to Borrelia burgdorferi involves Kupffer cells and iNKT cells. Nat Immunol. 2010 Apr;11(4):295-302. Epub 2010 Mar 14. PMID:20228796

Lefas G, Chaconas G. High-throughput screening identifies three inhibitor classes of the telomere resolvase from the lyme disease spirochete. Antimicrob Agents Chemother. 2009 Oct;53(10):4441-9. Epub 2009 Jul 13. PMID:19596868

Lenčáková DH, Schulte-Spechtel U, Fingerle V, Pet'ko B, Wilske B. Detection of a large linear plasmid in Borrelia spielmanii isolate. Can J Microbiol. 2011 Apr;57(4):343-6. PMID:21491987

Lenormand C, Jaulhac B, De Martino S, Barthel C, Lipsker D. Species of Borrelia burgdorferi complex that cause borrelial lymphocytoma in France. Br J Dermatol. 2009 Jul;161(1):174-6. Epub 2009 Mar 19. PMID:19302068

Leonhard S, Jensen K, Salkeld DJ, Lane RS. Distribution of the Lyme disease spirochete Borrelia burgdorferi in naturally and experimentally infected western gray squirrels (Sciurus griseus). Vector Borne Zoonotic Dis. 2010 Jun;10(5):441-6. PMID:20017717

Leschnik MW, Kirtz G, Khanakah G, Duscher G, Leidinger E, Thalhammer JG, Joachim A, Stanek G. Humoral immune response in dogs naturally infected with Borrelia burgdorferi sensu lato and in dogs after immunization with a Borrelia vaccine. Clin Vaccine Immunol. 2010 May;17(5):828-35. Epub 2010 Mar 10. PMID:20219882

Letts RM. Commentary on an article by Matthew D. Milewski, MD, et al.: "Lyme Arthritis in Children Presenting with Joint Effusions". J Bone Joint Surg Am. 2011 Feb 2;93(3):e11. PMID:21266634

Levy E, Morruzzi C, Barbarini A, Sordet C, Cribier B, Jaulhac B, Lipsker D. Clinical images: toe dactylitis revealing late Lyme borreliosis. Arthritis Rheum. 2012 Apr;64(4):1293. Epub 2012 Jan 24. PMID:22275216

Li C, Xu H, Zhang K, Liang FT. Inactivation of a putative flagellar motor switch protein FliG1 prevents Borrelia burgdorferi from swimming in highly viscous media and blocks its infectivity. Mol Microbiol. 2010 Mar;75(6):1563-76. Epub 2010 Feb 18. PMID:20180908

Li X, McHugh GA, Damle N, Sikand VK, Glickstein L, Steere AC. Burden and viability of Borrelia burgdorferi in skin and joints of patients with erythema migrans or lyme arthritis. Arthritis Rheum. 2011 Aug;63(8):2238-47. PMID:21590753

Lidar M, Lipschitz N, Langevitz P, Shoenfeld Y. The infectious etiology of vasculitis. Autoimmunity. 2009 Aug;42(5):432-8. PMID:19811260

Ligor M, Olszowy P, Buszewski B. Application of medical and analytical methods in Lyme borreliosis monitoring. Anal Bioanal Chem. 2012 Mar;402(7):2233-48. Epub 2011 Oct 21. PMID:22015476

Lim S, Irwin PJ, Lee S, Oh M, Ahn K, Myung B, Shin S. Comparison of selected canine vector-borne diseases between urban animal shelter and rural hunting dogs in Korea. Parasit Vectors. 2010 Apr 8;3(1):32. PMID:20377869

Lin T, Gao L, Edmondson DG, Jacobs MB, Philipp MT, Norris SJ. Central role of the Holliday junction helicase RuvAB in vlsE recombination and infectivity of Borrelia burgdorferi. PLoS Pathog. 2009 Dec;5(12):e1000679. Epub 2009 Dec 4. PMID:19997622

Lipińiska-Ojrzanowska A, Wittczak T, Krzyczmanik D, Pałczyński C, Walusiak-Skorupa J. [Invasion by trichinae in the patient hospitalized with suspicion of occupational borreliosis: a case report].[Article in Polish]. Med Pr. 2011;62(1):73-6. PMID:21748886

Lisbôa RS, Teixeira RC, Rangel CP, Santos HA, Massard CL, Fonseca AH. Avian spirochetosis in chickens following experimental transmission of Borrelia anserina by Argas (Persicargas) miniatus. Avian Dis. 2009 Jun;53(2):166-8. PMID:19630219

Little SE, Heise SR, Blagburn BL, Callister SM, Mead PS. Lyme borreliosis in dogs and humans in the USA. Trends Parasitol. 2010 Apr;26(4):213-8. Epub 2010 Mar 6. PMID:20207198

Liu H, Fitzgerald D, Gran B, Leong JM, Alugupalli KR. Induction of distinct neurologic disease manifestations during relapsing fever requires T lymphocytes. J Immunol. 2010 May 15;184(10):5859-64. Epub 2010 Apr 9. PMID:20382883

Liu N, Belperron AA, Booth CJ, Bockenstedt LK. The caspase 1 inflammasome is not required for control of murine Lyme borreliosis. Infect Immun. 2009 Aug;77(8):3320-7. Epub 2009 Jun 1. PMID:19487481

Liveris D, Schwartz I, Bittker S, Cooper D, Iyer R, Cox ME, Wormser GP. Improving the yield of blood cultures from patients with early Lyme disease. J Clin Microbiol. 2011 Jun;49(6):2166-8. Epub 2011 Apr 13. PMID:21490189

Liveris D, Schwartz I, McKenna D, Nowakowski J, Nadelman R, Demarco J, Iyer R, Bittker S, Cooper D, Holmgren D, Wormser GP. Comparison of five diagnostic modalities for direct detection of Borrelia burgdorferi in patients with early Lyme disease. Diagn Microbiol Infect Dis. 2012 May 7. [Epub ahead of print]. PMID:22571973

Liveris D, Schwartz I, McKenna D, Nowakowski J, Nadelman RB, Demarco J, Iyer R, Cox ME, Holmgren D, Wormser GP. Quantitation of cell-associated borrelial DNA in the blood of Lyme disease patients with erythema migrans. Eur J Clin Microbiol Infect Dis. 2012 May;31(5):791-5. Epub 2011 Aug 16. PMID:21842448

Livey I, O'Rourke M, Traweger A, Savidis-Dacho H, Crowe BA, Barrett PN, Yang X, Dunn JJ, Luft BJ. A new approach to a Lyme disease vaccine. Clin Infect Dis. 2011 Feb;52 Suppl 3:s266-70. PMID:21217174

Ljøstad U, Mygland A. Remaining complaints 1 year after treatment for acute Lyme neuroborreliosis; frequency, pattern and risk factors. Eur J Neurol. 2010 Jan;17(1):118-23. Epub 2009 Jul 23. PMID:19645771

Ljøstad U, Mygland A. The phenomenon of 'chronic Lyme'; an observational study. Eur J Neurol. 2012 Mar 15. [Epub ahead of print]. PMID:22416947

Lobato E, Pearce-Duvet J, Staszewski V, Gómez-Díaz E, González-Solís J, Kitaysky A, McCoy KD, Boulinier T. Seabirds and the circulation of Lyme borreliosis bacteria in the North Pacific. Vector Borne Zoonotic Dis. 2011 Dec;11(12):1521-7. Epub 2011 Sep 15. PMID:21919724

Lommano E, Bertaiola L, Dupasquier C, Gern L. Infections and co-infections of questing Ixodes ricinus ticks by emerging zoonotic pathogens in Western Switzerland. Appl Environ Microbiol. 2012 Apr 20. [Epub ahead of print]. PMID:22522688

Londoño D, Cadavid D. Bacterial lipoproteins can disseminate from the periphery to inflame the brain. Am J Pathol. 2010 Jun;176(6):2848-57. Epub 2010 Apr 29. PMID:20431027

Lopez JE, Mccoy BN, Krajacich BJ, Schwan TG. Acquisition and subsequent transmission of Borrelia hermsii by the soft tick Ornithodoros hermsi. J Med Entomol. 2011 Jul;48(4):891-5. PMID:21845950

Lopez JE, Porcella SF, Schrumpf ME, Raffel SJ, Hammer CH, Zhao M, Robinson MA, Schwan TG. Identification of conserved antigens for early serodiagnosis of relapsing fever Borrelia. Microbiology. 2009 Aug;155(Pt 8):2641-51. Epub 2009 May 14. PMID:19443544

Lopez JE, Schrumpf ME, Nagarajan V, Raffel SJ, McCoy BN, Schwan TG. A novel surface antigen of relapsing fever spirochetes can discriminate between relapsing fever and Lyme borreliosis. Clin Vaccine Immunol. 2010 Apr;17(4):564-71. Epub 2010 Feb 10. PMID:20147497

Lorch M, Teach SJ. Facial nerve palsy: etiology and approach to diagnosis and treatment. Pediatr Emerg Care. 2010 Oct;26(10):763-9; quiz 770-3. PMID:20930602

Lotric-Furlan S, Ruzic-Sabljic E, Strle F. Concomitant human granulocytic anaplasmosis and Lyme neuroborreliosis. Clin Microbiol Infect. 2009 Dec;15 Suppl 2:28-9. Epub 2009 Mar 26. PMID:19416290

Lotric-Furlan S, Strle F. Peripheral facial palsy in patients with tick-borne encephalitis. Clin Microbiol Infect. 2011 Nov 12. [Epub ahead of print]. PMID:22192120

Lovrich SD, Jobe DA, Kowalski TJ, Policepatil SM, Callister SM. Expansion of the Midwestern focus for human granulocytic anaplasmosis into the region surrounding La Crosse, Wisconsin. J Clin Microbiol. 2011 Nov;49(11):3855-9. Epub 2011 Sep 14. PMID:21918026

Lowe AM. [Lyme disease. A tick bite, no panic! Emerging zoonoses in Quebec].[Article in French]. Perspect Infirm. 2011 May-Jun;8(3):25-7. PMID:21612076

Łuczaj W, Moniuszko A, Rusak M, Pancewicz S, Zajkowska J, Skrzydlewska E. Lipid peroxidation products as potential bioindicators of Lyme arthritis. Eur J Clin Microbiol Infect Dis. 2011 Mar;30(3):415-22. Epub 2010 Nov 6. PMID:21057969

Lundqvist J, Larsson C, Nelson M, Andersson M, Bergström S, Persson C. Concomitant infection decreases the malaria burden but escalates relapsing fever borreliosis. Infect Immun. 2010 May;78(5):1924-30. Epub 2010 Feb 9. PMID:20145098

Lybecker MC, Abel CA, Feig AL, Samuels DS. Identification and function of the RNA chaperone Hfq in the Lyme disease spirochete Borrelia burgdorferi. Mol Microbiol. 2010 Nov;78(3):622-35. Epub 2010 Sep 27. PMID:20815822

Ma Y, Miller JC, Crandall H, Larsen ET, Dunn DM, Weiss RB, Subramanian M, Weis JH, Zachary JF, Teuscher C, Weis JJ. Interval-specific congenic lines reveal quantitative trait Loci with penetrant lyme arthritis phenotypes on chromosomes 5, 11, and 12. Infect Immun. 2009 Aug;77(8):3302-11. Epub 2009 Jun 1. PMID:19487472

Macauda MM, Erickson P, Miller J, Mann P, Closter L, Krause PJ. Long-term Lyme disease antibiotic therapy beliefs among New England residents. Vector Borne Zoonotic Dis. 2011 Jul;11(7):857-62. Epub 2011 Mar 21. PMID:21417921

Mackensen F, Zimmermann S, Alle W, Max R, Jakob E, Becker MD, Thiemeyer D. Difficulties of interpreting Borrelia serology in patients with uveitis. Ocul Immunol Inflamm. 2011 Aug;19(4):227-31. PMID:21770797

Maczka I, Chmielewski T, Walczak E, Rózański J, Religa G, Tylewska-Wierzbanowska S. Tick-borne infections as a cause of heart transplantation. Pol J Microbiol. 2011;60(4):341-3. PMID:22390070

Madagi S, Patil VM, Sadegh S, Singh AK, Garwal B, Banerjee A, Talambedu U, Bhattacharjee B. Identification of membrane associated drug targets in Borrelia burgdorferi ZS7- subtractive genomics approach. Bioinformation. 2011;6(9):356-9. Epub 2011 Jul 19. PMID:21814395

Maggi RG, Reichelt S, Toliver M, Engber B. Borrelia species in Ixodes affinis and Ixodes scapularis ticks collected from the coastal plain of North Carolina. Ticks Tick Borne Dis. 2010 Dec;1(4):168-71. Epub 2010 Oct 20. PMID:21771524

Magnarelli LA, Norris SJ, Fikrig E. Serum antibodies to whole-cell and recombinant antigens of Borrelia burgdorferi in cottontail rabbits. J Wildl Dis. 2012 Jan;48(1):12-20. PMID:22247369

Magnarelli LA, Williams SC, Fikrig E. Seasonal prevalence of serum antibodies to whole cell and recombinant antigens of Borrelia burgdorferi and Anaplasma phagocytophilum in white-tailed deer in Connecticut. J Wildl Dis. 2010 Jul;46(3):781-90. PMID:20688684

Magnaval JF, Tolou H, Gibert M, Innokentiev V, Laborde M, Melnichuk O, Grandadam M, Crubézy E, Alekseev A. Seroepidemiology of nine zoonoses in Viljujsk, Republic of Sakha (Northeastern Siberia, Russian Federation). Vector Borne Zoonotic Dis. 2011 Feb;11(2):157-60. Epub 2010 Jun 24. PMID:20575641

Maher B, Murday D, Harden SP. Cardiac MRI of Lyme disease myocarditis. Heart. 2012 Feb;98(3):264. Epub 2011 Nov 14. PMID:22082689

Mak S, Morshed M, Henry B. Ecological niche modeling of lyme disease in British Columbia, Canada. J Med Entomol. 2010 Jan;47(1):99-105. PMID:20180315

Makhani N, Morris SK, Page AV, Brophy J, Lindsay LR, Banwell BL, Richardson SE. A twist on Lyme: the challenge of diagnosing European Lyme neuroborreliosis. J Clin Microbiol. 2011 Jan;49(1):455-7. Epub 2010 Nov 10. PMID:21068272

Makris GC, Makris MC, Wilmot VV, Geroulakos G, Falagas ME. The role of infection in carotid plaque pathogenesis and stability: the clinical evidence. Curr Vasc Pharmacol. 2010 Nov;8(6):861-72. PMID:20180770

Maloney EL. Article shed no light. Minn Med. 2010 Jan;93(1):6-7. PMID:20191722

Maloney EL. The management of Ixodes scapularis bites in the upper Midwest. WMJ. 2011 Apr;110(2):78-81; quiz 85. PMID:21560562

Mannelli A, Bertolotti L, Gern L, Gray J. Ecology of Borrelia burgdorferi sensu lato in Europe: transmission dynamics in multi-host systems, influence of molecular processes and effects of climate change. FEMS Microbiol Rev. 2011 Nov 1. [Epub ahead of print]. PMID:22091928

Mantovani E, Marangoni RG, Gauditano G, Bonoldi VL, Yoshinari NH. Amplification of the flgE gene provides evidence for the existence of a Brazilian borreliosis. Rev Inst Med Trop Sao Paulo. 2012 Jun;54(3):153-8. PMID:22634887

Manzoor K, Aftab W, Choksi S, Khan IA. Lyme carditis: sequential electrocardiographic changes in response to antibiotic therapy. Int J Cardiol. 2009 Oct 2;137(2):167-71. Epub 2008 Aug 5. PMID:18684533

Maraspin V, Ogrinc K, Ružić-Sabljić E, Lotrič-Furlan S, Strle F. Isolation of Borrelia burgdorferi sensu lato from blood of adult patients with borrelial lymphocytoma, Lyme neuroborreliosis, Lyme arthritis and acrodermatitis chronica atrophicans. Infection. 2011 Feb;39(1):35-40. Epub 2010 Dec 10. PMID:21153429

Maraspin V, Ružić-Sabljić E, Pleterski-Rigler D, Strle F. Pregnant women with erythema migrans and isolation of borreliae from blood: course and outcome after treatment with ceftriaxone. Diagn Microbiol Infect Dis. 2011 Dec;71(4):446-8. Epub 2011 Sep 13. PMID:21917394

Marchal C, Schramm F, Kern A, Luft BJ, Yang X, Schuijt TJ, Hovius JW, Jaulhac B, Boulanger N. Antialarmin effect of tick saliva during the transmission of Lyme disease. Infect Immun. 2011 Feb;79(2):774-85. Epub 2010 Dec 6. PMID:21134970

Marchal CM, Luft BJ, Yang X, Sibilia J, Jaulhac B, Boulanger NM. Defensin is suppressed by tick salivary gland extract during the in vitro interaction of resident skin cells with Borrelia burgdorferi. J Invest Dermatol. 2009 Oct;129(10):2515-7. Epub 2009 Apr 2. PMID:19340008

Marcsisin RA, Campeau SA, Lopez JE, Barbour AG. Alp, an arthropod-associated outer membrane protein of borrelia species that cause relapsing Fever. Infect Immun. 2012 May;80(5):1881-90. Epub 2012 Feb 21. PMID:22354035

Marcu A, Uzzell D, Barnett J. Making sense of unfamiliar risks in the countryside: the case of Lyme disease. Health Place. 2011 May;17(3):843-50. Epub 2011 Apr 13. PMID:21514209

Margos G, Castillo-Ramírez S, Hoen AG. Phylogeography of Lyme borreliosis-group spirochetes and methicillin-resistant Staphylococcus aureus. Parasitology. 2012 May 23:1-14. [Epub ahead of print]. PMID:22617338

Margos G, Fish D. Klaus Kurtenbach--a tribute to his life. Ticks Tick Borne Dis. 2010 Mar;1(1):69-72. PMID:21894640

Margos G, Vollmer SA, Cornet M, Garnier M, Fingerle V, Wilske B, Bormane A, Vitorino L, Collares-Pereira M, Drancourt M, Kurtenbach K. A new Borrelia species defined by multilocus sequence analysis of housekeeping genes. Appl Environ Microbiol. 2009 Aug;75(16):5410-6. Epub 2009 Jun 19. PMID:19542332

Margos G, Vollmer SA, Ogden NH, Fish D. Population genetics, taxonomy, phylogeny and evolution of Borrelia burgdorferi sensu lato. Infect Genet Evol. 2011 Oct;11(7):1545-63. Epub 2011 Aug 5. PMID:21843658

Marinopoulos SS, Coylewright M, Auwaerter PG, Flynn JA. Clinical problem-solving. More than meets the ear. N Engl J Med. 2010 Apr 1;362(13):1228-33. PMID:20357286

Markeljević J, Sarac H, Rados M. Tremor, seizures and psychosis as presenting symptoms in a patient with chronic lyme neuroborreliosis (LNB). Coll Antropol. 2011 Jan;35 Suppl 1:313-8. PMID:21648354

Marks DH. Neurological complications of vaccination with outer surface protein A (OspA). Int J Risk Saf Med. 2011;23(2):89-96. PMID:21673416

Marques A, Brown MR, Fleisher TA. Natural killer cell counts are not different between patients with post-Lyme disease syndrome and controls. Clin Vaccine Immunol. 2009 Aug;16(8):1249-50. Epub 2009 Jun 10. PMID:19515868

Marques AR. Lyme disease: a review. Curr Allergy Asthma Rep. 2010 Jan;10(1):13-20. PMID:20425509

Marre ML, Darcy CT, Yinh J, Akira S, Uematsu S, Steere AC, Hu LT. Role of adrenomedullin in Lyme disease. Infect Immun. 2010 Dec;78(12):5307-13. Epub 2010 Oct 4. PMID:20921145

Marre ML, Petnicki-Ocwieja T, DeFrancesco AS, Darcy CT, Hu LT. Human integrin α(3)β(1) regulates TLR2 recognition of lipopeptides from endosomal compartments. PLoS One. 2010 Sep 22;5(9):e12871. PMID:20877569

Marsot M, Sigaud M, Chapuis JL, Ferquel E, Cornet M, Vourc'h G. Introduced Siberian chipmunks (Tamias sibiricus barberi) harbor more-diverse Borrelia burgdorferi sensu lato genospecies than native bank voles (Myodes glareolus). Appl Environ Microbiol. 2011 Aug 15;77(16):5716-21. Epub 2011 Jun 24. PMID:21705536

Martzolff L, Bouhala M, Dukic R, Saraceni O, Wilhelm JM, Bombaron P, Kieffer P. [Recurrent nerve palsy due to Lyme disease: report of two cases].[Article in French]. Rev Med Interne. 2010 Mar;31(3):229-31. Epub 2010 Jan 15. PMID:20079561

Matalliotakis IM, Cakmak H, Ziogos MD, Kalogeraki A, Kappou D, Arici A. Endometriosis-associated Lyme disease. J Obstet Gynaecol. 2010 Feb;30(2):184-6. PMID:20143981

Mathers A, Smith RP, Cahill B, Lubelczyk C, Elias SP, Lacombe E, Morris SR, Vary CP, Parent CE, Rand PW. Strain diversity of Borrelia burgdorferi in ticks dispersed in North America by migratory birds. J Vector Ecol. 2011 Jun;36(1):24-9. PMID:21635638

Mattéi J, Pélissier P, Richard O, Manoli P, Girod JP, Cazorla C, Bru JP, Stéphan JL. [Lyme uveitis: 2 case reports].[Article in French]. Arch Pediatr. 2011 Jan;18(1):49-53. Epub 2010 Dec 8. PMID:21144716

Mattsson N, Bremell D, Anckarsäter R, Blennow K, Anckarsäter H, Zetterberg H, Hagberg L. Neuroinflammation in Lyme neuroborreliosis affects amyloid metabolism. BMC Neurol. 2010 Jun 22;10:51. PMID:20569437

Matusková V, Vyslouzilová D. [The possibility of the treatment of bilateral macular edema without the anti VEGF treatment--a case report].[Article in Czech]. Cesk Slov Oftalmol. 2010 Feb;66(1):30-5. PMID:20521508

Maurizi L, Marié JL, Aoun O, Courtin C, Gorsane S, Chal D, Davoust B. Seroprevalence survey of equine Lyme borreliosis in France and in sub-Saharan Africa. Vector Borne Zoonotic Dis. 2010 Jun;10(5):535-7. PMID:19877821

Mavin S, Evans R, Milner RM, Chatterton JM, Ho-Yen DO. Local Borrelia burgdorferi sensu stricto and Borrelia afzelii strains in a single mixed antigen improves western blot sensitivity. J Clin Pathol. 2009 Jun;62(6):552-4. Epub 2009 Feb 23. PMID:19240047

Mavin S, McDonagh S, Evans R, Milner RM, Chatterton JM, Ho-Yen DO. Interpretation criteria in Western blot diagnosis of Lyme borreliosis. Br J Biomed Sci. 2011;68(1):5-10. PMID:21473255

Mayne PJ. Emerging incidence of Lyme borreliosis, babesiosis, bartonellosis, and granulocytic ehrlichiosis in Australia. Int J Gen Med. 2011;4:845-52. Epub 2011 Dec 16. PMID:22267937

Mazepa AW, Kidd LB, Young KM, Trepanier LA. Clinical presentation of 26 anaplasma phagocytophilum-seropositive dogs residing in an endemic area. J Am Anim Hosp Assoc. 2010 Nov-Dec;46(6):405-12. PMID:21041333

Mc Causland FR, Niedermaier S, Bijol V, Rennke HG, Choi ME, Forman JP. Lyme disease-associated glomerulonephritis. Nephrol Dial Transplant. 2011 Sep;26(9):3054-6. Epub 2011 Jul 12. PMID:21750163

McCall JW, Baker CF, Mather TN, Chester ST, McCall SD, Irwin JP, Young SL, Cramer LG, Pollmeier MG. The ability of a topical novel combination of fipronil, amitraz and (S)-methoprene to protect dogs from Borrelia burgdorferi and Anaplasma phagocytophilum infections transmitted by Ixodes scapularis. Vet Parasitol. 2011 Jul 15;179(4):335-42. PMID:21777736

McCown M, Grzeszak B. Zoonotic and infectious disease surveillance in Central America: Honduran feral cats positive for toxoplasma, trypanosoma, leishmania, rickettsia, and Lyme disease. J Spec Oper Med. 2010 Summer;10(3):41-3. PMID:21049434

McKay G, Gill I, Chauhan S. Lyme disease: an unusual case of peripheral nerve palsy. J Bone Joint Surg Br. 2010 May;92(5):713-5. PMID:20436011

Mead P, Goel R, Kugeler K. Canine serology as adjunct to human Lyme disease surveillance. Emerg Infect Dis. 2011 Sep;17(9):1710-2. PMID:21888800

Medrano MS, Policastro PF, Schwan TG, Coburn J. Interaction of Borrelia burgdorferi Hbb with the p66 promoter. Nucleic Acids Res. 2010 Jan;38(2):414-27. Epub 2009 Nov 12. PMID:19910373

Meirelles Richer L, Aroso M, Contente-Cuomo T, Ivanova L, Gomes-Solecki M. Reservoir targeted vaccine for lyme borreliosis induces a yearlong, neutralizing antibody response to OspA in white-footed mice. Clin Vaccine Immunol. 2011 Nov;18(11):1809-16. Epub 2011 Sep 14. PMID:21918116

Melby KK, Skar AG. [Borrelia--serologic tests for benefit and problems].[Article in Norwegian]. Tidsskr Nor Laegeforen. 2009 Oct 22;129(20):2135. PMID:19855457

Mener DJ, Mener AS, Daubert JP, Fong M. Tick tock. Am J Med. 2011 Apr;124(4):306-8. PMID:21435420

Mervine P. Don't deny treatment. Minn Med. 2009 Dec;92(12):6. PMID:20092159

Meyer JM, Ejendal KF, Watts VJ, Hill CA. Molecular and pharmacological characterization of two D(1)-like dopamine receptors in the Lyme disease vector, Ixodes scapularis. Insect Biochem Mol Biol. 2011 Aug;41(8):563-71. Epub 2011 Mar 30. PMID:21457782

Middelveen MJ, Stricker RB. Filament formation associated with spirochetal infection: a comparative approach to Morgellons disease. Clin Cosmet Investig Dermatol. 2011;4:167-77. Epub 2011 Nov 14. PMID:22253541

Mietze A, Strube C, Beyerbach M, Schnieder T, Goethe R. Occurrence of Bartonella henselae and Borrelia burgdorferi sensu lato co-infections in ticks collected from humans in Germany. Clin Microbiol Infect. 2011 Jun;17(6):918-20. Epub 2010 Nov 10. PMID:21682805

Miklossy J. Alzheimer's disease - a neurospirochetosis. Analysis of the evidence following Koch's and Hill's criteria. J Neuroinflammation. 2011 Aug 4;8:90. PMID:21816039

Miklossy J. Emerging roles of pathogens in Alzheimer disease. Expert Rev Mol Med. 2011 Sep 20;13:e30. PMID:21933454

Milewski MD, Cruz AI Jr, Miller CP, Peterson AT, Smith BG. Lyme arthritis in children presenting with joint effusions. J Bone Joint Surg Am. 2011 Feb 2;93(3):252-60. PMID:21266639

Milhano N, de Carvalho IL, Alves AS, Arroube S, Soares J, Rodriguez P, Carolino M, Núncio MS, Piesman J, de Sousa R. Coinfections of Rickettsia slovaca and Rickettsia helvetica with Borrelia lusitaniae in ticks collected in a Safari Park, Portugal. Ticks Tick Borne Dis. 2010 Dec;1(4):172-7. PMID:21771525

Miller JC, Maylor-Hagen H, Ma Y, Weis JH, Weis JJ. The Lyme disease spirochete Borrelia burgdorferi utilizes multiple ligands, including RNA, for interferon regulatory factor 3-dependent induction of type I interferon-responsive genes. Infect Immun. 2010 Jul;78(7):3144-53. Epub 2010 Apr 19. PMID:20404081

Miller NJ, Thomas WA, Mather TN. Evaluating a deer-targeted acaricide applicator for area-wide suppression of blacklegged ticks, Ixodes scapularis (Acari: Ixodidae), in Rhode Island. Vector Borne Zoonotic Dis. 2009 Aug;9(4):401-6. PMID:19650734

Milner RM, Mavin S, Ho-Yen DO. Lyme borreliosis in Scotland is different. J Infect. 2009 Aug;59(2):146-7. Epub 2009 May 29. PMID:19535148

Mir A, Tlougan B, O'Reilly K, Tzu J, Meehan S, Kamino H, Franks AG Jr. Morphea with discoid lupus erythematosus. Dermatol Online J. 2011 Oct 15;17(10):10. PMID:22031636

Mircean V, Dumitrache MO, Györke A, Pantchev N, Jodies R, Mihalca AD, Cozma V. Seroprevalence and Geographic Distribution of Dirofilaria immitis and Tick-Borne Infections (Anaplasma phagocytophilum, Borrelia burgdorferi sensu lato, and Ehrlichia canis) in Dogs from Romania. Vector Borne Zoonotic Dis. 2012 May 18. [Epub ahead of print]. PMID:22607068

Misić Majerus L, Daković Rode O, Ruzić Sabljić E. [Post-encephalitic syndrome in patients with tick-borne encephalitis].[Article in Croatian]. Acta Med Croatica. 2009 Oct;63(4):269-78. PMID:20034327

Mladenović J, Cekanac R, Stajković N, Krstić M. [Risk of Lyme disease development after a tick bite].[Article in Serbian]. Vojnosanit Pregl. 2010 May;67(5):369-74. PMID:20499729

Moemenbellah-Fard MD, Benafshi O, Rafinejad J, Ashraf H. Tick-borne relapsing fever in a new highland endemic focus of western Iran. Ann Trop Med Parasitol. 2009 Sep;103(6):529-37. PMID:19695158

Molin S, Ruzicka T, Prinz JC. Bell's palsy during etanercept treatment caused by neuroborreliosis. Br J Dermatol. 2010 Jul;163(1):228-30. Epub 2010 Apr 9. PMID:20408829

Molin S, Ruzicka T, Prinz JC. Borreliosis mimicking lupus-like syndrome during infliximab treatment. Clin Exp Dermatol. 2010 Aug;35(6):631-3. Epub 2010 Feb 20. PMID:20184613

Moniuszko A, Gińdzieńska-Sieśkiewicz E, Pancewicz SA, Czupryna P, Zajkowska J, Sierakowski S. Evaluation of skin thickness lesions in patients with Lyme disease measured by modified Rodnan total skin score. Rheumatol Int. 2011 Sep 30. [Epub ahead of print]. PMID:21960047

Moravcová L, Pícha D, Vanousová D, Hercogová J. [Detection of borrelia DNA from patients with neuroborreliosis and erythema migrans].[Article in Czech]. Klin Mikrobiol Infekc Lek. 2009 Oct;15(5):160-5. PMID:19916154

Moreno MA. Advice for patients. Lyme disease in children and adolescents. Arch Pediatr Adolesc Med. 2011 Jan;165(1):96. PMID:21199990

Mori A, Konnai S, Yamada S, Hidano A, Murase Y, Ito T, Takano A, Kawabata H, Onuma M, Ohashi K. Two novel Salp15-like immunosuppressant genes from salivary glands of Ixodes persulcatus Schulze tick. Insect Mol Biol. 2010 Jun 1;19(3):359-65. Epub 2010 Feb 26. PMID:20201978

Moriarty TJ, Chaconas G. Identification of the determinant conferring permissive substrate usage in the telomere resolvase, ResT. J Biol Chem. 2009 Aug 28;284(35):23293-301. Epub 2009 Jun 26. PMID:19561077

Moser MM. Treatment for a 14-year-old girl with Lyme disease using therapeutic exercise and gait training. Phys Ther. 2011 Sep;91(9):1412-23. Epub 2011 Jul 7. PMID:21737523

Motaleb MA, Pitzer JE, Sultan SZ, Liu J. A novel gene inactivation system reveals altered periplasmic flagellar orientation in a Borrelia burgdorferi fliL mutant. J Bacteriol. 2011 Jul;193(13):3324-31. Epub 2011 Mar 25. PMID:21441522

Motaleb MA, Sultan SZ, Miller MR, Li C, Charon NW. CheY3 of Borrelia burgdorferi is the key response regulator essential for chemotaxis and forms a long-lived phosphorylated intermediate. J Bacteriol. 2011 Jul;193(13):3332-41. Epub 2011 Apr 29. PMID:21531807

Müllegger RR, Glatz M. [Skin infections in pregnancy].[Article in German]. Hautarzt. 2010 Dec;61(12):1034-9. PMID:21079901

Müller I, Freitag MH, Poggensee G, Scharnetzky E, Straube E, Schoerner Ch, Hlobil H, Hagedorn HJ, Stanek G, Schubert-Unkmeir A, Norris DE, Gensichen J, Hunfeld KP. Evaluating frequency, diagnostic quality, and cost of Lyme borreliosis testing in Germany: a retrospective model analysis. Clin Dev Immunol. 2012;2012:595427. Epub 2011 Dec 27. PMID:22242037

Mulić R, Petković B, Klismanić Z, Jeroncić I. [Tick-borne diseases in the Republic of Croatia].[Article in Croatian]. Lijec Vjesn. 2011 Mar-Apr;133(3-4):89-95. PMID:21612103

Munson E, Nardelli DT, Du Chateau BK, Callister SM, Schell RF. Hamster and murine models of severe destructive Lyme arthritis. Clin Dev Immunol. 2012;2012:504215. Epub 2012 Feb 22. PMID:22461836

Murdock JH, Yabsley MJ, Little SE, Chandrashekar R, O'Connor TP, Caudell JN, Huffman JE, Langenberg JA, Hollamby S. Distribution of antibodies reactive to Borrelia lonestari and Borrelia burgdorferi in white-tailed deer (Odocoileus virginianus) populations in the eastern United States. Vector Borne Zoonotic Dis. 2009 Dec;9(6):729-36. PMID:19874183

Murillo G, Ramírez B, Romo LA, Muñoz-Sanz A, Hileeto D, Calonge M. Oculopalpebral Borreliosis as an Unusual Manifestation of Lyme Disease. Cornea. 2012 Apr 10. [Epub ahead of print]. PMID:22495033

Murray K, Helgason KO. Positive Borrelia burgdorferi serology secondary to intravenous immunoglobulin therapy. J Infect. 2012 Jan;64(1):117-8. Epub 2011 Oct 21. PMID:22037548

Murray TS, Shapiro ED. Lyme disease. Clin Lab Med. 2010 Mar;30(1):311-28. PMID:20513553

Mwirigi NW, Rodriguez-Porcel M. 31-year-old man with fever, palpitations, and generalized rash. Mayo Clin Proc. 2010 Apr;85(4):e13-6. PMID:20360288

Myers TA, Kaushal D, Philipp MT. Microglia are mediators of Borrelia burgdorferi-induced apoptosis in SH-SY5Y neuronal cells. PLoS Pathog. 2009 Nov;5(11):e1000659. Epub 2009 Nov 13. PMID:19911057

Mygland A, Ljøstad U, Fingerle V, Rupprecht T, Schmutzhard E, Steiner I; European Federation of Neurological Societies. EFNS guidelines on the diagnosis and management of European Lyme neuroborreliosis. Eur J Neurol. 2010 Jan;17(1):8-16, e1-4. Epub 2009 Nov 23. PMID:19930447

Mygland A. [When red flag flips, but blood tests and MR are normal]. [Article in Norwegian]. Tidsskr Nor Laegeforen. 2011 May 20;131(9-10):961. PMID:21606996

Mylonas I. Borreliosis during pregnancy: a risk for the unborn child? Vector Borne Zoonotic Dis. 2011 Jul;11(7):891-8. Epub 2010 Oct 6. PMID:20925520

Nadolny RM, Wright CL, Hynes WL, Sonenshine DE, Gaff HD. Ixodes affinis (Acari: Ixodidae) in southeastern Virginia and implications for the spread of Borrelia burgdorferi, the agent of Lyme disease. J Vector Ecol. 2011 Dec;36(2):464-7. PMID:22129422

Naesens R, Vermeiren S, Van Schaeren J, Jeurissen A. False positive Lyme serology due to syphilis: report of 6 cases and review of the literature. Acta Clin Belg. 2011 Jan-Feb;66(1):58-9. PMID:21485767

Nafeev AA, Fefelova EV. [Causes affecting the incidence of Ixodes tick-borne borreliosis].[Article in Russian]. Med Parazitol (Mosk). 2009 Jul-Sep;(3):42-4. PMID:19827516

Nafeev AA, Klimova LV. [Clinical manifestations of neuroborreliosis in the Volga region].[Article in Russian]. Ter Arkh. 2010;82(11):68-70. PMID:21381354

Nafeev AA, Vinogradova IB, Tishina LV, Ladanova RK. [Cutaneous manifestations of the late stage of Lyme's disease].[Article in Russian]. Klin Med (Mosk). 2011;89(2):59-60. PMID:21574447

Nafeev AA. [Quality assessment of antiepidemic measures in feral herd infections].[Article in Russian]. Med Parazitol (Mosk). 2011 Jan-Mar;(1):55-6. PMID:21476263

Nardelli DT, Luedtke JO, Munson EL, Warner TF, Callister SM, Schell RF. Significant differences between the Borrelia-infection and Borrelia-vaccination and -infection models of Lyme arthritis in C3H/HeN mice. FEMS Immunol Med Microbiol. 2010 Oct;60(1):78-89. PMID:20662925

Nazzi F, Martinelli E, Del Fabbro S, Bernardinelli I, Milani N, Iob A, Pischiutti P, Campello C, D'Agaro P. Ticks and Lyme borreliosis in an alpine area in northeast Italy. Med Vet Entomol. 2010 Sep;24(3):220-6. Epub 2010 May 30. PMID:20534008

Nefedova VV, Korenberg EI, Gorelova NB. [Genetic variants of Borrelia garinii, a widely spread Eurasian pathogen of ixodic tick borreliosis].[Article in Russian]. Mol Gen Mikrobiol Virusol. 2010;(3):7-12. PMID:20882770

Nefedova VV, Korenberg EI, Gorelova NB. [Genotyping some Borrelia burgdorferi sensu lato isolates from Ixodes ricinus ticks in Russia and Ukraine].[Article in Russian]. Mol Gen Mikrobiol Virusol. 2010;(1):21-6. PMID:20364477

Network to Reduce Lyme Disease in School-Aged Children. You can make a difference to a child by reducing risk of Lyme disease. NASN Sch Nurse. 2010 May;25(3):110-3. PMID:20486444

Nghiem PP, Schatzberg SJ. Conventional and molecular diagnostic testing for the acute neurologic patient. J Vet Emerg Crit Care (San Antonio). 2010 Feb;20(1):46-61. PMID:20230434

Nieto NC, Holmes EA, Foley JE. Survival rates of immature Ixodes pacificus (Acari: Ixodidae) ticks estimated using field-placed enclosures. J Vector Ecol. 2010 Jun;35(1):43-9. PMID:20618646

Nieto NC, Leonhard S, Foley JE, Lane RS. Coinfection of western gray squirrel (Sciurus griseus) and other sciurid rodents with Borrelia burgdorferi sensu stricto and Anaplasma phagocytophilum in California. J Wildl Dis. 2010 Jan;46(1):291-6. PMID:20090047

Niu Q, Guan G, Yang J, Fu Y, Xu Z, Li Y, Ma M, Liu Z, Liu J, Liu A, Ren Q, Jorgensen W, Luo J, Yin H. Detection and differentiation of Borrelia burgdorferi sensu lato in ticks collected from sheep and cattle in China. BMC Vet Res. 2011 Apr 29;7:17. Retraction in: BMC Vet Res. 2011;7:56. PMID:21529349

No authors listed. [Borreliosis. Questionable diagnoses, questionable therapies].[Article in German]. MMW Fortschr Med. 2009 Aug 20;151(34-35):20-1. PMID:19771783

No authors listed. [The proof of antineural antibodies in patients with neuroborreliosis].[Article in Czech]. Klin Mikrobiol Infekc Lek. 2011 Aug;17(4):141-3. PMID:22052101

No authors listed. First aid for coping with summer pests. Consum Rep. 2009 Jul;74(7):12. PMID:19697480

No authors listed. How can I tell if my joint pain is Lyme arthritis or Lyme disease and is the treatment any different for either condition? Duke Med Health News. 2009 Dec;15(12):8. PMID:20120512

No authors listed. It's time to really get the ticks off. The coming months are the prime time for getting tick-borne Lyme disease. Harv Health Lett. 2010 Apr;35(6):4-5. PMID:20513146

No authors listed. Risk of Lyme disease higher than previously thought. Vet Rec. 2012 Jan;170(4):88. PMID:22287388

No authors listed. Treatment of Lyme disease. Med Lett Drugs Ther. 2010 Jul 12;52(1342):53-4. PMID:20622805

Nogueira SV, Smith AA, Qin JH, Pal U. A surface enolase participates in Borrelia burgdorferi-plasminogen interaction and contributes to pathogen survival within feeding ticks. Infect Immun. 2012 Jan;80(1):82-90. Epub 2011 Oct 24. PMID:22025510

Nordberg M, Forsberg P, Johansson A, Nyman D, Jansson C, Ernerudh J, Ekerfelt C. Cytotoxic mechanisms may play a role in the local immune response in the central nervous system in neuroborreliosis. J Neuroimmunol. 2011 Mar;232(1-2):186-93. Epub 2010 Nov 5. PMID:21056912

Norris SJ, Howell JK, Odeh EA, Lin T, Gao L, Edmondson DG. High-throughput plasmid content analysis of Borrelia burgdorferi B31 by using Luminex multiplex technology. Appl Environ Microbiol. 2011 Feb;77(4):1483-92. Epub 2010 Dec 17. PMID:21169439

Norris SJ, Lin T. Out of the woods: the remarkable genomes of the genus Borrelia. J Bacteriol. 2011 Dec;193(24):6812-4. Epub 2011 Oct 14. PMID:22001507

Nowakowski J, McKenna D, Nadelman RB, Bittker S, Cooper D, Pavia C, Holmgren D, Visintainer P, Wormser GP. Blood cultures for patients with extracutaneous manifestations of Lyme disease in the United States. Clin Infect Dis. 2009 Dec 1;49(11):1733-5. PMID:19886794

O'Connell S. Lyme borreliosis: current issues in diagnosis and management. Curr Opin Infect Dis. 2010 Jun;23(3):231-5. PMID:20407371

Ogden NH, Bouchard C, Kurtenbach K, Margos G, Lindsay LR, Trudel L, Nguon S, Milord F. Active and passive surveillance and phylogenetic analysis of Borrelia burgdorferi elucidate the process of Lyme disease risk emergence in Canada. Environ Health Perspect. 2010 Jul;118(7):909-14. Epub 2010 Mar 25. PMID:20421192

Ogden NH, Lindsay LR, Morshed M, Sockett PN, Artsob H. The emergence of Lyme disease in Canada. CMAJ. 2009 Jun 9;180(12):1221-4. PMID:19506281

Ogden NH, Margos G, Aanensen DM, Drebot MA, Feil EJ, Hanincová K, Schwartz I, Tyler S, Lindsay LR. Investigation of genotypes of Borrelia burgdorferi in Ixodes scapularis ticks collected during surveillance in Canada. Appl Environ Microbiol. 2011 May;77(10):3244-54. Epub 2011 Mar 18. PMID:21421790

Ogden NH, Tsao JI. Biodiversity and Lyme disease: dilution or amplification? Epidemics. 2009 Sep;1(3):196-206. Epub 2009 Jun 21. PMID:21352766

Ogłodek E, Moś D, Araszkiewicz A. [Coexisting of borreliosis, depression and psoriasis--case report].[Article in Polish]. Pol Merkur Lekarski. 2010 Jan;28(163):53-5. PMID:20369726

Oliveira A, Fonseca AH, Costa CM, Mantovani E, Yoshinari NH. Growth, cysts and kinetics of Borrelia garinii (Spirochaetales: Spirochaetacea) in different culture media. Mem Inst Oswaldo Cruz. 2010 Aug;105(5):717-9. PMID:20835623

Onder O, Humphrey PT, McOmber B, Korobova F, Francella N, Greenbaum DC, Brisson D. OspC is a potent plasminogen-receptor on the surface of Borrelia burgdorferi. J Biol Chem. 2012 Mar 20. [Epub ahead of print]. PMID:22433849

Oosting M, Berende A, Sturm P, Ter Hofstede HJ, de Jong DJ, Kanneganti TD, van der Meer JW, Kullberg BJ, Netea MG, Joosten LA. Recognition of Borrelia burgdorferi by NOD2 is central for the induction of an inflammatory reaction. J Infect Dis. 2010 Jun 15;201(12):1849-58. PMID:20441518

Oosting M, Ter Hofstede H, Sturm P, Adema GJ, Kullberg BJ, van der Meer JW, Netea MG, Joosten LA. TLR1/TLR2 heterodimers play an important role in the recognition of Borrelia spirochetes. PLoS One. 2011;6(10):e25998. Epub 2011 Oct 5. PMID:21998742

Oosting M, ter Hofstede H, van de Veerdonk FL, Sturm P, Kullberg BJ, van der Meer JW, Netea MG, Joosten LA. Role of interleukin-23 (IL-23) receptor signaling for IL-17 responses in human Lyme disease. Infect Immun. 2011 Nov;79(11):4681-7. Epub 2011 Sep 6. PMID:21896776

Oosting M, van de Veerdonk FL, Kanneganti TD, Sturm P, Verschueren I, Berende A, van der Meer JW, Kullberg BJ, Netea MG, Joosten LA. Borrelia species induce inflammasome activation and IL-17 production through a caspase-1-dependent mechanism. Eur J Immunol. 2011 Jan;41(1):172-81. Epub 2010 Dec 9. PMID:21182088

Ostendorf GM. [No work disability in supposed post-borreliosis syndrome. On the decision of the OLG Saarbrücken of 19 May 2010]. [Article in German]. Versicherungsmedizin. 2011 Jun 1;63(2):106-7. PMID:21698949

Oteiza-Olaso J, Tiberio-López G, Martínez de Artola V, Belzunegui-Otano T. [Seroprevalence of Lyme disease in Navarra, Spain].[Article in Spanish]. Med Clin (Barc). 2011 Mar 26;136(8):336-9. Epub 2010 Sep 29. PMID:20880560

Ouyang Z, Deka RK, Norgard MV. BosR (BB0647) controls the RpoN-RpoS regulatory pathway and virulence expression in Borrelia burgdorferi by a novel DNA-binding mechanism. PLoS Pathog. 2011 Feb 10;7(2):e1001272. PMID:21347346

Ouyang Z, Kumar M, Kariu T, Haq S, Goldberg M, Pal U, Norgard MV. BosR (BB0647) governs virulence expression in Borrelia burgdorferi. Mol Microbiol. 2009 Dec;74(6):1331-43. Epub 2009 Nov 2. PMID:19889086

Ouyang Z, Narasimhan S, Neelakanta G, Kumar M, Pal U, Fikrig E, Norgard MV. Activation of the RpoN-RpoS regulatory pathway during the enzootic life cycle of Borrelia burgdorferi. BMC Microbiol. 2012 Mar 23;12:44. PMID:22443136

Pachner AR. Do we need to broaden the spectrum of Lyme neuroborreliosis? J Neurol Sci. 2010 Aug 15;295(1-2):8-9. Epub 2010 Jun 8. PMID:20621799

Padgett KA, Bonilla DL. Novel exposure sites for nymphal Ixodes pacificus within picnic areas. Ticks Tick Borne Dis. 2011 Dec;2(4):191-5. Epub 2011 Sep 25. PMID:22108011

Padgett KA, Casher LE, Stephens SL, Lane RS. Effect of prescribed fire for tick control in California chaparral. J Med Entomol. 2009 Sep;46(5):1138-45. PMID:19769046

Palecek T, Kuchynka P, Hulinska D, Schramlova J, Hrbackova H, Vitkova I, Simek S, Horak J, Louch WE, Linhart A. Presence of Borrelia burgdorferi in endomyocardial biopsies in patients with new-onset unexplained dilated cardiomyopathy. Med Microbiol Immunol. 2010 May;199(2):139-43. Epub 2010 Jan 6. PMID:20052487

Palmen C, Jamblin P, Florkin B, Hoyoux C. [Borrelia-associated lymphocytoma cutis].[Article in French]. Arch Pediatr. 2010 Aug;17(8):1159-61. Epub 2010 Jun 22. PMID:20573489

Palmer GH, Bankhead T, Lukehart SA. 'Nothing is permanent but change'-antigenic variation in persistent bacterial pathogens. Cell Microbiol. 2009 Dec;11(12):1697-705. Epub 2009 Aug 25. PMID:19709057

Panelius J, Ranki A, Meri T, Seppälä I, Meri S. Expression and sequence diversity of the complement regulating outer surface protein E in Borrelia afzelii vs. Borrelia garinii in patients with erythema migrans or neuroborreliosis. Microb Pathog. 2010 Dec;49(6):363-8. Epub 2010 Aug 9. PMID:20603210

Panic G, Stanulovic V, Popov T. Atrio-ventricular block as the first presentation of disseminated Lyme disease. Int J Cardiol. 2011 Aug 4;150(3):e104-6. Epub 2010 Mar 11. PMID:20226549

Pantchev N, Schaper R, Limousin S, Norden N, Weise M, Lorentzen L. Occurrence of Dirofilaria immitis and tick-borne infections caused by Anaplasma phagocytophilum, Borrelia burgdorferi sensu lato and Ehrlichia canis in domestic dogs in France: results of a countrywide serologic survey. Parasitol Res. 2009 Aug;105 Suppl 1:S101-14. PMID:19575231

Pappas CJ, Iyer R, Petzke MM, Caimano MJ, Radolf JD, Schwartz I. Borrelia burgdorferi requires glycerol for maximum fitness during the tick phase of the enzootic cycle. PLoS Pathog. 2011 Jul;7(7):e1002102. Epub 2011 Jul 7. PMID:21750672

Paradowska-Stankiewicz I, Chrześcijańska I. [Lyme borreliosis in Poland in 2009].[Article in Polish]. Przegl Epidemiol. 2011;65(2):279-80. PMID:21913475

Parola P, Diatta G, Socolovschi C, Mediannikov O, Tall A, Bassene H, Trape JF, Raoult D. Tick-borne relapsing fever borreliosis, rural senegal. Emerg Infect Dis. 2011 May;17(5):883-5. PMID:21529402

Parola P, Ryelandt J, Mangold AJ, Mediannikov O, Guglielmone AA, Raoult D. Relapsing fever Borrelia in Ornithodoros ticks from Bolivia. Ann Trop Med Parasitol. 2011 Jul;105(5):407-11. PMID:21929883

Parveen N, Cornell KA. Methylthioadenosine/S-adenosylhomocysteine nucleosidase, a critical enzyme for bacterial metabolism. Mol Microbiol. 2011 Jan;79(1):7-20. Epub 2010 Nov 18. PMID:21166890

Pasareanu AR, Mygland Å, Kristensen Ø. A woman in her 50s with manic psychosis.[Article in English, Norwegian]. Tidsskr Nor Laegeforen. 2012 Mar 6;132(5):537-9. PMID:22398772

Pascucci I, Cammà C. Lyme disease and the detection of Borrelia burgdorferi genospecies in Ixodes ricinus ticks from central Italy. [Article in English, Italian]. Vet Ital. 2010 Apr-Jun;46(2):173-80, 181-8. PMID:20560127

Patil N, Bariola JR, Saccente M, Vyas KS, Bradsher RW Jr. A clinical review of Lyme disease in Arkansas. J Ark Med Soc. 2010 Feb;106(8):186-8. PMID:20218039

Paton M. Just a tick. Interview by Mary-Claire Mason. Nurs Stand. 2010 May 5-11;24(35):25. PMID:20509377

Patton TG, Dietrich G, Brandt K, Dolan MC, Piesman J, Gilmore RD Jr. Saliva, salivary gland, and hemolymph collection from Ixodes scapularis ticks. J Vis Exp. 2012 Feb 21;(60). pii: 3894. PMID:22371172

Patton TG, Dietrich G, Dolan MC, Piesman J, Carroll JA, Gilmore RD Jr. Functional analysis of the Borrelia burgdorferi bba64 gene product in murine infection via tick infestation. PLoS One. 2011 May 3;6(5):e19536. PMID:21559293

Patton TG, Dietrich G, Gilmore RD Jr. Detection of Borrelia burgdorferi DNA in tick feces provides evidence for organism shedding during vector feeding. Vector Borne Zoonotic Dis. 2011 Mar;11(3):197-200. Epub 2010 Oct 6. PMID:20925527

Pereyra-Rodríguez JJ, Bernabeu-Wittel J, Cañas E, Conejo-Mir J. [Slowly enlarging erythematous macule].[Article in Spanish]. Enferm Infecc Microbiol Clin. 2011 Jan;29(1):68-9. Epub 2010 Dec 30. PMID:21194805

Pérez D, Kneubühler Y, Rais O, Gern L. Seasonality of Ixodes ricinus Ticks on Vegetation and on Rodents and Borrelia burgdorferi sensu lato Genospecies Diversity in Two Lyme Borreliosis-Endemic Areas in Switzerland. Vector Borne Zoonotic Dis. 2012 May 18. [Epub ahead of print]. PMID:22607074

Pérez D, Kneubühler Y, Rais O, Jouda F, Gern L. Borrelia afzelii ospC genotype diversity in Ixodes ricinus questing ticks and ticks from rodents in two Lyme borreliosis endemic areas: contribution of co-feeding ticks. Ticks Tick Borne Dis. 2011 Sep;2(3):137-42. Epub 2011 Aug 19. PMID:21890066

Pérez López A, Bandiera Geb Popowa D, Padilla Esteba E, Beinbrech B. [Facial palsy in a 7-year-old German tourist].[Article in Spanish]. An Pediatr (Barc). 2009 Jun;70(6):601-2. Epub 2009 May 14. PMID:19446508

Peterhans E, Peterhans E. ["Lyme disease" as a possible cause for lameness in the cat].[Article in German]. Schweiz Arch Tierheilkd. 2010 Jun;152(6):295-7. PMID:20533203

Petnicki-Ocwieja T, DeFrancesco AS, Chung E, Darcy CT, Bronson RT, Kobayashi KS, Hu LT. Nod2 suppresses Borrelia burgdorferi mediated murine Lyme arthritis and carditis through the induction of tolerance. PLoS One. 2011 Feb 28;6(2):e17414. PMID:21387014

Petranović D, Duletić-Nacinović A, Skarpa-Prpić I, Batinac T, Marić J, Kardum M, Vukić-Troselj B. Gorski Kotar--an endemic region for primary gastric non-hodgkin lymphoma? Coll Antropol. 2010 Sep;34(3):877-80. PMID:20977076

Petzke MM, Brooks A, Krupna MA, Mordue D, Schwartz I. Recognition of Borrelia burgdorferi, the Lyme disease spirochete, by TLR7 and TLR9 induces a type I IFN response by human immune cells. J Immunol. 2009 Oct 15;183(8):5279-92. Epub 2009 Sep 30. PMID:19794067

Pfister HW. [Clinical aspects of neuroborreliosis].[Article in German]. MMW Fortschr Med. 2010 Jul 1;152(25-27):31-4; quiz 35. PMID:20672660

Pfister HW. [Infectious neurological diseases. Diagnostic confirmation from the cerebrospinal fluid].[Article in German]. MMW Fortschr Med. 2010 Jul 1;152(25-27):30. PMID:20672659

Piesman J, Hojgaard A. Protective value of prophylactic antibiotic treatment of tick bite for Lyme disease prevention: An animal model. Ticks Tick Borne Dis. 2012 Mar 13. [Epub ahead of print]. PMID:22421585

Pietikäinen J, Meri T, Blom AM, Meri S. Binding of the complement inhibitor C4b-binding protein to Lyme disease Borreliae. Mol Immunol. 2010 Mar;47(6):1299-305. Epub 2009 Dec 21. PMID:20022381

Pignataro L, Torretta S, Capaccio P, Esposito S, Marchisio P. Unusual otolaryngological manifestations of certain systemic bacterial and fungal infections in children. Int J Pediatr Otorhinolaryngol. 2009 Dec;73 Suppl 1:S33-7. PMID:20114153

Pistone D, Pajoro M, Fabbi M, Vicari N, Marone P, Genchi C, Novati S, Sassera D, Epis S, Bandi C. Lyme borreliosis, Po River Valley, Italy. Emerg Infect Dis. 2010 Aug;16(8):1289-91. PMID:20678327

Pitzer JE, Sultan SZ, Hayakawa Y, Hobbs G, Miller MR, Motaleb MA. Analysis of the Borrelia burgdorferi cyclic-di-GMP-binding protein PlzA reveals a role in motility and virulence. Infect Immun. 2011 May;79(5):1815-25. Epub 2011 Feb 28. PMID:21357718

Platonov AE, Karan LS, Kolyasnikova NM, Makhneva NA, Toporkova MG, Maleev VV, Fish D, Krause PJ. Humans infected with relapsing fever spirochete Borrelia miyamotoi, Russia. Emerg Infect Dis. 2011 Oct;17(10):1816-23. PMID:22000350

Platonov AE, Maleev VV, Karan' LS. [Relapsing borrelioses fevers: forgotten and new ones].[Article in Russian]. Ter Arkh. 2010;82(11):74-80. PMID:21381356

Plotkin SA. Correcting a public health fiasco: The need for a new vaccine against Lyme disease. Clin Infect Dis. 2011 Feb;52 Suppl 3:s271-5. PMID:21217175

Podsiadły E, Chmielewski T, Karbowiak G, Kędra E, Tylewska-Wierzbanowska S. The occurrence of spotted fever rickettsioses and other tick-borne infections in forest workers in Poland. Vector Borne Zoonotic Dis. 2011 Jul;11(7):985-9. Epub 2010 Nov 17. PMID:21083370

Pohlit AM, Rezende AR, Lopes Baldin EL, Lopes NP, Neto VF. Plant extracts, isolated phytochemicals, and plant-derived agents which are lethal to arthropod vectors of human tropical diseases--a review. Planta Med. 2011 Apr;77(6):618-30. Epub 2011 Mar 22. PMID:21432748

Poland GA. Vaccines against Lyme disease: What happened and what lessons can we learn? Clin Infect Dis. 2011 Feb;52 Suppl 3:s253-8. PMID:21217172

Polat E, Turhan V, Aslan M, Müsellim B, Onem Y, Ertuğrul B. [First report of three culture confirmed human Lyme cases in Turkey].[Article in Turkish]. Mikrobiyol Bul. 2010 Jan;44(1):133-9. PMID:20455410

Policastro PF, Raffel SJ, Schwan TG. Cotransmission of divergent relapsing fever spirochetes by artificially infected Ornithodoros hermsi. Appl Environ Microbiol. 2011 Dec;77(24):8494-9. Epub 2011 Sep 30. PMID:21965393

Poljak A, Comstedt P, Hanner M, Schüler W, Meinke A, Wizel B, Lundberg U. Identification and characterization of Borrelia antigens as potential vaccine candidates against Lyme borreliosis. Vaccine. 2011 Nov 18. [Epub ahead of print]. PMID:22100635

Ponirovskiĭ EN, Podbornov VM. [Nikolai Ivanovich Latyshev (on the occasion of 125th anniversary of his birth)].[Article in Russian]. Med Parazitol (Mosk). 2011 Oct-Dec;(4):57-60. PMID:22308718

Popko J, Olszewski S, Guszczyn T, Zwierz K, Pancewicz S. Glycoconjugate markers of joint diseases. Biochem Soc Trans. 2011 Jan;39(1):331-5. PMID:21265798

Poponnikova TV, Bedareva TIu, Vakhrameeva TN, Galieva GIu. [The cytokine profile in the acute period of tick-borne neuroinfections in children].[Article in Russian]. Zh Nevrol Psikhiatr Im S S Korsakova. 2010;110(5 Pt 1):9-12. PMID:21322819

Porwancher RB, Hagerty CG, Fan J, Landsberg L, Johnson BJ, Kopnitsky M, Steere AC, Kulas K, Wong SJ. Multiplex immunoassay for Lyme disease using VlsE1-IgG and pepC10-IgM antibodies: improving test performance through bioinformatics. Clin Vaccine Immunol. 2011 May;18(5):851-9. Epub 2011 Mar 2. PMID:21367982

Pound JM, Miller JA, George JE, Fish D. The United States Department Of Agriculture Northeast Area-wide Tick Control Project: history and protocol. Vector Borne Zoonotic Dis. 2009 Aug;9(4):365-70. PMID:19650730

Pozsgay V, Kubler-Kielb J, Coxon B, Marques A, Robbins JB, Schneerson R. Synthesis and antigenicity of BBGL-2 glycolipids of Borrelia burgdorferi, the causative agent of Lyme disease. Carbohydr Res. 2011 Sep 6;346(12):1551-63. Epub 2011 May 3. PMID:21601180

Pratt JW, Meyer DR, Wroblewski D, Carlson JA. Orbital inflammation and lyme disease. Ophthalmology. 2011 Sep;118(9):1892.e1-2. PMID:21889662

Priest HL, Irby NL, Schlafer DH, Divers TJ, Wagner B, Glaser AL, Chang YF, Smith MC. Diagnosis of Borrelia-associated uveitis in two horses. Vet Ophthalmol. 2012 Feb 23. [Epub ahead of print]. PMID:22360730

Probst C, Ott A, Scheper T, Meyer W, Stöcker W, Komorowski L. N-terminal disulfide-bridging of Borrelia outer surface protein C increases its diagnostic and vaccine potentials. Ticks Tick Borne Dis. 2012 Feb;3(1):1-7. Epub 2011 Nov 25. PMID:22309852

Promnares K, Kumar M, Shroder DY, Zhang X, Anderson JF, Pal U. Borrelia burgdorferi small lipoprotein Lp6.6 is a member of multiple protein complexes in the outer membrane and facilitates pathogen transmission from ticks to mice. Mol Microbiol. 2009 Oct;74(1):112-25. Epub 2009 Aug 24. PMID:19703109

Pukhovskaia NM, Rar VA, Ivanov LI, Vysochina NP, Igolkina IaP, Fomenko NV, Zaraĭchenkova NV, Plashkova VV, Oreshkina SG, Mal'tseva IP, Chistov VA, Chechikova VA. [PCR detection of the causative agents of infections transmitted by ticks on the Kamchatka Peninsula].[Article in Russian]. Med Parazitol (Mosk). 2010 Oct-Dec;(4):36-9. PMID:21400710

Pulzova L, Kovac A, Mucha R, Mlynarcik P, Bencurova E, Madar M, Novak M, Bhide M. OspA-CD40 dyad: ligand-receptor interaction in the translocation of neuroinvasive Borrelia across the blood-brain barrier. Sci Rep. 2011;1:86. Epub 2011 Sep 8. PMID:22355605

Quine CP, Barnett J, Dobson AD, Marcu A, Marzano M, Moseley D, O'Brien L, Randolph SE, Taylor JL, Uzzell D. Frameworks for risk communication and disease management: the case of Lyme disease and countryside users. Philos Trans R Soc Lond B Biol Sci. 2011 Jul 12;366(1573):2010-22. PMID:21624921

Qureshi M, Bedlack RS, Cudkowicz ME. Lyme disease serology in amyotrophic lateral sclerosis. Muscle Nerve. 2009 Oct;40(4):626-8. PMID:19697382

Radolf JD, Caimano MJ, Stevenson B, Hu LT. Of ticks, mice and men: understanding the dual-host lifestyle of Lyme disease spirochaetes. Nat Rev Microbiol. 2012 Jan 9;10(2):87-99. PMID:22230951

Ragagli C, Bertolotti L, Giacobini M, Mannelli A, Bisanzio D, Amore G, Tomassone L. Transmission dynamics of Borrelia lusitaniae and Borrelia afzelii among Ixodes ricinus, lizards, and mice in Tuscany, central Italy. Vector Borne Zoonotic Dis. 2011 Jan;11(1):21-8. Epub 2010 May 19. PMID:20482342

Raizman EA, Holland JD, Keefe LM, Moro MH. Forest and surface water as predictors of Borrelia burgdorferi and its vector Ixodes scapularis (Acari: Ixodidae) in Indiana. J Med Entomol. 2010 May;47(3):458-65. PMID:20496594

Rajaguru S, Havlichek D, Khalife W, Kalra A. A 20-year-old man with fever, headache, and neck stiffness. Neuroborreliosis with tick-borne relapsing fever. Clin Infect Dis. 2011 Jan 15;52(2):218, 271-2. PMID:21288847

Raju BV, Esteve-Gassent MD, Karna SL, Miller CL, Van Laar TA, Seshu J. Oligopeptide permease A5 modulates vertebrate host-specific adaptation of Borrelia burgdorferi. Infect Immun. 2011 Aug;79(8):3407-20. Epub 2011 May 31. PMID:21628523

Ramesh G, Benge S, Pahar B, Philipp MT. A possible role for inflammation in mediating apoptosis of oligodendrocytes as induced by the Lyme disease spirochete Borrelia burgdorferi. J Neuroinflammation. 2012 Apr 23;9(1):72. [Epub ahead of print]. PMID:22524232

Ramesh G, Borda JT, Gill A, Ribka EP, Morici LA, Mottram P, Martin DS, Jacobs MB, Didier PJ, Philipp MT. Possible role of glial cells in the onset and progression of Lyme neuroborreliosis. J Neuroinflammation. 2009 Aug 25;6:23. PMID:19706181

Rand PW, Lacombe EH, Elias SP, Cahill BK, Lubelczyk CB, Smith RP Jr. Multitarget test for emerging Lyme disease and anaplasmosis in a serosurvey of dogs, Maine, USA. Emerg Infect Dis. 2011 May;17(5):899-902. PMID:21529407

Rand PW, Lacombe EH, Elias SP, Lubelczyk CB, St Amand T, Smith RP Jr. Trial of a minimal-risk botanical compound to control the vector tick of Lyme disease. J Med Entomol. 2010 Jul;47(4):695-8. PMID:20695287

Randolph SE, Dobson AD. Pangloss revisited: a critique of the dilution effect and the biodiversity-buffers-disease paradigm. Parasitology. 2012 Feb 16:1-17. [Epub ahead of print]. PMID:22336330

Randolph SE. Tick-borne disease systems emerge from the shadows: the beauty lies in molecular detail, the message in epidemiology. Parasitology. 2009 Oct;136(12):1403-13. Epub 2009 Apr 14. PMID:19366480

Ranki A, Hyry H, Klimenko T, Laukkala T, Majamaa H, Mäkelä M, Syrjänen J, Vuopio J; Suomalaisen Lääkäriseuran Duodecimin; Suomen Ihotautilääkäriyhdistys RY:N; Asettama Työryhmä. [Update on current care guidelines. Bacterial skin infections].[Article in Finnish]. Duodecim. 2010;126(24):2883-4. PMID:21268910

Raya AI, Afonso JC, Perez-Ecija RA, Blanco B, Martín-de Las Mulas J, Carrasco L, Cortade LE, Gomez-Laguna J. Orbital myositis associated with Lyme disease in a dog. Vet Rec. 2010 Oct 23;167(17):663-4. PMID:21257469

Rego RO, Bestor A, Rosa PA. Defining the plasmid-borne restriction-modification systems of the Lyme disease spirochete Borrelia burgdorferi. J Bacteriol. 2011 Mar;193(5):1161-71. Epub 2010 Dec 30. PMID:21193609

Reirden DH, Menchise AN, Knox B, Gereige R, Howard T, Thomas EL, Connelly R, Tyler S, McPeak K. Index of suspicion. Pediatr Rev. 2009 Sep;30(9):357-63. PMID:19726702

Reisen WK. Landscape epidemiology of vector-borne diseases. Annu Rev Entomol. 2010;55:461-83. PMID:19737082

Reller ME, Clemens EG, Schachterle SE, Mtove GA, Sullivan DJ, Dumler JS. Multiplex 5' nuclease-quantitative PCR for diagnosis of relapsing fever in a large Tanzanian cohort. J Clin Microbiol. 2011 Sep;49(9):3245-9. Epub 2011 Jul 20. PMID:21775542

Rey V, Du Pasquier R, Muehl A, Péter O, Michel P. [Multiple ischemic strokes due to Borrelia garinii meningovasculitis].[Article in French]. Rev Neurol (Paris). 2010 Nov;166(11):931-4. PMID:20434741

Reye AL, Arinola OG, Hübschen JM, Muller CP. Pathogen prevalence in ticks collected from the vegetation and livestock in Nigeria. Appl Environ Microbiol. 2012 Apr;78(8):2562-8. Epub 2012 Feb 10. PMID:22327584

Reye AL, Hübschen JM, Sausy A, Muller CP. Prevalence and seasonality of tick-borne pathogens in questing Ixodes ricinus ticks from Luxembourg. Appl Environ Microbiol. 2010 May;76(9):2923-31. Epub 2010 Mar 12. PMID:20228110

Rhee H, Cameron DJ. Lyme disease and pediatric autoimmune neuropsychiatric disorders associated with streptococcal infections (PANDAS): an overview. Int J Gen Med. 2012;5:163-74. Epub 2012 Feb 22. PMID:22393303

Rhodes RG, Atoyan JA, Nelson DR. The chitobiose transporter, chbC, is required for chitin utilization in Borrelia burgdorferi. BMC Microbiol. 2010 Jan 26;10:21. PMID:20102636

Ricaud X, Rozenbaum JP, Landowski S, Baudouin C, Labbé A. Abnormal corneal nerves in a patient with Lyme disease. Eye (Lond). 2011 Nov;25(11):1524-5. Epub 2011 Aug 19. PMID:21852805

Richter D, Debski A, Hubalek Z, Matuschka FR. Absence of Lyme disease spirochetes in larval Ixodes ricinus ticks. Vector Borne Zoonotic Dis. 2012 Jan;12(1):21-7. Epub 2011 Sep 16. PMID:21923267

Richter D, Matuschka FR. "Candidatus Neoehrlichia mikurensis," Anaplasma phagocytophilum, and lyme disease spirochetes in questing european vector ticks and in feeding ticks removed from people. J Clin Microbiol. 2012 Mar;50(3):943-7. Epub 2012 Jan 11. PMID:22205824

Richter D, Matuschka FR. Differential risk for Lyme disease along hiking trail, Germany. Emerg Infect Dis. 2011 Sep;17(9):1704-6. PMID:21888798

Richter D, Matuschka FR. Elimination of lyme disease spirochetes from ticks feeding on domestic ruminants. Appl Environ Microbiol. 2010 Nov;76(22):7650-2. Epub 2010 Sep 24. PMID:20870789

Richter D, Schlee DB, Matuschka FR. Reservoir competence of various rodents for the lyme disease Spirochete Borrelia spielmanii. Appl Environ Microbiol. 2011 Jun;77(11):3565-70. Epub 2011 Apr 1. PMID:21460106

Rigó K, Gyuranecz M, Tóth AG, Földvári G. Detection of Borrelia burgdorferi Sensu Lato and Anaplasma phagocytophilum in small mammals and ectoparasites in Hungary. Vector Borne Zoonotic Dis. 2011 Nov;11(11):1499-501. Epub 2011 Jul 7. PMID:21736488

Riley LK. Lyme disease warning. Br Dent J. 2009 Nov 28;207(10):466. PMID:19942875

Ritzman AM, Hughes-Hanks JM, Blaho VA, Wax LE, Mitchell WJ, Brown CR. The chemokine receptor CXCR2 ligand KC (CXCL1) mediates neutrophil recruitment and is critical for development of experimental Lyme arthritis and carditis. Infect Immun. 2010 Nov;78(11):4593-600. Epub 2010 Sep 7. PMID:20823213

Rizzoli A, Hauffe H, Carpi G, Vourc H G, Neteler M, Rosa R. Lyme borreliosis in Europe. Euro Surveill. 2011 Jul 7;16(27). pii: 19906. PMID:21794218

Rodríguez I, Fernández C, Sánchez L, Martínez B, Siegrist HH, Lienhard R. Prevalence of antibodies to Borrelia burgdorferi sensu stricto in humans from a Cuban village. Braz J Infect Dis. 2012 Jan-Feb;16(1):82-5. PMID:22358362

Rogers EA, Abdunnur SV, McDowell JV, Marconi RT. Comparative analysis of the properties and ligand binding characteristics of CspZ, a factor H binding protein, derived from Borrelia burgdorferi isolates of human origin. Infect Immun. 2009 Oct;77(10):4396-405. Epub 2009 Jul 20. PMID:19620346

Ronn S. In the lymelight: law and clinical practice guidelines. South Med J. 2009 Jun;102(6):626-30. PMID:19434013

Ropper AH. Thoracoabdominal paralysis after walking in the brush. J Clin Neurosci. 2010 Dec;17(12):1541, 1608. PMID:21058442

Rorat M, Kuchar E, Szenborn L, Małyszczak K. [Growing boreliosis anxiety and its reasons].[Article in Polish]. Psychiatr Pol. 2010 Nov-Dec;44(6):895-904. PMID:21449171

Rosenfeld LE. Temporary permanent or permanent temporary pacing? Pacing Clin Electrophysiol. 2011 Jun;34(6):670-1. Epub 2011 Mar 31. PMID:21453335

Rosenlund S, Bækgaard N, Menné T. [Acrodermatitis chronica atrophicans can be difficult to diagnose].[Article in Danish]. Ugeskr Laeger. 2011 Dec 12;173(50):3272-3. PMID:22153213

Rostoff P, Gajos G, Konduracka E, Gackowski A, Nessler J, Piwowarska W. Lyme carditis: epidemiology, pathophysiology, and clinical features in endemic areas. Int J Cardiol. 2010 Oct 8;144(2):328-33. Epub 2009 Mar 28. PMID:19328565

Rudenko N, Golovchenko M, Grubhoffer L, Oliver JH Jr. Updates on Borrelia burgdorferi sensu lato complex with respect to public health. Ticks Tick Borne Dis. 2011 Sep;2(3):123-8. Epub 2011 May 27. PMID:21890064

Rudenko N, Golovchenko M, Lin T, Gao L, Grubhoffer L, Oliver JH Jr. Delineation of a new species of the Borrelia burgdorferi Sensu Lato Complex, Borrelia americana sp. nov. J Clin Microbiol. 2009 Dec;47(12):3875-80. Epub 2009 Oct 21. PMID:19846628

Rudolf I, Sikutová S, Kopecký J, Hubálek Z. Salivary gland extract from engorged Ixodes ricinus (Acari: Ixodidae) stimulates in vitro growth of Borrelia burgdorferi sensu lato. J Basic Microbiol. 2010 Jun;50(3):294-8. PMID:20143350

Ruef C. Borrelia burgdorferi bacteremia. Infection. 2011 Feb;39(1):1. PMID:21311945

Ruiz AM, Alcaraz LG, Fructuoso JR, Miguélez SA. [Peripheral facial palsy caused by Lyme disease].[Article in Spanish]. An Pediatr (Barc). 2009 Oct;71(4):369-70. Epub 2009 Sep 2. PMID:19729353

Rupprecht TA, Plate A, Adam M, Wick M, Kastenbauer S, Schmidt C, Klein M, Pfister HW, Koedel U. The chemokine CXCL13 is a key regulator of B cell recruitment to the cerebrospinal fluid in acute Lyme neuroborreliosis. J Neuroinflammation. 2009 Dec 30;6:42. PMID:20042073

Rydzewski J, Mateus-Pinilla N, Warner RE, Hamer S, Weng HY. Ixodes scapularis and Borrelia burgdorferi among diverse habitats within a natural area in east-central Illinois. Vector Borne Zoonotic Dis. 2011 Oct;11(10):1351-8. Epub 2011 Jun 20. PMID:21688974

Ryelandt J, Noireau F, Lazzari CR. A multimodal bait for trapping blood-sucking arthropods. Acta Trop. 2011 Feb;117(2):131-6. Epub 2010 Nov 27. PMID:21114956

Rymaszewska A, Adamska M. Molecular evidence of vector-borne pathogens coinfecting dogs from Poland. Acta Vet Hung. 2011 Jun;59(2):215-23. PMID:21665575

Sabino GJ, Hwang SJ, McAllister SC, Mena P, Furie MB. Interferon-γ influences the composition of leukocytic infiltrates in murine lyme carditis. Am J Pathol. 2011 Oct;179(4):1917-28. Epub 2011 Aug 5. PMID:21820995

Sabourin G. [Lyme disease. The carrier tick has settled in Quebec]. [Article in French]. Perspect Infirm. 2009 Sep-Oct;6(5):18-9. PMID:20120304

Safdie G, Farrah IY, Yahia R, Marva E, Wilamowski A, Sawalha SS, Wald N, Schmiedel J, Moter A, Göbel UB, Bercovier H, Abdeen Z, Assous MV, Fishman Y. Molecular characterization of Borrelia persica, the agent of tick borne relapsing fever in Israel and the Palestinian Authority. PLoS One. 2010 Nov 24;5(11):e14105. PMID:21124792

Sahay B, Patsey RL, Eggers CH, Salazar JC, Radolf JD, Sellati TJ. CD14 signaling restrains chronic inflammation through induction of p38-MAPK/SOCS-dependent tolerance. PLoS Pathog. 2009 Dec;5(12):e1000687. Epub 2009 Dec 11. PMID:20011115

Sahay B, Singh A, Gnanamani A, Patsey RL, Blalock JE, Sellati TJ. CD14 signaling reciprocally controls collagen deposition and turnover to regulate the development of lyme arthritis. Am J Pathol. 2011 Feb;178(2):724-34. PMID:21281805

Salkeld DJ, Lane RS. Community ecology and disease risk: lizards, squirrels, and the Lyme disease spirochete in California, USA. Ecology. 2010 Jan;91(1):293-8. PMID:20380218

Salman-Dilgimen A, Hardy PO, Dresser AR, Chaconas G. HrpA, a DEAH-box RNA helicase, is involved in global gene regulation in the Lyme disease spirochete. PLoS One. 2011;6(7):e22168. Epub 2011 Jul 26. PMID:21814569

Salo J, Loimaranta V, Lahdenne P, Viljanen MK, Hytönen J. Decorin binding by DbpA and B of Borrelia garinii, Borrelia afzelii, and Borrelia burgdorferi sensu Stricto. J Infect Dis. 2011 Jul 1;204(1):65-73. PMID:21628660

Samimi S, Salah S, Bonicel P. [Acquired nystagmus in a 12-year-old boy as initial presentation of Lyme disease].[Article in French]. J Fr Ophtalmol. 2011 May;34(5):325.e1-3. Epub 2011 Apr 14. PMID:21496946

Samuels DS, Radolf JD. Who is the BosR around here anyway? Mol Microbiol. 2009 Dec;74(6):1295-9. Epub 2009 Nov 25. PMID:19943896

Samuels DS. Gene regulation in Borrelia burgdorferi. Annu Rev Microbiol. 2011;65:479-99. PMID:21801026

Sanjuan E, Esteve-Gassent MD, Maruskova M, Seshu J. Overexpression of CsrA (BB0184) alters the morphology and antigen profiles of Borrelia burgdorferi. Infect Immun. 2009 Nov;77(11):5149-62. Epub 2009 Sep 8. PMID:19737901

Santino I, Comite P, Gandolfo GM. Borrelia burgdorferi, a great chameleon: know it to recognize it! Neurol Sci. 2010 Apr;31(2):193-6. Epub 2009 Nov 6. PMID:19894021

Santino I, Longobardi V. Clinical and serological features of patients with suspected Lyme borreliosis. Int J Immunopathol Pharmacol. 2011 Jul-Sep;24(3):797-801. PMID:21978712

Santos M, Haddad Júnior V, Ribeiro-Rodrigues R, Talhari S. Lyme borreliosis.[Article in English, Portuguese]. An Bras Dermatol. 2010 Dec;85(6):930-8. PMID:21308327

Santos M, Ribeiro-Rodrigues R, Lobo R, Talhari S. Antibody reactivity to Borrelia burgdorferi sensu stricto antigens in patients from the Brazilian Amazon region with skin diseases not related to Lyme disease. Int J Dermatol. 2010 May;49(5):552-6. PMID:20534091

Santos M, Ribeiro-Rodrigues R, Talhari C, Ferreira LC, Zelger B, Talhari S. Presence of Borrelia burgdorferi "Sensu Lato" in patients with morphea from the Amazonic region in Brazil. Int J Dermatol. 2011 Nov;50(11):1373-8. PMID:22004491

Sapi E, Kaur N, Anyanwu S, Luecke DF, Datar A, Patel S, Rossi M, Stricker RB. Evaluation of in-vitro antibiotic susceptibility of different morphological forms of Borrelia burgdorferi. Infect Drug Resist. 2011;4:97-113. Epub 2011 May 3. PMID:21753890

Sarih M, Garnier M, Boudebouch N, Bouattour A, Rihani A, Hassar M, Gern L, Postic D, Cornet M. Borrelia hispanica relapsing fever, Morocco. Emerg Infect Dis. 2009 Oct;15(10):1626-9. PMID:19861058

Sarkar A, Hayes BM, Dulebohn DP, Rosa PA. Regulation of the virulence determinant OspC by bbd18 on linear plasmid lp17 of Borrelia burgdorferi. J Bacteriol. 2011 Oct;193(19):5365-73. Epub 2011 Jul 22. PMID:21784941

Sauer A, Hansmann Y, Jaulhac B, Bourcier T, Speeg-Schatz C. [Ocular Lyme disease occurring during childhood: five case reports].[Article in French]. J Fr Ophtalmol. 2012 Jan;35(1):17-22. Epub 2011 Jun 22. PMID:21696850

Savely V. Lyme disease: a diagnostic dilemma. Nurse Pract. 2010 Jul;35(7):44-50. PMID:20555245

Savić S, Vidić B, Lazić S, Lako B, Potkonjak A, Lepsanović Z. Borrelia burgdorferi in ticks and dogs in the province of Vojvodina, Serbia. Parasite. 2010 Dec;17(4):357-61. PMID:21275243

Schicht S, Junge S, Schnieder T, Strube C. Prevalence of Anaplasma phagocytophilum and coinfection with Borrelia burgdorferi sensu lato in the hard tick Ixodes ricinus in the city of Hanover (Germany). Vector Borne Zoonotic Dis. 2011 Dec;11(12):1595-7. Epub 2011 Sep 15. PMID:21919727

Schmidt C, Plate A, Angele B, Pfister HW, Wick M, Koedel U, Rupprecht TA. A prospective study on the role of CXCL13 in Lyme neuroborreliosis. Neurology. 2011 Mar 22;76(12):1051-8. PMID:21422457

Schmit VL, Patton TG, Gilmore RD Jr. Analysis of Borrelia burgdorferi Surface Proteins as Determinants in Establishing Host Cell Interactions. Front Microbiol. 2011;2:141. Epub 2011 Jul 1. PMID:21747816

Schoen RT. A case revealing the natural history of untreated Lyme disease. Nat Rev Rheumatol. 2011 Mar;7(3):179-84. Epub 2010 Dec 21. PMID:21173795

Schröder J, Kirch W. [Lyme borreliosis: How should erythema migrans be treated in pregnant women?].[Article in German]. Dtsch Med Wochenschr. 2009 Nov;134(46):2354. Epub 2009 Nov 5. PMID:19894205

Schuijt TJ, Coumou J, Narasimhan S, Dai J, Deponte K, Wouters D, Brouwer M, Oei A, Roelofs JJ, van Dam AP, van der Poll T, Van't Veer C, Hovius JW, Fikrig E. A tick mannose-binding lectin inhibitor interferes with the vertebrate complement cascade to enhance transmission of the lyme disease agent. Cell Host Microbe. 2011 Aug 18;10(2):136-46. PMID:21843870

Schuijt TJ, Hovius JW, van der Poll T, van Dam AP, Fikrig E. Lyme borreliosis vaccination: the facts, the challenge, the future. Trends Parasitol. 2011 Jan;27(1):40-7. Epub 2010 Jun 30. PMID:20594913

Schulze RJ, Chen S, Kumru OS, Zückert WR. Translocation of Borrelia burgdorferi surface lipoprotein OspA through the outer membrane requires an unfolded conformation and can initiate at the C-terminus. Mol Microbiol. 2010 Jun 1;76(5):1266-78. Epub 2010 Apr 14. PMID:20398211

Schulze TL, Jordan RA, Hung RW, Schulze CJ. Effectiveness of the 4-Poster passive topical treatment device in the control of Ixodes scapularis and Amblyomma americanum (Acari: Ixodidae) in New Jersey. Vector Borne Zoonotic Dis. 2009 Aug;9(4):389-400. PMID:19650733

Schulze TL, Jordan RA, White JC, Roegner VE, Healy SP. Geographical distribution and prevalence of selected Borrelia, Ehrlichia, and Rickettsia infections in Amblyomma americanum (Acari: Ixodidae) in New Jersey. J Am Mosq Control Assoc. 2011 Sep;27(3):236-44. PMID:22017087

Schutzer SE, Angel TE, Liu T, Schepmoes AA, Clauss TR, Adkins JN, Camp DG, Holland BK, Bergquist J, Coyle PK, Smith RD, Fallon BA, Natelson BH. Distinct cerebrospinal fluid proteomes differentiate post-treatment lyme disease from chronic fatigue syndrome. PLoS One. 2011 Feb 23;6(2):e17287. PMID:21383843

Schutzer SE, Fraser-Liggett CM, Casjens SR, Qiu WG, Dunn JJ, Mongodin EF, Luft BJ. Whole-genome sequences of thirteen isolates of Borrelia burgdorferi. J Bacteriol. 2011 Feb;193(4):1018-20. Epub 2010 Oct 8. PMID:20935092

Schutzer SE, Fraser-Liggett CM, Qiu WG, Kraiczy P, Mongodin EF, Dunn JJ, Luft BJ, Casjens SR. Whole-genome sequences of Borrelia bissettii, Borrelia valaisiana, and Borrelia spielmanii. J Bacteriol. 2012 Jan;194(2):545-6. PMID:22207749

Schwan TG, Raffel SJ, Schrumpf ME, Gill JS, Piesman J. Characterization of a novel relapsing fever spirochete in the midgut, coxal fluid, and salivary glands of the bat tick Carios kelleyi. Vector Borne Zoonotic Dis. 2009 Dec;9(6):643-7. PMID:19281412

Schwan TG, Raffel SJ, Schrumpf ME, Schrumpf ME, Webster LS, Marques AR, Spano R, Rood M, Burns J, Hu R. Tick-borne relapsing fever and Borrelia hermsii, Los Angeles County, California, USA. Emerg Infect Dis. 2009 Jul;15(7):1026-31. PMID:19624916

Schwanz LE, Brisson D, Gomes-Solecki M, Ostfeld RS. Linking disease and community ecology through behavioural indicators: immunochallenge of white-footed mice and its ecological impacts. J Anim Ecol. 2011 Jan;80(1):204-14. Epub 2010 Aug 26. PMID:20796206

Schwanz LE, Voordouw MJ, Brisson D, Ostfeld RS. Borrelia burgdorferi has minimal impact on the Lyme disease reservoir host Peromyscus leucopus. Vector Borne Zoonotic Dis. 2011 Feb;11(2):117-24. Epub 2010 Jun 23. PMID:20569016

Schwarzová K, Kost'anová Z, Holecková K, Spitalská E, Boldis V. Direct detection of Borrelia burgdorferi spirochetes in patients with early disseminated Lyme borreliosis. Cent Eur J Public Health. 2009 Dec;17(4):179-82. PMID:20377044

Schwarzwalder A, Schneider MF, Lydecker A, Aucott JN. Sex differences in the clinical and serologic presentation of early Lyme disease: Results from a retrospective review. Gend Med. 2010 Aug;7(4):320-9. PMID:20869632

Scott JD, Anderson JF, Durden LA. Widespread dispersal of Borrelia burgdorferi-infected ticks collected from songbirds across Canada. J Parasitol. 2012 Feb;98(1):49-59. Epub 2011 Aug 24. PMID:21864130

Scott JD, Lee MK, Fernando K, Durden LA, Jorgensen DR, Mak S, Morshed MG. Detection of Lyme disease spirochete, Borrelia burgdorferi sensu lato, including three novel genotypes in ticks (Acari: Ixodidae) collected from songbirds (Passeriformes) across Canada. J Vector Ecol. 2010 Jun;35(1):124-39. PMID:20618658

Scott JD. Borrelia burgdorferi. J Med Entomol. 2012 Mar;49(2):237; author reply 237. PMID:22493839

Scott MC, Rosen ME, Hamer SA, Baker E, Edwards H, Crowder C, Tsao JI, Hickling GJ. High-prevalence Borrelia miyamotoi infection among [corrected] wild turkeys (Meleagris gallopavo) in Tennessee. J Med Entomol. 2010 Nov;47(6):1238-42. PMID:21175079

Seemanapalli SV, Xu Q, McShan K, Liang FT. Outer surface protein C is a dissemination-facilitating factor of Borrelia burgdorferi during mammalian infection. PLoS One. 2010 Dec 31;5(12):e15830. PMID:21209822

Seifter A, Schwarzwalder A, Geis K, Aucott J. The utility of "Google Trends" for epidemiological research: Lyme disease as an example. Geospat Health. 2010 May;4(2):135-7. PMID:20503183

Sekeyova Z, Subramanian G, Mediannikov O, Diaz MQ, Nyitray A, Blaskovicova H, Raoult D. Evaluation of clinical specimens for Rickettsia, Bartonella, Borrelia, Coxiella, Anaplasma, Franciscella and Diplorickettsia positivity using serological and molecular biology methods. FEMS Immunol Med Microbiol. 2012 Feb;64(1):82-91. Epub 2011 Dec 13. PMID:22098390

Seling A, Siegel C, Fingerle V, Jutras BL, Brissette CA, Skerka C, Wallich R, Zipfel PF, Stevenson B, Kraiczy P. Functional characterization of Borrelia spielmanii outer surface proteins that interact with distinct members of the human factor H protein family and with plasminogen. Infect Immun. 2010 Jan;78(1):39-48. Epub 2009 Oct 26. PMID:19858303

Semmler D, Blank R, Rupprecht H. Complete AV block in Lyme carditis: an important differential diagnosis. Clin Res Cardiol. 2010 Aug;99(8):519-26. Epub 2010 May 13. PMID:20464556

Sen E, Uchishima Y, Okamoto Y, Fukui T, Kadosaka T, Ohashi N, Masuzawa T. Molecular detection of Anaplasma phagocytophilum and Borrelia burgdorferi in Ixodes ricinus ticks from Istanbul metropolitan area and rural Trakya (Thrace) region of north-western Turkey. Ticks Tick Borne Dis. 2011 Jun;2(2):94-8. Epub 2011 May 25. PMID:21771542

Senel M, Rupprecht TA, Tumani H, Pfister HW, Ludolph AC, Brettschneider J. The chemokine CXCL13 in acute neuroborreliosis. J Neurol Neurosurg Psychiatry. 2010 Aug;81(8):929-33. Epub 2009 Dec 3. PMID:19965843

Seppänen M. [Insect-borne diseases and insect bites in Finland].[Article in Finnish]. Duodecim. 2011;127(13):1393-400. PMID:21834346

Seriburi V, Ndukwe N, Chang Z, Cox ME, Wormser GP. High frequency of false positive IgM immunoblots for Borrelia burgdorferi in Clinical Practice. Clin Microbiol Infect. 2011 Dec 7. [Epub ahead of print]. PMID:22369185

Seugé L, Fischbach M, Laugel V, Lipsker D. [Children Lyme Borreliosis: retrospective study of 16 cases].[Article in French]. Presse Med. 2011 Sep;40(9 Pt 1):e359-64. Epub 2011 May 5. PMID:21549553

Seward RJ, Drouin EE, Steere AC, Costello CE. Peptides presented by HLA-DR molecules in synovia of patients with rheumatoid arthritis or antibiotic-refractory Lyme arthritis. Mol Cell Proteomics. 2011 Mar;10(3):M110.002477. Epub 2010 Nov 16. PMID:21081667

Sewnaik A, Kamarashev J, Peters NS, van Rijswijk JB. A non-traumatic, blue-purple auricle: case report. J Laryngol Otol. 2010 Jul;124(7):804-6. Epub 2009 Dec 11. PMID:20003592

Shah PM. Higher dosage at later stages. Dtsch Arztebl Int. 2009 Jul;106(31-32):524-5; author reply 525. Epub 2009 Aug 3. PMID:19730722

Sharma A, Jaimungal S, Basdeo-Maharaj K, Chalapathi Rao AV, Teelucksingh S. Erythema migrans-like illness among Caribbean islanders. Emerg Infect Dis. 2010 Oct;16(10):1615-7. PMID:20875293

Sharma V, Biswas S. Self-limiting fourth and sixth cranial nerve palsy after Lyme disease. J Pediatr Ophthalmol Strabismus. 2010 Mar-Apr;47(2):114-6. PMID:19645376

Shaw DK, Hyde JA, Skare JT. The BB0646 protein demonstrates lipase and haemolytic activity associated with Borrelia burgdorferi, the aetiological agent of Lyme disease. Mol Microbiol. 2012 Jan;83(2):319-34. Epub 2011 Dec 11. PMID:22151008

Shen AK, Mead PS, Beard CB. The Lyme disease vaccine--a public health perspective. Clin Infect Dis. 2011 Feb;52 Suppl 3:s247-52. PMID:21217171

Shen S, Shin JJ, Strle K, McHugh G, Li X, Glickstein LJ, Drouin EE, Steere AC. Treg cell numbers and function in patients with antibiotic-refractory or antibiotic-responsive Lyme arthritis. Arthritis Rheum. 2010 Jul;62(7):2127-37. PMID:20506317

Shi C, Sahay B, Russell JQ, Fortner KA, Hardin N, Sellati TJ, Budd RC. Reduced immune response to Borrelia burgdorferi in the absence of $\gamma\delta$ T cells. Infect Immun. 2011 Oct;79(10):3940-6. Epub 2011 Jul 18. PMID:21768278

Shin JJ, Strle K, Glickstein LJ, Luster AD, Steere AC. Borrelia burgdorferi stimulation of chemokine secretion by cells of monocyte lineage in patients with Lyme arthritis. Arthritis Res Ther. 2010;12(5):R168. Epub 2010 Sep 9. PMID:20828409

Shtannikov AV, Reshetniak TV, Repolovskaia TV, Panfertsev EA, Perovskaia ON, Gutova VP, Vasil'eva IS, Ershova AS, Prilipov AG, Biketov SF, Zeidner N. [Search for protective antigens in Ixodes persulcatus (ixodidae) salivary gland extracts].[Article in Russian]. Med Parazitol (Mosk). 2010 Apr-Jun;(2):36-9. PMID:20608183

Sigal LH. Musculoskeletal features of Lyme disease: understanding the pathogenesis of clinical findings helps make appropriate therapeutic choices. J Clin Rheumatol. 2011 Aug;17(5):256-65. PMID:21778908

Sigurdsson MI, Gudnason T, Thorgrímsson S. [Case of the month: A boy with a notable skin rash].[Article in Icelandic]. Laeknabladid. 2011 Jan;97(1):35-6. PMID:21217198

Sikutová S, Halouzka J, Mendel J, Knoz J, Rudolf I. Novel spirochetes isolated from mosquitoes and black flies in the Czech Republic. J Vector Ecol. 2010 Jun;35(1):50-5. PMID:20618647

Silva L, Sampaio L, Pinto J, Ventura FS. [Arthritis and clinical history]. [Article in Portuguese]. Acta Med Port. 2011 Jul;24(4):629-32. Epub 2011 Dec 12. PMID:22521022

Silva R, Botelho C, Cadinha S, Lisboa C, Azevedo I, Cernadas JR. Possible DRESS syndrome in a child with borreliosis. Allergol Immunopathol (Madr). 2012 Mar-Apr;40(2):129-31. Epub 2011 May 5. PMID:21549496

Siva N. China to scale up collaborations in infectious disease research. Nat Med. 2010 Sep;16(9):938. PMID:20823854

Sjöwall J, Fryland L, Nordberg M, Sjögren F, Garpmo U, Jansson C, Carlsson SA, Bergström S, Ernerudh J, Nyman D, Forsberg P, Ekerfelt C. Decreased Th1-type inflammatory cytokine expression in the skin is associated with persisting symptoms after treatment of erythema migrans. PLoS One. 2011 Mar 31;6(3):e18220. PMID:21483819

Skogman BH, Ekerfelt C, Ludvigsson J, Forsberg P. Seroprevalence of Borrelia IgG antibodies among young Swedish children in relation to reported tick bites, symptoms and previous treatment for Lyme borreliosis: a population-based survey. Arch Dis Child. 2010 Dec;95(12):1013-6. Epub 2010 Aug 10. PMID:20702388

Skogman BH, Hellberg S, Ekerfelt C, Jenmalm MC, Forsberg P, Ludvigsson J, Bergström S, Ernerudh J. Adaptive and innate immune responsiveness to Borrelia burgdorferi sensu lato in exposed asymptomatic children and children with previous clinical Lyme borreliosis. Clin Dev Immunol. 2012;2012:294587. Epub 2011 Dec 5. PMID:22190976

Skotarczak B. Adaptation factors of Borrelia for host and vector. Ann Agric Environ Med. 2009 Jun;16(1):1-8. PMID:19572471

Slack GS, Mavin S, Yirrell D, Ho-Yen DO. Is Tayside becoming a Scottish hotspot for Lyme borreliosis? J R Coll Physicians Edinb. 2011 Mar;41(1):5-8. PMID:21365058

Smetanick MT, Zellis SL, Ermolovich T. Acrodermatitis chronica atrophicans: a case report and review of the literature. Cutis. 2010 May;85(5):247-52. PMID:20540415

Smith BG, Cruz AI Jr, Milewski MD, Shapiro ED. Lyme disease and the orthopaedic implications of lyme arthritis. J Am Acad Orthop Surg. 2011 Feb;19(2):91-100. PMID:21292932

Smith FD, Ballantyne R, Morgan ER, Wall R. Estimating Lyme disease risk using pet dogs as sentinels. Comp Immunol Microbiol Infect Dis. 2012 Mar;35(2):163-7. Epub 2012 Jan 16. PMID:22257866

Smith IS, Rechlin DP. Delayed diagnosis of neuroborreliosis presenting as bell palsy and meningitis. J Am Osteopath Assoc. 2010 Aug;110(8):441-4. PMID:20805550

Smith MP, Ponnusamy L, Jiang J, Ayyash LA, Richards AL, Apperson CS. Bacterial pathogens in ixodid ticks from a Piedmont County in North Carolina: prevalence of rickettsial organisms. Vector Borne Zoonotic Dis. 2010 Dec;10(10):939-52. Epub 2010 May 10. PMID:20455778

Sno HN. [Signs and significance of a tick-bite: psychiatric disorders associated with Lyme disease].[Article in Dutch]. Tijdschr Psychiatr. 2012;54(3):235-43. PMID:22422416

Socolovschi C, Mediannikov O, Raoult D, Parola P. Update on tick-borne bacterial diseases in Europe. Parasite. 2009 Dec;16(4):259-73. PMID:20092057

Sonderegger FL, Ma Y, Maylor-Hagan H, Brewster J, Huang X, Spangrude GJ, Zachary JF, Weis JH, Weis JJ. Localized production of IL-10 suppresses early inflammatory cell infiltration and subsequent development of IFN-γ-mediated Lyme arthritis. J Immunol. 2012 Feb 1;188(3):1381-93. Epub 2011 Dec 16. PMID:22180617

Song X, Lasanajak Y, Xia B, Heimburg-Molinaro J, Rhea JM, Ju H, Zhao C, Molinaro RJ, Cummings RD, Smith DF. Shotgun glycomics: a microarray strategy for functional glycomics. Nat Methods. 2011 Jan;8(1):85-90. Epub 2010 Dec 5. PMID:21131969

Sorge F. [Prevention with repellent in children].[Article in French]. Arch Pediatr. 2009 Oct;16 Suppl 2:S115-22. PMID:19836673

Souayah N, Ajroud-Driss S, Sander HW, Brannagan TH, Hays AP, Chin RL. Small fiber neuropathy following vaccination for rabies, varicella or Lyme disease. Vaccine. 2009 Dec 9;27(52):7322-5. Epub 2009 Oct 4. PMID:19808027

Spirin NN, Baranova NS, Fadeeva OA, Shipova EG, Stepanov IO. [Differential aspects of multiple sclerosis and chronic borrelial encephalomyelitis].[Article in Russian]. Zh Nevrol Psikhiatr Im S S Korsakova. 2011;111(7):8-12. PMID:21947065

Spitalská E, Literák I, Kocianová E, Taragel'ová V. The importance of Ixodes arboricola in transmission of Rickettsia spp., Anaplasma phagocytophilum, and Borrelia burgdorferi sensu lato in the Czech Republic, Central Europe. Vector Borne Zoonotic Dis. 2011 Sep;11(9):1235-41. Epub 2011 May 25. PMID:21612531

Spolidorio MG, Labruna MB, Machado RZ, Moraes-Filho J, Zago AM, Donatele DM, Pinheiro SR, Silveira I, Caliari KM, Yoshinari NH. Survey for tick-borne zoonoses in the state of Espirito Santo, southeastern Brazil. Am J Trop Med Hyg. 2010 Jul;83(1):201-6. PMID:20595502

Srivastava SY, de Silva AM. Characterization of Borrelia burgdorferi aggregates. Vector Borne Zoonotic Dis. 2009 Jun;9(3):323-9. PMID:19499997

Sroka J, Szymanska J, Wojcik-Fatla A. The occurrence of Toxoplasma gondii and Borrelia burgdorferi sensu lato in Ixodes ricinus ticks from east Poland with the use of pcr. Ann Agric Environ Med. 2009 Dec;16(2):313-9. PMID:20047269

Stafford KC 3rd, Denicola AJ, Pound JM, Miller JA, George JE. Topical treatment of white-tailed deer with an acaricide for the control of Ixodes scapularis (Acari: Ixodidae) in a Connecticut Lyme borreliosis hyperendemic Community. Vector Borne Zoonotic Dis. 2009 Aug;9(4):371-9. PMID:19650731

Stanek G, Fingerle V, Hunfeld KP, Jaulhac B, Kaiser R, Krause A, Kristoferitsch W, O'Connell S, Ornstein K, Strle F, Gray J. Lyme borreliosis: clinical case definitions for diagnosis and management in Europe. Clin Microbiol Infect. 2011 Jan;17(1):69-79. PMID:20132258

Stanek G, Reiter M. The expanding Lyme Borrelia complex—clinical significance of genomic species? Clin Microbiol Infect. 2011 Apr;17(4):487-93. PMID:21414082

Stanek G, Strle F. Lyme borreliosis: a European perspective on diagnosis and clinical management. Curr Opin Infect Dis. 2009 Oct;22(5):450-4. PMID:19571749

Stanek G, Wormser GP, Gray J, Strle F. Lyme borreliosis. Lancet. 2012 Feb 4;379(9814):461-73. Epub 2011 Sep 6. PMID:21903253

Steere AC, Drouin EE, Glickstein LJ. Relationship between immunity to Borrelia burgdorferi outer-surface protein A (OspA) and Lyme arthritis. Clin Infect Dis. 2011 Feb;52 Suppl 3:s259-65. PMID:21217173

Steffen A, Hagenah J, Wollenberg B, Brüggemann N. A case of central sleep apnea strictly dependent upon REM-sleep. J Neurol. 2010 Jan;257(1):143-5. PMID:19756821

Stolarska U, Gergont A, Swierczyńska A, Biedroń A. [The influence of child's behaviour on the course of neurological diagnosis].[Article in Polish]. Przegl Lek. 2010;67(11):1223-7. PMID:21442981

Stollery N. Bites and stings. Practitioner. 2009 Sep;253(1721):35-7. PMID:19873858

Stonehouse A, Studdiford JS, Henry CA. An update on the diagnosis and treatment of early Lyme disease: "focusing on the bull's eye, you may miss the mark". J Emerg Med. 2010 Nov;39(5):e147-51. Epub 2007 Oct 18. PMID:17945460

Stricker RB, Delong AK, Green CL, Savely VR, Chamallas SN, Johnson L. Benefit of intravenous antibiotic therapy in patients referred for treatment of neurologic Lyme disease. Int J Gen Med. 2011;4:639-46. Epub 2011 Sep 6. PMID:21941449

Stricker RB, Frismodt C, Schwarzbach A. [Reply to a feature article defending Danish Borrelia diagnostics].[Article in Danish]. Ugeskr Laeger. 2010 Aug 30;172(35):2405; author reply 2405. PMID:20848688

Stricker RB, Green CL, Savely VR, Chamallas SN, Johnson L. Safety of intravenous antibiotic therapy in patients referred for treatment of neurologic Lyme disease. Minerva Med. 2010 Feb;101(1):1-7. PMID:20228716

Stricker RB, Johnson L. "Lyme literacy" and physicians in Connecticut. J Pediatr. 2011 Mar;158(3):518-9; author reply 519-20. Epub 2011 Jan 13. PMID:21232763

Stricker RB, Johnson L. Gender bias in chronic lyme disease. J Womens Health (Larchmt). 2009 Oct;18(10):1717-8; author reply 1719-20. PMID:19857097

Stricker RB, Johnson L. Letter to the editor re "Anti-neural antibody reactivity in patients with a history of Lyme borreliosis and persistent symptoms" by Chandra et al. Brain Behav Immun. 2010 Aug;24(6):1025; author reply 1026. Epub 2010 Apr 24. PMID:20417704

Stricker RB, Johnson L. Long-term outcomes in patients with early lyme disease: more false hope? Clin Infect Dis. 2010 Jun 15;50(12):1683-4; author reply 1684. PMID:20482263

Stricker RB, Johnson L. Lyme disease diagnosis and treatment: lessons from the AIDS epidemic. Minerva Med. 2010 Dec;101(6):419-25. PMID:21196901

Stricker RB, Johnson L. Lyme disease: the next decade. Infect Drug Resist. 2011;4:1-9. Epub 2011 Jan 7. PMID:21694904

Stricker RB, Johnson L. Persistent symptoms following treatment of early Lyme disease: false hope? Am J Med. 2010 Aug;123(8):e25; author reply e27-8. PMID:20670707

Stricker RB, Johnson L. 'Rare' infections mimicking multiple sclerosis: consider Lyme disease. Clin Neurol Neurosurg. 2011 Apr;113(3):259-60. Epub 2010 Dec 18. PMID:21168953

Stricker RB, Johnson L. The Infectious Diseases Society of America Lyme guidelines: poster child for guidelines reform. South Med J. 2009 Jun;102(6):565-6. PMID:19434025

Stricker RB, Johnson L. The Lyme disease chronicles, continued. Chronic Lyme disease: in defense of the patient enterprise. FASEB J. 2010 Dec;24(12):4632-3; author reply 4633-4. PMID:21123300

Stricker RB, Johnson L. The pain of chronic Lyme disease: moving the discourse backward? FASEB J. 2011 Dec;25(12):4085-7. PMID:22131364

Stricker RB, Winger EE. Natural killer cells in chronic Lyme disease. Clin Vaccine Immunol. 2009 Nov;16(11):1704; author reply 1704-6. PMID:19880717

Strle F, Ružić-Sabljić E, Logar M, Maraspin V, Lotrič-Furlan S, Cimperman J, Ogrinc K, Stupica D, Nadelman RB, Nowakowski J, Wormser GP. Comparison of erythema migrans caused by Borrelia burgdorferi and Borrelia garinii. Vector Borne Zoonotic Dis. 2011 Sep;11(9):1253-8. Epub 2011 May 25. PMID:21612533

Strle K, Drouin EE, Shen S, Khoury JE, McHugh G, Ruzic-Sabljic E, Strle F, Steere AC. Borrelia burgdorferi stimulates macrophages to secrete higher levels of cytokines and chemokines than Borrelia afzelii or Borrelia garinii. J Infect Dis. 2009 Dec 15;200(12):1936-43. PMID:19909078

Strle K, Jones KL, Drouin EE, Li X, Steere AC. Borrelia burgdorferi RST1 (OspC type A) genotype is associated with greater inflammation and more severe Lyme disease. Am J Pathol. 2011 Jun;178(6):2726-39. PMID:21641395

Strle K, Shin JJ, Glickstein LJ, Steere AC. Association of a toll-like receptor 1 polymorphism with heightened Th1 inflammatory responses and antibiotic-refractory Lyme arthritis. Arthritis Rheum. 2012 May;64(5):1497-507. PMID:22246581

Strube C, Montenegro VM, Epe C, Eckelt E, Schnieder T. Establishment of a minor groove binder-probe based quantitative real time PCR to detect Borrelia burgdorferi sensu lato and differentiation of Borrelia spielmanii by ospA-specific conventional PCR. Parasit Vectors. 2010 Aug 10;3:69. PMID:20698952

Strube C, Schicht S, Schnieder T. Borrelia burgdorferi sensu lato and Rickettsia spp. infections in hard ticks (Ixodes ricinus) in the region of Hanover (Germany). Berl Munch Tierarztl Wochenschr. 2011 Nov-Dec;124(11-12):512-7. PMID:22191173

Strunk T, Hetzer S, Homey B, Reifenberger J. [Anetoderma with positive Borrelia serology].[Article in German]. Hautarzt. 2011 Oct;62(10):720-2. PMID:21915730

Struthers S. Bell's palsy and Lyme disease. Br J Gen Pract. 2009 Oct;59(567):779. PMID:19843426

Stübs G, Fingerle V, Zähringer U, Schumann RR, Rademann J, Schröder NW. Acylated cholesteryl galactosides are ubiquitous glycolipid antigens among Borrelia burgdorferi sensu lato. FEMS Immunol Med Microbiol. 2011 Oct;63(1):140-3. Epub 2011 Jun 27. PMID:21635569

Stübs G, Rupp B, Schumann RR, Schröder NW, Rademann J. Chemoenzymatic synthesis of a glycolipid library and elucidation of the antigenic epitope for construction of a vaccine against Lyme disease. Chemistry. 2010 Mar 15;16(11):3536-44. PMID:20143357

Stupica D, Lusa L, Cerar T, Ružić-Sabljić E, Strle F. Comparison of post-Lyme Borreliosis symptoms in erythema migrans patients with positive and negative Borrelia burgdorferi sensu lato skin culture. Vector Borne Zoonotic Dis. 2011 Jul;11(7):883-9. Epub 2010 Nov 17. PMID:21083376

Stupica D, Lusa L, Ruzic-Sabljic E, Cerar T, Strle F. Treatment of Erythema Migrans With Doxycycline for 10 Days Versus 15 Days. Clin Infect Dis. 2012 Apr 20. [Epub ahead of print]. PMID:22523260

Sultan P, Green C, Riley E, Carvalho B. Spinal anaesthesia for caesarean delivery in a parturient with babesiosis and Lyme disease. Anaesthesia. 2012 Feb;67(2):180-3. PMID:22251109

Sultan SZ, Pitzer JE, Boquoi T, Hobbs G, Miller MR, Motaleb MA. Analysis of the HD-GYP domain cyclic dimeric GMP phosphodiesterase reveals a role in motility and the enzootic life cycle of Borrelia burgdorferi. Infect Immun. 2011 Aug;79(8):3273-83. Epub 2011 Jun 13. PMID:21670168

Sultan SZ, Pitzer JE, Miller MR, Motaleb MA. Analysis of a Borrelia burgdorferi phosphodiesterase demonstrates a role for cyclic-di-guanosine monophosphate in motility and virulence. Mol Microbiol. 2010 Jul 1;77(1):128-42. Epub 2010 Apr 27. PMID:20444101

Sundin M, Hansson ME, Engman ML, Orvell C, Lindquist L, Wide K, Lidefelt KJ. Pediatric tick-borne infections of the central nervous system in an endemic region of Sweden: a prospective evaluation of clinical manifestations. Eur J Pediatr. 2012 Feb;171(2):347-52. Epub 2011 Aug 13. PMID:21842178

Susta L, Uhl EW, Grosenbaugh DA, Krimer PM. Synovial lesions in experimental canine lyme borreliosis. Vet Pathol. 2012 May;49(3):453-61. Epub 2011 Nov 10. PMID:22075774

Svihrova V, Hudeckova H, Jesenak M, Schwarzova K, Kostanova Z, Ciznar I. Lyme borreliosis--analysis of the trends in Slovakia, 1999-2008. Folia Microbiol (Praha). 2011 May;56(3):270-5. Epub 2011 May 24. PMID:21607749

Swei A, Meentemeyer R, Briggs CJ. Influence of abiotic and environmental factors on the density and infection prevalence of Ixodes pacificus (Acari:Ixodidae) with Borrelia burgdorferi. J Med Entomol. 2011 Jan;48(1):20-8. PMID:21337944

Swei A, Ostfeld RS, Lane RS, Briggs CJ. Effects of an invasive forest pathogen on abundance of ticks and their vertebrate hosts in a California Lyme disease focus. Oecologia. 2011 May;166(1):91-100. Epub 2010 Oct 13. PMID:20941513

Swei A, Ostfeld RS, Lane RS, Briggs CJ. Impact of the experimental removal of lizards on Lyme disease risk. Proc Biol Sci. 2011 Oct 7;278(1720):2970-8. Epub 2011 Feb 16. PMID:21325326

Switaj K, Olszynska-Krowicka M, Zarnowska-Prymek H, Zaborowski P. Tularaemia after tick exposure - typical presentation of rare disease misdiagnosed as atypical presentation of common diseases: a case report. Cases J. 2009 Jul 31;2:7954. PMID:19830027

Sze CW, Li C. Inactivation of bb0184, which encodes carbon storage regulator A, represses the infectivity of Borrelia burgdorferi. Infect Immun. 2011 Mar;79(3):1270-9. Epub 2010 Dec 20. PMID:21173314

Sze CW, Morado DR, Liu J, Charon NW, Xu H, Li C. Carbon storage regulator A (CsrA(Bb)) is a repressor of Borrelia burgdorferi flagellin protein FlaB. Mol Microbiol. 2011 Nov;82(4):851-64. Epub 2011 Oct 18. PMID:21999436

Sze CW, Zhang K, Kariu T, Pal U, Li C. Borrelia burgdorferi needs chemotaxis to establish infection in mammals and to accomplish its enzootic cycle. Infect Immun. 2012 Apr 16. [Epub ahead of print]. PMID:22508862

Takano A, Goka K, Une Y, Shimada Y, Fujita H, Shiino T, Watanabe H, Kawabata H. Isolation and characterization of a novel Borrelia group of tick-borne borreliae from imported reptiles and their associated ticks. Environ Microbiol. 2010 Jan;12(1):134-46. Epub 2009 Sep 16. PMID:19758349

Takano A, Muto M, Sakata A, Ogasawara Y, Ando S, Hanaoka N, Tsurumi M, Sato F, Nakamura N, Fujita H, Watanabe H, Kawabata H. Relapsing fever spirochete in seabird tick, Japan. Emerg Infect Dis. 2009 Sep;15(9):1528-30. PMID:19788834

Takano A, Nakao M, Masuzawa T, Takada N, Yano Y, Ishiguro F, Fujita H, Ito T, Ma X, Oikawa Y, Kawamori F, Kumagai K, Mikami T, Hanaoka N, Ando S, Honda N, Taylor K, Tsubota T, Konnai S, Watanabe H, Ohnishi M, Kawabata H. Multilocus sequence typing implicates rodents as the main reservoir host of human-pathogenic Borrelia garinii in Japan. J Clin Microbiol. 2011 May;49(5):2035-9. Epub 2011 Mar 16. PMID:21411595

Talhari S, de Souza Santos MN, Talhari C, de Lima Ferreira LC, Silva RM Jr, Zelger B, Massone C, Ribeiro-Rodrigues R. Borrelia Burgdorferi "sensu lato" in Brazil: Occurrence confirmed by immunohistochemistry and focus floating microscopy. Acta Trop. 2010 Sep;115(3):200-4. Epub 2010 Mar 6. PMID:20211144

Tauber SC, Ribes S, Ebert S, Heinz T, Fingerle V, Bunkowski S, Kugelstadt D, Spreer A, Jahn O, Eiffert H, Nau R. Long-term intrathecal infusion of outer surface protein C from Borrelia burgdorferi causes axonal damage. J Neuropathol Exp Neurol. 2011 Sep;70(9):748-57. PMID:21865883

Teglas MB, Mapes S, Hodzic E, Nieto NC. Co-infection of Ornithodoros coriaceus with the relapsing fever spirochete, Borrelia coriaceae, and the agent of epizootic bovine abortion. Med Vet Entomol. 2011 Sep;25(3):337-43. Epub 2011 Mar 16. PMID:21410735

Telford SR 3rd, Cunningham JA, Waltari E, Hu L. Nest box-deployed bait for delivering oral vaccines to white-footed mice. Ticks Tick Borne Dis. 2011 Sep;2(3):151-5. Epub 2011 Aug 2. PMID:21890068

Temmesfeld M. Veterinary medical research. Dtsch Arztebl Int. 2009 Jul;106(31-32):524; author reply 525. Epub 2009 Aug 3. PMID:19730723

Terhorst D, Kalali BN, Ollert M, Ring J, Mempel M. The role of toll-like receptors in host defenses and their relevance to dermatologic diseases. Am J Clin Dermatol. 2010;11(1):1-10. PMID:20000870

Thai PT, Collins CC, Fortner KA, Koenig A, Hayes SM, Budd RC. Increased caspase activity primes human Lyme arthritis synovial $\gamma\delta$ T cells for proliferation and death. Hum Immunol. 2011 Dec;72(12):1168-75. Epub 2011 Sep 22. PMID:21983117

Thalmann H, Müller JB. [Suspected borreliosis: therapy is incompatible with the French sun].[Article in German]. MMW Fortschr Med. 2009 Oct 8;151(41):5. PMID:19891174

Tijsse-Klasen E, Jacobs JJ, Swart A, Fonville M, Reimerink JH, Brandenburg AH, van der Giessen JW, Hofhuis A, Sprong H. Small risk of developing symptomatic tick-borne diseases following a tick bite in The Netherlands. Parasit Vectors. 2011 Feb 10;4:17. PMID:21310036

Tillett T. Tracking the deer tick: emerging lyme disease threat in Canada. Environ Health Perspect. 2010 Jul;118(7):A305. PMID:20601318

Tilly K, Bestor A, Dulebohn DP, Rosa PA. OspC-independent infection and dissemination by host-adapted Borrelia burgdorferi. Infect Immun. 2009 Jul;77(7):2672-82. Epub 2009 Apr 27. PMID:19398538

Tjernberg I, Carlsson M, Ernerudh J, Eliasson I, Forsberg P. Mapping of hormones and cortisol responses in patients after Lyme neuroborreliosis. BMC Infect Dis. 2010 Feb 5;10:20. PMID:20137075

Tjernberg I, Henningsson AJ, Eliasson I, Forsberg P, Ernerudh J. Diagnostic performance of cerebrospinal fluid chemokine CXCL13 and antibodies to the C6-peptide in Lyme neuroborreliosis. J Infect. 2011 Feb;62(2):149-58. Epub 2010 Nov 16. PMID:21087629

Tjernberg I, Sillanpää H, Seppälä I, Eliasson I, Forsberg P, Lahdenne P. Antibody responses to borrelia IR(6) peptide variants and the C6 peptide in Swedish patients with erythema migrans. Int J Med Microbiol. 2009 Aug;299(6):439-46. Epub 2009 Jan 9. PMID:19138558

Tokarz R, Jain K, Bennett A, Briese T, Lipkin WI. Assessment of polymicrobial infections in ticks in New York state. Vector Borne Zoonotic Dis. 2010 Apr;10(3):217-21. PMID:19725770

Toledo A, Anda P, Escudero R, Larsson C, Bergstrom S, Benach JL. Phylogenetic analysis of a virulent Borrelia species isolated from patients with relapsing fever. J Clin Microbiol. 2010 Jul;48(7):2484-9. Epub 2010 May 12. PMID:20463158

Toledo A, Coleman JL, Kuhlow CJ, Crowley JT, Benach JL. The enolase of Borrelia burgdorferi is a plasminogen receptor released in outer membrane vesicles. Infect Immun. 2012 Jan;80(1):359-68. Epub 2011 Nov 14. PMID:22083700

Tomanović S, Radulović Z, Masuzawa T, Milutinović M. Coexistence of emerging bacterial pathogens in Ixodes ricinus ticks in Serbia. Parasite. 2010 Sep;17(3):211-7. PMID:21073144

Tory HO, Zurakowski D, Sundel RP. Outcomes of children treated for Lyme arthritis: results of a large pediatric cohort. J Rheumatol. 2010 May;37(5):1049-55. Epub 2010 Apr 1. PMID:20360182

Träisk F, Andersson M, Svenungsson E. Three cases of neuroborreliosis misdiagnosed as giant cell arteritis. Scand J Rheumatol. 2012;41(2):158-60. PMID:22420373

Travinsky B, Bunikis J, Barbour AG. Geographic differences in genetic locus linkages for Borrelia burgdorferi. Emerg Infect Dis. 2010 Jul;16(7):1147-50. PMID:20587192

Troxell B, Xu H, Yang XF. Borrelia burgdorferi, a pathogen that lacks iron, encodes a manganese-dependent superoxide dismutase essential for resistance to streptonigrin. J Biol Chem. 2012 Apr 12. [Epub ahead of print]. PMID:22500025

Tsao K, Fish D, Galvani AP. Predicted Outcomes of Vaccinating Wildlife to Reduce Human Risk of Lyme Disease. Vector Borne Zoonotic Dis. 2012 Jan 17. [Epub ahead of print]. PMID:22251312

Tuerlinckx D, Glupczynski Y. Lyme neuroborreliosis in children. Expert Rev Anti Infect Ther. 2010 Apr;8(4):455-63. PMID:20377339

Tumani H, Cadavid D. Are high CSF levels of CXCL13 helpful for diagnosis of Lyme neuroborreliosis? Neurology. 2011 Mar 22;76(12):1034-5. PMID:21422454

Tunev SS, Hastey CJ, Hodzic E, Feng S, Barthold SW, Baumgarth N. Lymphoadenopathy during lyme borreliosis is caused by spirochete migration-induced specific B cell activation. PLoS Pathog. 2011 May;7(5):e1002066. Epub 2011 May 26. PMID:21637808

Tuuminen T, Hedman K, Söderlund-Venermo M, Seppälä I. Acute parvovirus B19 infection causes nonspecificity frequently in Borrelia and less often in Salmonella and Campylobacter serology, posing a problem in diagnosis of infectious arthropathy. Clin Vaccine Immunol. 2011 Jan;18(1):167-72. Epub 2010 Nov 24. PMID:21106777

Tvarůzková Z, Pavlová S, Doubek M, Mayer J, Pospísilová S. [Lymphoproliferative disease in patients with autoimmune and inflammatory diseases: significance of antigenic stimulation and inflammatory processes].[Article in Czech]. Cas Lek Cesk. 2011;150(3):161-8. PMID:21560455

Tveitnes D, Natås OB, Skadberg Ø, Øymar K. Lyme meningitis, the major cause of childhood meningitis in an endemic area: a population based study. Arch Dis Child. 2012 Mar;97(3):215-20. Epub 2012 Jan 13. PMID:22247243

Tzipory N, Crawford PC, Levy JK. Prevalence of Dirofilaria immitis, Ehrlichia canis, and Borrelia burgdorferi in pet dogs, racing greyhounds, and shelter dogs in Florida. Vet Parasitol. 2010 Jul 15;171(1-2):136-9. Epub 2010 Mar 17. PMID:20399018

Uggeldahl PE, Peltomaa M. [Skin manifestation of Lyme borreliosis].[Article in Finnish]. Duodecim. 2010;126(10):1151-61. PMID:20597345

Václav R, Ficová M, Prokop P, Betáková T. Associations between coinfection prevalence of Borrelia lusitaniae, Anaplasma sp., and Rickettsia sp. in hard ticks feeding on reptile hosts. Microb Ecol. 2011 Feb;61(2):245-53. Epub 2010 Aug 14. PMID:20711724

Valančienė G, Jasaitienė D, Valiukevičienė S. Pathogenesis and treatment modalities of localized scleroderma. Medicina (Kaunas). 2010;46(10):649-56. PMID:21393982

Van Bortel W, Versteirt V, Van Gompel F, Coosemans M. [Climate change and emerging diseases: a complex interplay of factors].[Article in French]. J Pharm Belg. 2009 Jun;(2):48-53. PMID:19739528

van Burgel ND, Bakels F, Kroes AC, van Dam AP. Discriminating Lyme neuroborreliosis from other neuroinflammatory diseases by levels of CXCL13 in cerebrospinal fluid. J Clin Microbiol. 2011 May;49(5):2027-30. Epub 2011 Mar 2. PMID:21367992

van Burgel ND, Balmus NC, Fikrig E, van Dam AP. Infectivity of Borrelia burgdorferi sensu lato is unaltered in C3-deficient mice. Ticks Tick Borne Dis. 2011 Mar;2(1):20-6. Epub 2010 Nov 26. PMID:21771533

van Burgel ND, Brandenburg A, Gerritsen HJ, Kroes AC, van Dam AP. High sensitivity and specificity of the C6-peptide ELISA on cerebrospinal fluid in Lyme neuroborreliosis patients. Clin Microbiol Infect. 2011 Oct;17(10):1495-500. Epub 2011 Mar 7. PMID:21375653

van Burgel ND, Kraiczy P, Schuijt TJ, Zipfel PF, van Dam AP. Identification and functional characterisation of Complement Regulator Acquiring Surface Protein-1 of serum resistant Borrelia garinii OspA serotype 4. BMC Microbiol. 2010 Feb 10;10:43. PMID:20146822

van Burgel ND, Oosterloo M, Kroon FP, van Dam AP. Severe course of Lyme neuroborreliosis in an HIV-1 positive patient; case report and review of the literature. BMC Neurol. 2010 Nov 30;10:117. PMID:21118561

Van den Enden E, Vlieghe E, Demeester R, Ieven G, Jansens H, Van den Hauwe L. A traveler with neurobrucellosis. Travel Med Infect Dis. 2009 Jul;7(4):215-8. Epub 2009 Jun 13. PMID:19717103

van der Giessen J, Overgaauw P. [Working together on occupational zoonoses].[Article in Dutch]. Tijdschr Diergeneeskd. 2012 Jan;137(1):64-5. PMID:22372067

van Egmond ME, Luijckx GJ, Kramer H, Benne CA, Slebos DJ, van Assen S. Diaphragmatic weakness caused by neuroborreliosis. Clin Neurol Neurosurg. 2011 Feb;113(2):153-5. Epub 2010 Oct 20. PMID:20965650

van Erp WS, Bakker NA, Aries MJ, Vroomen JP. Opsoclonus and multiple cranial neuropathy as a manifestation of neuroborreliosis. Neurology. 2011 Sep 6;77(10):1013-4. Epub 2011 Aug 24. PMID:21865581

van Vugt M, Wetsteyn JC, Haverkort M, Kolader M, Verhaar N, Spanjaard L, Grobusch MP, Bart A, van Gool T. New England souvenirs. J Travel Med. 2011 Nov-Dec;18(6):425-6. Epub 2011 Oct 12. PMID:22017722

Vanthomme K, Bossuyt N, Boffin N, Van Casteren V. Incidence and management of presumption of Lyme borreliosis in Belgium: recent data from the sentinel network of general practitioners. Eur J Clin Microbiol Infect Dis. 2012 Mar 6. [Epub ahead of print]. PMID:22391757

Varis A, Oksi J, Järveläinen H. [Central nervous system infection--tick-borne encephalitis, neuroborreliosis or both?].[Article in Finnish]. Duodecim. 2011;127(1):75-9. PMID:21442877

Vatne A, Mygland A, Ljøstad U. Multiple sclerosis in Vest-Agder County, Norway. Acta Neurol Scand. 2011 Jun;123(6):396-9. PMID:21492097

Vaughn MF, Sloane PD, Knierim K, Varkey D, Pilgard MA, Johnson BJ. Practice-Based Research Network Partnership with CDC to acquire clinical specimens to study the etiology of southern tick-associated rash illness (STARI). J Am Board Fam Med. 2010 Nov-Dec;23(6):720-7. PMID:21057067

Verma A, Brissette CA, Bowman A, Stevenson B. Borrelia burgdorferi BmpA is a laminin-binding protein. Infect Immun. 2009 Nov;77(11):4940-6. Epub 2009 Aug 24. PMID:19703983

Vermeersch P, Resseler S, Nackers E, Lagrou K. The C6 Lyme antibody test has low sensitivity for antibody detection in cerebrospinal fluid. Diagn Microbiol Infect Dis. 2009 Jul;64(3):347-9. Epub 2009 Apr 18. PMID:19376674

Vieira ML, de Morais ZM, Gonçales AP, Romero EC, Vasconcellos SA, Nascimento AL. Lsa63, a newly identified surface protein of Leptospira interrogans binds laminin and collagen IV. J Infect. 2010 Jan;60(1):52-64. Epub 2009 Oct 30. PMID:19879894

Villeneuve A, Goring J, Marcotte L, Overvelde S. Seroprevalence of Borrelia burgdorferi, Anaplasma phagocytophilum, Ehrlichia canis, and Dirofilaria immitis among dogs in Canada. Can Vet J. 2011 May;52(5):527-30. PMID:22043075

Vitorino L, Margos G, Zé-Zé L, Kurtenbach K, Collares-Pereira M. Plasmid profile analysis of Portuguese Borrelia lusitaniae strains. Ticks Tick Borne Dis. 2010 Sep;1(3):125-8. Epub 2010 Aug 30. PMID:21771519

Volkman D. Letter to the editor re "Anti-neural antibody reactivity in patients with a history of Lyme borreliosis and persistent symptoms" by Chandra et al. Brain Behav Immun. 2010 Aug;24(6):1027; author reply 1028. Epub 2010 May 1. PMID:20434537

Volkman DJ. Comment on: Efficacy of antibiotic prophylaxis for the prevention of Lyme disease: an updated systematic review and meta-analysis. J Antimicrob Chemother. 2010 Oct;65(10):2271; author reply 2271-3. Epub 2010 Jun 15. PMID:20551218

Volkman DJ. Recommendation for management of I. scopularis bites draws mixed reactions. WMJ. 2011 Jun;110(3):100. PMID:21751473

Vollmer SA, Bormane A, Dinnis RE, Seelig F, Dobson AD, Aanensen DM, James MC, Donaghy M, Randolph SE, Feil EJ, Kurtenbach K, Margos G. Host migration impacts on the phylogeography of Lyme Borreliosis spirochaete species in Europe. Environ Microbiol. 2011 Jan;13(1):184-92. Epub 2010 Aug 16. PMID:20722696

von Rosen JF. [Physicians, who will still "treat"].[Article in German]. MMW Fortschr Med. 2009 Jul 23;151(30-33):7. PMID:19722449

Vuyyuru R, Liu H, Manser T, Alugupalli KR. Characteristics of Borrelia hermsii infection in human hematopoietic stem cell-engrafted mice mirror those of human relapsing fever. Proc Natl Acad Sci U S A. 2011 Dec 20;108(51):20707-12. Epub 2011 Dec 5. PMID:22143787

Waespe N, Steffen I, Heininger U. Etiology of aseptic meningitis, peripheral facial nerve palsy, and a combination of both in children. Pediatr Infect Dis J. 2010 May;29(5):453-6. PMID:19934789

Wagner B, Freer H, Rollins A, Erb HN, Lu Z, Gröhn Y. Development of a multiplex assay for the detection of antibodies to Borrelia burgdorferi in horses and its validation using Bayesian and conventional statistical methods. Vet Immunol Immunopathol. 2011 Dec 15;144(3-4):374-81. Epub 2011 Aug 17. PMID:21890217

Wagner B, Freer H, Rollins A, Erb HN. A fluorescent bead-based multiplex assay for the simultaneous detection of antibodies to B. burgdorferi outer surface proteins in canine serum. Vet Immunol Immunopathol. 2011 Apr 15;140(3-4):190-8. Epub 2010 Dec 10. PMID:21208663

Wagner B, Freer H, Rollins A, Garcia-Tapia D, Erb HN, Earnhart C, Marconi R, Meeus P. Antibodies to Borrelia burgdorferi OspA, OspC, OspF, and C6 antigens as markers for early and late infection in dogs. Clin Vaccine Immunol. 2012 Apr;19(4):527-35. Epub 2012 Feb 15. PMID:22336289

Wagner V, Zima E, Gellér L, Merkely B. [Acute atrioventricular block in chronic Lyme disease].[Article in Hungarian]. Orv Hetil. 2010 Sep 26;151(39):1585-90. PMID:20840915

Wang J, Li Y, Kinjo Y, Mac TT, Gibson D, Painter GF, Kronenberg M, Zajonc DM. Lipid binding orientation within CD1d affects recognition of Borrelia burgorferi antigens by NKT cells. Proc Natl Acad Sci U S A. 2010 Jan 26;107(4):1535-40. Epub 2009 Dec 30. PMID:20080535

Wang W, Zeng JS, Qian SY. [Lyme disease complicated with human granulocytic anaplasmosis in a case].[Article in Chinese]. Zhonghua Er Ke Za Zhi. 2010 Nov;48(11):867-8. PMID:21215035

Warnet S. [Ticks and Lyme disease].[Article in French]. Rev Infirm. 2010 Apr;(159):51. PMID:20432858

Warshafsky S, Lee DH, Francois LK, Nowakowski J, Nadelman RB, Wormser GP. Efficacy of antibiotic prophylaxis for the prevention of Lyme disease: an updated systematic review and meta-analysis. J Antimicrob Chemother. 2010 Jun;65(6):1137-44. Epub 2010 Apr 9. PMID:20382722

Weber K. Is juvenile localized scleroderma related to Lyme borreliosis? J Am Acad Dermatol. 2009 Nov;61(5):901. PMID:19836648

Welc-Falęciak R, Hildebrandt A, Siński E. Co-infection with Borrelia species and other tick-borne pathogens in humans: two cases from Poland. Ann Agric Environ Med. 2010 Dec;17(2):309-13. PMID:21186774

Welc-Faleciak R, Rodo A, Siński E, Bajer A. Babesia canis and other tick-borne infections in dogs in Central Poland. Vet Parasitol. 2009 Dec 23;166(3-4):191-8. Epub 2009 Sep 26. PMID:19837515

Werner U. [Apparent and real sequelae of a tick bite. Unbelievable what is on this "market"].[Article in German]. MMW Fortschr Med. 2009 Oct 1;151(40):7. PMID:19927907

Wetter DA, Ruff CA. Erythema migrans in Lyme disease. CMAJ. 2011 Aug 9;183(11):1281. Epub 2011 May 30. PMID:21624904

Widhe M, Ekerfelt C, Jarefors S, Skogman BH, Peterson EM, Bergström S, Forsberg P, Ernerudh J. T-cell epitope mapping of the Borrelia garinii outer surface protein A in lyme neuroborreliosis. Scand J Immunol. 2009 Aug;70(2):141-8. PMID:19630920

Willen C, Mullen GR, Yee J, Read RW. Conjunctival attachment of a tick: clinicopathologic report of a case. J Emerg Med. 2011 Mar;40(3):e41-4. Epub 2008 Jun 2. PMID:18514466

Williams S, Matthews M, Barnett T. Lyme disease update: 30 years after the first cases, the clinical picture remains cloudy. Adv NPs PAs. 2011 Jul;2(7):27-8, 30-2, 38. PMID:21834353

Wodecka B, Leońska A, Skotarczak B. A comparative analysis of molecular markers for the detection and identification of Borrelia spirochaetes in Ixodes ricinus. J Med Microbiol. 2010 Mar;59(Pt 3):309-14. Epub 2009 Dec 10. PMID:20007765

Wodecka B, Rymaszewska A, Sawczuk M, Skotarczak B. Detectability of tick-borne agents DNA in the blood of dogs, undergoing treatment for borreliosis. Ann Agric Environ Med. 2009 Jun;16(1):9-14. PMID:19572472

Wojciechowska-Koszko I, Mączyńska I, Szych Z, Giedrys-Kalemba S. Serodiagnosis of borreliosis: indirect immunofluorescence assay, enzyme-linked immunosorbent assay and immunoblotting. Arch Immunol Ther Exp (Warsz). 2011 Feb;59(1):69-77. Epub 2011 Jan 22. PMID:21258869

Wójcik-Fatla A, Szymańska J, Wdowiak L, Buczek A, Dutkiewicz J. Coincidence of three pathogens (Borrelia burgdorferi sensu lato, Anaplasma phagocytophilum and Babesia microti) in Ixodes ricinus ticks in the Lublin macroregion. Ann Agric Environ Med. 2009 Jun;16(1):151-8. PMID:19630205

Wolańska-Klimkiewicz E, Szymańska J, Bachanek T. Orofacial symptoms related to boreliosis--case report. Ann Agric Environ Med. 2010 Dec;17(2):319-21. PMID:21186776

Wolf GK, Frakes MA, Gallagher M, Allan CK, Wedel SK. Management of suspected myocarditis during critical-care transport. Pediatr Emerg Care. 2010 Jul;26(7):512-7. PMID:20622634

Wong SS, Teng JL, Poon RW, Choi GK, Chan KH, Yeung ML, Hui JJ, Yuen KY. Comparative evaluation of a point-of-care immunochromatographic test SNAP 4Dx with molecular detection tests for vector-borne canine pathogens in Hong Kong. Vector Borne Zoonotic Dis. 2011 Sep;11(9):1269-77. Epub 2011 May 25. PMID:21612526

Woodman ME, Cooley AE, Avdiushko R, Bowman A, Botto M, Wooten RM, van Rooijen N, Cohen DA, Stevenson B. Roles for phagocytic cells and complement in controlling relapsing fever infection. J Leukoc Biol. 2009 Sep;86(3):727-36. Epub 2009 May 20. PMID:19458267

Wormser GP, Daniels TJ, Bittker S, Cooper D, Wang G, Pavia CS. Failure of topical antibiotics to prevent disseminated Borrelia burgdorferi infection following a tick bite in C3H/HeJ mice. J Infect Dis. 2012 Mar;205(6):991-4. Epub 2011 Sep 19. PMID:21930606

Wormser GP, O'Connell S. Treatment of infection caused by Borrelia burgdorferi sensu lato. Expert Rev Anti Infect Ther. 2011 Feb;9(2):245-60. PMID:21342072

Wormser GP, Schwartz I. Antibiotic treatment of animals infected with Borrelia burgdorferi. Clin Microbiol Rev. 2009 Jul;22(3):387-95. PMID:19597005

Wormser GP, Shapiro ED. Implications of gender in chronic Lyme disease. J Womens Health (Larchmt). 2009 Jun;18(6):831-4. PMID:19514824

Wright DJ, Maria B. Ich bin ein Berliner*. Clin Microbiol Infect. 2011 Apr;17(4):484-6. PMID:21414081

Wright SA, Tucker JR, Donohue AM, Castro MB, Kelley KL, Novak MG, Macedo PA. Avian hosts of Ixodes pacificus (Acari: Ixodidae) and the detection of Borrelia burgdorferi in larvae feeding on the Oregon junco. J Med Entomol. 2011 Jul;48(4):852-9. PMID:21845945

Wu J, Weening EH, Faske JB, Höök M, Skare JT. Invasion of eukaryotic cells by Borrelia burgdorferi requires β(1) integrins and Src kinase activity. Infect Immun. 2011 Mar;79(3):1338-48. Epub 2010 Dec 20. PMID:21173306

Wutte N, Berghold A, Krainberger I, Aberer E. Serum CXCL13 chemokine is not a marker for active Lyme borreliosis. Acta Derm Venereol. 2011 Oct;91(6):724-5. PMID:21879246

Wywial E, Haven J, Casjens SR, Hernandez YA, Singh S, Mongodin EF, Fraser-Liggett CM, Luft BJ, Schutzer SE, Qiu WG. Fast, adaptive evolution at a bacterial host-resistance locus: the PFam54 gene array in Borrelia burgdorferi. Gene. 2009 Sep 15;445(1-2):26-37. Epub 2009 Jun 6. PMID:19505540

Xiao S, Kumar M, Yang X, Akkoyunlu M, Collins PL, Samal SK, Pal U. A host-restricted viral vector for antigen-specific immunization against Lyme disease pathogen. Vaccine. 2011 Jul 18;29(32):5294-303. Epub 2011 May 19. PMID:21600949

Xu H, Caimano MJ, Lin T, He M, Radolf JD, Norris SJ, Gherardini F, Wolfe AJ, Yang XF. Role of acetyl-phosphate in activation of the Rrp2-RpoN-RpoS pathway in Borrelia burgdorferi. PLoS Pathog. 2010 Sep 16;6(9):e1001104. PMID:20862323

Xu H, He M, He JJ, Yang XF. Role of the surface lipoprotein BBA07 in the enzootic cycle of Borrelia burgdorferi. Infect Immun. 2010 Jul;78(7):2910-8. Epub 2010 Apr 26. PMID:20421380

Xu H, He M, Pang X, Xu ZC, Piesman J, Yang XF. Characterization of the highly regulated antigen BBA05 in the enzootic cycle of Borrelia burgdorferi. Infect Immun. 2010 Jan;78(1):100-7. Epub 2009 Oct 12. PMID:19822648

Xu H, Raddi G, Liu J, Charon NW, Li C. Chemoreceptors and flagellar motors are subterminally located in close proximity at the two cell poles in spirochetes. J Bacteriol. 2011 May;193(10):2652-6. Epub 2011 Mar 25. PMID:21441520

Xu Q, McShan K, Liang FT. Two regulatory elements required for enhancing ospA expression in Borrelia burgdorferi grown in vitro but repressing its expression during mammalian infection. Microbiology. 2010 Jul;156(Pt 7):2194-204. Epub 2010 Apr 15. PMID:20395273

Yabsley MJ, Parsons NJ, Horne EC, Shock BC, Purdee M. Novel relapsing fever Borrelia detected in African penguins (Spheniscus demersus) admitted to two rehabilitation centers in South Africa. Parasitol Res. 2012 Mar;110(3):1125-30. Epub 2011 Aug 26. PMID:21870246

Yakimchuk K, Roura-Mir C, Magalhaes KG, de Jong A, Kasmar AG, Granter SR, Budd R, Steere A, Pena-Cruz V, Kirschning C, Cheng TY, Moody DB. Borrelia burgdorferi infection regulates CD1 expression in human cells and tissues via IL1-β. Eur J Immunol. 2011 Mar;41(3):694-705. Epub 2011 Jan 18. PMID:21246541

Yalcin EB, Stangl H, Pichu S, Mather TN, King RS. Monoamine neurotransmitters as substrates for novel tick sulfotransferases, homology modeling, molecular docking, and enzyme kinetics. ACS Chem Biol. 2011 Feb 18;6(2):176-84. Epub 2010 Nov 15. PMID:21043483

Yang J, Liu Z, Guan G, Che R, Niu Q, Li Y, Liu J, Ma M, Ren Q, Liu A, Luo J, Yin H. Evaluation of molecular methods for detection of Borrelia burgdorferi senso lato in ticks. Diagn Microbiol Infect Dis. 2012 Apr 9. [Epub ahead of print]. PMID:22494560

Yang X, Lenhart TR, Kariu T, Anguita J, Akins DR, Pal U. Characterization of unique regions of Borrelia burgdorferi surface-located membrane protein 1. Infect Immun. 2010 Nov;78(11):4477-87. Epub 2010 Aug 9. PMID:20696833

Yegutkin GG, Hytönen J, Samburski SS, Yrjänäinen H, Jalkanen S, Viljanen MK. Disordered lymphoid purine metabolism contributes to the pathogenesis of persistent Borrelia garinii infection in mice. J Immunol. 2010 May 1;184(9):5112-20. Epub 2010 Mar 31. PMID:20357256

Yoshinari NH, Mantovani E, Bonoldi VL, Marangoni RG, Gauditano G. [Brazilian lyme-like disease or Baggio-Yoshinari syndrome: exotic and emerging Brazilian tick-borne zoonosis].[Article in English, Portuguese]. Rev Assoc Med Bras. 2010 May-Jun;56(3):363-9. PMID:20676548

Younger DS, Orsher S. Lyme Neuroborreliosis: Preliminary Results from an Urban Referral Center Employing Strict CDC Criteria for Case Selection. Neurol Res Int. 2010;2010:525206. Epub 2010 Jun 23. PMID:21188224

Yrjänäinen H, Hytönen J, Hartiala P, Oksi J, Viljanen MK. Persistence of borrelial DNA in the joints of Borrelia burgdorferi-infected mice after ceftriaxone treatment. APMIS. 2010 Sep 1;118(9):665-73. PMID:20718718

Zajkowska J, Czupryna P, Pancewicz SA, Kondrusik M, Moniuszko A. Acrodermatitis chronica atrophicans. Lancet Infect Dis. 2011 Oct;11(10):800. PMID:21958583

Zajkowska JM, Kułakowska A, Tarasiuk J, Pancewicz SA, Drozdowski W. [Peripheral neuropathies in Lyme borreliosis].[Article in Polish]. Pol Merkur Lekarski. 2010 Aug;29(170):115-8. PMID:20842825

Zajkowska JM, Owłasiuk P, Pancewicz SA, Swierzbińska R, Kondrusik M, Grygorczuk S, Moniuszko A, Czupryna P. [Presence of antibodies against gangliosides among patients with Lyme borreliosis--preliminary study].[Article in Polish]. Pol Merkur Lekarski. 2010 Feb;28(164):108-11. PMID:20369737

Zajkowska JM. [Transmission and circulation of tick borne pathogens (TBE and Lyme borreliosis) and the role of changing environment].[Article in Polish]. Przegl Epidemiol. 2010;64(4):525-31. PMID:21473069

Zákovská A, Kučerová H, Nejezchlebová H, Bartoňková N, Rašovská T, Norek A. [Monitoring the prevalence of pathogenic Borrelia burgdorferi sensu lato in ticks in two Brno locations].[Article in Czech]. Klin Mikrobiol Infekc Lek. 2011 Oct;17(5):179-83. PMID:22161755

Zhan L, Chu CY, Zuo SQ, Wu XM, Dumler JS, Jia N, Jiang BG, Yang H, Cao WC. Anaplasma phagocytophilum and Borrelia burgdorferi in rabbits from southeastern China. Vet Parasitol. 2009 Jun 10;162(3-4):354-6. Epub 2009 Mar 13. PMID:19345508

Zhang F, Gong Z, Zhang J, Liu Z. Prevalence of Borrelia burgdorferi sensu lato in rodents from Gansu, northwestern China. BMC Microbiol. 2010 May 28;10:157. PMID:20509909

Zhang K, Tong BA, Liu J, Li C. A single-domain FlgJ contributes to flagellar hook and filament formation in the Lyme disease spirochete Borrelia burgdorferi. J Bacteriol. 2012 Feb;194(4):866-74. Epub 2011 Dec 9. PMID:22155773

Zhang L, Zhang Y, Adusumilli S, Liu L, Narasimhan S, Dai J, Zhao YO, Fikrig E. Molecular interactions that enable movement of the Lyme disease agent from the tick gut into the hemolymph. PLoS Pathog. 2011 Jun;7(6):e1002079. Epub 2011 Jun 9. PMID:21695244

Zhang X, Yang X, Kumar M, Pal U. BB0323 function is essential for Borrelia burgdorferi virulence and persistence through tick-rodent transmission cycle. J Infect Dis. 2009 Oct 15;200(8):1318-30. PMID:19754308

Zheng W, Chen H, Liu X, Guo X, Fu R. Severe tick infestation in a hare and potential risk for transmitting pathogens to humans. Korean J Parasitol. 2011 Dec;49(4):419-22. Epub 2011 Dec 16. PMID:22355211

Ziemer M, Eisendle K, Müller H, Zelger B. Lymphocytic infiltration of the skin (Jessner-Kanof) but not reticular erythematous mucinosis occasionally represents clinical manifestations of Borrelia-associated pseudolymphoma. Br J Dermatol. 2009 Sep;161(3):583-90. Epub 2009 May 26. PMID:19486001

Zinecker S. [Enlarged lymph nodes, fever, abdominal cramps, numbness in arm and leg. Deciding evidence in the gluteal fold].[Article in German]. MMW Fortschr Med. 2009 Jun 4;151(23):5. PMID:19591341

Zollinger T, Mertz KD, Schmid M, Schmitt A, Pfaltz M, Kempf W. Borrelia in granuloma annulare, morphea and lichen sclerosus: a PCR-based study and review of the literature. J Cutan Pathol. 2010 May;37(5):571-7. Epub 2009 Dec 10. PMID:20015188

Dr. Schaller has been published in:

Journal of the American Medical Association

Journal of Clinical Neuroscience

Medscape (Academic Journal of WebMD)

Journal of the American Society of Child and Adolescent Psychiatry

American Journal of Psychiatry

European Journal of Child and Adolescent Psychiatry

Compounding Pharmaceuticals: Triad

Fleming Revell Press (Four Languages)

Internal Medicine News

Family Practice News

Spire Mass Market Books

Internet Journal of Family Medicine

Greenwood Press

Child and Adolescent Psychiatry Drug Alerts

Hope Academic Press

Clinical Psychiatry News

Psychiatric Drug Alerts

Townsend Journal

OB/GYN News

AMA News

Currents

A Sample of Other Books by Dr. Schaller

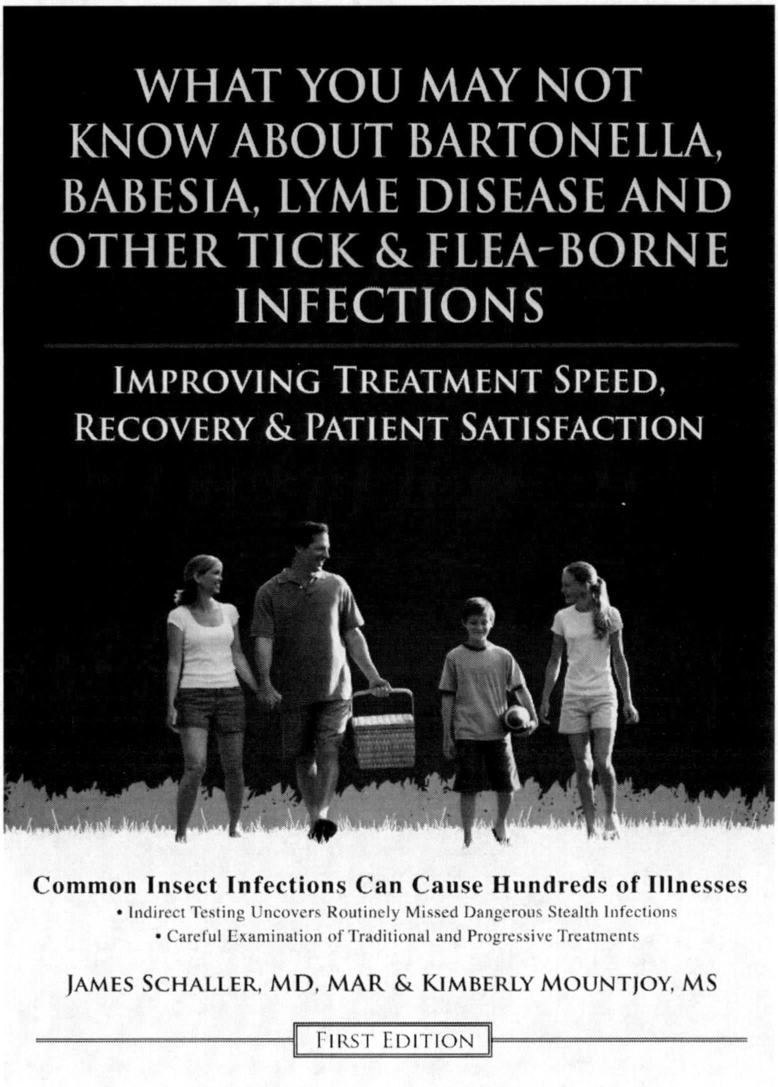

This 800 page book contains a hundred useful treatment testing and treatment pearls. However, it does not give one size fits all "mill medicine" treatments. It also includes advanced and comprehensive diagnostic checklists to prevent health care workers from missing Bartonella, Babesia and Lyme disease. Veteran physicians and functional medicine practitioners report they are learning a great deal from this book. It also shows that very few healers are able to read full time to reach tomorrow's medical care now, and Dr. Schaller shows he is one of them by clear broad thinking and thousands of references. His primary clinical pearls are in the first 200 pages.

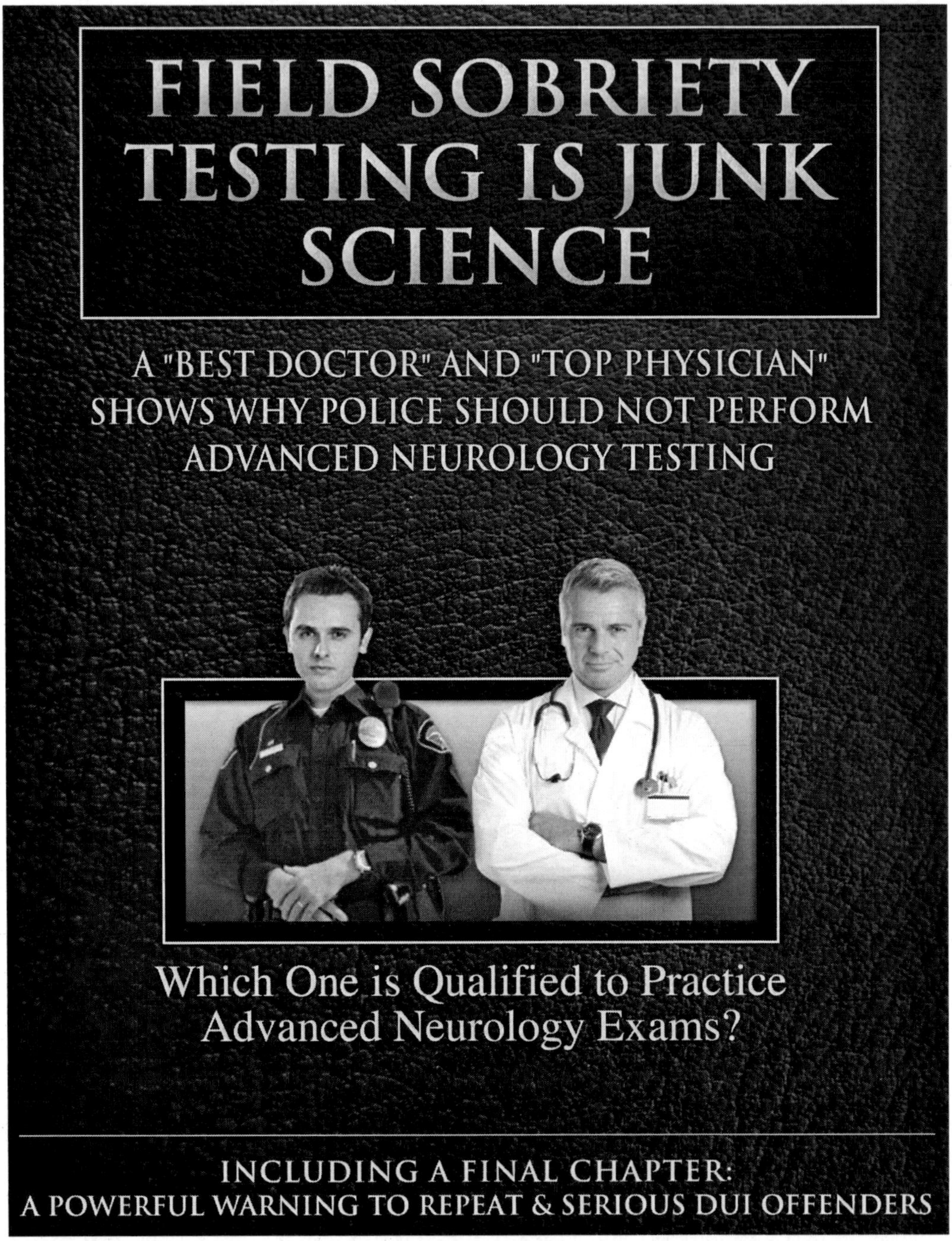

This fascinating book appeals to all peace officers, legislatures, and concerned citizens to rethink the science of these super medical examinations which help save lives, **but also often allow for many to be placed under arrest for over 500 medical problems.**

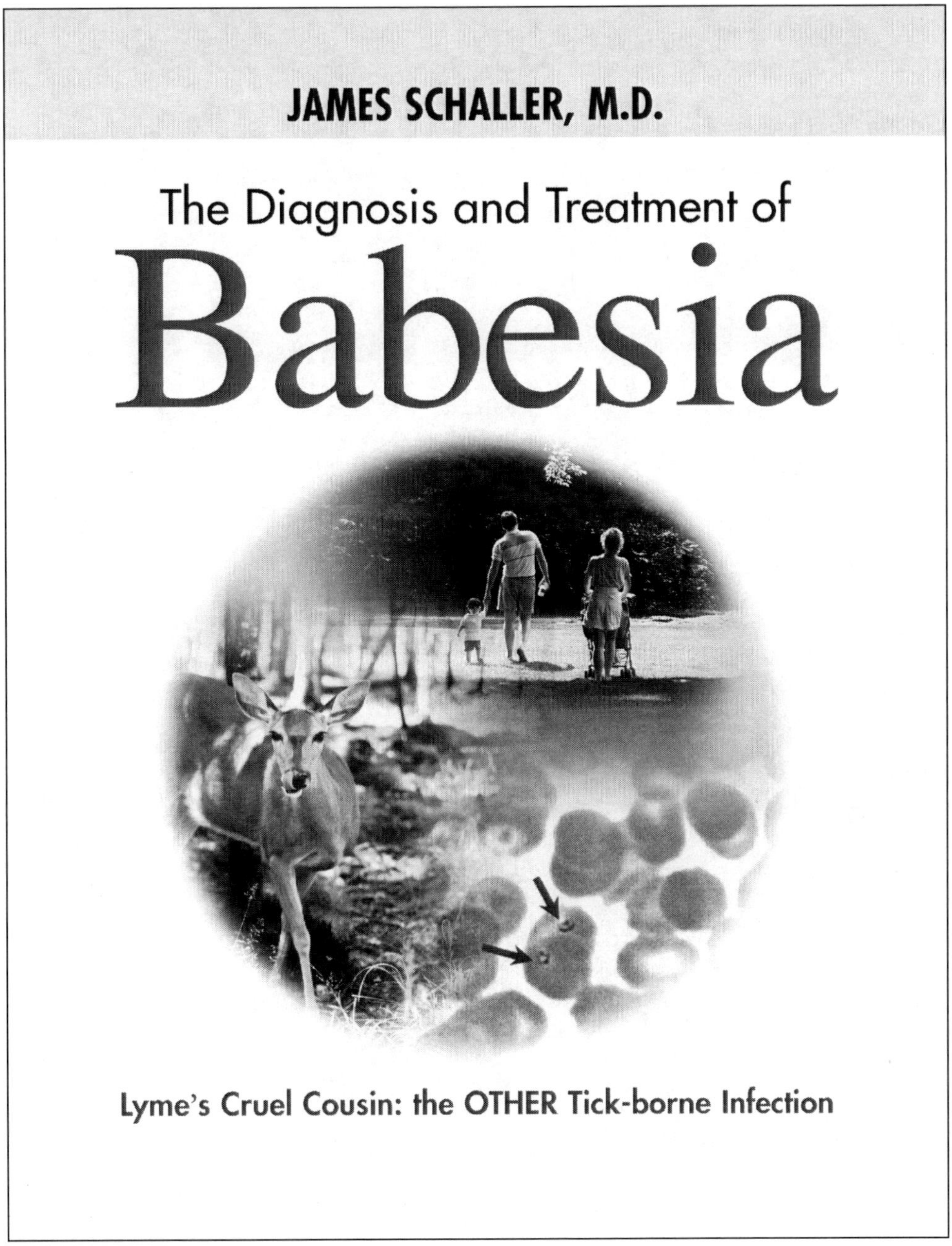

This large textbook is clear and easy to read. It is really three books. While some points are partially outdated since 2006, much would be considered new to most readers.

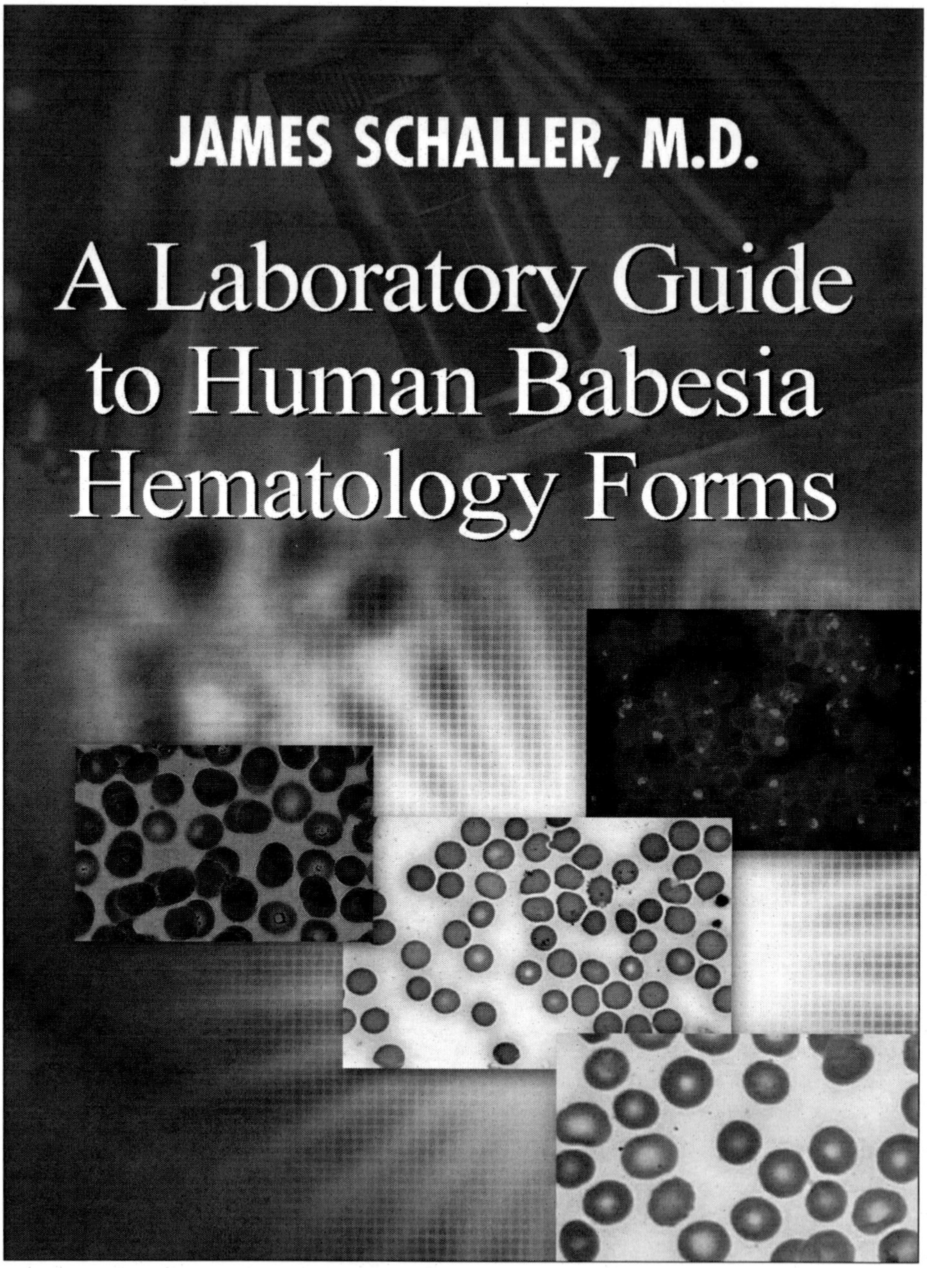

The only hematology book exclusively dedicated to Babesia.

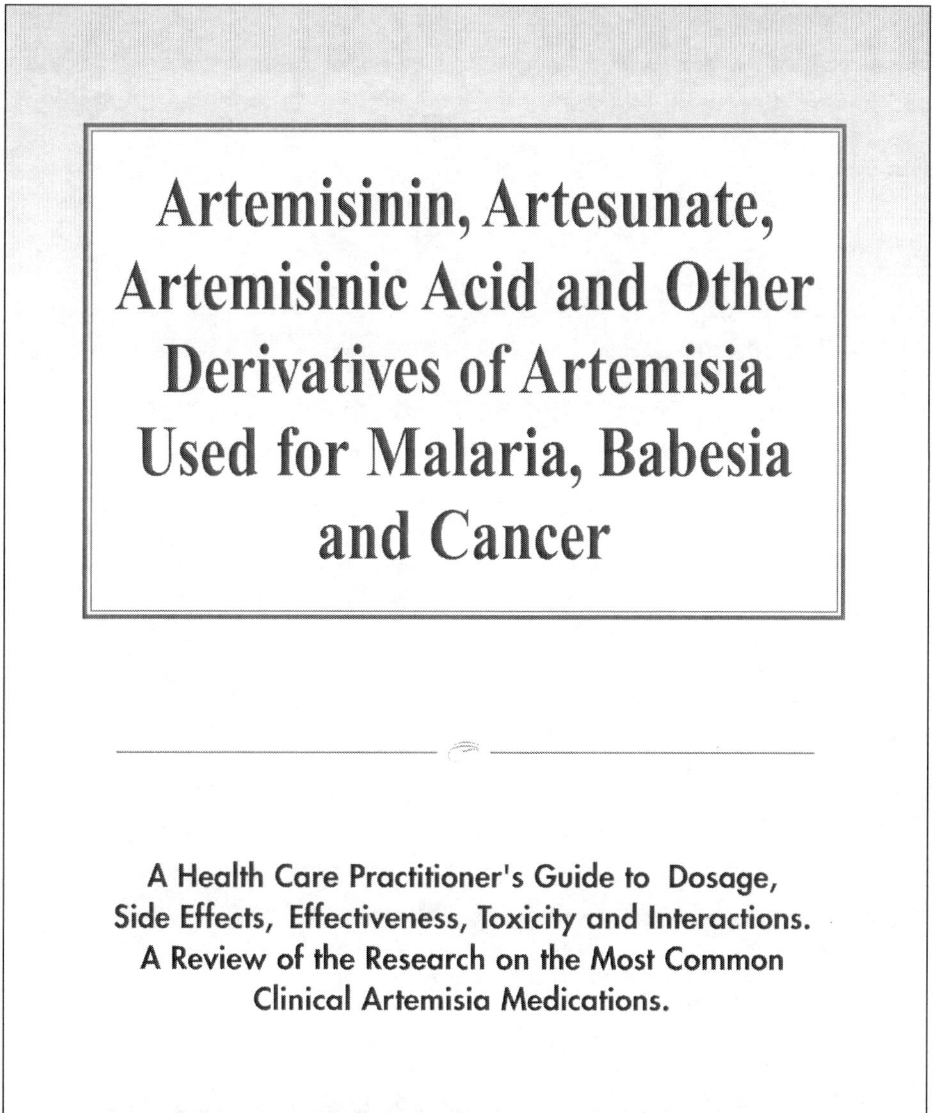

The most up-to-date academic and patient-centered book on practical Artemisia Babesia issues.

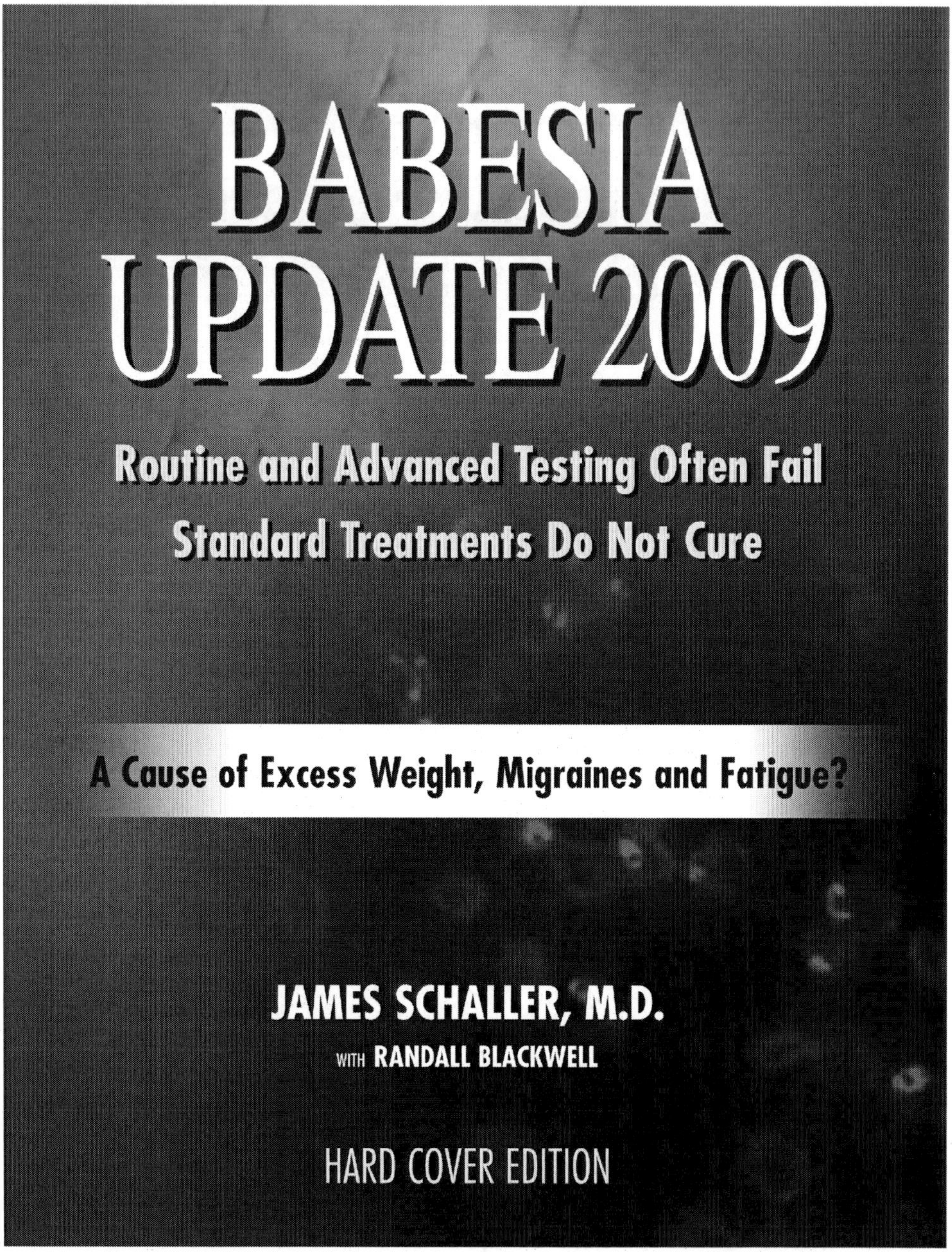

A book with advanced research based information, that moves Babesia medicine into a new decade. It presents highly practical information on ways to detect Babesia that are not mere IgM/G titer tests. Learn how to detect new species being discovered routinely and which seriously undermine function. This text also discusses why some individuals do not experience the easy and fast cure promised in other writings.

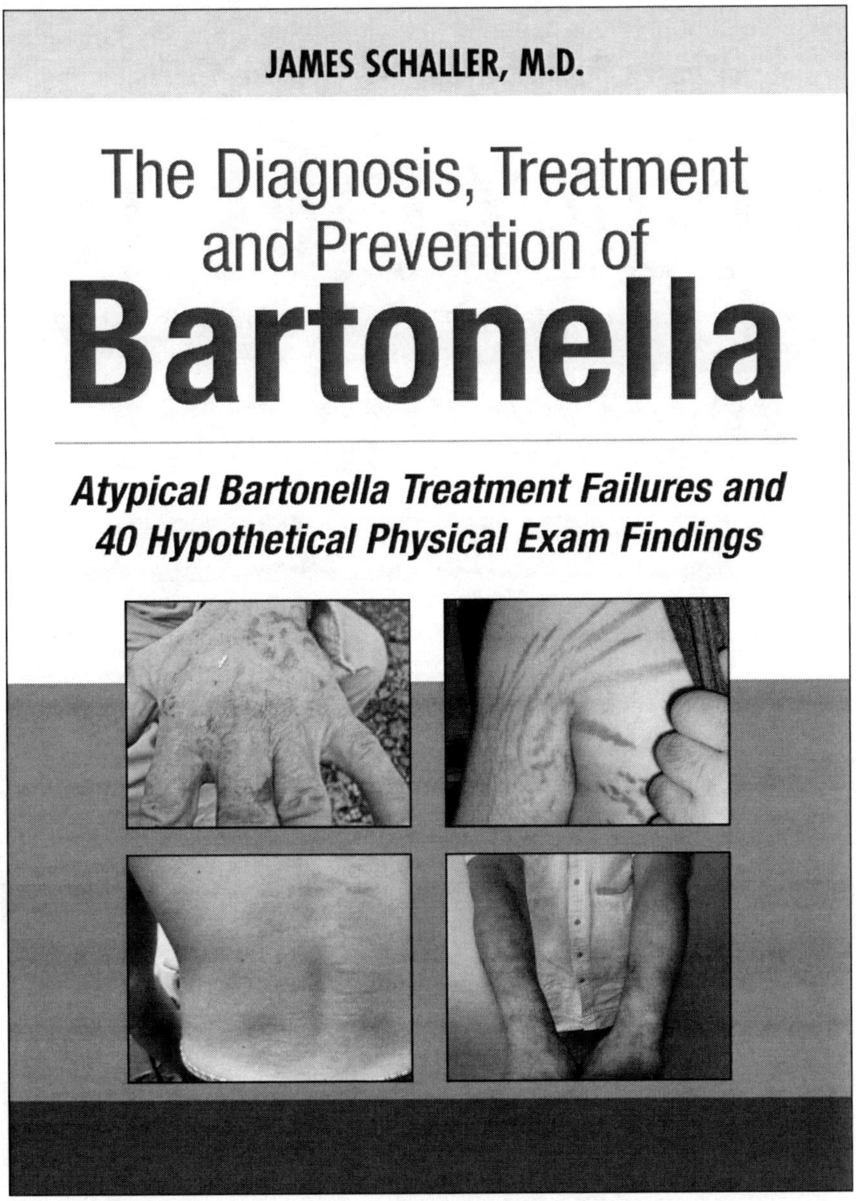

Bartonella diagnosis is very complex. This current text creatively uses a new set of tools to assist in diagnosis based on solid research of blood vessel and skin augmentation chemicals created by Bartonella. It literally creates a new Bartonella physical exam. This book helps with limited basic lab testing, and **prevents the use of routinely relapsing or poor treatments promoted in both traditional and integrative medicine.** No other book on this topic is based on over a thousand top research articles, and no one has published anything remotely close to replacing this work in over five years. **In summary, Bartonella is carried by more vectors than any infection on earth with one top specialist saying most testing and treatment is very poor.**

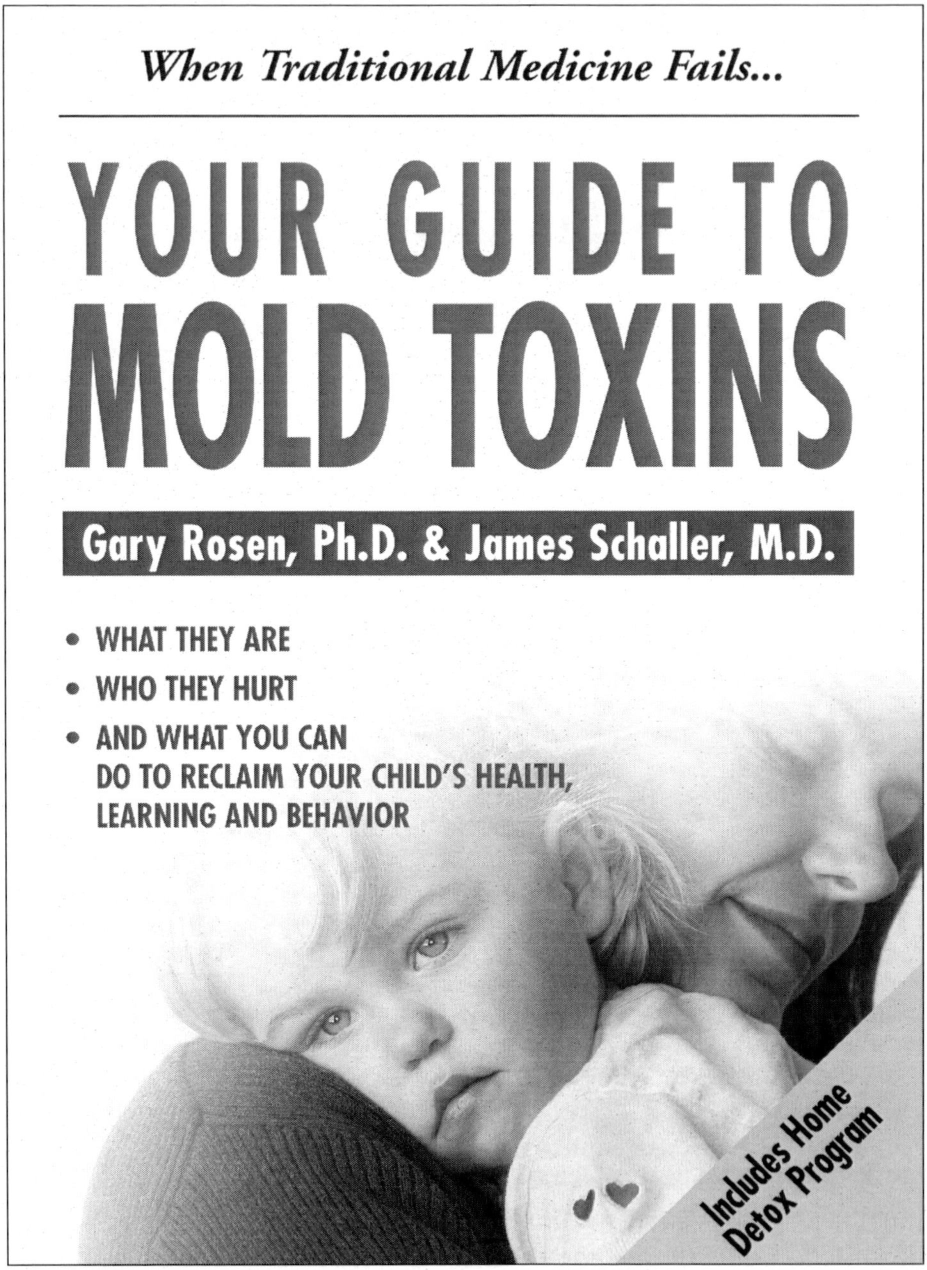

Dr. Schaller is a Certified Mold Investigator and a Certified Mold Remediator. Here is a practical and readable mold mycotoxin book.

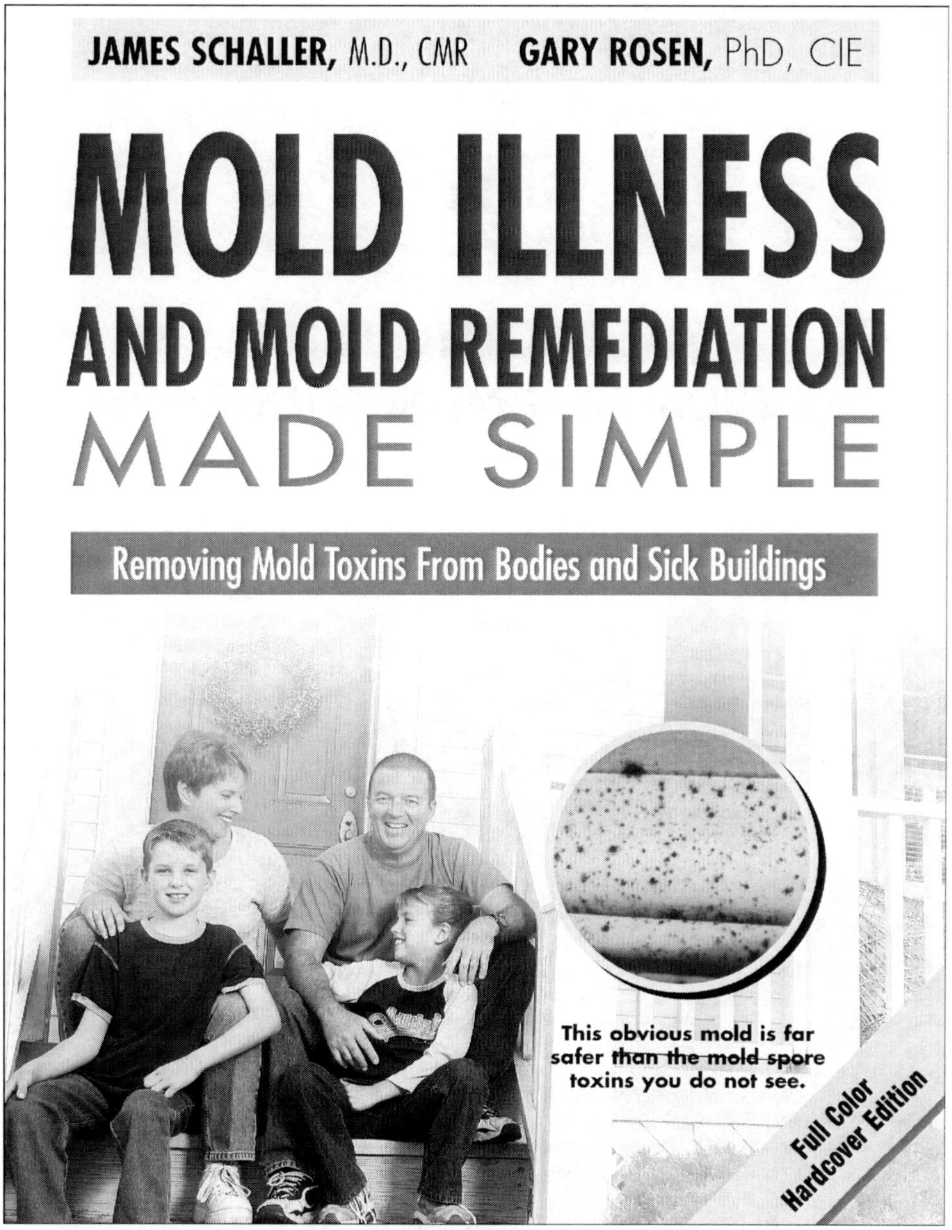

This book is helpful for people who are ill, or have trouble thinking and reading science materials. This is very practical and shows the clean-up errors made by 95% of experienced and expensive licensed mold remediators and renovation workers. Just reading ten pages from this book has shown people why they are not getting better. And this text helps you spot poor remediators after simply reading 40 easy to understand comics. Most remediations fail and most building hygiene actions are flawed. See why fast. **The six best mycotoxin binders cannot cure you if you are still in a "sick" home or moldy work location.**

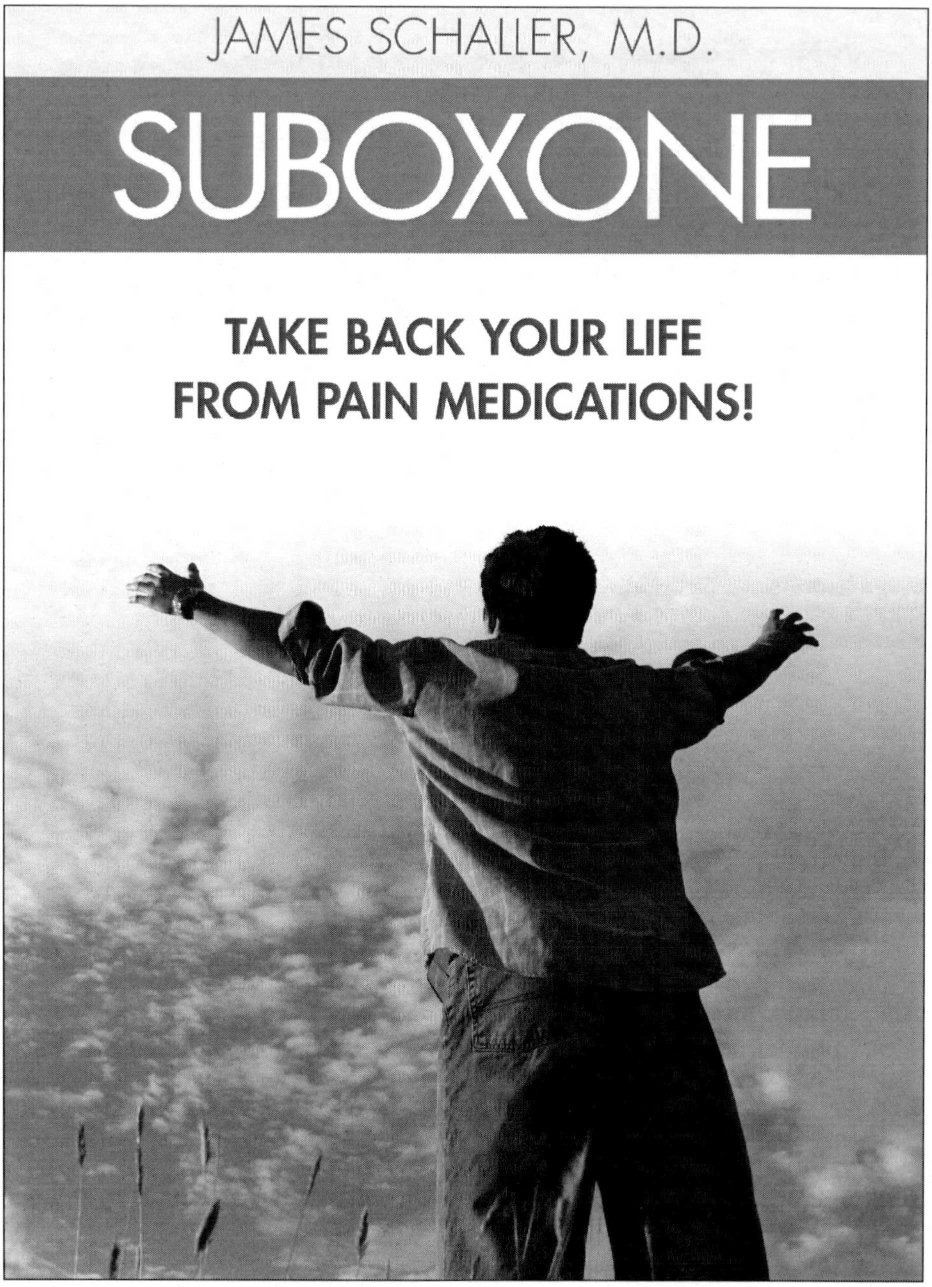
JAMES SCHALLER, M.D.
SUBOXONE
TAKE BACK YOUR LIFE
FROM PAIN MEDICATIONS!

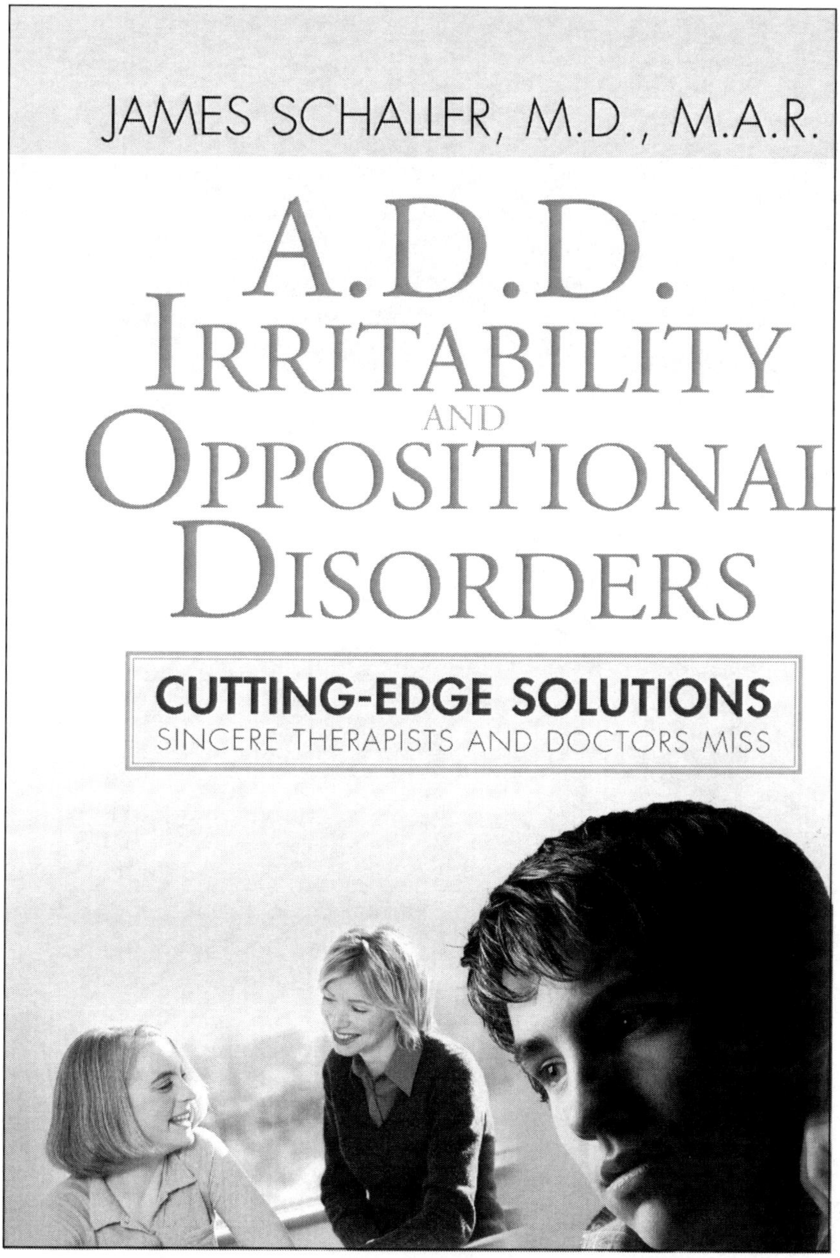

The many missed **medical and neurological** causes of poor focus and bad behaviors can no longer be ignored. This unique text advances medicine and shows how much in youth psychiatry has medical roots that are ignored or unknown even in solid child and adolescent psychiatry practices.

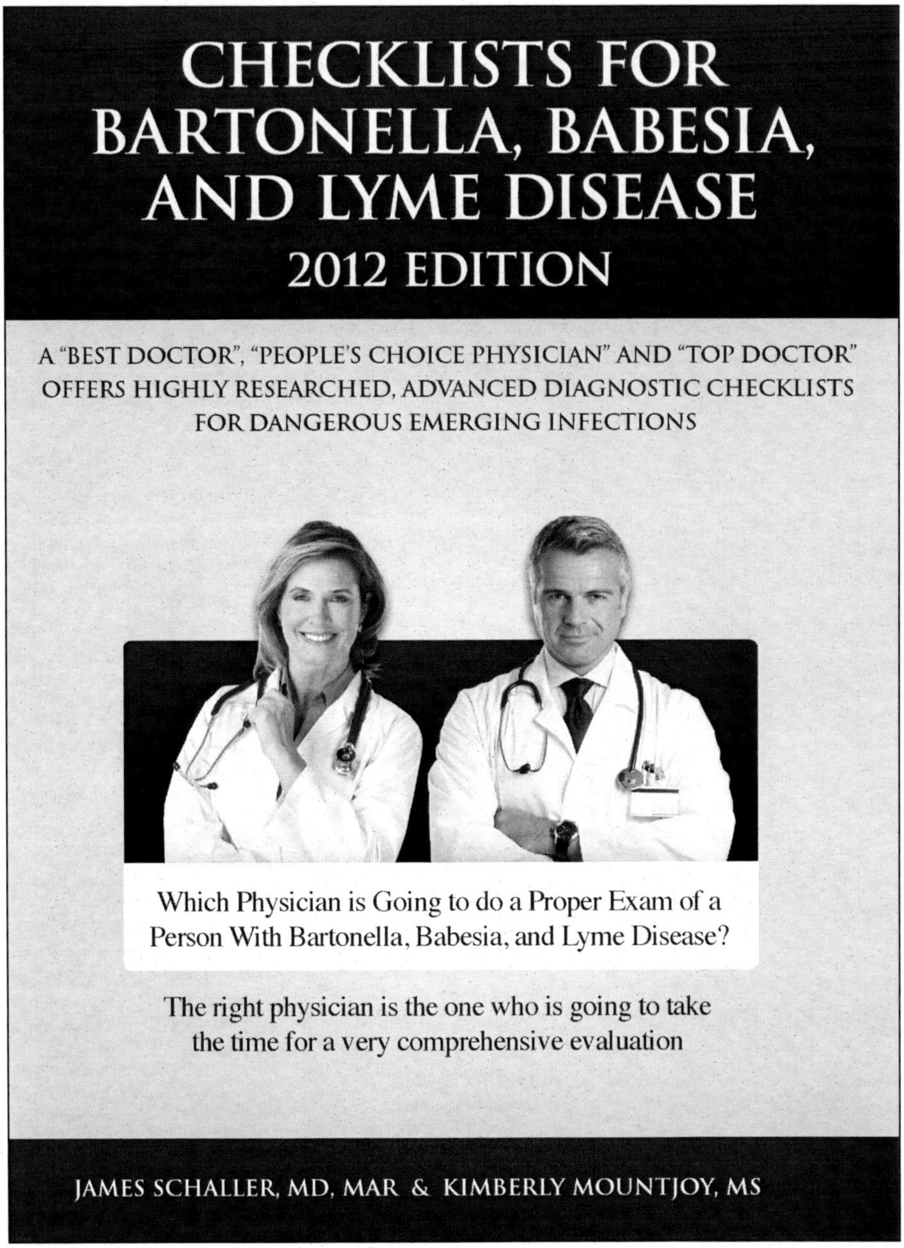
CHECKLISTS FOR
BARTONELLA, BABESIA,
AND LYME DISEASE
2012 EDITION
A "BEST DOCTOR", "PEOPLE'S CHOICE PHYSICIAN" AND "TOP DOCTOR"
OFFERS HIGHLY RESEARCHED, ADVANCED DIAGNOSTIC CHECKLISTS
FOR DANGEROUS EMERGING INFECTIONS
Which Physician is Going to do a Proper Exam of a
Person With Bartonella, Babesia, and Lyme Disease?
The right physician is the one who is going to take
the time for a very comprehensive evaluation
JAMES SCHALLER, MD, MAR & KIMBERLY MOUNTJOY, MS

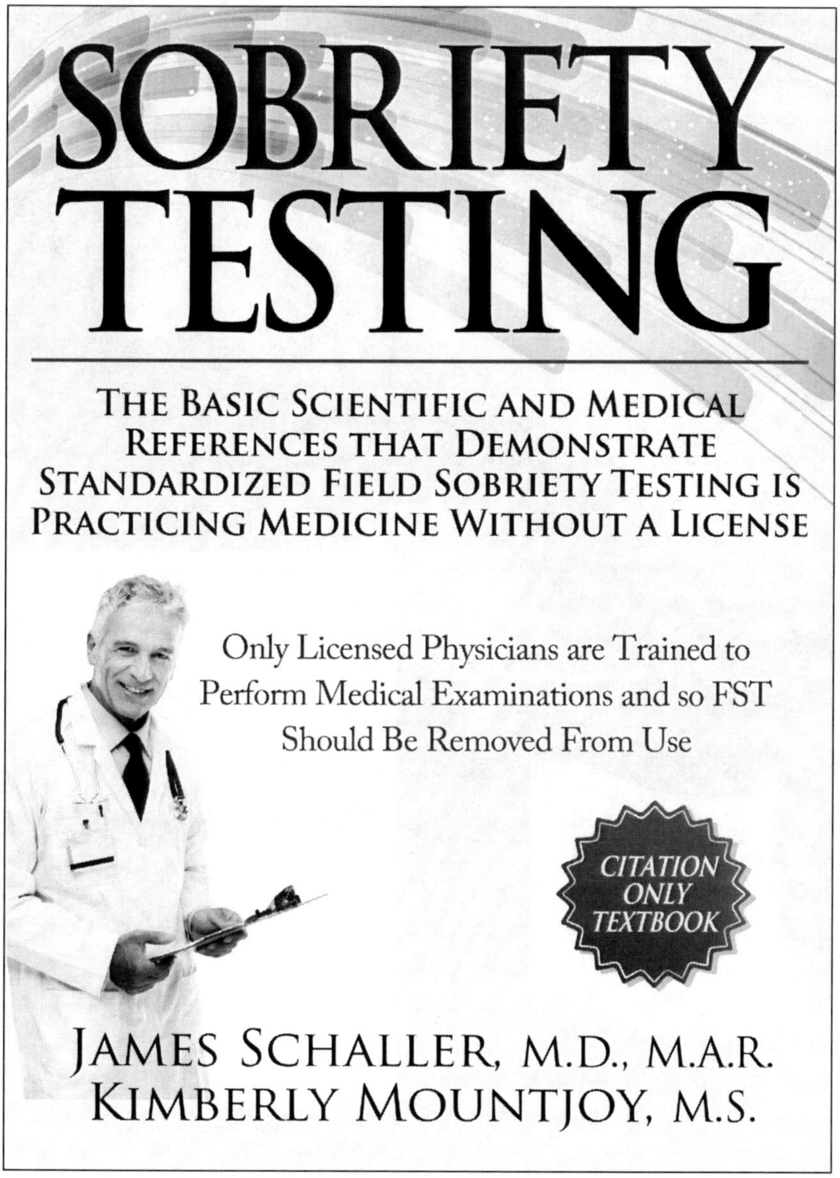

This firm book is a strong appeal for all involved in preventing impaired driving, which often causes profound disability and death, to appreciate the medical testing done on dark sidewalks or streets is a practice of advanced medical testing. FST has hundreds of routinely missed medical troubles which cause false positive tests. All civilized societies must lower the many arrests based on a lack of knowledge in human physiology and human pathology.

Further, the simplistic teaching that field sobriety testing is very easy for sober people is wrong. How many adults can walk on a balance beam a mere few feet off the ground?

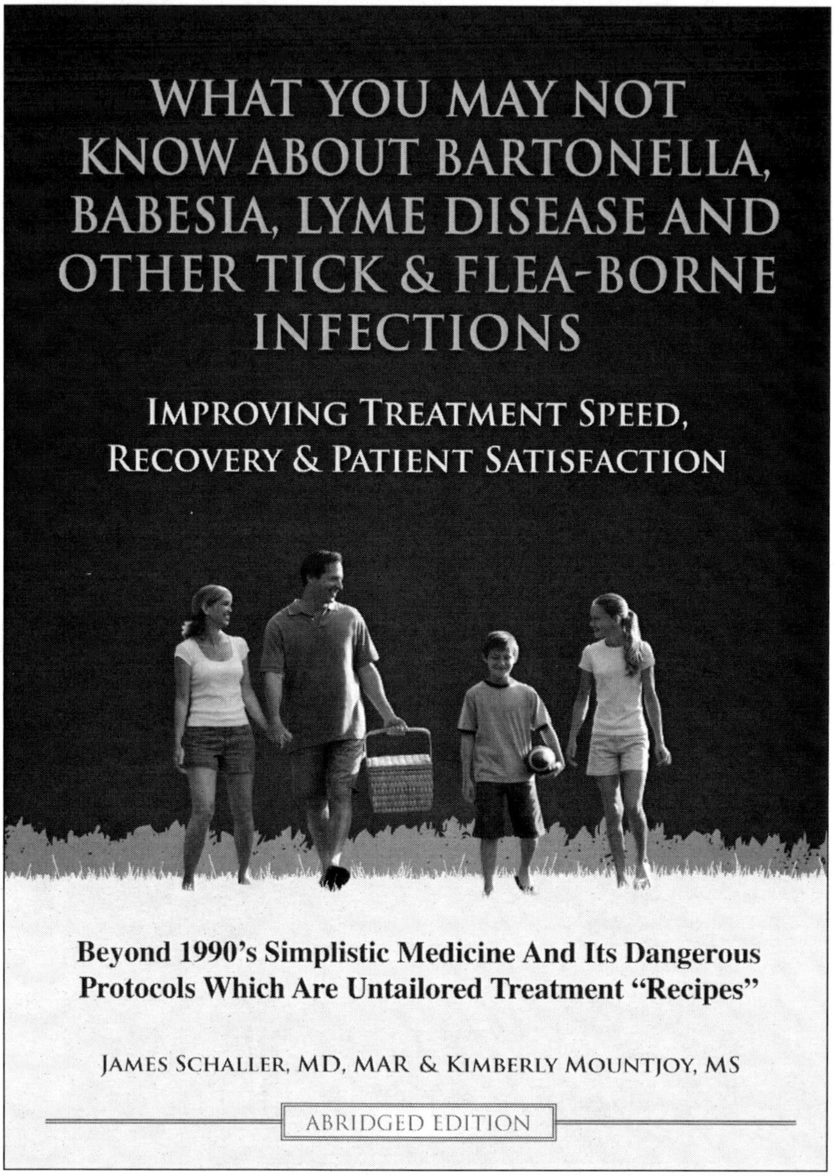

This powerful book is from one of the highest rated physicians doing research on all major tick infections. He only treats people who have failed to be cured by a number of previous smart healers. It is a book of ideas proposing reasons you do not feel recovered and back to normal. This book has over 90% of its references removed which are still in the first edition if you are a researcher who is ill or have family, friends or doctors mocking your careful science reflections.

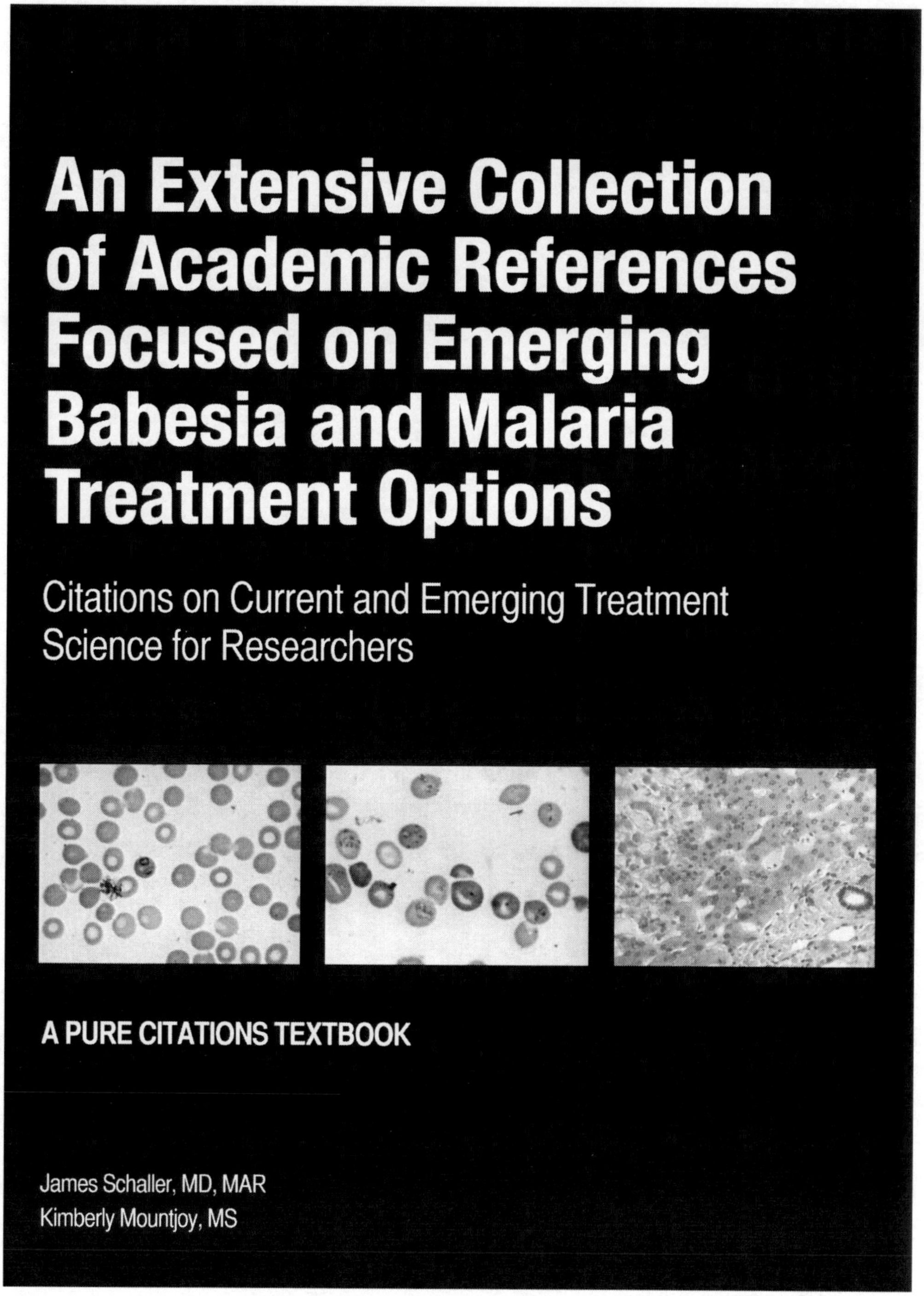

The is a researcher's textbook for M.D.'s, DO.'s, Ph.D.'s and Master's of Science working directly in Babesia and malaria research. It has no use for patients, unless they also are full-time researchers in this exact area of advanced academic research.

Disclaimer

Dr. Schaller is not a specialist in infectious disease medicine. He is also not a pathologist. Both of these specialties have over 2,000 diseases to treat and study. Dr. Schaller is only interested in four infections and has read and published on only these four. The medical ideas, health thoughts, health comments, products and any claims made about specific illnesses, diseases, and causes of health problems in this book are purely speculative, hypothetical, and are not meant to be authoritative in any setting. No comment or image has been evaluated by the FDA, CDC, NIH, IDSA or the AMA. Never assume any United States medical body, society, or the majority of American physicians endorse any comment in this book. No comment in this book is approved by any government agency, medical body or medical society. Nothing in this book is to be used to diagnose, treat, cure or prevent disease. The information provided in this book is for educational purposes only. It is not intended as a substitute for the advice from your physician or other health care professionals.

No patient should use the information in this book for the diagnosis or treatment of any health problem, or for prescription of any medication or other treatment. You should consult with a health care professional before deciding on any diagnosis, or initiating any treatment plan of any kind. Dr. Schaller does not claim to be an expert in any illness, disease or treatment. In this book, he is merely sharing one of his interests. Please do not start any diet, exercise or supplementation program, or take any type of nutrient, herb, or medication, without clear consultation with your licensed health care provider.

Infection diagnosis or treatment comments and reports of possible positive or negative treatment outcomes are hypothetical. No treatment should be rejected or embraced by anyone, based on the preliminary research and study in this book.

Contacting Dr. Schaller

Should you wish to talk to Dr. Schaller, he offers individualized education phone consults, which can be arranged by calling 239-263-0133. Please leave all your phone numbers, a working email and a fax number. These consults are typically in 15 minute units and can last as long as you wish. All that is required is the completion of a short informed consent form.

If you would like a full diagnostic consult or to see Dr. Schaller as a patient, know he treats patients from all over the USA and from outside the country. He meets with you first and then does follow-up care with you by phone.

If you would like to fly in to see Dr. Schaller, his staff are very familiar with all the closest airports and hotels.

Made in United States
North Haven, CT
04 November 2026

21728199R00396